CONTEMPORARY PSYCHOANALYSIS IN AMERICA

Leading Analysts Present Their Work

CONTEMPORARY PSYCHOANALYSIS IN AMERICA

Leading Analysts Present Their Work

Edited by

ARNOLD M. COOPER, M.D.

American Psychiatric Publishing, Inc.

Washington, DC
London, England

Note: The authors have worked to ensure that all information in this book is accurate at the time of publication and consistent with general psychiatric and medical standards. Therapeutic standards may change. Moreover, specific situations may require a specific therapeutic response not included in this book. We recommend that readers follow the advice of physicians directly involved in their care or the care of a member of their family.

Manufactured in the United States of America on acid-free paper
10 09 08 07 06 5 4 3 2 1
First Edition

Typeset in Adobe's Palatino and Futura.

American Psychiatric Publishing, Inc.
1000 Wilson Boulevard
Arlington, VA 22209-3901
www.appi.org

Library of Congress Cataloging-in-Publication Data
Contemporary psychoanalysis in America: leading analysts present their work / edited by Arnold M. Cooper.—1st ed.
p. ; cm.
Includes bibliographical references and index.
ISBN 1-58562-232-X (hardcover : alk. paper)
1. Psychoanalysis—United States. 2. Psychoanalysts—United States—Biography. I. Cooper, Arnold M. II. American Psychiatric Publishing.
[DNLM: 1. Psychoanalysis—United States—Collected Works. 2. Psychoanalysis—United States—Personal Narratives. 3. Psychoanalytic Theory—United States—Collected Works. 4. Psychoanalytic Theory—United States—Personal Narratives. WM 460 C67 2006]
RC504.P757 2006
616.89'17--dc22

2005032042

British Library Cataloguing in Publication Data
A CIP record is available from the British Library.

CONTENTS

CONTRIBUTORS

CHARLES BRENNER, M.D.
New York, New York

PHILIP M. BROMBERG, PH.D.
New York, New York

FRED BUSCH, PH.D.
New York, New York

NANCY J. CHODOROW, PH.D.
Cambridge, Massachusetts

ARNOLD M. COOPER, M.D.
New York, New York

ROBERT N. EMDE, M.D.
Denver, Colorado

PETER FONAGY, PH.D., F.B.A.
London, England

LAWRENCE FRIEDMAN, M.D.
New York, New York

GLEN O. GABBARD, M.D.
Houston, Texas

ARNOLD GOLDBERG, M.D.
Chicago, Illinois

JAY R. GREENBERG, PH.D.
New York, New York

WILLIAM I. GROSSMAN, M.D.
Tenafly, New Jersey

IRWIN Z. HOFFMAN, PH.D.
Chicago, Illinois

THEODORE J. JACOBS, M.D.
New York, New York

JUDY L. KANTROWITZ, PH.D.
Brookline, Massachusetts

OTTO F. KERNBERG, M.D.
White Plains, New York

EDGAR A. LEVENSON, M.D.
Hastings-on-Hudson, New York

LESTER LUBORSKY, PH.D.
Philadelphia, Pennsylvania

ROBERT MICHELS, M.D.
New York, New York

THOMAS H. OGDEN, M.D.
San Francisco, California

PAUL H. ORNSTEIN, M.D.
Brookline, Massachusetts

ETHEL SPECTOR PERSON, M.D.
New York, New York

FRED PINE, PH.D.
New York, New York

OWEN RENIK, M.D.
San Francisco, California

ROY SCHAFER, PH.D.
New York, New York

EVELYNE ALBRECHT SCHWABER, M.D.
Brookline, Massachusetts

THEODORE SHAPIRO, M.D.
New York, New York

HENRY F. SMITH, M.D.
Cambridge, Massachusetts

DANIEL N. STERN, M.D.
Geneva, Switzerland

ROBERT D. STOLOROW, PH.D.
Santa Monica, California

ROBERT S. WALLERSTEIN, M.D.
Belvedere, California

PREFACE

THE PHRASE *theoretical pluralism* has become a cliché in discussions of American psychoanalysis. It is the intent of this volume to provide authoritative presentations, in each analyst's own words, of the views of leading figures representing the major schools, movements, or trends in American psychoanalysis today. After half a century of dominance, it is widely accepted today that ego psychology—with its scientistic attention to energies, forces, and quantities, and its clinical insistence on the analyst's neutrality, objectivity, and anonymity—has run its course and that no single psychodynamic conception has replaced it. Instead, we have versions of object relations theory, self psychology, interpersonal and relational psychoanalysis, hermeneutics, derivatives of infant observation, and updated versions of ego psychology, all competing for allegiance on what is now a fairly level playing field.

Several developments within psychoanalysis have fostered this flowering of new ideas. The maturation of psychoanalysis and the acceptance of the death of Freud have surely been important in our willingness to consider and sometimes embrace new ideas and new research efforts. In addition, the agreement of the American Psychoanalytic Association to accept nonmedical persons into analytic training and the related decision of the International Psychoanalytical Association to accept into membership individuals and institutes in the United States that are not linked to the American Psychoanalytic Association have released a great burst of creativity. The pace of theoretical and clinical change in the conduct of psychoanalysis has been rapid. As a result, the breadth of the field is now enormous. In this climate, and in marked contrast to the situation not long ago, it is extremely difficult if not impossible for someone interested in American psychoanalysis to be expert on the variety of viewpoints that are now part of the mainstream.

The magnitude of innovation and experimentation that is now acceptable is in sharpest contrast to the so-called orthodoxy of the not so distant past. Ideas and practices that were considered heretical just a few years ago are today accepted or at least seriously considered within the mainstream. Some examples include self-disclosure, enactments, the significant role of preoedipal development, the many ramifications of object relations theory, a central role for the analyst's subjectivity, changing definitions of the unconscious—the list could go on. The rise, and perhaps subsequent fall, of postmodernism has had a powerful effect on psychoanalytic thinking, influencing our concepts of objectivity—including the possibility of "accurately" observing the patient—and raising countertransference to new significance in any attempt to understand the patient's psychoanalytic behavior. I hope that one important use of this volume will be to dispel preexisting biases and provide us a much broader notion of contemporary psychoanalysis.

This burgeoning of new ideas and new research has led to an intense reawakening of interest in psychoanalysis from neighboring disciplines ranging from the humanities to neuroscience and including the nonanalytic psychotherapies. The analytic literature is now vast, and few of us can keep up with the journals of the many different groups that are contributing to this vibrant scene. In the analytic world that I am describing, it is obviously desirable to have a reasonably clear conception of what the major theorists and practitioners themselves think. While some degree of theoretical confusion may be inevitable or even desirable, it should at least be a confusion based on the actual ideas of the authors, rather than on second-hand interpretations.

All of the authors represented here are established leaders in the field, and each is generally regarded as representing a major point of view. The authors were asked to contribute the paper that each thought best represented his or her current thinking and his or her major contribution to psychoanalysis. I believe they have done so. Moreover, these papers are quite free of professional jargon, offer vivid clinical vignettes, and will be readily accessible to anyone with an interest in psychoanalysis. While it is convenient to think of analytic contributors as falling under certain rubrics—interpersonal, object-relational, ego-psychological, and so forth—it is striking in reading these authors' works to find how much some of them have in common, especially in clinical practice, as well as the sharp differences that we might expect. Nonetheless, despite efforts at unity around such topics as intersubjectivity, narrative cohesion, and the relevance of countertransference, these authors do represent significantly different viewpoints. Together they can be regarded as reflecting the spectrum of psychoanalysis as it currently exists in the United States. My hope is that the reader will be better able to participate in the dialogue concerning the varieties of theory after hearing from these authors in their own voices.

I thought a good deal about how to divide these papers into sections. An attempt to do so by schools fails, since many of the authors publicly identified as representing a "school" have submitted papers that belie that description. I also found it difficult to section the book by clinical, theoretical, or research contribution, since many of the papers cross these boundaries. It has therefore seemed best to present the papers alphabetically by author. In the chapter introductions, the authors briefly explain why they have chosen this particular paper from among their many significant works. The papers are also preceded by a short autobiographical or biographical summary (the latter written by me) of the author's place in the analytic firmament.

I have struggled to make this volume as broadly representative as possible, but I am quite aware that someone else doing this job might feel that some highly significant figures have been omitted. Anyone following the American psychoanalytic scene could suggest the names of important analysts who might appropriately have been included in the book. The publisher and I decided, however, that for the book to be most useful it would be important to keep it to a reasonable size and to accept the inevitability of errors of omission. I do believe, however, that no significant current of analytic thought has been omitted. I requested papers from 30 authors, including myself (on the insistence of the publisher), and it has been deeply gratifying that each author responded enthusiastically and promptly to the request for a contribution.

I am grateful to many people for their invaluable help in compiling this collection. The book owes its very existence to the enthusiastic cooperation of each of the contributing authors. I cannot adequately express my deep gratitude to them for their papers, their encouragement, and their good ideas. Peter Fonagy took time from his brilliant researches and prodigious publications to write a masterful introduction that with deep insight and clarity describes the position of each of the authors and brings an intellectual order to the collection that I could not. The idea for the volume arose from a conversation with my friend Stanley Moss, poet and publisher, who suggested a psychoanalytic anthology. Bob Hales and his entire staff at American Psychiatric Publishing, Inc., have been spectacularly supportive and helpful and a joy to work with. My successive assistants, Emily Tucker and Melanie Benvenue, put up with me and my endless demands, and the book could not exist without them. My wife, Katherine Addleman, has been the loving and relentless critic that I needed, both to begin and to complete this volume.

Arnold M. Cooper, M.D.

INTRODUCTION

Walking Among Giants

WALKING AMONG GIANTS is what preparing this introduction felt like. Thirty great people whom I have respected, admired, and sometimes disagreed with offered their favorite papers for this volume. The best of the best. "This is true super-league stuff," I thought. I also thought, "Perhaps a little focused on the past rather than the present." But, as I quickly discovered as I worked my way through the collection, I was quite wrong. As I read the papers, I became increasingly aware of (and awed by) the significance of this volume. In selecting specific papers for the collection, the most significant contributors to North American psychoanalysis were identifying what they perceived as their own most important contribution to the field as it is today. Thus in selecting papers they did so far less with an eye to the past but rather to the present and, perhaps even more, to the future. Perhaps this should have surprised me less than it did because the authors selected here, perhaps more than any other 30 individuals, have been instrumental in defining the present and future of psychoanalysis in the United States.

What this selection represents is the cutting edge of North American psychoanalytic writing. It is far from the European caricature of American psychoanalytic writing, dense with metapsychology, rigid and narrow in its conceptualization, light on clinical detail, and very experience distant. The papers selected by the authors as their favorites not surprisingly also are invariably highly accessible, are almost always built around clinical illustrations, are explicitly suspicious of pseudoscientific models, tend to embrace aspects of postmodernism, incorporate concepts with Kleinian and other European lineage, include sometimes painful examinations of the analyst's subjectivity, and are open to a broad set of disciplinary influences while retaining an unwavering commitment to clinical psychoanalysis.

The papers, or chapters for this reader, divide neatly into two types. About half the contributors nominated papers that aim at the systematization of theory, making distinctions and identifying convergences for the most part in relatively general terms, with a smaller number focusing on specific developmental, cultural, and clinical concerns. The second set of papers are more clearly focused on practice, either in terms of pointing to elements of the therapeutic, including the psychoanalytic therapeutic context, or more specifically are occupied with elaborating the psychoanalyst's position within the analytic relationship. It seems to me that this reflects where the growing points of the subject are: in reconstructing the theoretical framework of psychoanalysis and, closely related to this point, reconstructing our understanding of the therapeutic situation.

SYSTEMATIZING THEORIES

Distinctions and Taxonomies

Two of the contributions concern a direct mapping of psychoanalytic theories, in the sense of offering taxonomy as much as integration. There is a certain kind of integrative paper that clearly demands to be written but once clearly put can be referred to again and again. Fred Pine's paper (Chapter 22) on the four psychologies of psychoanalysis is a prime example of this type. The psychology of drives allows us to ask questions about our patients concerning wishes, unconscious fantasies, and defenses against them. The psychology of the ego provides a way of looking at patients in whom the tools for adaptation have failed to develop (e.g., failures of affect regulation). The psychology of object relations invites questions about the role the patient experiences playing in relation to the analyst or in interpersonal relations that may be illuminated by childhood relationships. The psychology of the self points to experiential questions in relation to boundaries, internalizations, and self-esteem.

The four psychologies suggest different types of interpretive work. Drive psychology suggests interpreting unconscious wishes and conflicts, whereas object-relation interpretations aim to free the patient to meet new experience for what it is rather than as part of an old drama. The psychology of ego deficit and of the self dictate care and caution in interpretation, emphasizing description, explanation, and reconstruction, but in common with all interpretation aiming to touch on something that is within the patient's range of experience. The four psychologies underscore different aspects of the therapeutic relationship, potentially mediating change. The key point here is that all four have a role. Thus the relationship with the analyst frequently serves to soften the superego (drive), provide a corrective interpersonal experience (object relations), address ego deficits in a developmental way, and create an opportunity for the self to be mirrored. True psychoanalysis, Pine maintains, requires all four sets of theoretical approaches and all four sets of technical interventions.

The taxonomy is broadened in Otto Kernberg's analysis (Chapter 15). In a sense it is not fair that Kernberg's remarkable productivity over the past half century of North American analysis is represented by a single paper. However, his creative solution to the limitation imposed on him by the editor was to nominate a paper that is in itself a breathtaking overview of the entire post-Freudian field of psychoanalytic scholarship that must perforce include all of his own contributions. The paper collects the threads of psychoanalytic writings on technique, identifying major contributions while remaining respectful of important differences. From this history, Kernberg weaves a veritable Bayeux Tapestry of the state of psychoanalysis at the end of the twentieth century.

Kernberg's paper is daunting in its depth of presentation of present-day analysis in North America as well as in Europe. Postwar psychoanalysis, with its more than 30,000 learned papers, is classified into three traditions: 1) a convergence of Freudian, Kleinian, and independent traditions that represents "the mainstream"; 2) the intersubjective relational approaches; and 3) the French psychoanalytic approach.

This paper sets the stage for everything else that could be included in this volume. Although as in any summative introduction the reader may quibble with what the author has chosen to highlight, the fundamental oppositions between these traditions are as real and palpable as any meeting of a regional or national psychoanalytic organization.

Convergences

The centripetal force of theorization aims to identify the critical feature that contains within it the key element of all psychoanalysis. In many ways all the contributions struggle to identify the single theory. Charles Brenner (Chapter 1) does a better job of this effort than most. Brenner is one of the great educators of North American psychoanalysis, a role that he achieved through an unmatched capacity to state complex ideas in simple, compelling, and definitive ways. His addressing of the common ground question is the simple, yet profound assertion that common ground does indeed exist and is defined by the continuation into adulthood of childhood wishes that are invariably conflict ridden and require the formation of endless compromises.

The compromise between pleasure and "unpleasure" is ubiquitous to every form of mental life. The sexual and aggressive wishes of the second 3 years of life are fateful for the adult mental world. The timetable is set by neural development. Earlier experiences may have a role but are not appropriate foci for analytic work because their impact is through their effects on sexual and aggressive conflicts and compromise formations in the 3- to 6-year period. The coherence and simplicity of this view gives it depth. It becomes a beacon in the troubled seas of clinical encounter, not only through providing a framework that minimizes distraction from the multiplicity of current psychoanalytic ideas but also in setting a model of a psychoanalytic thinker able to let go of cherished assumptions (of structural theory) when faced with persuasive evidence.

William Grossman (Chapter 11) is another contributor who looks at the justification for a plurality of psychoanalytic approaches and finds it wanting. Grossman's paper addresses one of the key historical dichotomies of psychoanalytic thought. Do we need two theories to capture self-experience? Is there a genuine lack in the ego psychological approach when it comes to a clinical phenomenological account? The paper elegantly maps the struggle between the two facets of psychoanalytic thinking: explanations in terms of reasons and causes (clinical theory) and metapsychology. Grossman shows that the self is at the fulcrum of these perspectives. He suggests that all Freudian metapsychology contains within it a subjective element and thus the self is not qualitatively different from the rest of metapsychology. He contends that the self is a "concept-fantasy-theory" that happens to have significance to the patient.

Grossman is thus able to incorporate the self within an ego psychological point of view. He argues persuasively that problems of addressing the self within analyses do not suggest the need for a new theory but rather increased attention to timing, dosage, and tact. The concept of self is made complicated because the fantasy of the self includes within it the complex meanings that others observing the self have attributed to it before its full formation. In this sense the self is always a social fantasy. Grossman is able to incorporate a relational post-Cartesian perspective into his ego psychological model (see Stolorow's contribution).

Arnold Goldberg (Chapter 9) addresses the same question but moves the center of gravity somewhat further toward the newfound emphasis on the experiential world. Psychoanalytic theory, according to Goldberg's 1997 plenary address to the American Psychoanalytic Association, is at the cusp between empathy and judgment, between first- and third-person perspectives, and between the traditions of Heinz Hartmann and Heinz Kohut. He contends that the analytic focus on unconscious content derivable from the past must be balanced by the analytic empathic stance that enables the patient to own that which has been vertically split. The essay included in this volume is deeply integrative, bringing together the classical with the self psychological but in the context of a relational dialectical perspective. Goldberg contends that clinical psychoanalyses are coauthored; they are autobiographies written by two people.

This distinction offers both a theoretical and a clinical frame for psychoanalysis and illustrates how the space between the first- and third-person perspectives may be used to understand practice as well as the specific clinical problems that clinicians encounter. The dichotomy, for example, illuminates isolated behavioral problems such as the dishonest acts of an otherwise honest person. Empathy is required to deal with the vertical split that separates the part of us that does unacceptable things. The same dichotomy illuminates therapeutic action as the analyst whose very presence heals is the analyst who interprets the past unconscious. Being empathic is being able to judge both what we mean to (transference from the past) and what we have brought (analyst as a real object) to our patient. Both the interpretive and the empathic stance are required of the clinical analyst, and neither should be privileged within our theoretical accounts.

Other contributors have promoted convergences that are beyond the dichotomy that Goldberg and Grossman address in their papers. Roy Schafer's candidate for the most important of his many significant contributions (Chapter 24) brings us closer to what many other contributors refer to as the hermeneutic tradition within North American psychoanalysis. Schafer's chapter on narration is remarkable for the simultaneous profound contributions it makes to theory and technique. By conceptualizing psychoanalytic theory as a narrative, he places theory in a particular place alongside storytellings: the Kleinian story about a mad infant, the Kohutian story about a frail depleted self, neglected and misunderstood, and so on. Of course the analyst's retelling of the patient's story influences how the patient tells his or her story. This is beyond the trite statement that theory influences the content of clinical analysis. To some extent the theory writes the analysis. The analytic narration is jointly constructed.

There can be as many retellings as there are psychoanalyses. But most psychoanalytic stories, Schafer demonstrates, have sexual and aggressive modes of action with defensive measures adopted to disguise, displace, deemphasize, or compromise. The narration often involves infancy, bodily zones, and body products, with stories concerning losses, illnesses, abuse, neglect, and real or imagined parental conflicts. These elements are repetitively introduced by the analysand into the dialogue and gradually elaborated by the analyst.

Considering psychoanalysis as narration changes the status of constructs such as drives, resistance, reality testing, and psychic reality. These constructs are no longer entities that can cause things. The explanation they provided was a masquerade of redescription. Drive just describes wishing, resistance is resisting. Analytic life histories (case histories) are second-order histories. The first-order history is the analysis. Analysis is not reductive nor is it mysterious; it is merely a commonsensical alternative way of looking at a life situation.

Not all contributors to the volume, however, welcome or indeed agree with the introduction of a hermeneutic stance. Theodore Shapiro's timely contribution on reminiscences (Chapter 26) notes the shift in North American psychoanalysis away from a theory of mind toward increasing concern with technical issues, particularly those that address the process of analytic understanding. His chapter is explicitly designated as a reaction against the narrativization of psychoanalysis by underscoring the power of memory to "cause."

Shapiro, with masterful command of psychiatric as well as psychoanalytic knowledge, marshals evidence consistent with his claim that memories cause posttraumatic stress disorder, that memories of childhood influence the mother's relationship with the infant, that experience of deprivation has irreversible effects on brain development, and so on. Shapiro is unhappy with the hermeneutic approach that avoids problems of probity. Shapiro's contribution reflects the increasing scientific interest in determining how past events determine current actions. He offers a robust defense of the Freudian analyst who is sophisticated about the nature of memory but knows that ultimately the patient is his or her past, that interactions can be remembered without objects, and that persuasive interpretations are persuasive in a clinical setting because the analyst's interpretative words connect with the way that the past was incorporated in the patient's mind.

Shapiro formulates psychoanalysis as offering an opportunity for the patient to reiterate significant constellations of psychological organization in symbolic representations that the analyst (with the patient) discovers and puts into words. This articulation helps the patient to understand the motives for current behavior and offers the opportunity for change.

Taking the volume as a whole, the most popular current convergence in North American psychoanalysis appears to be around relational ideas. Nowhere are these ideas more succinctly and clearly exposed than in the exquisite contribution of Robert Stolorow (Chapter

29). Stolorow asks, "What is left of the unconscious in a post-Cartesian relational psychoanalysis?" If topography has become metaphor and the structural model is incompatible with a phenomenological approach, what is left from Freud's second Copernican revolution? Stolorow's answer is that all psychoanalytic approaches have in common the notion that "there is always something more than meets the eye" and further that this is central to understanding what ails us.

Within the classical Freudian model, consciousness is an epiphenomenon. The unconscious is what is psychically real. The analyst is thought to possess crucial knowledge of that which is repressed and creates distortions in the experience of living and enlightens the patient about this home of decontextualized ahistorical evil. Stolorow suggests that this model of the unconscious is defensively omnipotent. Freud posited inner badness as an account for the neuroses to avoid awareness of disappointing aspects of his relationship with his mother. Stolorow rejects the layered self-awareness approach entailed by both the topographical and the structural model of the unconscious.

The relational unconscious is not an isolated part of the mind with sharp structural distinctions in types of activity (repression, splitting, dissociation, denial, disavowal). It does not involve a subject-object bifurcation or a cognition-affect split. Rather unconsciousness is seen as evolving from situations of massive maltreatment. This may have involved the child's experiences not being responded to so that they felt unwelcome or dangerous. Alternatively experiences may never become articulated because of the absence of validating intersubjective context. Stolorow offers a beautiful case illustration initially presented using the classical psychoanalytic model, then reformulated so that symptoms can be seen as the consequence of repression when aspects of subjective experience were not allowed by the parent to enter the child's experiential world. The analytic situation provided an ideal setting for asking questions that loosen the control of calcified fantasies and nameless dread.

Daniel Stern (Chapter 28) adds a further dimension to the relational approach: that of developmental psychology. His innovative integrative contribution provides a developmental psychological framework for relational psychoanalysis. He contends that our nervous systems were designed to be captured by the nervous system of others so that we should be able to experience others as if we were within their skin at the same time as feeling within our own. The differentiated self is just a special state of intersubjectivity.

The self is non-Cartesian with a permeable boundary. Stern marshals considerable evidence consistent with this proposition, including the discovery of mirror neurons, the role of adaptive oscillators (timers) in interpersonal interactions, the primary other person orientation of infants, the imitation of others while interpreting their intention, the pathology of the nonsharing mind of the autistic individual, and so on.

Stern's paper also spells out in broad terms the implications of this developmental relational approach for psychoanalysis. Epistemologically it is no longer possible for the mind to be considered as open to objective inquiry as a singular entity. The treatment itself yields "emergent properties" that are co-created and therefore unpredictable, and resist linear and causal analysis except with the benefit of hindsight. Echoing Sidney Blatt's (2004) formulation of development and psychopathology, Stern considers attachment and separation-individuation to be continuous tasks that need to be concurrently performed. Psychodynamic meaning can be carried, enacted, and expressed through nonsymbolizing processes. Relationally embedded meanings are exchanged through rapid communication in lived experience. These communications organize and direct our actions. Language and abstract thought are rooted in this earlier form of meaning, but although these are nonsymbolic, they are not superseded by the symbolic. Stern directs the attention of the clinician to this nonsymbolic, nonconscious aspect of the mind, the implicit way of being with the other. It is the deepest level of meaning from which other meanings emerge. It is the home of unconscious fantasy, the level of lived engagement with others.

The Status of Theories

A theme that runs through many of the contributions concerns the status of theory in psychoanalysis. Three contributions, however, speak directly to this most thorny of issues. Robert Wallerstein (Chapter 30) has made a remarkable contribution in identifying at least a potential for shared psychoanalytic discourse within the international psychoanalytic movement as well as in our approaches to our conceptual work. There are few papers in the psychoanalytic literature that have given rise to a universally recognized phrase across the whole profession, but Wallerstein's "common ground" paper is one. The starting point of this impressive review is the still applicable observation that psychoanalysts have never dealt with Freud's death, that our manner of dealing with new ideas evidenced the fantasized continuation of Freud's life. New ideas for up to 35 years after Freud's death, particularly in North America, were frequently dealt with by exclusion rather than the British/European tendency toward integration. This paper offers a report card on North American psychoanalysis that is well reflected in the present volume (self psychology, ego psychological object relations theory, hermeneutic phenomenological approaches).

The burden of the paper, however, is pointing to common ground in the plurality of international psychoanalysis in claiming that experience-near clinical theory is all the theory that psychoanalysis needs or can test. The common ground corresponds to what Sandler and Sandler (1987) have placed in the domain of the present unconscious. Wallerstein identifies discourse concerning the patient's present unconscious as what is common and should be common to all approaches. Within clinical theory, distinct pragmatic approaches are testable. Models of the past unconscious that are beyond the probity of clinical evidence can be dramatically different across different models. But these are mere sources of metaphors for clinical discourse, all of which are apt in the domain of the present unconscious. Discrepancies need concern neither the clinician nor the patient.

Robert Michels (Chapter 18) also takes a "metapsychoanalytic" position. Michels is probably without peer (or challenger) as an evaluator and discussant of psychoanalytic ideas in North America. What better person to comment on the entire body of psychoanalytic theories? He offers a vast vista, first a historical model that takes psychoanalysis from a biology through a basic psychology to a set of semi-independent clinical theories. Then he adopts another vector: subject matter. He distinguishes bridging theories that trace mental phenomena to a domain outside of mental life, psychological theories that stay within the mental domain but are restricted to a description of the mental phenomena under scrutiny offering illusorily causal accounts, and clinical problem–oriented theories that forgo the ambition of offering a general psychology but directly address the clinical situation.

Michels's major intellectual contribution is in specifying the function of a theory in relation to practice. He points to three key functions: 1) enriching the analyst's association to the patient's material creating generative interpretations, 2) influencing the analyst's stance (attitude or manner toward the patient), and 3) comforting both analyst and patient. In relation to the second of these functions Michels highlights the crucial fact that theory orients the analyst to a particular facet of the patient's material (e.g., conflict theory to omissions, object relations theory to self-other relationships). Teaching and research also have use for theory, although in the latter case theoretically informed discourse often masquerades as the discovery of new facts.

Lester Luborsky's contribution (Chapter 17) is an implicit reply to the question of the epistemological status of psychoanalytic theorization. There is a point of view that is represented in some of the contributions to the volume (e.g., Shapiro, Kernberg, Stern) that extraclinical data is required for establishing the validity of alternative psychoanalytic formulations. Luborsky devoted his intellect and creativity to the task of quantifying psychoanalytic constructs, particularly the nature of the therapeutic process. In this paper he introduces the reader to an extremely influential method of analyzing relationship representations, the core conflictual relationship theme (CCRT). The CCRT categorizes relationship episodes according to 1) the predominant wishes, needs, and intentions; 2) the response of others; and 3) the response of the self. The frequency with which a particular configuration of these three elements emerges is considered to characterize the dominant mental structure of the individual.

CCRT depicts conflicts. The conflicts can be between wishes or between the wish and a response. The response of the self is often a symptom. Thus the CCRT offers a way of approaching psychopathology. The paper included in this volume is remarkable in several ways. First, it is the sole empirical paper in the entire collection. Second, it demonstrates that something as subtle as patterns of transference or object relationships is open to empirical enquiry. Third, the paper is one of the first in the literature to show the value of combined qualitative and quantitative empirical research methodologies in illuminating the psychoanalytic process. Luborsky is the great pioneer of psychoanalytic psychotherapeutic research, and many of the greatest innovations in this field originate with him.

The Application of Theory to Problems of Development and Culture

Two papers in this collection focus on addressing social phenomena that speak to our entire culture, way beyond our rather inward-turning psychoanalytic community. A literary critic as well as psychoanalyst by profession, Nancy Chodorow (Chapter 4) takes a welcome developmental perspective. Her paper makes a staggering observation: psychoanalysis does not have a developmental account of heterosexuality. Perhaps psychoanalysts have considered it so core, so readily reducible to evolutionary pressures that no special account seemed necessary. Yet as Chodorow's scholarly, powerful text demonstrates, the diversity of heterosexuality cannot be reduced to biology. The absence of satisfactory developmental accounts is in stark contrast to the comprehensive theories and rich clinical accounts of deviant sexuality.

Heterosexuality, Chodorow demonstrates, is as much the consequence of defenses and compromise formations as homosexuality. It is as driven, as complex, as potentially narrow a psychic state as deviant sexuality, but the passion, intensity, and oftentimes addictive quality of heterosexuality is not to be explained away as perversion. Addiction and compulsion are ingredients in all intense sexual experience and fantasy. Chodorow considers the pathologizing of deviant sexualities in terms of early deficits and conflicts unhelpful because heterosexual behavior can characterize the most disturbed individual.

This paper contains a well-argued rejection of heterosexuality as the only adequate resolution of oedipal conflicts. For example, she draws attention to the unquestioning acceptance of the assumption that gender difference is coterminous with sexual orientation. We are forced to conclude that homosexuality cannot be more pathological, more symptomatic than heterosexuality without better accounts of heterosexuality. Ultimately we have to agree with Chodorow that given the current state of psychoanalytic knowledge we have no grounds on which to differentiate homosexuality and heterosexuality. The approach that Chodorow contributed to overturning had probably reified gender and sexual difference and contributed to sustaining sexual inequality.

Ethel Person (Chapter 21) has cast her net even wider, taking on a critical facet of the social system: that of authority. It is at least ironical if not an outright paradox to challenge authority with a paper that illuminates our general willingness to acquiesce to interpersonal authority. Person's paper about our limited ability to be disobedient certainly challenges received truth. Person brings together a subtle and beautifully constructed set of insightful conjectures in what is an outstandingly intelligent treatment of a pervasive and most dangerous social issue.

At the heart of the paper is the compellingly illustrated universal fantasy of attaching ourselves to power through submissiveness and obedience. The need to deny our powerlessness in early life is only part of the story. Anxieties, perhaps even more powerful, are generated throughout life related to our ultimate fate: death and oblivion. It is in the face of death that a thirst for obedience is created that goes beyond that accounted for by the transference to a family romance or by a wish to defy parental authority. The motivator of the fantasy is what Freud regarded as the phenomenon in need of explanation to join in an "ant heap" of shared belief: a transcendent group. Participation in the group mind assuages the fear of meaninglessness rather than the in any case questionable terrors of childhood. This paper is of particular importance at the present time in helping understand the potency of fundamentalism and, beyond the violence inflicted on us, the violence we find ourselves inflicting on others.

Two papers in this volume bring lasting insight to specific clinical conditions, both from a developmental standpoint. Arnold Cooper's writings on masochism are a marker of the shifting center of gravity of North American psychoanalysis. He starts his paper (Chapter 5) by providing a thumbnail sketch of the contemporary shift toward the preoedipal in the understanding of neurosogenesis. Any shift in culture creates an opportunity for new ideas to emerge. Cooper briefly reviews Freud's accounts of masochism that included the neurophysiological (excess of stimulation), the primarily instinctual (death instinct), the secondarily instinctual (reversal of aggression), the excessive harshness of the superego, and masochism as part of feminine passivity or as a ransom to be paid to have access to pleasure. The very richness of these accounts suggests a problem with the adequacy of each. Acknowledging in a scholarly way the contributions of diverse authors such as Bergler, Hermann, and Lewin, Cooper offers a comprehensive and radical revision of our theory of masochism as an extension of normal painful ways of achieving gratifying self-definition.

He suggests that pain is necessary for the achievement of selfhood and that separation-individuation inevitably damages self-esteem. Putting these together, he argues that self-esteem may be restored through making suffering ego-syntonic. In individuals in whom early narcissistic humiliation was excessive, ego-syntonic self-harm becomes the preferred mode. Rejection is under one's own control, acceptance is not. Pleasure is normally derived from self-presentation. Those with masochistic character unconsciously provoke disaffection and are then indignant and pseudo-aggressive about this, provoking further rejection and defeat, thereby generating self-pity. Beyond the self-harm and the self-pity of masochism is the masochist's recovery of his or her sense of self through the experience of suffering. The underlying pathology is a deadened capacity to feel, muted pleasure, hypersensitive self-esteem, and the inability to derive satisfaction from or sustain a pleasurable relationship. Cooper thus recasts masochism as part of a mechanism available and at various times made use of probably by all for maintaining an adequate sense of self.

Philip Bromberg's contribution (Chapter 2) addresses a related clinical problem, eating disorder, but does so in the context of offering what is almost an entirely new psychoanalytic model of the structure of personality and the nature of psychoanalytic therapy. His serious and subtle clinical essay provides a framework for understanding and helping the so-called difficult patient. The paper explores the nature of the effects of trauma within a relational frame of reference. It shows us how symptoms linked with trauma force the analyst to proceed slowly and to be patient because underlying the patient's symptoms is an organized system of self-experience that we commonly label dissociation. Bromberg shows that trauma impedes an intrinsic self-righting capacity of the mind that is normally found through interpersonal relationships. Analogous to mother-infant interaction, intimate relationships such as the one between patient and analyst can normally be reparative, following interactive errors that demonstrate to both protagonists that miscommunication is neither permanent nor catastrophic. When the other is potentially traumatizing, recovery from such errors can no longer be the source of a sense of self-efficacy and a reaffirmation of the other as an object of trust.

This closely argued and wonderfully illustrated presentation describes the subjective experience of the analyst as well as that of the traumatized patient. The analyst's countertransference of dissociation together with the patient's experience can coexist as perceived events as they both stand in the spaces between previously unbridgeable self states. With regard to eating disorder, the dissociated state created in the analyst is desire. Desire dominates the patient's mental life (for food), and desire for cure can similarly come to dominate and undermine the analytic intent of the treater.

FOCUSING ON PRACTICE

Elements of the Therapeutic

Three of the contributions to this volume have taken the delineation of the therapeutic aspect of psychoanalytic treatment as their focus. Although this question is addressed in various ways and in a range of contexts, these three papers provide valuable complementary perspectives on the therapeutic. There can be few more helpful clinical papers in the psychoanalytic corpus than Fred Busch's contribution, "'In the Neighborhood'" (Chapter 3). First, as many of the papers in this volume, the paper includes a historical overview that is in itself a tour de force, focusing our attention on how psychoanalysts could overlook something as obvious and as experience near as the conscious ego. The implicit critique of a psychoanalytic past that excluded a phenomenological perspective was timely, is timeless, and beautifully delivered. The conscious readiness to grasp the hidden meaning of an experience is the essence of interpretive work. This is more than just timing. This perspective is also essential to adequate formulation.

The attitude to working near the conscious ego, the layeredness of psychoanalytic work, is a key guiding principle of analytic thinking. Cognitive-behavioral therapy perhaps rediscovered the conscious ego and stole a march on psychoanalysis by claiming something that was, as Busch's essay so clearly illustrates, by right "ours." No doubt there is resistance to "working in the neighborhood" in the regressive relationship of analyst and patient. Yet self-control, a central aim of analytic work, is evidently enhanced by the gradual enlargement of consciousness rather than its forced enlightenment through "deep interpretations."

A second essential principle of the therapeutic is identified and beautifully analyzed by Robert Emde (Chapter 6). Emde focuses his breathtaking integrative essay on empathy. He traces the concept with exemplary scholarship to major psychoanalytic contributors (Loewald, Greenson, Kohut, and many others) and to constructs from developmental psychology such as Vygotsky's zone of proximal development, the processes of affect regulation, and pioneering work on social referencing.

Of course many of the developmental discoveries that he cites are his own, although Emde remains the modest scholar to a fault. He leads the reader through all the stages of the analytic process to show how fundamental modes of development are mobilized by the background sense of mutuality, an affective as well as cognitive executive "we" and the sense of reciprocity that early moral internalization reflected in empathy entails. An important implication of Emde's argument is the legitimization of a creative, playful analytic process. Role responsiveness, mirroring, and the scaffolding of analytic work serve as examples in which developmental research and ideas concerning therapeutic process can be seamlessly integrated.

A different but nevertheless equally ubiquitous aspect of clinical work is pointed to by Edgar Levenson (Chapter 16). Levenson's masterful paper starts with a deconstruction of a relational experience, an interpersonal interaction in what seems like an ordinary analysis. But the implications he draws from this meticulous scrutiny are far from ordinary. In his attempt at identifying "common ground" across the plurality of psychoanalytic theorization, Levenson first of all points to the indeterminacy inherent to the search for meaning within analytic material, fantasy, or relational experience, whether in terms of a horizontal broadening (linking to other current situations) or a vertical extension (to past experience). Levenson's key insight is that the common ground is to be found not in the breakdown of defenses or the finding of a common emerging narrative, but rather the deliberate and purposeful fragmentation of the patient's fictionalization of his or her life.

Forcing a story onto a story by interpretation is the key method of psychoanalysis. It allows new meanings to emerge from a chaotic flux of meanings in the crucible of the transference. This is not the same as the notion of narrative truth; it is not the compelling persuasive narrative that wins the day. The only truth Levenson maintains in line with postmodernists (i.e., Eco, Norris, and Derrida) is the very play of deconstruction. It mobilizes and captures the healing process of the patient, although what this process is remains a mystery. However, in passing he offers an important clarification between relational theory (of which this is a part) and relational therapy (the curative power of the analytic relationship). Relationship may be the curative element even if the analytic aim is simply that of interpretation.

Countertransference and the Analytic Context

Three excellent contributions have as their central concern the context within which treatment takes place. The context of course is defined by the analyst's person.

Most of the countertransference literature in this field deals with the analyst's reaction as a key to the patient's current state. The work of Judy Kantrowitz (Chapter 14) highlights an alternative aspect of countertransference: not what has been put into the analyst but rather what was there in the first place. Kantrowitz's work has established a system for considering the extent to which patient and analyst overlap in terms of attitudes, values, beliefs, cognitive and defensive style, and general strategies for adaptation. Her work has clearly established how blind spots can be created by the analyst's character. Similarity between patient and analyst may distance the analyst from the problem in an effort to resist empathic identification. Alternatively, a match can create too great an immersion undermining exploration of similarities. Looking for similarities can help the analyst and patient find an effective way of working together, creating a feeling of affective resonance. But at another phase of the analysis it can impede the work by, for example, unhelpfully protecting the patient from an emotional experience of isolation.

Kantrowitz is clear and eloquent on the subject in suggesting a solution to the clinical problems that are brought into focus through the examination of the match. There is need for outside input. Consultation, supervision, and continuous case discussions with peers are all potentially helpful if they can focus specifically on identifying the nature and extent of the match between patient and analyst. In fairness she points out that continuing discussion groups can be troubled by the same issues of match as individual patient-analyst pairs. Ideally psychoanalytic training at all levels should incorporate this perspective.

The importance of supervision and external consultation is highlighted also by the acknowledged master of the kinds of difficult clinical situations which we tend to bring for consultation. Glen Gabbard's paper on boundary violations (Chapter 8) has all the qualities that a plenary address to the International Psychoanalytical Association should have. It provides a remarkable illumination of countertransference phenomena in cases in which boundary violation occurs. The sensitively presented but profoundly unsettling clinical material shows how our improved understanding of the mechanism of borderline personality disorder is helpful in seeing why all of us may be vulnerable to the kinds of self-deception that can derail a psychoanalysis, a professional life, and a patient's right to be healed.

The importance of Gabbard's description is in bringing the experience of dramatic violations into the realm of everyday clinical work. The predictable destruction of our capacity to think with suicidal patients, originating from the mismanagement of aggression and hatred, creates the vulnerability from which a treatment may not recover. The analyst's unconscious anxieties about his sadism triggered by the patient's suicidality generating a folie à deux in the treatment setting is part of our daily work. Gabbard's contribution by allowing us to hate as well as love our clinical work perhaps succeeds in obviating the risk that patient and analyst can represent for each other.

The analytic frame and the rituals that surround it normally create the boundary that protects the patient (and analyst) from the risk of maltreatment. Yet as Irwin Hoffman (Chapter 12) points out, the frame is complex and not in all ways in the patient's best interests. Hoffman addresses the subjective experience of the frame for patient and analyst. In an enormously helpful and practical paper, he points to the dialectic interplay between ritual and spontaneity at every moment of every analysis. There is a dialectic between what is given and what is created. But there is an interdependence between what he terms the analytic ritual (the frame) and the spontaneity that can occur within it.

While accepting the need for the frame, Hoffman also points to its pathological malignant aspects. Ultimately he links the frame to something that helps us buttress our belief in the worthwhileness of life in the face of the certainty of death. Frequently the analyst is called on to act without the luxury of thinking, and although transgressing the ritual is rarely a deliberate act, it is invariably the product of a struggle between ritual and spontaneity that permits something new to emerge from the shadows of something old.

While recognizing the role of the patient in creating these situations, Hoffman believes that acceding to a patient's request that might violate the frame can paradoxically facilitate the patient's feeling that it is unnecessary for him or her to pressure the analyst in this way. Somewhat contrasting with Gabbard, who highlights the risks of caving in to internal pressures to accede to requests, Hoffman considers noncatastrophic transgressions to be helpful in creating an experience for the patient in which the analyst is seen to be owning part of the patient's subjective experience, for example his or her drives. This rich and insightful paper also foreshadows and complements Thomas Ogden's contribution (Chapter 19) in that Hoffman describes what Ogden termed an analytic object, something that neither the patient nor the analyst owned but was created by their joint subjectivities.

The Analyst's Basic Attitude

Reading the selections, I was fascinated to see that the largest group of papers was focused on reviewing the analyst's position, what may be called the basis of a psychoanalytic attitude. Traditionally of course we consider ourselves benignly neutral with respect to our patients. However, many of the previous papers in this collection and all the ones to follow are consistent in repudiating this now apparently somewhat disingenuous point of view. The scene is set by Lawrence Friedman's paper (Chapter 7), which highlights the adversarial character of the analytic attitude. Friedman's paper is not only brilliant, it is a joy to read. The combination of intelligence and humor seduces the reader almost to overlook the profound penetration Friedman achieves into the psychoanalytic unconscious, the story behind our story as practicing psychoanalysts. The paper aims to illuminate the analytic attitude, Freud's and ours, and explain changing foci and technique in terms of the demand characteristics of the analyst's situation. Friedman focuses on the implicit adversarial stance opted for by most Freudian analysts. It originates, he believes, in the intolerability of our dependency on our patients.

Friedman gently leads us through the development of psychoanalysis as a therapeutic technique in Freud's hands and shows components of this attitude. For example, all analysts know that patients only reveal things in order to conceal something more important. The adversarial attitude toward the patient of course also pervades interprofessional discourse. Being collusive with the patient is the most common critique of clinical presentations, and analysts determined to present a more human face (e.g., Loewald and Kohut) are treated with suspicion in case the necessary alertness to possible collusion may have been diluted. Echoing Levenson, Friedman sees the deconstruction of the patient's presentation as essential to freeing the analyst's imagination. Freud's adversarial attitude is neutralized by his focus on mental mechanisms to which we cannot attribute malevolent intent, only dysfunction. But Friedman shows how moralizing keeps drifting back into therapy with the patient as the guilty party. He illuminates analytic attitudes and finds them ultimately dull and lacking in affection and drama. However, he finds this both necessary and desirable because the attitude itself is the source of that most ephemeral of contexts, a psychoanalytic treatment and a laboratory of the special paradoxes of humanness.

Four of the selected favorite articles have grappled with the problem of disclosure. Three of these argue the merits or even the essential quality of disclosure of countertransference experience. Paul Ornstein's contribution (Chapter 20) comes upon this issue somewhat indirectly. Ornstein presents Kohut's ideas on narcissistic rage with a clear purpose and focus. He accepts Kohut's assertion that all types of destructive aggression are a manifestation of narcissistic rage because they all involve an insistence on perfection in the idealized selfobject and the limitless power of the grandiose self. These are rooted in traumatic injuries to the grandiose self or obstacles to merger with the parental imago. This beautiful paper provides a phenomenological framework to narcissistic rage that cannot progress to self-assertiveness because it is the self structure that is enfeebled and vulnerable. The clinical focus needs to be on the self-defining, self-bolstering function of rage.

Ornstein's purpose in giving this account, however, is to illuminate the appropriate clinical stance with individuals whose limited experience of selfhood includes the incapacity to fully experience rage. This can create an analytic stance of withholding that will have a negative impact on the patient. He describes a clinical context within which an analytic reserve against providing mirroring transference is sensed by such a patient who feels that he requires acceptance without reservation. Exposing this aspect of countertransference is found to help, but it is the change in attitude to the initial demands that is seen as preventing the negative reactions. If emotional recognition is there but not experienced by the patient it is likely that a countertransference reticence was present.

Evelyn Schwaber (Chapter 25) also recommends sensitive disclosures of the countertransference when indicated by difficulties in listening. Schwaber's chapter is immensely rich in clinical detail, which is essential given her important intent to elaborate the challenges inherent to the basic analytic task of listening. In this paper she takes as her focus the common experience of attempting to disguise our "actual" attitude from our patients. She identifies that such disguise relinquishes our basic position of collaboration. Further, disguising our real attitudes imposes uncertainty on the patient about what he or she perceives.

Schwaber recommends asking ourselves and attempting to answer the question of why we might wish to present ourselves in a way that disguises our real feelings. She also points to instances when slight differences emerge between how the analyst and the patient describe a specific experience. These and other countertransference phenomena are an indication that the analyst is trying to move the patient in his or her direction, toward his or her assumptions of meaning, whereas the patient may have something else to tell us.

A central concern of the paper is with listening while not knowing, providing sufficient space for the patient to discover a way of being through listening to the patient who is set adrift from his or her history but resisting the temptation of knowing for him or her. In this context Schwaber confronts but does not attempt to resolve the complex problem of reconstruction. The paper ends with a beautiful epigrammatic analogy for psychoanalysis of Oliver Sacks's blind patient who is a sought-after traveling companion for sighted people because she asks them questions: "then they look, and see things they wouldn't otherwise." But as the title of the paper states, it is a struggle for most of us to accept the role of the blind traveling companion.

Theodore Jacobs (Chapter 13) was one of the courageous pioneers who mapped the clinical use of the analyst's subjective experience. In this painstakingly self-exploratory paper he discusses the unspoken frame that defines what is and is not acceptable in a clinical situation with a specific patient. The frame is set jointly by patient and analyst but outside the awareness of each and is maintained through a degree of collusion. This way of seeing the frame brings it far more into the realm of what is co-constructed than conceiving of the frame as a set of rituals imposed by a psychoanalytic superego.

This allows Jacobs to explore the value of experiencing with the patient his own subjectivity but at the same time to consider the risks this brings. He considers risks in the use of the countertransference that can entail inadvertent aggression, frequently with the aim of protecting the analyst's self-esteem, maintaining his or her autonomy and superiority, or hiding his or her sexual feelings or dependency. The analyst's countertransference here as elsewhere is a response to the patient's unconscious mind, frequently marked by resonances indicated by nonverbal behaviors. The analyst's error, whether or not triggered by the patient, in making use of his or her countertransference is best then shared with the patient. In Jacobs's view suppressing something the patient knows occurred outside of their shared frame is demanding collusion only to bolster the analyst's self-esteem.

Whereas the previous three contributions discuss specific situations that call for countertransference disclosure, or indeed the risks that such disclosure can carry that are nevertheless best met by being open with the patient, Owen Renik (Chapter 23) brings a very radical solution, making disclosure a "default position." Renik combines clarity of thought and expression with a dramatic message. He has done more than most to make relational technique in general and self-disclosure in particular acceptable to mainstream psychoanalysis. Everything an analyst does is self-disclosing in some way, and even a purposeful effort to self-disclose will obscure some things. Renik argues for intentional self-disclosure to be an element of the psychoanalytic method. This means, for example, to respond to inquiries as constructive requests for information. The analyst should be nonselective in his or her disclosure; in other words disclosure should not be a special response as Jacobson and Schwaber suggest. Disclosure should be the default position, but it must exclude instances when normal discourse would not demand disclosure.

Renik argues that making the analyst's experience of clinical events constantly available for the patient is choosing the patient's welfare over the analyst's comfort and in this he echoes Jacobson. Allowing the patient access to the analyst as subject is seen as desirable because it reduces excessive focus on the analyst where this is at the expense of the patient. Further, it avoids the wasteful "guess what is on my mind" game and in general increases profitable self-investigation. In addition, disclosure establishes the analyst as fallible and an appropriate subject for collaborative investigation. In this way it may enhance the analyst's as well as the patient's self-awareness. Renik identifies limitations to the method of consultation recommended, for example, by Kantrowitz and Gabbard and advocates calling the patient in as consultant. He argues that idealization is neither undermined nor unduly encouraged in such a process.

Intersubjective Models of the Clinical Process

Three wonderful papers round off this powerful collection for me, with major contributions to the understanding of intersubjectivity in the clinical setting from three points of view that together fairly encompass the current North American clinical perspective. Apparently closest to the perceived tradition is Henry Smith's beautiful and original essay (Chapter 27) that may hide its revolutionary colors. Smith sees countertransference as all pervasive and the logical consequence of the self-evident truth that as all mental activity is the product of compromise formation the analyst's listening to the patient must also be inherently conflictual. Thus all reactions to patients must involve the analyst's unconscious fantasies. The analysts' observations about their patients and themselves in relation to the patients will always be processed through such compromise formations and analytic work then can be seen to serve a defensive function for the analyst.

The analytic attitude, a willing suspension of disbelief, permits a simultaneous identification with the patient (concordant countertransferences) and the patient's objects (complementary countertransferences). In relation to these experiences, Smith eschews the retrospective self-disclosure we have considered previously in this introduction, which in his view frequently has a compliant felicitous quality that attempts to reduce or simplify countertransference. Any example of disclosure represents just another phase in what in reality is just a moment in a continuous process of enactment.

Smith offers an example of a background of irritation at a patient's resistance as being a form of benign negative countertransference, illustrating how the analyst's and the patient's experience together constitute the transference. In this way, Smith's contribution is the definition of the analytic object relationship as a co-creation that must at all times be the central focus of the analyst's work. The clinical illustration beautifully and precisely illustrates the phenomenon, although how to deal with it remains in the realm of art.

Jay Greenberg's contribution (Chapter 10) is equally evocative and original as he also tries to find the voice of clinical intersubjectivity. Of the many dichotomies that psychoanalysts have identified to help organize analytic theory as well as their patients' material, Greenberg chose the active-passive opposition for his beautiful philologically inspired paper. It is Greenberg's dissatisfaction with the subject-object dichotomy that brings him to the discovery of the "middle voice," a voice between active and passive known to Ancient Greeks but lost to current Indo-European grammar. Greenberg's expansion of relational theory links Freud's difficulties with being the object of others' wishes and intentions (a theme we also saw in Friedman's chapter) to the common experience of an incomplete sense of agency. We all sense the danger of being trapped by our own decisions. We have agency but so do others who share our world.

Traditional psychoanalytic theory of wish fulfillment, Greenberg suggests, is inadequate in depicting the unconscious experience of being acted on by other people. The clinical material that Greenberg brings illustrates that extending a patient's sense of agency to an unconscious part of his or her mind is sometimes neither clarifying nor therapeutic. The middle voice is a much closer approximation to the subjective experience of all tragic heroes and the rest of us, aware of the need to act while being aware of living out a history of being acted on and irreducibly uncertain how we will be acted on in the future.

And finally, Thomas Ogden's paper (Chapter 19) is a superlative exposition of the intersubjective aspects of the clinical process, using the concept of projective identification with the virtuosity of the master theoretician that he undoubtedly is. The analytic setting for Ogden must include two subjectivities whose subtle interplay he shows us creates the analytic third that is simultaneously within and outside the unconscious intersubjectivities of analyst and analysand. His theory, which is meticulously drawn out with the aesthetic qualities of a Dürer etching, shows how through projective identification the subjectivity of both patient and analyst are subjugated by a third unconscious that has to be overcome, and the individual subjectivities reappropriated for analysis to succeed.

But the paper is not about abstractions; it is more hands on and practical than the vast bulk of clinical analytic writing. In illustrating his model of process, Ogden shows how analysts must hold on to lapses of attention, test and retest their intuition about connections between their own and their patient's subjectivity, and discard that which feels shallow, self-serving, or clichéd. Ogden's phenomenological description has staggering richness and texture. In exploring his own subjectivity, he shows how recognizing fresh aspects of mundane rumination in the course of a session identifies the stray thought as an analytic object created through analytic intersubjectivity. It is not new material, thought, or interpretation that drives the process but rather the change of subjective experience for both patient and analyst. The analyst speaks of this from a position outside it but drawing on images created by the intersubjective experience.

What Ogden elaborates requires an openness to experience that is very different from free-floating attention. He treads on private sacred ground made available to the analytic process. He advances a Hegelian model in showing how projective identification entails disowning the self either into the other, whereas the other disowns the self to become the projector or to become what is projected. Either entails mutual creation, negation, and the preservation of dialectic subjects, each of which is subjugated by the other and only freed through discourse from the third position. Ogden's model of analytic experience achieves great subtlety and complexity but retains all clarity and coherence.

CONCLUSION

This book opens a gateway to the current thinking of the greatest North American psychoanalysts. It presents an exciting picture, a vibrant discipline, in ferment, in the process of radical transformation, finding new ideas, and developing inspiring and challenging integrations. Freud was unnecessarily concerned about the fate of psychoanalysis in the context of the predominantly pragmatic North American culture. Historically psychoanalysis thrived in the United States more than anywhere else in the world. The bias toward pragmatism is still there in twenty-first century American psychoanalysis, but it is massively enriched by, as indeed it enriches, the clinical focus founded in the Berlin-Budapest rather than the Vienna prewar psychoanalytic tradition. Readers interested in acquiring a comprehensive and authoritative as well as entertaining guide to current North American psychoanalytic thinking need look no further than Arnold Cooper's collection of master papers.

Peter Fonagy, Ph.D., F.B.A.

REFERENCES

Blatt SJ: Experiences of Depression: Theoretical, Clinical, and Research Perspectives. Washington, DC, American Psychological Association, 2004

Sandler J, Sandler AM: The past unconscious, the present unconscious, and the vicissitudes of guilt. Int J Psychoanal 68:331–341, 1987

1

CHARLES BRENNER, M.D.

INTRODUCTION

Charles Brenner, M.D., graduated from Harvard College and Harvard Medical School in Cambridge, Massachusetts. He did residencies in medicine, psychiatry, and neurology and was a member of the faculty of neurology at Harvard and later at the Columbia University College of Physicians and Surgeons in New York. He graduated from the New York Psychoanalytic Institute, where he is a Training and Supervising Analyst, and has served as President of the New York Psychoanalytic Society and Chair of the Program Committee of the American Psychoanalytic Association and subsequently its President. He is Clinical Professor of Psychiatry at the University of the State of New York in Brooklyn. He has been one of the most prominent analysts on the American psychoanalytic scene for the past half century.

Dr. Brenner's many honors include the Mary S. Sigourney Award for Contributions to the Field of Psychoanalysis, the award of the American Psychoanalytic Association for Distinguished Contributions to Psychoanalytic Education, and both the establishment of the Charles Brenner Award for Outstanding Contributions to Psychoanalytic Education by the New York Psychoanalytic Institute and the Charles Brenner Visiting Professorship in Psychoanalysis of the Milwaukee Psychoanalytic Foundation and the Medical College of Wisconsin. He is an honorary member of five of the constituent societies of the American Psychoanalytic Association. He has held numerous visiting professorships and is the author of 100 papers and four books: *An Elementary*

Textbook of Psychoanalysis, Psychoanalytic Concepts and the Structural Theory (with Dr. Jacob A. Arlow), *Psychoanalytic Technique and Psychic Conflict*, and *The Mind in Conflict.*

Dr. Brenner's career has been notable in many respects, but mostly for his courageous willingness on more than one occasion to alter accepted psychoanalytic paradigms. His 1959 article on masochistic character gave new meaning to Robert Waelder's concept of multiple function, which Dr. Brenner continued to enlarge. In the 1970s he hugely expanded our concept of conflict and defense by emphasizing that depressive affect is a motivator of defense on a par with anxiety. He has, throughout his writings, emphasized that conflict and consequent compromise formation are ubiquitous in all mental functioning, both normal and neurotic. In recent years he has taken the further step, which he considers to be logically necessary, of suggesting that the mind is better understood in terms of conflict and compromise formation rather than in terms of separate structures: id, ego, and superego.

Perhaps Dr. Brenner's greatest influence was achieved as author of *An Elementary Textbook of Psychoanalysis,* which was published in 1955 and, amazingly, is still in print. It has been translated into a dozen languages and has sold more than one million copies. It has been an introduction to the field for generations of Americans, both psychoanalysts and nonpsychoanalysts.

Dr. Brenner has been a model of productivity and scholarship and of original contributions to psychoanalysis throughout his lifetime, and he continues in this mode. Where many would have been content to rest on early laurels, he has continued to excite interest and controversy through continued innovation.

He has said of himself,

> I don't quite know how to respond to your question about my ideas about my role in the psychoanalytic scene. I was president of both the American Psychoanalytic Association and the New York Psychoanalytic Society and was appointed a Training and Supervising Analyst of the New York Psychoanalytic Institute in 1957. I was also Chair of the Program Committee of the American Psychoanalytic Association for 7 years and Secretary of the New York Psychoanalytic Society for 3 years, which involved being in charge of arranging its programs of scientific sessions during that time. As such, I had much to do with the evolution of the program format of the American into the form its meetings had for many years.
>
> I'm sure my most significant influence was as author of *An Elementary Textbook of Psychoanalysis....* Many colleagues have told me that their interest in psychoanalysis stemmed from reading it in college or graduate school.

When I turned 60, in 1973, I felt I could look back on a professional career that I felt proud of as being more than usually successful. I never imagined at that time that what I consider to be my major contributions to psychoanalysis were yet to come. It has been both a surprise and a great source of satisfaction that that's the way it turned out.

WHY I CHOSE THIS PAPER

Charles Brenner, M.D.

I chose "Conflict, Compromise Formation, and Structural Theory" for inclusion in this volume because it contains what I judge to be the most useful and valuable contribution I have been able to make to the field of psychoanalysis. The changes Freud made in his so-called topographic theory, that resulted in what is commonly called his structural theory, substantially altered psychoanalytic practice as well. They, plus Anna Freud's "The Ego and the Mechanisms of Defence" and Fenichel's "Problems of Psychoanalytic Technique," were responsible for the realization that defenses are to be analyzed rather than dealt with in some other way, as had been mostly the case previously.

In this paper I suggest that the recognition of the fact that compromise formation resulting from conflict over the sexual and aggressive wishes of early childhood is universal and ubiquitous, rather than occasional and limited to psychopathology, also substantially alters psychoanalytic practice as well as the psychoanalytic theory of how the mind works. It makes explicit the idea that every thought and action, rather than just the ones judged to be pathological, is potential grist for the analytic mill.

CONFLICT, COMPROMISE FORMATION, AND STRUCTURAL THEORY

CHARLES BRENNER, M.D.

FREUD'S FIRST PUBLISHED EXPOSITION of a theory of the mind—or to use his preferred term, of the mental apparatus—is contained in the seventh chapter of *The Interpretation of Dreams* (Freud 1900). There he suggested that the mind is composed of three systems, for which he suggested the names *Cs.* (= Conscious), *Pcs.* (= Preconscious), and *Ucs.* (= Unconscious). Although he changed the names and the definitions of the systems into which he proposed to divide the mind, the idea that the mind is best understood as a group of functionally identifiable systems, agencies, or structures (the three words are synonymous in this context) is one that he held to throughout his life (Arlow and Brenner 1964; Brenner 1994).

The fact that these systems and structures are, moreover, an aspect of psychoanalytic theory that has won general and unchallenged acceptance by psychoanalysts is attested to by the currency of the terms that Freud introduced at various times to designate the various systems: the conscious, the preconscious, the unconscious, the ego, the id, the superego. But despite the fact that the idea (= theory) that the mind is best understood as a group of functionally identifiable and separable structures has achieved general acceptance, I believe it is not a valid theory and should be discarded (Brenner 1994, 1998). In the present paper, I propose to present evidence that I believe further supports my view. I shall also include some comments on both the nature and the origin of conflict and compromise formation in mental life.

"Conflict, Compromise Formation, and Structural Theory," by Charles Brenner, M.D., was first published in © The Psychoanalytic Quarterly, 2002, *The Psychoanalytic Quarterly,* Volume 71, Number 3, pages 397–417. Used with permission.

CONFLICT AND COMPROMISE FORMATION

The related ideas of conflict and compromise formation were what suggested to Freud in the first place that different parts of the mind can be opposed to one another. He discovered very early in his analytic work with patients that psychogenic symptoms have meaning (Freud 1894, 1896). His early observations persuaded him that such patients want to gratify some sexual wish(es) of childhood origin that are inaccessible to consciousness in adult life and at the same time, they want to deny, disavow, or suppress those wishes. To explain these findings, he proposed the theory that one part of the mind, inaccessible to consciousness, is bent on gratifying such wishes and another, conscious or accessible to consciousness, is opposed to their gratification. Mental conflict and symptom formation are then explainable as results of conflict between different systems or structures within the mind.

To summarize very briefly, the one system or structure, called first the Ucs. and later the id, was understood to be concerned with the achievement of pleasurable gratification of sexual and aggressive wishes of childhood origin without delay and to function without regard to the demands and limitations imposed by the environment (=external reality). Another structure, or group of related functions, called first the Cs.-Pcs. and later the ego, was understood to take account of and conform to those very demands and limitations. It was credited with serving the function of controlling—and when necessary, opposing—the sexual and aggressive wishes of the id. A third structure, the superego, was understood to serve the function of erecting and enforcing each individual's moral code of beliefs and behavior. Thus, the clinically observable data of mental conflict are to be explained, according to Freud, by the assumption that the mind is composed of functionally definable and separable structures (= systems, = agencies) that may, by their very nature, be opposed to one another.

The fundamental importance attributed to this theoretical concept is attested by the fact that analysts customarily use it to designate the whole of psychoanalytic theory. Its first version, which divides the mind into Cs., Pcs., and Ucs., gave rise to the term *topographic theory,* a term generally used by psychoanalysts to designate the whole of psychoanalytic theory as it existed prior to 1923, when Freud published *The Ego and the Id.* The second version, which divided the mind into ego, superego, and id, gave rise to the term *structural theory,* which, in its turn, has generally been used to designate the whole of psychoanalytic theory as it has developed subsequent to the publication of *The Ego and the Id.*

The truth is, however, that the theoretical concept that divides the mind into structures, systems, or agencies is but one part of psychoanalytic theory, a part that has been, to be sure, an important and enduring one until now. It is only that part that I am calling into question at the present time. I am not suggesting that one call into question such aspects of psychoanalytic theory as, for example, psychic causality, or the role of unconscious mental processes, or that dreams and symptoms have meaning, or that psychosexual life begins in early childhood, to name but a few of its tenets. I assert only that mental functioning in general and mental conflict and compromise formation in particular are not best explained by the theory that the mind is composed of three functionally definable and separable structures (= systems or agencies) called ego, superego, and id.

It should be added that Freud attributed additional distinguishing characteristics to the systems or structures into which he proposed to divide the mind. These will be merely mentioned here, since I assume they are familiar to most readers.[1] Freud believed that what he called the *id* functions according to what he proposed to call the *primary process.* The id is concerned solely with achieving prompt and full gratification of pleasure-seeking wishes of childhood origin. In its functioning (= primary process), it takes no account of external reality, disregards rules of logic, tolerates mutually contradictory ideas, is unconcerned with temporal restraints or demands, and so on. Its way of functioning can be aptly described as being in accord with the demand, "I want what I want and I want it right now!" The id, Freud believed, is a part of the mind that serves the drives and ignores the environment.

The ego, by contrast, was conceived to be as tied to external reality as the id is tied to each individual's pleasure-seeking wishes. The ego, Freud proposed, functions according to the *secondary process.* It obeys the rules of logic, is cognizant of the demands and constraints of the environment and attempts to conform to them, does not tolerate mutually contradictory ideas, is concerned with temporal constraints, and so on. In addition, Freud postulated that what goes on in the id, following the primary process, is nonverbal, while what goes on in the ego, following the secondary process, is verbal. As is evident from even such a very brief summary as this, the theory of mental agencies embodies Freud's conclusion that what he had discovered about the role of conflict in mental life is best understood if one assumes that one part of the mind functions in an infantile way while another part functions in a more mature way.

---

[1]A fuller discussion can be found in Arlow and Brenner 1964.

EVALUATING FREUD'S SYSTEMS/STRUCTURES OF THE MIND

How consonant is this theory or assumption with the observable facts? Let's start with the id. What can be observed of the sexual drives of each individual are that individual's wishes for pleasurable sexual satisfaction (Brenner 1976, 1982). From the very earliest time of life at which such wishes can be observed, they are anchored in reality. They never—so far as can be observed with the help of the psychoanalytic method—ignore external reality as perceived and understood by the individual at the time of life in question. A child aged 3 years or thereabouts wants satisfaction from its parent, i.e., from a particular person, and it wants a particular form of physical contact with that person. It does not want only oral gratification, for example; it wants to suck or swallow a particular person's penis or breast. Its wishes are realistic ones, given its state of mental development. They are determined by its experiences and by its thoughts about those experiences. It wants to do or to have done to it what it has observed and/or fantasied being done to or by one or more of the persons of its environment. However illogical and unrealistic its wishes may be by adult standards, they are quite in accord with what the child in question understands of the real world in which it lives. Associated competitive, murderous and/or castrative wishes are similarly determinatively influenced by the persons and events of the external world.

Furthermore, such sexual and aggressive wishes cannot be said to be nonverbal. All of them can be formulated in words and are so formulated by each individual, however primitive and immature its verbal capacities may be. All young children certainly have wishes that are irrational and/or unrealistic by adult standards, and that appear so when they persist—as they so often do—into adult life, whether consciously or unconsciously. They were not, however, either irrational or unrealistic at their time of origin. To say that there is a part of the mind that strives for sexual gratification with no concern for external reality is wholly at odds with the observable data.

The same is true for the theory that a part of the mind exists that is reality bound, that strives to be mature and logical, that is more concerned with its relation to the external world than with achieving pleasurable sexual gratification. Every aspect of mental functioning attributable to what Freud proposed to call the *ego* is, in fact, a compromise formation that serves the purpose of gratifying pleasure-seeking wishes of childhood origin, as well as the purpose of defending against them (Brenner 1968, 1982, 1994, 1997). There is no part of the mind that functions in a mature, logical, realistic way simply because that is the way that part of the mind is designed to function, which is what the structural theory maintains is the case. To be mature in one's thinking, to be logical, to be consistent, to take account of the demands and constraints of the environment are all behaviors that express conflict and compromise formation originating in the pleasure-seeking wishes of childhood. The most intelligent of persons may believe religious myths that are obviously unsupported by observable data. Millions of individuals in time of war are united in attributing to the enemy the least acceptable of their own wishes. There is no part of the mind that functions as the ego is supposed to do. Being logical, mature, and realistic in one's thinking has a pleasure premium. It may gratify childhood wishes to be as omniscient as one's parents seem to every child to be, to win their praise, or to compete with them or with brothers and sisters. Like all compromise formations, such attitudes and behaviors have a defensive function as well; they may reassure that one is not castrated or otherwise defective, or that one is reasonable and obedient and not rebelliously antagonistic.

THE UBIQUITY OF COMPROMISE FORMATIONS

Whatever its origins may be, a mature, logical, and realistic attitude is in every case a compromise formation, as can be demonstrated whenever analysis is possible. Analytic and other data do not support the conclusion that secondary process mentation occurs due to the fact that a part of the mind, the ego, operates by its very nature in a mature, logical, and realistic way. For the mind to operate in the way that Freud called the primary process is often perfectly ego-syntonic (Brenner 1968).

The compromise formations that result from conflict over the pleasure-seeking (= libidinal and aggressive) wishes of childhood are not necessarily pathological, as Freud believed to be the case. His belief was that conflict—or, more precisely, compromise formation—and pathology (in mental life) are synonymous. Normal, adult mental functioning, he believed, is not conflictual. It is, as Hartmann (1964) later put it, conflict free. Witness the idea, still widely current, that psychoanalysis and/or psychoanalytic psychotherapy, when successful, resolve conflicts. "The patient's conflicts over childhood libidinal and aggressive wishes were resolved and the symptoms (= compromise formations) disappeared" is the customary formulation.

Freud recognized very early—almost from the start of his psychoanalytic work—that psychogenic symptoms are compromise formations.

It was not long before he realized that the same is true for the slips and errors of daily life, and for dreams as well. But he never recognized that nearly all aspects of mental life that are of interest to analysts—thoughts, plans, fantasies, dreams, actions, to name but a few—are, in fact, compromise formations that are determinatively influenced by the same childhood wishes and conflicts that give rise to symptoms of mental origin (Brenner 1982). Mental functioning, both in childhood and in adult life, is governed by the pleasure/unpleasure principle.

The difference between what is customarily called *normal* and what is called *pathological* in mental functioning is not that the one of these is a compromise formation, while the other is not (Brenner 1982); in fact, both are compromise formations. If a compromise formation allows for enough in the way of pleasurable gratification, if it is not accompanied by too much unpleasure in the form of anxiety and/or depressive affect, if there is not too much inhibition of function as a result of the defenses at work and not too much by way of self-punishing and/or self-destructive tendencies, the compromise formation, whatever its nature, is classified as *normal*. If, on the other hand, a compromise formation allows for too little in the way of pleasurable gratification, if it involves too much unpleasure in the form of anxiety and/or depressive affect, if there is too much inhibition of function and too many self-destructive and/or self-injurious tendencies, that compromise formation is classified as *pathological* (Brenner 1982).

Whether normal or pathological, the dynamics of every thought, fantasy, and so forth are the same: all are determinatively influenced by childhood conflicts in accordance with the pleasure/unpleasure principle. Every mind works at all times to gain as much by way of pleasure through the gratification of childhood sexual and aggressive wishes as it can and, at the same time, to avoid as much unpleasure as possible. The problem is not to satisfy the need of some mental agency or structure to be reasonable, mature, and realistic, while simultaneously pressed by the desire of another agency to achieve immediate pleasurable gratification of childhood sexual and aggressive wishes; rather, the problem is how to achieve as much pleasurable gratification as possible, while avoiding as much associated unpleasure as possible.

To put the matter as succinctly as possible, when one wishes for something that is intensely pleasurable, either in fact or fantasy, and that is at the same time associated with intense unpleasure, what results is what Freud (1894, 1896) called a *compromise formation*. That is to say, Freud discovered that every obsessional or hysterical symptom is at the same time both the gratification of a childhood, pleasure-seeking wish and the defense against and/or punishment for gratifying that same wish. It is, he discovered, a mixture of gratification and defense and/or self-punishment. More recently, it has become clear that the same is true not just for obsessional and hysterical symptoms, but for every aspect of mental life. Conflict and compromise formation are ubiquitous and normal, not exceptional and pathological (Brenner 1982).

In the light of our newer knowledge we can say that what *compromise formation* means today is that the human mind always functions so as to achieve as much pleasurable gratification as it can, while at the same time avoiding as much as possible of any associated unpleasure. When a pleasure-seeking wish is associated with unpleasure, the mind is in conflict. What one observes in thought and behavior in situations of conflict is *compromise formation.* Conflict and compromise formation characterize all of mental life. Everything we observe that is of interest to us as analysts is a compromise formation.

MENTAL CONFLICTS IN EARLY CHILDHOOD

The conflicts that are the most intense and fateful for mental functioning throughout the course of an individual's life are those that center on the sexual and aggressive wishes of early childhood (Freud 1905, 1926). They make their first identifiable appearance in mental life at about the age of 3 years. The pleasure-seeking wishes in question are essentially the same as those that characterize the sexual lives of adults. Children of that age yearn for the attention of other persons, usually their parents, and for the stimulating pleasure of physical contact with them. They are jealous of any rival. They intensely resent any evidence of infidelity, lack of interest, or neglect on the part of the person they yearn for. They desire revenge, whether on a successful rival, the faithless loved one, or both. Being ignorant, they are curious about what adult sexual partners do with and to each other, and wish to do the same themselves. They wonder where babies come from and want to make them. Being relatively small, weak, ignorant, and unintelligent, they feel inferior, humiliated, and, in turn, miserable, desperate, and enraged at being made to feel so. They intensely desire to be grown-up sexual men and women who are as clever, wise, and sexually successful as the adults around them seem to them to be.

The gratification of these sexual and aggressive wishes, in fact or fantasy, is associated with intense pleasure. Efforts to achieve their gratification persist as fundamental motives in thought and behavior throughout life, though disavowed and disguised after the first few years of childhood. The period of life during which they appear relatively undisguised lasts approximately from ages 3 to 6 years. Analysts customarily refer to the wishes themselves as *oedipal wishes* and to the period of life between the ages of 3 to 6 years as the *oedipal period.*

This customary terminology, introduced by Freud, has dramatic and didactic value. King Oedipus, in the play written more than two thousand years ago, murdered his father, married his mother, and had children by her. But in addition to its obvious value, it is a usage that has disadvantages as well. Emerging sexual and aggressive wishes during this time of life include much that the legend of Oedipus did not even hint at, at least in the form in which it has come down to us. For example, jealous and rivalrous sexual wishes are as important and as characteristic a feature of the development of girls as of boys. Why designate them with a male name? Moreover, the sexual wishes in question are never exclusively heterosexual. They are, as far as one can judge from experience to date, always bisexual. Young boys have wishes to be girls or women, just as young girls have wishes to be boys or men. Calling these sexual and aggressive wishes *oedipal* has, therefore, often led to misunderstanding, as though to imply that the sexual and aggressive wishes that are identifiable at ages 3 to 6 are limited to the crimes attributed to Oedipus in the play.

What the terms *oedipal wishes* and *oedipal period* actually mean when used by analysts, in most cases, is much better described as the *sexual and aggressive wishes that usually appear in identifiable form at about ages 3 to 6 years.* Such wishes vary from person to person, and always include far more than just killing father and marrying mother. The reader must constantly be alert to this ambiguity whenever the term *oedipal wishes* appears and substitute for it, where indicated, the more accurate term *sexual and aggressive wishes that are first identifiable at about age 3,* and must similarly substitute *ages 3 to 6 years* for *oedipal period.*

The reasons why these wishes give rise to conflict that is both so intense and so long-lasting in its effects are not far to seek. Children at that age are not independent creatures. They are dependent on their caregivers—usually parents—not only physically, but emotionally as well. Parental love, physical contact, approval, admiration, protection, and all that go with them are of utmost importance to children as sources of pleasure before, during, and after ages 3 to 6. Children long for and seek them all. Contrariwise, anything that—in a child's mind—forfeits or threatens to forfeit parental love and approval, anything that the child feels has turned or will turn one or both parents against the child, becomes a source of intense unpleasure to the child. High on the list of those sources of intense unpleasure are the child's own pleasure-seeking, sexual wishes, many of which are directed toward and/or against its parents. In addition to being sources of great pleasure, they become associated with intensely unpleasurable ideas of disapproval, rejection, abandonment, retribution, and punishment by the parents. It is that association, that inevitable concatenation of pleasure and unpleasure, that is the essence of conflict in mental life.

From then on, throughout the course of life, people's minds strive to achieve pleasurable gratification of the sexual and aggressive wishes in question, and at the same time, to avoid the associated unpleasure. Every thought, plan, fantasy, action, and so on is a compromise between these two imperatives, and every thought, plan, fantasy, and action must be understood as such. Mental activity forevermore is governed by the simultaneous opposing efforts to gain pleasure and to avoid unpleasure in connection with the sexual and aggressive wishes that are so clearly identifiable beginning at about 3 years of age. Mental functioning, beginning then and forever after, is always a compromise between the two. Compromise formation has become the rule in mental life.

But why at ages 3 to 6 years? It is obvious to the most casual observer that mental activity—what we call *mind*—begins long before age 3, and that, from its beginnings, the mind seeks pleasure and avoids unpleasure. Why should the period from 3 to 6 be of such crucial importance in mental development? Is mental functioning so different then from what it was before? If so, what are the differences and what causes them?

Physiological Development of the Brain

Mind is one aspect of the functioning of the brain. In humans, the brain is far from fully developed at birth. Both anatomically and functionally, it continues to grow and change until well into adolescence. Evidences of this are legion. For one example, the electroencephalogram of a normal neonate is very different from that of an older child or adult; in fact, it could easily be mistaken for that of a comatose adult. As another example, many children cannot coordinate eye movements until several weeks after birth, with each eye moving independently of the other. The neurons that will later coordinate the movements of the two eyes develop their full functioning in these infants only a few weeks after birth. As still another example, certain postural reflexes are normally present at birth, while a day or two later, the brain has changed and the reflexes in question have disappeared.

To give one more example, the cells of the precentral gyrus, the so-called motor cortex, do not control movements of the limbs until months after birth. In fact, the normal plantar reflex of babies a few months old is the same as the abnormal plantar reflex of an older child or adult whose leg has become paralyzed as the result of a stroke or other damage to the neuronal fibers that have their origin in the motor cortex. It is not until about the age of a year that the brain has developed to the stage at which the plantar reflex is of the normal, adult type and motor control is mediated through the axons of the cells of the precentral gyrus.

Equally striking and more directly to the point are the progressive changes in language capacity that result from the growth and development of the brain in the months and years after birth. During the first several months of infancy, the human brain is not yet an organ that can acquire language. Some individuals develop the capacity for acquiring language earlier than others, but none has ever been known to have the capacity at birth. The median age for developing the capacity is, roughly speaking, about a year after birth. Before that time, language is literally impossible; the brain is not capable of it. It is not a matter of the need for time, experience, and practice to acquire language, but rather, the human brain cannot acquire language before a certain stage of development, a stage that is never reached until several months after birth. And even then it takes months and years for the capacity for language acquisition to develop fully. No child can learn to read or write, for example, until long after it has the capacity to speak and to understand spoken words.

A brain so immature that it has no capacity for language is capable of only very simple thoughts. Before the age of 3, or thereabouts, the average child cannot have the relatively complex, language-dependent thoughts that constitute the pleasure-seeking sexual and aggressive wishes that give rise to the conflicts and compromise formations that play so large a part in mental functioning from ages 3 to 6 and ever after. What makes the period from 3 to 6 of such crucial importance in mental development is the fact that at that age, the brain has matured sufficiently so that thoughts not previously possible appear—thoughts expressing sexual and aggressive wishes and their real and fantasied consequences. There is no reason to believe that children aged 3 to 6 are any more (or less) driven to seek pleasure and avoid unpleasure than when they are younger. What change are the specificity and complexity of their pleasure-seeking wishes, as well as the association between those very wishes and highly unpleasurable perceptions, memories, and fantasies. Those are the changes that lead inevitably to conflict and compromise formation. No child on the road from infancy to adulthood can escape such conflicts; they are part of human development.

Childhood Sexual Wishes

The pleasure-seeking childhood wishes that give rise to conflict are, as Freud (1905) emphasized, associated with pleasurable sensations in various parts of the body—not only the genitals, but the mouth, anus, skin, and organs of special sense as well. As he and many subsequent authors have noted, these wishes also have to do with the persons in the child's environment. Childhood sexual wishes, and the accompanying rivalrous and vengeful, aggressive ones, are reality bound. They have to do with each child's current life experiences and environment, as was noted earlier. It is not possible to separate a child's wish for sexual pleasure from its knowledge of the world about it. Furthermore, the importance of pleasurable sensations in the genitals and other parts of the body must not be ignored or underestimated. Both thoughts and perceptions of its own body and thoughts and perceptions of its environment are essential elements of every child's sexual and aggressive wishes. The pleasure and unpleasure associated with each motivates everyone from childhood on.

What is of fateful importance for every child during the years from ages 3 to 6 is that he or she is but a child. Whatever the rare exceptions may be, it is certainly the rule that children cannot woo and win the adult(s) they yearn for, nor can they destroy or otherwise avenge themselves on those whom they perceive as rivals or as faithless. A 3- to 6-year-old child cannot be the sexually and otherwise physically mature adult it wishes to be. It is scant comfort to a child to be told that some day it, too, will be grown up and have all the pleasures it longs for now. To a child, *someday* is too far off; it is the same as *never.* Even tomorrow is very distant in the mind of a 3-year-old.

In addition, as noted earlier, children are extremely dependent on the adults (parental figures) whom they love and hate—dependent both physically and emotionally. And the parental figures in a child's life are, the child believes, both omniscient and omnipotent. How to combat such an adversary? How to imagine making an enemy of such a loved one? One has only to imagine oneself in a child's position to realize how inevitable it is that the pleasure-seeking sexual and aggressive wishes of a 3- to 6-year-old child must give rise to intense conflict.

It was the application of the psychoanalytic method to the psychoanalytic treatment of adults and children that led to the discovery of the importance in mental life of the sexual wishes and conflicts of early childhood (Freud 1905, 1926). This discovery was soon observed to be supported by a wide variety of nonclinical data, beginning with the *Gradiva* paper (Freud 1907).[2] As I have noted elsewhere (Brenner 2000), the available, pertinent evidence, both clinical and nonclinical, compels one to conclude that the conflicts and compromise formations that begin at about age 3 have a determinative effect on all subsequent mental activity—an effect that can be explained by assuming that the mind functions according to the pleasure/unpleasure principle, i.e., to achieve pleasure and to avoid unpleasure. In this case, the pleasure and unpleasure are those associated with the sexual and aggressive wishes of childhood. To assume the existence of mental agencies or structures that are often at odds with one another is not only unnecessary, it is often misleading, since it obscures the fact that conflict and compromise formation are ubiquitous in mental life. They are not merely occasional or pathological, but are ever present and normal.

The Preoedipal Period

What has been said about conflict and compromise formation having their origins at ages 3 to 6 has been criticized as ignoring or minimizing the importance of earlier events in the mental lives of children—events in the so-called *preoedipal period.* I see no reason to doubt the importance of the events of the first 3 years of life for mental development. How a child deals with the conflicts of the second 3 years of life must, it seems to me, be profoundly influenced by at least some of the experiences of the first 3. The earlier events, however, do not affect mental functioning in later childhood and adult life independently of the conflicts of the second 3 years of life. Whatever a patient's symptoms (= compromise formations) may be in adult life, they are never simply or directly a consequence of psychologically unfavorable events (= psychic traumas) that occurred in the first 3 years of life. The way the mind functions in later childhood and in adult life is the outcome of the conflicts and compromise formations of the second 3 years of life, influenced and shaped as they have been by whatever went on during the first 3 years as well.

This view is not accepted by all analysts. Some separate symptoms into those they believe to be preoedipal in origin and those they believe to be of oedipal origin. The former include symptoms showing much evidence of separation anxiety or depressive affect associated with separation, as well as symptoms with evidence of wishes to merge with a loved and/or hated person. Ideas of dissolution, fragmentation, and

---

[2]A fairly full account of their nature can be found in the last chapter of *The Mind in Conflict* (Brenner 1982).

unreality are also often classified as preoedipal. My own experience is that in every such case, if one reserves judgment and pays attention to the patient's associations to the symptoms described, one discovers that such a classification is incorrect. Though they may not be immediately apparent, sexual and aggressive wishes—and the conflicts and compromise formations associated with them—are as much the determinants of such so-called preoedipal conflicts and symptoms as they are of any other.

A good example would be an adult patient with symptoms of depression, whose mother was emotionally unavailable during the patient's first and second years of life. Analysis—i.e., attention to the patient's associations and behavior—will show in every such case that the patient's reactions to mother's absence can be understood only when the conflicts of the second 3 years of life are taken into account. Such a patient may be convinced, for example, that mother did not love her/him because of the patient's "bad" sexual wishes, or because of his/her "bad" murderous impulses or jealousy, and that his/her punishment and/or penance included castration—wishes and fears that arose and flowered in the patient's mind during the ages of 3 to 6 years.

To repeat, I see no reason to doubt the significance of what happens in the earliest years, but the evidence available to us at present supports the view that its importance lies in its effects upon the sexual conflicts and compromise formations that characterize the ages of 3 to 6 years.

Effects of Psychological Trauma

It is not unusual for the orderly sequence of mental development to be interrupted by an event in a child's life that exacerbates conflict and produces long-lasting consequences in development and functioning. Common examples are absence, illness, or death of a member of the child's immediate family, birth of a sibling, serious physical disability and/or illness, physical abuse, and sexual seduction or overstimulation. Analysts are accustomed to finding evidence of such psychologically traumatic events in patients' histories, and recognize that they produce discontinuity in mental development to a greater or lesser degree. Things are not the same after the event as they were before it; the course of development and the way the individual's mind functions have been altered. I believe that the developmental changes in brain anatomy and physiology that make it possible to acquire language and to have language-dependent thoughts have consequences for mental development and functioning that are similar in kind and in degree to the consequences of the psychic traumas of which I have given examples. The greatly increased ability to think that is characteristic of the second 3 years of life results in a discontinuity in mental development. Things are not the same afterwards as they were before. Mental functioning has changed forever.

To be sure, the term *psychological trauma* implies that the resulting changes are undesirable and disadvantageous, and in making the above comparison, I do not wish to imply that the same is true of the changes in mental development and functioning to which I refer. In any case, such value judgments are beside the point here. The point is that it is commonplace for events to occur that result in discontinuities in development, and that one such event which is universal is the change that regularly occurs during the second 3 years of life in that aspect of brain functioning that is called the *mind.* One of its consequences is the greatly increased role of conflict and compromise formation associated with sexual and aggressive wishes. I believe that is why that period of life is a crucial one for mental development and for all subsequent mental functioning.[3]

SUMMARY

To summarize, the mind is not best understood in terms of structures or agencies. It is better understood in terms of conflict and compromise formation in accordance with the pleasure/unpleasure principle. There is no mental structure or agency that ignores external reality, nor is there any that by its nature is bound to external reality. What the term *mental conflict* refers to is a situation in which one wants some pleasurable satisfaction and is at the same time frightened and/or made miserable by the idea of achieving it. One wants it because it is so pleasurable, and at the same time does not want it because of the frightening and/or miserable consequences associated with the idea of achieving it. The earliest identifiable conflicts of this sort develop during the ages of 3 to 6 years, in connection with the pleasure-seeking sexual and aggressive wishes characteristic of that period of life. The reasons for these con-

---

[3]It is of interest to note that the period of the second 3 years of life is not the only one regularly marked by an exacerbation of mental conflict. Another such period is puberty, when general physical maturity, and especially sexual maturity, is attained. Still another is the time when sexual functioning wanes: in women, the time of menopause; in men, the time of the less obvious male climacteric.

flicts have to do with the physical and emotional immaturity of children of that age and with their dependence on parental figures. The reasons for the flowering of conflict during those years have to do with the functional development of the brain, which is the organ of the mind, and especially with the development of the capacity for language-dependent thought. Other periods of life in which conflict related to these wishes is regularly exacerbated are puberty and climacterium.

I wish to add the following, on a personal note. It was no easy matter for me to consider giving up the familiar and useful concepts of id, ego, and superego. It took me a dozen years to convince myself that it is valid and useful to do so. Even then, I doubt if I should have expressed this conclusion so directly in the public forum without encouragement from my colleagues, Drs. Yale Kramer and Arnold D. Richards (Brenner 1994, p. 473n). It has become evident to me during the course of the years that have elapsed since I published my first paper on the subject (Brenner 1994) that most of my analytic colleagues are today as reluctant to discard the concepts under discussion as I myself was for many years. I am convinced that my own reluctance was due to the continuing influence of conflicts arising from childhood sexual and aggressive wishes. It was important to me to continue to believe in the concepts of ego, superego, and id, even in the face of what seems to me now to be convincing evidence that those concepts constitute an invalid theory. That the same may be true for others is indicated by the following anecdote.

In the course of discussion with a colleague well versed in analytic theory, and with long experience of analytic practice, the colleague raised the following objection to my suggestion that the concepts ego, id, and superego should be given up.

"The ego," said my colleague, "is an integrating agency. It makes compromises among conflicting demands of the mind. Compromise formation is an aspect of ego functioning according to the structural theory. The idea that compromise formation is ubiquitous is perfectly consistent with the concept of an ego as part of psychoanalytic theory."

I objected that this formulation asserts that symptom formation is a function of the ego and is thus at odds with the structural theory, which explains symptom formation not as an ego function, but as a result of conflict between id and ego in which ego gives way. My colleague promptly agreed and suggested that, as was the case for me for so many years, so also for my colleague it was more important to cling to the concepts of ego, id, and superego than to draw the conclusion that there are important and obvious facts that render those concepts invalid.

REFERENCES

Arlow JA, Brenner C: Psychoanalytic Concepts and the Structural Theory. Madison, CT, International Universities Press, 1964

Brenner C: Archaic features of ego functioning. Int J Psychoanal 49:426–430, 1968

Brenner C: An Elementary Textbook of Psychoanalysis, 2nd Edition. Madison, CT, International Universities Press, 1973

Brenner C: Psychoanalytic Technique and Psychic Conflict. Madison, CT, International Universities Press, 1976

Brenner C: The Mind in Conflict. Madison, CT, International Universities Press, 1982

Brenner C: The mind as conflict and compromise formation. J Clin Psychoanal 3:473–488, 1994

Brenner C: Environmental factors in the development of reality testing, chapter 20 in The Perverse Transference and Other Matters. Edited by Ahumada JL et al. Northvale, NJ, Jason Aronson, 1997

Brenner C: Beyond the ego and the id revisited. J Clin Psychoanal 7:165–180, 1998

Brenner C: Observations on some aspects of current psychoanalytic theories. Psychoanal Q 69:597–632, 2000

Freud S: The neuro-psychoses of defence (1894), in The Standard Edition of the Complete Psychological Works of Sigmund Freud [SE], Vol 3. Translated and edited by Strachey J. London, Hogarth Press, 1962, pp 45–61

Freud S: Further remarks on the neuro-psychoses of defence (1896). SE, 3:159–185, 1962

Freud S: The Interpretation of Dreams (1900). SE, 4–5 (Chap 7), 1953

Freud S: Three essays on the theory of sexuality (1905). SE, 7:125–243, 1953

Freud S: Delusions and dreams in Jensen's *Gradiva* (1907). SE, 9:1–95, 1959

Freud S: The Ego and the Id (1923). SE, 19:3–59, 1961

Freud S: Inhibitions, Symptoms and Anxiety (1926). SE, 20:77–175, 1959

Hartmann H: Essays in Ego Psychology. Madison, CT, International Universities Press, 1964

2

PHILIP M. BROMBERG, PH.D.

INTRODUCTION

Philip Bromberg was awarded the Ph.D. in Clinical Psychology from New York University and a Certificate in Psychoanalysis from the William Alanson White Institute. He is the author of many papers on the therapeutic action of psychoanalysis and the analytic relationship from a postclassical perspective, with special focus on working with "difficult" patients. He is a Training and Supervising Analyst and faculty member of the William Alanson White Psychoanalytic Institute and recipient of their Distinguished Service Award. A Fellow of the American Psychological Association, Dr. Bromberg is a Clinical Professor of Psychology and Supervisor of Psychoanalysis at the New York University Postdoctoral Program. Dr. Bromberg is Joint Editor-in-Chief (with Donnel Stern) of the journal *Contemporary Psychoanalysis* and is on the editorial boards of several other analytic journals, including *Psychoanalytic Dialogues, Psychoanalytic Inquiry,* and *The Journal of the American Academy of Psychoanalysis.* In addition to his numerous articles and book chapters, Dr. Bromberg is most widely known as the author of *Standing in the Spaces: Essays on Clinical Process, Trauma, and Dissociation* (The Analytic Press, 1998). A second volume of his work on clinical process, *Awakening the Dreamer: Clinical Journeys,* is to be released shortly by The Analytic Press.

His statement concerning his role in American psychoanalysis follows:

I believe that my writings over the past 25 years have contributed significantly to a postclassical perspective on human mental development as a nonlinear process. This understanding emphasizes self-organization, states of consciousness, dissociation, and multiple self states that can change suddenly from one to another when a parameter value crosses a critical threshold. I have argued for a view of the mind as a configuration of discontinuous, shifting states of consciousness with varying degrees of access to perception and cognition. When the acquired, developmentally adaptive illusion of being a unitary self is traumatically threatened with unavoidable, precipitous disruption, its very cohesiveness becomes a liability because that cohesiveness is in jeopardy of being overwhelmed by a trauma that it cannot process symbolically. In such situations, the mind, if able, will enlist its dissociative ability as a protective solution to ensure continuity and coherence of selfhood—its own survival.

This means that there are important ways in which the seemingly unitary self that we meet in our patients is incapable of true dialogic engagement and, in other important ways, incapable of the experience of intrapsychic conflict. It is the unanticipated eruption of the patient's internal relational world, with its push-pull impact on the analyst's effort to maintain a therapeutic stance, that makes possible the deepest and most therapeutically fruitful type of analytic experience. This, in turn, has contributed to an increased understanding of the central role of dissociation and enactment in the analytic process and the value of an overarching focus on the analyst's own dissociated emotional experience as a means of connecting the patient with the affective core of his or her unconscious processes.

I have further suggested that the psychoanalytic understanding of character pathology needs to be revamped to take into account the inherent dissociative structure of the mind. I have proposed that the concept of personality "disorder" might usefully be defined as the characterological outcome of the inordinate use of dissociation in the schematization of self-other mental representation, and that independent of type (narcissistic, schizoid, borderline, paranoid, etc.), it reflects a mental structure organized in part as a proactive protection against the potential repetition of early trauma. Thus, the distinctive personality traits of each type of personality disorder are embodied within a mental structure that allows each trait to be always "on call" for the trauma that is seen as inevitable. All in all, I could be seen as having done the following:

1. Extended psychoanalytic theory beyond Freud in terms of the psychoanalytic relationship in general, and particularly, with regard to treating the "difficult patient." I have argued that the most relevant clinical question is not "What technique should be applied?" but rather, "What are the necessary and sufficient conditions to support an analytic process?" The latter question is more rooted in gestalt field theory, chaos theory, and nonlinear dynamic systems theory than in the 19th-century positivism that shaped Freud's thinking. When Freud dismissed the phe-

nomenon of dissociation, he formulated a belief system which posited that (except for the most seriously disturbed patients) his concepts of "repetition compulsion" and "interpretation of resistance to unconscious conflict" constituted sufficient foundation on which to build a theory of clinical technique.

2. Expanded Sullivan's formulation that the mental development of every human being is shaped by a set of discrete, more or less overlapping schemata of who he is and that each schema is organized around a core self-other configuration that originated early in life.
3. Developed Ferenczi's pioneering work into a contemporary analytic view that regressive reliving of early traumatic experience in the analytic transference is to some degree curative in itself because it encourages active mastery of the traumatic past through use of the here-and-now analytic relationship. From this perspective, psychological trauma can be defined as the precipitous disruption of self-continuity through the invalidation of early attachment patterns of interaction that give meaning to "who one is."

WHY I CHOSE THIS PAPER

Philip M. Bromberg, Ph.D.

This paper puts into particular high relief the core elements of my clinical contribution. It shows the intrinsic relationship between dissociation and character formation whether or not symptoms are present, and it demonstrates that both symptoms and character pathology are the end result of prolonged necessity in infancy to control traumatic dysregulation of affect. Most of all, the paper makes it particularly vivid that "trauma work" is not all about accessing memories of massive trauma, but that it is a process tied to the ubiquitous and more subtle presence of developmental trauma. The essence of the clinical work is to facilitate the patient's surrender of his or her own "self-cure"—the dissociative mental structure that plunders the present and future of its vitality and spontaneity as a protection against past trauma whose return it is designed to anticipate. It can be observed here that symptoms, because they have voices of their own, can be addressed relationally as self-expressive parts of the patient whose particular functions must be comprehended and validated before they can be surrendered. As this takes place, the patient's ability to safely experience internal conflict is increased, and the potential for resolution of conflict is in turn increased. This paper, through its emphasis on symptoms as relational phenomena, helps to show how analytic work with every patient becomes most powerful when it provides an experience-near perspective from which to engage dissociation clinically and why concepts such as "intractable resistance" and "therapeutic stalemates" merit reconsideration from this vantage point.

TREATING PATIENTS WITH SYMPTOMS— AND SYMPTOMS WITH PATIENCE

Reflections on Shame, Dissociation, and Eating Disorders

PHILIP M. BROMBERG, PH.D.

MY OVERARCHING AIM as a psychoanalytic author has been to explore the clinical and conceptual implications of viewing the human mind as a relationally configured, self-organizing system. I've argued that personality functioning, normal and pathological, is best understood as an ongoing, nonlinear repatterning of self-state configurations, and that this process is mediated at the brain level by a continuing dialectic between dissociation and conflict. Normal dissociation, a hypnoid brain mechanism that is intrinsic to everyday mental functioning, ensures that the mind functions as creatively as possible, selecting whichever self-state configuration is most adaptive to the moment. Johnson (2004) compared this to Edelman's (1989, 1992, 2004) view that the internal mechanisms of both the brain and the immune system run miniversions of natural selection:

> Think of those modules in your brain as species competing for precious resources—in some cases they're competing for control of the entire organism; in others, they're competing for your attention. Instead of struggling to pass their genes on to the next generation, they're struggling to pass their message on to other groups of neurons, including groups that shape your conscious sense of self. Picture yourself walking down a crowded urban street. As you walk, your brain is filled with internal

---

"Treating Patients With Symptoms—and Symptoms With Patience: Reflections on Shame, Dissociation, and Eating Disorders," by Philip M. Bromberg, Ph.D., was first published in *Psychoanalytic Dialogues,* 11:891–912, 2001.

> voices all competing for your attention. At any given moment, a few of them are selected, while most go unheeded. (Johnson 2004, p. 199)

When dissociation is enlisted as a defense against trauma, the brain utilizes its hypnoid function to limit self-state communication, thereby insulating the mental stability of each separate state. Self-continuity is thus preserved *within* each state, but self-coherence *between* states is sacrificed and replaced by a dissociative mental structure that forecloses the possibility of *conflictual* experience. Clinically, the phenomenon of dissociation, though observable at many points in *every* treatment, comes into highest relief during enactments, requiring an analyst's close attunement to unacknowledged affective shifts in his own and his patient's self-states. Through the joint cognitive processing of enactments played out interpersonally and intersubjectively between the "not-me" experiences of patient and analyst, a patient's sequestered self-states come alive as a "remembered present" (Edelman 1989) that can affectively and cognitively reconstruct a remembered past. Because the ability to safely *experience* conflict is increased, the potential for *resolution* of conflict is in turn increased for *all* patients. It allows one's work with so-called good analytic patients to become more powerful because it provides a more experience-near perspective from which to engage clinical phenomena that are immune to interpretation, such as "intractable resistance" and "therapeutic stalemate." Further, it puts to rest the notion of "analyzability" and allows analysts to use their expertise with a wide spectrum of personality disorders often considered "difficult" or unanalyzable, such as those encountered in individuals diagnosed as borderline, schizoid, narcissistic, or dissociative.

In the present paper, I discuss how this treatment perspective can be especially useful in working with individuals for whom symptoms are a central feature of their personalities, such as patients with eating disorders. I offer the view that the symptom picture found in most patients with eating disorders, as well as the symptomatology of many other so-called difficult patients, is the end result of prolonged necessity in infancy to control traumatic dysregulation of affect. I propose that the central issue for an eating-disordered patient is that because she is at the mercy of her own physiologic and affective states and lacks an experience of human relatedness and its potential for reparation that mediates self-regulation, she is enslaved by her felt inability to contain desire as a regulatable affect. Trauma compromises trust in the reparability of relationship, and for symptoms to be surrendered, trust in reparability must be simultaneously restored. I discuss the inevitability of the analyst's own dissociative reactions in response to the patient's enacted internal war over desire and control, as well as the different types of interpersonal enactments into which an analyst is drawn. Illustrating with clinical vignettes, I show how analyst and patient slip in and out of a constantly shifting array of self-states and thereby have an opportunity to co-construct a transitional reality within which the patient's impaired faith in the reliability of human relatedness can be restored and eating can become linked to appetite rather than to control.

TO THINE OWN SELVES BE TRUE

Virginia Woolf (1928), with characteristically understated perceptiveness, casually observed in her novel *Orlando* that "these selves of which we are built up, one on top of another, as plates are piled on a waiter's hand, have... little constitutions and rights of their own."

> One will only come if it is raining, another [will emerge only] in a room with green curtains, another when Mrs. Jones is not there, another if you can promise it a glass of wine—and so on.... [E]verybody can multiply from his own experience the different terms which his different selves have made with him—and some are too wildly ridiculous to be mentioned in print at all. (pp. 308–309)

I've quoted this passage because rarely has the wondrous nature of the self been portrayed with such matter-of-fact honesty and simplicity. Woolf's evocative description is easily embraced by the reader with feelings of pleasurable recognition, and even her use of the phrase "different selves" has a felt rightness to it that is accepted without resistance. Perhaps her language, so personal and down-to earth, allows her such a warmly congenial relationship with the reader that it helps overcome the potential for discontent that sometimes can be evoked by the notion that we each comprise different selves. As Popeye put it, flexing his muscles belligerently, "I yam what I yam and that's all that I yam," and any idea that suggests otherwise, whether offered by an analyst to a patient or by a writer to a reader, feels "right" only if presented in a manner that simultaneously supports one's basic experience of self-continuity. It is when an analyst fails to provide such support that he is most apt to experience his patient as "difficult."

If we were to place our "difficult" patients into one group and our so-called good patients (more and more difficult to find these days) into a second group, there is one particular characteristic of most patients in the first group that transcends the individual personality traits that we use in making differential diagnoses *between* the members of this group.

Put simply, the thing our "difficult" patients most require from their therapists for growth to occur is, paradoxically, the same thing that is most difficult for the therapist to provide—interpersonal engagement that combines affective authenticity and affective safety. Although it is certainly true that this same combination is needed by patients in the second group, with that group its provision is part of the natural give-and-take of the relationship and is often unnoticeable except as "background music."

For patients in the "difficult" group, this natural give-and-take is minimal, sometimes totally absent. Most of them, with good reason, have come to mistrust signs of genuine relatedness from another person as though these signs were "really" omens of potential betrayal. Such patients *are* difficult, and they *feel* difficult to a therapist because they deprive a therapist of what he most counts on in order to sustain hope—a working relationship that will grow in depth and security as the work progresses. With these individuals, such a relationship does not as a rule exist, at least for a long time, because their mental structure has been shaped too extensively or for too long by the effects of trauma and dissociation. Their capacity to trust a human relationship must first be slowly restored—in some cases, built for the first time—and without this taking place, any attempt at psychoanalysis from an interpretive stance results, at best, in "pseudoanalysis."

If such a person is ever to truly feel recognized within a relationship, the therapist must comprehend that when his patient behaves as if the only self that she feels is "really" her is the one that is there at the moment, she is not being capricious, inconsistent, or worse, resistant. The therapist's task is to allow himself to slowly discover all her selves or self-states and to form relationships with each, allowing that each holds a different version of "truth" and its own agenda for treatment.

HYSTERIA, DISSOCIATION, AND SYMPTOMS

The title of this chapter, "Treating Patients With Symptoms—and Symptoms With Patience," is one I used originally (Bromberg 1995b) at a conference celebrating the centennial of Freud's publication of *Studies on Hysteria* (Breuer and Freud 1893–1895). In that paper, I discussed Freud's treatment of his famous patient Frau Emmy von N, from a vantage point 100 years later. Freud's refreshingly honest assessment was that "the therapeutic success on the whole was considerable; but it was not a lasting one" and that "the patient's tendency to fall ill in a similar way under the impact of fresh traumas was not got rid of" (pp. 101–

102). From my perspective (Bromberg 1996), the symptoms that Freud called hysteric are more usefully seen as dissociative, and the reason Emmy was still susceptible to falling ill was that her need to maintain the dissociative structure of her mind was kept alive by the present, as much as by the past, and thus remained untouched. Like any trauma survivor, she protected herself against the future by treating the present as if it were nothing but a replica of the past. In this context, her "illness" was not represented only by her symptoms, but perhaps even more by the plundering of her life—a foreclosure of the "here and now" on behalf of the "there and then," effectively preventing her from living life with spontaneity, pleasure, or immediacy. In other words, to understand why Emmy's cure was not a lasting one is also to understand that we do not treat patients such as Emmy to cure them of something that was done to them in the past; rather, we are trying to cure them of what they still do to themselves (and to others) in order to *cope* with what was done to them in the past.

All in all, I've come to accept that our success as clinicians in treating patients with symptoms lies, at least in part, in our ability and willingness to treat symptoms with patience—a conclusion that is brought into especially high relief with regard to symptoms associated with eating (which, by the way, Emmy manifested to no small degree). Eating disorder symptoms, in an unusually concrete way, highlight the basic adaptational function of dissociation. They foreclose the mental chaos of needing to hold in a single state of consciousness two incompatible modes of relating. As Freud put it, "it is impossible to eat with disgust and pleasure at the same time" (Breuer and Freud 1893–1895, p. 89). In its most general form, the person is protected from the destabilizing impossibility of trying to respond self-reflectively with feelings of fear and security toward the same object at the same moment.

DISSOCIATION, SYMPTOMS, AND EATING DISORDERS

Kathryn Zerbe, a psychoanalyst affiliated with the Menninger Clinic and a specialist in eating disorders, wrote: "Given the frequency with which dissociative states and eating disorders may occur together, it behooves clinicians to keep an open eye to making both diagnoses if one or the other is found" (Zerbe 1993, p. 321). Everill and colleagues (1995) put it that "a temporary cognitive narrowing is experienced during a binge as the bulimic refocuses attention on to the immediate stimulus. This refocusing allows a reduction in negative affect or a general reduction in self-awareness" (p. 155). On the basis of my own clinical observations and those of others (e.g., Everill et al. 1995; Gleaves et al. 1996; Katz and Gleaves 1996; McCallum et al. 1992), I offer the view that most of the symptoms associated with eating disorders can be most usefully understood as an intrinsic outcome of dissociation, whereby the ability to act from a coherent sense of self-agency is "repackaged" in unlinked states of mind, leading to a personality dynamic wherein certain self-states are stubbornly intractable and others are inhibited but simultaneously "on alert."

Freud never followed through on the early insights he achieved in his hypnotic work with Emmy von N, and in his subsequent war with Janet[1] he ended up minimizing the significance of trauma and dissociation in human mental functioning. In this context, Havens (1973), in *Approaches to the Mind,* had some things to say about Janet and Freud that are highly relevant:

> It was obvious to both Janet and Freud that the *conscious* ideas of the patients did not encompass the phenomenon of hysteria. Freud then searched, first by hypnosis and later by the method of free associations, for unconscious ideas and was led forward to the idea of unconscious yearnings, attitudes, convictions, and expectations. Janet searched for what besides ideas was dissociated, and in what ways. He left behind the old conception of single ideas, resulting from trauma, and splitting off from mental life, for that of dissociated functions or systems within which many sensations, acts, fears, and ideas were included—separate, organized centers of attention, receiving impressions and able to be communicated with; in control of the personality (as in the somnambulisms and fugue states) or capturing a leg, arm, or the function of eating.... Each hysterical function had its own consciousness, organizing principles, and capacities for communication. (pp. 59–60)

With regard to patients suffering from eating disorders, this issue is particularly salient, as was Janet's contribution. For the anorectic, wrote Janet (1907), the act of eating is an amnesia, "a somnambulistic phenomenon which can only be effected in the somnambulistic state...[and] is lost to the normal and waking consciousness" (p. 243). The most powerful and enduring significance of Janet's work in this area, Havens (1973) asserted, is not simply in recognizing the centrality of dissociation, but in demonstrating that dissociation involves an organized sys-

---

[1]See Louis Breger's breathtakingly honest biography *Freud: Darkness in the Midst of Vision* (2000) for the most comprehensive understanding of Freud's "anti-Janet" stand and its constricting effect on the evolution of psychoanalytic theory over the past 100 years.

tem of self-experience rather than just a single idea or sensation, and that in the case of anorexic illness this cut off system has captured and redefined the meaning and function of eating (pp. 49–50). It is a hypnoidally isolated complex of physiological events, fears, movements, sensations, and ideas which work together as a separate center of attention that is able to be communicated with, and is in control of the total personality when it needs to be.

DISSOCIATION, MULTIPLICITY, AND WHOLENESS

What Janet called a "system or complex" is what I see as a dissociated self-state or a self organized by its own dominant affect, its own view of social phenomena and human relationships, its own moral code, its own view of reality that is fiercely held as a truth, and, with patients suffering from eating disorders, its own relationship to food and to the body. In the contemporary analytic community, Janet's ideas have begun to take hold only during the last 10 to 15 years, influenced mainly by data provided from outside psychoanalysis. At this point in time, however, an increasing number of analytic clinicians, researchers, and theoreticians are themselves presenting evidence that the human personality begins and continues as a multiplicity of selves or self-states, each with its own dominant affect and sets of characteristics that are always shifting in configuration and moment-to-moment availability to one another. One's different states are subjectively linked together by the developmentally necessary illusion of being "*one* self," and, if all goes relatively well early in life, one's self-state shifts are normally as unobservable as the beating of one's heart, and self-continuity goes on without disruption. Most of us can access a broad range of self-states that can participate in even the most emotionally complex and psychologically conflicted situations. But not all are so lucky. In the face of trauma, self-continuity is threatened, and this threat, for most human beings, is met with an evolutionary survival response, dissociation, that is equivalent in survival priority to certain genetically coded response patterns of lower animals to a life-threatening attack by a predator.

For instance, there is a sea creature, the holothurian, that is known for its ability, when attacked, to divide itself into unlinked parts and to regenerate from that which escapes death. "Non omnis moriar"—I shall not wholly die! Consider the following excerpt from a poem by the Polish poet Wislawa Szymborska (1983). The title, "Autotomy," is the biological term for the capacity of certain living things to give up wholeness in order to preserve life:

> In danger the holothurian splits itself in two:
> it offers one self to be devoured by the world
> and in its second self escapes.
> In the middle of the holothurian's body a chasm opens
> and its edges immediately become alien to each other.
> On the one edge, death, on the other, life.
> Here despair, there, hope.
> To die as much as necessary, without overstepping
> the bounds. To grow again from a salvaged remnant.
> Here a heavy heart, there non omnis moriar,
> three little words only, like three little plumes ascending.
> (pp. 115–116)

I shall not wholly die! With these words in mind, now contemplate a piece of advice offered more than 140 years ago by George MacDonald (1858), the Scottish clergyman and author whom the writer C.S. Lewis acknowledged as the primary source from which his own capacity to bridge fantasy and reality was shaped. MacDonald wrote that "the best way to manage some kinds of painful thoughts is to dare them to do their worst, to let them lie and gnaw at your heart till they are tired, and you find you still have a residue of life they cannot kill" (p. 55). MacDonald's words sometimes come to me when hope seems far away with certain patients. But all too often it's just too damned difficult for *anyone* to do what MacDonald proposed. It's difficult even for individuals who haven't been seriously traumatized as children. But for a patient who has, trying to hold painful thoughts, letting them "gnaw at her heart till they are tired," and surviving without dissociating, is frequently an impossibility. Consider Laurie, for instance:

Laurie

Laurie, age 26, had been obese as a child and became bulimic during adolescence, at which point she shed most of her weight and for a brief period became anorectic. At the point when I first met her she appeared slightly underweight but not anorectically thin. Her older sister, who had also been obese as a child, remained that way, never having developed a bulimic solution. She became for Laurie the apotheosis of greed—an object of contempt and a constant reminder to Laurie of who she was *not*. Laurie entered treatment with a variety of symptoms along with the eating disorder. Some were classically dissociative, such as fugue states manifested in such things as her history of "forgotten" appointments, not going to class, not coming to work, all without awareness. She also suffered from flashbacks, traumatic nightmares, and a body experience sometimes blurred and always unstable. She would frequently start sessions by asking me either "What do I look like today?" or "Do you think I look different from last time?"

She was also prone to sudden state-shifts during sessions, preceded by attentional disturbances in which she seemed to "disappear" from whatever interaction was taking place between us. She also presented with other symptoms, less classically dissociative but often found to accompany the former. The major ones were migraine headaches so severe that they could virtually incapacitate her, and a compulsive "hair twirling" leading to "hair pulling" habit since age 14, at which age she also developed amenorrhea that lasted until she left home at age 20. The bingeing and hair pulling had both been described by her as reducing tension because they "make her mind a blank."

On this particular day she began her session, as she frequently did, sitting silently and staring, trance-like, into space. She then began to talk blandly and without affect about having pulled out her hair the night before. "I discovered I haven't stopped. *You* thought I had." As I listened to her I became aware of my own feelings—an odd blend of apathy and irritation. I might have ignored it and just launched into another dead-end inquiry about the details of what led to the hair pulling, except that I noticed her sitting back contentedly like someone settling in to watch a movie. I commented on this, and her response was to remember a dream she had had the night before about being at her sister's birthday party that was taking place in an insane asylum. "There was a big gooey birthday cake—my sister loves cake; I hate it—and she's getting mad at me because I don't want any. I finally start yelling at her to 'shove it.' I woke up just as I had my face up against hers, screaming 'I don't have that body, it's yours, not *mine*, you pig!'"

I asked her what thoughts she had about the dream and she said in an offhand manner, "None! I don't like to come up with ideas. I'd rather wait for *you* to have some. That way I can either agree or disagree and I don't have to risk being wrong." There was a look in her eye as she spoke that made me feel she was trying to pull me into a battle. But unlike earlier in the session, I could vaguely sense she was conscious of what was going on between us, at least to some extent. Contrary to the apathy and irritation I was feeling earlier, I was not put off by her manner this time. In fact, I was feeling kind of playful, and I found myself saying to her:

"Actually, what you usually do is agree *and* disagree at the same time, so I never can really be sure what you feel. It's like I slave over a hot couch all week [she in fact sits up, but she got the point]. I cook you my best interpretations. Do you eat them? No! You taste a piece here, a piece there. I throw out three quarters of what I cook. There are starving patients in Europe who would be grateful for what I throw away that you don't eat."

She began to laugh, and I could feel the atmosphere shift—lending some support to Lewis's (1995) observation that laughter is a mechanism by which shame can be reduced or eliminated. "Laughter," Lewis says, "especially laughter around one's transgression as it occurs in a social context, provides the opportunity for the transgressing person to join others in viewing the self. In this way, the self metaphorically moves from the site of the shame to the site of observing the shame with the other" (p. 130). In my own preferred idiom (since I don't see the shift as "metaphorical"), it allows more of one's selves to get into the act. A part of her that was lively, animated, and almost enthusiastic was now clearly participating.

I said to her that at this stage of our work the odds of each of us being wrong were pretty high because there's so much we don't know yet. But the odds get better when we compare notes about what each of us is feeling about what we are doing. It reduces the amount of guessing. After a moment of silence, she replied:

"I think the insane asylum was your office. Sometimes I feel you want to make me fat like my sister. All these interesting things you say to me make me afraid to hear more. Yeah, I guess I was sitting back like I was getting ready to take in a great movie—like a great meal I could have without getting fat because I didn't even know I was eating it. I think I know what made me start pulling my hair out again."

She then described an event that took place 2 days before this session: "I was walking to a restaurant with my father and he holds my hand in this weird way—he won't let go. I had to pretend I was fixing my hair to remove my hand." This was her first concrete association that could potentially shed some light on the "hair-twirling/pulling" behavior. Then, suddenly, in the voice of a preadolescent child: "He never touches mommy that way. I wonder sometimes if people who see us think I shrunk."

"Who would they see?" I asked her.

Now back in the other voice, "They'd see a 10-year-old girl walking with her father. My husband lives with her most of the time. Most of the time he likes it. But he doesn't like it when I change. He says, 'Why do you have to be different people on different days?' "

"Well, I'm glad I had a chance to meet her," I replied, "even if it was only very briefly."

"Yes," she said pointedly, "She *went away* again as soon as you asked me to *tell* you about her." A bit dazed as the hour approached the end, I mumbled what I hoped would be a supportive response and a "good" note on which to stop: "Maybe if I talk to her more directly she will stay longer. Do you think so?"

Naively anticipating that this would be our "marker" for next time, I was shocked when she ignored what I thought were my obvious cues that the time was up, and she began what felt like a nonstop monologue. She began to talk about how afraid she was of offending people at whom she secretly scoffed—people who think that what they say matters to her when it really doesn't. "It's so strange," she went on. "Even though some people don't seem to get angry about it, *I* crash when it's over. I'll go home and binge and vomit."

I felt paralyzed at this point. Even though I felt she was talking about *us* and about what it feels like for her after she leaves sessions, I also wanted to end the session. I kept hoping that if I gave her just a little more time I would think of the "right" thing to say, so I let her go on…and on…and on…hoping against hope that if I didn't stop her before she stopped herself it would end in the "right" way. Well, I finally abandoned that hope and stopped her 10 minutes past the end of the session.

She said, sounding a bit miffed, "I haven't finished yet." I replied, probably sounding a bit contrite, "I know, but our time is up for today, and I'd love for us to have a moment to reflect on what just happened here." She retorted, "I never reflect on what I'm saying when I'm like this." I answered, now a bit more composed, "But later when you get home, a different part of you does think about it—all alone. And then you decide you were horrible and end up bingeing and vomiting." At that moment something clicked into place for me, and I added, "But in a funny way you only did what I asked you to do, didn't you? Remember when I said, "Maybe if I talk to *her* more directly she'll stay longer? I just didn't expect it to happen *now*! But why wouldn't it?" And then, shifting realities, "After all, you were just being you. 'Longer' means until you've finished, right?" She, stood up, grinned and left. I breathed a grateful sigh of relief.

AFFECT-DYSREGULATION, SHAME, AND RESTORATION OF TRUST

In the preceding vignette, one can see the intricate relationship among trauma, dissociation, damaged capacity for affect-regulation, and the need for an analytic relationship in which growth and repair are inseparable components. As we know, successful interpersonal transactions between infant and caregiver mediate, at the brain level, the capacity for affect-regulation within an internal experience of secure human-relatedness. One could, if one wished, translate this into the language of attachment theory, whereby the phrase "attachment bonds" could substitute for the phrase "secure human relatedness." When these early patterns are relatively nondisruptive and, most importantly, reparable, they create a stable foundation for internal affect-regulation that is largely nonverbal and unconscious.

Tronick and Weinberg (1997), in a seminal paper on research into affect-regulation and the "architecture of mother-infant interactions," emphasized how disruptions in the mutual regulatory process create a break in the development of intersubjectivity. In the face of chronic failure to repair the interactions, the infant is unable to achieve social connectedness and develops dysregulated affective states that it is unable to control. An early coping style begins to develop in which most of the infant's activity is enlisted into stabilizing out-of-control affect. Most significant is Tronick and Weinberg's conclusion that

> reparation of interactive errors is the critical process of normal interactions that is related to developmental outcome rather than synchrony or positive affect per se. That is, reparation, its experience and extent, is the

> "social-interactive mechanism" that affects the infant's development...[because] the infant develops a representation of him- or herself as effective, of his or her interactions as positive and reparable, and of the caretaker as reliable and trustworthy (pp. 65–66).

Much adult psychopathology may thus be the end result of the individual's prolonged necessity in infancy to control physiologic and affective states while lacking an experience of human relatedness and trust in its potential for reparation. An early foundation of reparability in relationships allows for further successful negotiation of interpersonal transactions at increasingly higher levels of adult self-development and interpersonal maturity, not only affecting the richness of one's life, but determining the difficulty an individual will experience in attempting to negotiate and use a psychotherapeutic relationship (Sullivan 1953, 1954). Trauma creates the experience of nonreparability, and in those areas in which trauma has occurred, the experience of trust in the continuity of human relatedness must be restored.

With regard to those individuals for whom this state of affairs leads to an eating disorder, Boris (1984, 1986) offered the view that eating disorders arise when the dysregulation of desire is linked in infancy with the dysregulation of appetite. This leads to what Boris called "an unevolved state of mind," in which one wishes and hopes to have everything all the time—a state of mind commonly known as greed. Greed is a state that attempts to eliminate the potential for traumatic rupture in human relatedness by replacing relationship with food—a solution that is largely self-contained and thus not subject to betrayal by the "other." But it is by no means a perfect solution. The particular problem with greed is that its presence is inevitably tarnished by the existence of choice and the shadowy pressure of the need to make one. The realization of the need for choice, Boris wrote, either stimulates a refusal to endure it, leading to the decay of appetite back into greed and an experience of vast frustration, or stimulates the making of the choice, leading to the satisfaction of appetite but always accompanied by the feeling of profound loss of the thing not chosen. In Boris's (1986) words, "Appetite...makes manifest the infant's first encounter with actuality and, as such, makes actual experience for the first time a player in the process. The quality of the appetitive experience will now play a role in whether the feeling of loss is modulated by compensatory and consoling experience—or is not" (pp. 48–49).

Boris was saying, in other words, that the essence of the human condition is having to recognize one's insufficiency (see Becker 1973), and that the degree to which one draws satisfaction from human relatedness will keep him from seeking nonhuman solutions (such as food) as a means of compensating for the experience of loss associated with the thing not chosen. For some people, because the recognition of insufficiency is unbearable, choice becomes unbearable, and in the infant who later in life develops an eating disorder, the capacity to make a choice is impaired because the experience of loss connected to appetite is not modulated by the compensation and consolation of human relatedness. That is, what in adulthood could develop into appetite and healthy, regulatable desire, because it is denied the relational context on which that transformation depends, freezes the experience of being an affectively out-of-control infant, within a dissociated self-state that takes on an imperious life of its own. In the previous clinical vignette, it was this self-state of Laurie's that I unexpectedly engaged when I naively invited her to stay longer.

Boris (1984) wrote: "By the simple expedient of declaring 'less is more,' greed for the breast is metamorphosed into a gluttony for punishment, yearning into abstinence, retention into elimination (in bulimia) via each and every alimentary orifice, indeed, by exercise and sweating, through the very pores themselves" (p. 317). The renunciation of desire is what we see as the hallmark of anorexia, and in a different way, of bulimia. But at its core, it is a loss of trust in the reliability of human relatedness. I have found that in patients with eating disorders, the transmutation of desire into renunciation is most frequently mediated through the mechanism of dissociation. Sands (1994) suggested that "dissociative defenses serve to regulate relatedness to others" and that the dissociative patient "is attempting to stay enough in relationship with the human environment to survive the present while, at the same time, keeping the needs for more intimate relatedness sequestered but alive" (p. 149). In other words, dissociative defenses are not designed simply as an impermeable suit of armor, and no matter how walled-off the patient may be from intimate contact with others, the broadest purpose of a dissociative mental structure, including its place in most eating disorders, is not just insularity but regulation. It is above all else a dynamic mental organization designed for affective self-regulation—a mental structure tailored to anticipate trauma, but sufficiently permeable to be a potential doorway to therapeutic growth. Its *insularity* reflects the necessity to remain ready for danger at all times so that—as with the original traumatic experiences—it will never arrive unanticipated; its *permeability* reflects a capacity for authentic but highly regulated exchange with the outside world and similarly regulated spontaneity of self-experience (Bromberg 1995a). In the words of a patient with dissociative symptoms—someone who did *not* have an eating disorder:

> When I was little and I got scared—scared because mommy was going to beat me up—I'd stare at a crack in the ceiling or a spider web on a pane of glass—and pretty soon I'd go into this place where everything was kind of foggy and far away, and I was far away too, and safe. At first, I had to stare real hard to get to this safe place. But then one day mommy was really beating on me and without even trying I was there, and I wasn't afraid of her. I knew she was punching me, and I could hear her calling me names, but it didn't hurt and I didn't care. After that, anytime I was scared, I'd suddenly find myself in that place, out of danger and peaceful. I've never told anybody about it, not even Daddy. I was afraid to because I was afraid that if other people knew about it, the place might go away, and I wouldn't be able to get there when I really needed to.

DESIRE, DISSOCIATION, AND AFFECTIVE SAFETY

As treatment progresses, a patient will often reveal the existence of an inner life dominated by a never-ending war between parts of the self, each denouncing the other around the issue of appetite and desire—a war that more often than not manifests itself experientially through the presence of internal voices, often sadistic and unrelenting, that the patient desperately needs to quiet by finding ways to give each some of what it wants. Because desire is never far away, the war between self-states never ends, and for someone with an eating disorder it means that the quality of life is reduced to life imprisonment with periodic "time off for good behavior."

How does this internal war get expressed in treatment, and how does it relate to dissociation? In bulimia, for instance, bingeing and purging as a cohesive act is done, by and large, in a dissociated (not-me) state. Muller (1996) wrote that such patients "are attempting to set a marker at the edge of the self so that they can experience a limit and not become fragmented in a diffuse untamable scatter" (p. 85). This purpose could not be served if the bulimic were fully conscious because it would be a self-experience that was being done *by me to me,* and thereby useless in its ability to ward off autonomic hyperarousal of affect. The trance state, through dissociation, allows this "marker" to be set between areas of self that trauma has made incompatible. But this protection comes at a huge price because it forces the self to severely limit what can be experienced as "me" at any given moment. As Ciocca (1998) has put it, we must find the reasons for a patient's intolerance of a conflict related to being herself.

> The aim of every therapeutic encounter is to lead her to a meeting with herself, as that which she is, and that which she could become.... Fore-

> most in therapy is her impossibility to deal with the dissociation itself. In such a situation it is useful to highlight the way in which her mind works, and how it influences the way in which she is living. (p. 54)

If a therapist is to work with a patient's here-and-now fear of losing her affective safety while he is highlighting the way her mind works, it is essential that he be especially attuned to his patient's potential for dissociated hyperarousal of affect created by the relationship itself. By negotiation *within* the enactment, he must address each patient's ongoing experience of emotional safety as an intrinsic and inseparable part of the analytic interchange. For those patients where the effect of trauma on the organization of psychic structure has been most pervasive, the self-reflective ability to work in the here and now is least likely to be present at the beginning. These patients tend to use each session to process nonprocessible experience that has occurred in prior sessions. In other words, each session becomes for at least one part of the self a kind of commentary (through derivatives, dreams, and enactments) on the session or sessions that have occurred before it. The therapy proceeds that way, with part of the therapist's job being to assure that the processing of unsymbolized affect feels increasingly safe, so that the person's tolerance for potential affective flooding *also* increases—that is, her threshold for dissociative triggering gets higher. As this is accomplished, the processing of the here and now becomes more and more experientially connectable to the patient's past.

Whenever a patient attempts to talk *about* events that were traumatic, a dissociated pain experience is invariably evoked, because "talking about" trauma is inseparable from reliving it. The pain makes the "telling" a source of here-and-now shame that leads to further dissociation, making the patient's story sound bewilderingly impersonal. Enough data are usually revealed, however, to stimulate the therapist's curiosity, setting off a process in which the therapist's attempt to "excavate" details about which the patient has no narrative memory leads to an *enacted* reliving of the trauma into which the therapist is drawn like a moth into a flame. As the enactment continues, the patient's dissociated shame escalates, and the therapist finds himself feeling things about his patient and about own role that make him increasingly uncomfortable, often triggering his own dissociative processes. I believe this collision of subjectivities to be an inevitability, not a sign of a technical error. It draws the work into an experiential interface between the here and now and the there and then, allowing the mutual construction of a transitional reality. In this transitional reality, both the patient's and the analyst's dissociated experience have an opportunity to coexist as a *perceived* event different enough from the patient's *narrative "truth"* to permit internal repatterning to take place while the patient's reliance upon dissociation is gradually surrendered. Analyst and patient are at those moments "standing in the spaces" between formerly unbridgeable self-states. Enacted (as yet unprocessed) experience is allowed to interface perceptually with *episodic* memory, thus optimizing its potential for integration into *narrative* memory and, ultimately, enriching self-narrative, the goal of any form of treatment.

DR. JEKYLL AND MS. "HIDE"

The term "eating *disorder*" can become a real handicap to therapy if it is embraced unreflectively by the therapist as simply a handicap to the patient. The therapist must simultaneously recognize and respect, as an achievement, the means by which a patient has constructed her eating "disorder" through finding ways to preserve its dissociative structure, and thereby give each part of self *some* of what it wants without unbearable conflict. In a 1994 paper, I described a case being presented to me in ongoing consultation (Bromberg 1994). The patient was a woman who had been in treatment for quite a few years and who had made major changes in her life and her self-experience, except with regard to the thing that had brought her into treatment in the first place, her obesity. The analyst, having had as much as he could handle of "getting nowhere" no matter how hard he tried, stopped addressing the issue of her weight, hoping that she would eventually bring it up on her own. The war over desire was in a new phase. He allowed long silences to develop in which he hoped that she might ultimately put what she was feeling into words, which she did, but not in the way that he had hoped. As he was finding the silences increasingly hard to tolerate, she began to take him to task for his "failure" to mention her weight when she herself wasn't mentioning it. Without the least regard for logic, she told him he had no right to stop trying to find out what she was feeling. "What did you think you were doing?" "*You* ought to know," she insisted, "that when I'm talking about anything else as long as I'm still fat, it's only my good self that's talking and that I'm doing something self-destructive that you're not even caring about." It was in the course of their dealing with the apparent "no-win" quality of his "failure" that he was able to begin to find a small island of shared experience on which he could plant at least one of his feet.

"Only in my silence," she declared, "do I feel real. The only way I can get out of here [meaning her inner world] is to be silent for a year."

How could it make any sense that the only way she recognized that she could release herself from the trap of her dissociated mental structure was without words, by remaining silent for a year? The point she was making was not that silence itself mattered, but silence in the presence of her analyst. Why? Because her silence in his presence could have a communicative impact *as long as he hadn't given up trying.* The analyst has to get fed up; it is *important* that he get fed up; he *should* get fed up. But he shouldn't get *so* detached from his own "fed-upness" that he cannot perceive the retaliatory component of his behavior. If he is open to that, he will feel the communication from the patient as it is pressed into his soul through her silence as well as into his brain through her words. The patient was ultimately able to put into words this remarkable insight:

> When I'm not talking to you and you don't realize that my silence is talking, I feel like I'm hurting myself and you don't care. I hurt myself by being fat in order to call attention to the inside "me." And if you don't notice or seem not to, it's like you're mad that I'm still fat and will let me hurt myself because I'm fat instead of putting why I'm fat into words. But if I do talk, it's not my fat self that's talking. So you have to find her by noticing the fat and not pretending you don't. If I get thin, no one will ever look for her because if I stop calling attention to her existence you will settle for my good self which looks healthy because it is thin, and you will never know it isn't real to me. I'm like Dr. Jekyll and Mr. Hyde.

DISSOCIATION AS AN INTERPERSONAL PROCESS

An analyst becomes trapped in such a no-win situation because his own dissociative processes invariably are a part of any enactment. With a patient who suffers from an eating disorder, the type of situation described above is not all that unusual. When a patient's eating behavior is held by the therapist for too long a time as simply a piece of pathology to get rid of—and the patient, of course, makes it very easy for us to hold that view—nothing much changes, and what we have come to call "resistance" starts to fill up all the space. It becomes very easy to grow to *hate* your patient's eating disorder and then, without recognizing it, to hate that part of yourself that is trying but failing to "cure" it. The analyst begins to feel victimized by his own desire and then feels the patient's "pathology" as an adversary. The mortal enemy of an eating-disordered patient, as Boris (1984, 1986) cogently elaborated, is desire. Because she does not wish to want, her solution is to stimulate desire in the other, to become object, not subject; to become the object of the other's wants. Where this leads in treatment is to a situation with which we are all painfully familiar. The patient-therapist relationship is pulled into the patient's internal drama that has become a substitute for living. The war over who shall hold the desire is externalized as an interpersonal war and fought out dissociatively, calling into play a constantly shifting array of the patient's and the analyst's self-states. It is a war that, in one respect, the analyst has to lose in order to win. A transitional reality has to be constructed in which trust in human relatedness begins to become possible, and this can happen only through the analyst's recognition and use of his own dissociated self-experience.

In the preceding vignette, the analyst's piece of the enactment allowed him to "therapeutically" ignore his patient's fatness while dissociating his *personal* motivation for doing so—"I'm not addressing her weight," he told himself, "because it's better for her to have freedom and not feel pressured." However, as he was increasingly forced to perceive those aspects of himself he hadn't been able to own—"I *hate* her fatness because it's making me feel helpless, and I want nothing more to do with it"—the enacted parts of his *patient's* self to which his own dissociated self-states were linked began to be experienced by him. As the respective experiences of patient and analyst were put into words and shared, a transition began to take place that the patient evocatively described as a growing awareness of her "Mr. Hide." In general, the success of such a transition depends on the ability of a patient to destroy successfully her analyst's unilateral experience of what he tells himself this is "*really* all about." Her major symptom had become *his* personal enemy, and only when he became unable to dissociate this experience and able to confront his hate and helplessness could those parts of her that had no words make themselves known. Within her fatness "Ms. Hide" lived, and for her to be found, the patient had to dismantle her analyst's unilaterally defined image of her as a fat woman who *has* a symptom and recognize that she *is* her symptom. The biggest problem for any analyst as he goes through a process like this is that his *own* self-image is being destabilized in the process, and he must "survive" his patient's "object use" (Winnicott 1969) without putting his need to restabilize himself ahead of relational authenticity. This last point has been eloquently developed by Stechler (2003), who wrote:

> Beneficial change within self-organizing systems can be brought about by destabilizing old states and by biasing the creation of new states through the negotiation process (p. 725). Whether that new state will be a richer, more complex, and more appropriate foundation for further development, or is the less advantageous choice in the sense of narrowing through toxic adaptation, may depend on whether the partner in this self-organizing system biases it in one direction or the other. The more

> toxic adaptation can stem from an interactional partner who reacts as if his destabilization were toxic. That is, if the therapist's (or parent's) primary aim is to reduce his own destabilization and its accompanying anxiety as if it were toxic and intolerable, the partner's aim and choice will be biased in the same direction. If the therapist can stay connected with his own and with the patient's destabilization and can bias his own subsequent state choice toward openness and affective authenticity, then the patient's will be similarly biased. On the other hand, if the patient feels the freezing or the pretense of the therapist at those critical moments, the work of the therapy cannot proceed well. (p. 723)

What Stechler called openness and affective authenticity require an abiding respect not only for a patient's autonomy, but an equally abiding respect for what might be called, more poetically, a patient's *autotomy*—the dissociative unlinking of parts of the self in the face of potential trauma so that *non omnis moriar!*—"I shall not wholly die!"

REFERENCES

Becker E: The Denial of Death. New York, Free Press, 1973

Boris HN: The problem of anorexia nervosa. Int J Psychoanal 65:315–322, 1984

Boris HN: The "other" breast: greed, envy, spite and revenge. Contemp Psychoanal 22:45–59, 1986

Breger L: Freud: Darkness in the Midst of Vision. New York, Wiley, 2000

Breuer J, Freud S: Studies on hysteria (1893–1895), in The Standard Edition of the Complete Psychological Works of Sigmund Freud, Vol 2. Translated and edited by Strachey J. London, Hogarth Press, 1955, pp 1–319

Bromberg PM: "Speak! that I may see you": some reflections on dissociation, reality, and psychoanalytic listening (1994), in Standing in the Spaces: Essays on Clinical Process, Trauma and Dissociation. Hillsdale, NJ, Analytic Press, 1998, pp 241–266

Bromberg PM: Psychoanalysis, dissociation, and personality organization (1995a), in Standing in the Spaces: Essays on Clinical Process, Trauma and Dissociation. Hillsdale, NJ, Analytic Press, 1998, pp 189–204

Bromberg PM: Treating patients with symptoms—and symptoms with patients. Paper presented at New York University Postdoctoral Program in Psychotherapy and Psychoanalysis. New York, NY, May 1995b

Bromberg PM: Hysteria, dissociation, and cure (1996), in Standing in the Spaces: Essays on Clinical Process, Trauma and Dissociation. Hillsdale, NJ, Analytic Press, 1998, pp 223–237

Ciocca A: Psychosomatic dissociation and eating disorders, in Psychotherapeutic Issues on Eating Disorders. Edited by Bria P, Ciocca A, de Risio S. Rome, Società Editrice Universo, 1998, pp 49–55

Edelman GM: The Remembered Present: A Biological Theory of Consciousness. New York, Basic Books, 1989

Edelman GM: Bright Air, Brilliant Fire. New York, Basic Books, 1992

Edelman GM: Wider Than the Sky: The Phenomenal Gift of Consciousness. New Haven, CT, Yale University Press, 2004

Everill JT, Waller G, Macdonald W: Reported sexual abuse and bulimic symptoms: the mediating role of dissociation. Dissociation 8:155–159, 1995

Gleaves DH, May MC, Eberenz KP: Measuring and discriminating dissociative and borderline symptomatology among women with eating disorders. Dissociation 9:110–117, 1996

Havens LL: Approaches to the Mind. Boston, MA, Little, Brown, 1973

Janet P: The Major Symptoms of Hysteria. New York, Macmillan, 1907

Johnson S: Mind Wide Open: Your Brain and the Neuroscience of Everyday Life. New York, Scribner, 2004

Katz BE, Gleaves DH: Dissociative symptoms among patients with eating disorders: associated feature or artifact of a comorbid dissociative disorder? Dissociation 9:28–36, 1996

Lewis M: Shame: The Exposed Self. New York, Free Press, 1995

MacDonald G: Phantastes (1858). Grand Rapids, MI, Eeerdmans, 1981

McCallum KE, Lock J, Kulla M, Rorty M, Wetzel RD: Dissociative symptoms and disorders in patients with eating disorders. Dissociation 5:227–235, 1992

Muller JP: Beyond the Psychoanalytic Dyad. New York, Routledge, 1996

Sands SH: What is dissociated? Dissociation 7:145–152, 1994

Stechler G: Affect: the heart of the matter. Psychoanalytic Dialogues 13:711–726, 2003

Sullivan HS: The Interpersonal Theory of Psychiatry. New York, Norton, 1953

Sullivan HS: The Psychiatric Interview. New York, Norton, 1954

Szymborska W: Autotomy, in Postwar Polish Poetry, 3rd Edition. Edited and translated by Milosz C. Berkeley, University of California Press, 1983, pp 115–116

Tronick EZ, Weinberg MK: Depressed mothers and infants: failure to form dyadic states of consciousness (1997), in Postpartum Depression and Child Development. Edited by Murray L, Cooper P. New York, Guilford, 1997, pp 54–81

Winnicott DW: The use of an object and relating through identifications (1969), in Playing and Reality. New York, Basic Books, 1971, pp 86–94

Woolf V: Orlando. New York, Harcourt Brace, 1928

Zerbe KJ: Selves that starve and suffocate: the continuum of eating disorders and dissociative phenomena. Bull Menninger Clin 57:319–327, 1993

3

FRED BUSCH, PH.D.

INTRODUCTION

Fred Busch was educated at City College of New York, attained his Ph.D. from the University of Massachusetts in Amherst, and did postdoctoral work at the Reiss-David Child Study Center in Los Angeles, California. He is a graduate of the Michigan Psychoanalytic Institute, where he was a Training and Supervising Analyst. He currently resides in Boston, Massachusetts. He is a Training and Supervising Analyst at the Psychoanalytic Institute of New England, East, in Needham, Massachusetts, and he is the author of numerous papers on technique and theory and of two influential books: *The Ego as the Center of Clinical Technique* and *Rethinking Clinical Technique.* He has been on the editorial boards of numerous psychoanalytic journals and has edited two books for the book series of *The Journal of the American Psychoanalytic Association.*

Dr. Busch first came to prominence in American psychoanalysis through his collaboration with Paul Gray and their emphasis on the primacy of analysis of defenses, particularly defenses against aggression. More recently, Busch has moved from this earlier stance, and he has described his current analytic views very vividly in the following response to my request for a self-description:

> A label! Not an easy question. Bear with me, please, as I attempt to answer this question.
>
> I know how everyone else labels me....i.e., A Contemporary Ego Psychologist. I have labeled myself as such, at times, but I'm no longer

comfortable with the label. The label is associated with the important work of Paul Gray, but there are a number of ways that I conceptualize psychoanalytic treatment differently than he did. For example,

1. I don't believe in the aggressive drive (I believe in aggression), and I see defenses occurring against self-states, internalized object relations, and sexual fantasies (i.e., fears of abandonment, disintegration, loss of love, castration, etc.).
2. I believe in the centrality of using one's countertransference in understanding certain patients much of the time, and with all patients some of the time.
3. I believe simply interpreting defenses is insufficient for helping patients to figure out what unconscious fears, fantasies, and disturbing self- and object states they are dealing with.
4. I believe we need to approach the wider-scope patient flexibly.
5. I would characterize my work in the following way: I use multiple perspectives to understand my patients. However, in conveying what I believe I understand in a way that I think patients may best use, I am constantly monitoring the patient's preconscious readiness to take in what I say in a meaningful way. This position, and the various ways to think about this, is my version of ego psychology. Also, I believe an appreciation for working with unconscious ego defenses is central to the patient's readiness to hear and take in interpretation.

In short, I see myself as part of an evolving American psychoanalysis that is attempting to integrate knowledge that has accrued from various sources, with a body of knowledge loosely known as American Ego Psychology. This is in contrast to those psychoanalysts who seem more interested in promoting their views as a new paradigm, leaving to the side much of what we've discovered in the past 60 years.

WHY I CHOSE THIS PAPER

Fred Busch, Ph.D.

Without my realizing it at the time, this paper, "'In the Neighborhood,'" set the agenda for my writing and thinking for over a decade. Everything I've written since has been an elaboration of the ideas first expressed in this paper. As far as I can tell, it is my most-read paper, and it is the first paper I assign when teaching courses on psychoanalytic technique. For me, the paper established something new for us to think about when talking to patients (i.e., the role of the conscious ego). Along with the work of many others, it has led to our greater awareness of the concept of analytic surfaces.

Over the years, I've learned some things that I feel would lead to my writing a slightly different paper now. I've indicated where in footnotes added to the paper. Further, although the thinking of Paul Gray looms large over this work, I've since incorporated many other perspectives in looking at the same phenomenon—especially the role of interpreting content and not just resistance and the role of countertransference in understanding character resistances.

"IN THE NEIGHBORHOOD"

Aspects of a Good Interpretation and a "Developmental Lag" in Ego Psychology

FRED BUSCH, PH.D.

THE PHRASE "IN THE NEIGHBORHOOD" comes from Freud's (1910) paper "'Wild' Psycho-Analysis." In this paper Freud tells of a woman consulting him after having gone to a young physician for problems with anxiety after a recent divorce. The physician diagnosed the woman's problems as due to lack of sexual satisfaction and suggested various sexual activities as a remedy. Freud chided the physician for assuming that the woman's primary problem was a lack of information and that providing this would result in cure.

> If knowledge about the unconscious were as important for the patient as people inexperienced in psycho-analysis imagine, listening to lectures or reading books would be enough to cure him. Such measures, however, have as much influence on the symptoms of nervous illness as a distribution of menu-cards in a time of famine has upon hunger.... Since, however, psycho-analysis cannot dispense with giving this information, it lays down that this shall not be done before two conditions have been fulfilled. First, the patient must, through preparation, himself have reached the neighborhood of what he has repressed, and secondly, he must have formed a sufficient attachment (transference) to the physi-

---

"'In the Neighborhood': Aspects of a Good Interpretation and a 'Developmental Lag' in Ego Psychology," by Fred Busch, Ph.D., was originally published in *The Journal of the American Psychoanalytic Association,* 41:151–177, 1993. Used with permission. Abridged slightly for this publication. *Footnotes added 2004.*

> cian for his emotional relationship to him to make a fresh flight impossible. (pp. 225–226)

By introducing the concept of the analysand needing to be "in the neighborhood" Freud is noting the centrality, among the principles of clinical technique, of the conscious ego. The patient must be able to make some connection between what he is aware of thinking and saying, and the analyst's intervention. No matter how brilliant the analyst's reading of the unconscious, it is not useful data until it can be connected to something the patient can be consciously aware of. From this perspective the young physician Freud described did not consider what his patient might understand, let alone if she might find his intervention objectionable. The potential difficulties with this approach are succinctly captured by Freud (1910) in the following:

> Attempts to "rush" him at first consultation, by brusquely telling him the secrets which have been discovered by the physician, are technically objectionable. And they mostly bring their own punishment by inspiring a hearty enmity towards the physician on the patient's part and cutting him off from having any further influence. (p. 226)

While few analysts would disagree with the necessity of their comments being in the same neighborhood as the patient's thoughts, it is my impression this is a rule more honored in the breach. As with resistances, there is what Gray (1982) aptly describes as a "developmental lag" between our understanding of the concept at an intellectual level and an affective, clinically useful one. The analysand's fear of and unfamiliarity with unconscious thoughts and feelings (i.e., resistances), along with the importance of including the conscious ego in the working-through process, seem not to have been well integrated within our analytic empathy. Listening to discussions of the clinical process, one is impressed with how many interpretations seem based less on what the patient is capable of hearing, and more on what the analyst is capable of understanding. We too often confuse our ability to read the unconscious and the patient's ability to understand it. We are frequently not clear enough on the distinction between an unconscious communication and our ability to communicate with the patient's unconscious. What the patient can hear, understand, and effectively utilize—let alone the benefits of considering such an approach—are rarely in the foreground of our clinical discussions. Getting to the "real" unconscious fantasy still seems to be our primary therapeutic goal. This appears to be a remnant of the topographic theory we still struggle with.

Greenson is one of those psychoanalysts who offered generously of his clinical work. His wisdom and humanity were evident to all those fortunate enough to have heard his presentations, while his clinical examples elucidate and challenge us. It is in this spirit that I shall introduce an extended example from his work (Greenson 1967).

> In the first year of his analysis, a young man comes into a session angrily denouncing a professor who lectures "without thinking of whether the students can follow." As he continues in this vein, he slips and says that he hates "to have him treat—I mean, teach me." He then challenges Greenson with the comment, "I suppose you will make something of that." When the patient continues to complain about the professor, Greenson makes a semi-resistance interpretation (i.e., where the resistance is noted but the intent is not to explore it but to get to what is being resisted). Greenson asks him, "Aren't you trying to run away from your anger toward me?" The patient acquiesces with some expressed doubt, but returns with thoughts about feeling sorry for the professor because of rumors that this wife had recently committed suicide. He then returns to complaining about the professor as a "big shot," who "doesn't give a shit for me."
>
> Greenson intervenes with the following comment: "Aren't you angry with me for going on my vacation next week?" The patient angrily denies this, accusing Greenson of sounding like he looked this up in a book, and of making a universal analytic comment. Greenson notes his anger, but tells the patient his "real" anger is over his vacation. The patient reluctantly agrees, and presents some confirmatory data in a desultory fashion. (pp. 299–300)

From the beginning of this vignette, Greenson seems not to be taking into account what the patient may consciously accept. As with the analysand's complaint about his professor, he does not consider "whether the students can follow." The slip, which indicates the patient has already made the unconscious connection between his feelings about Greenson and the professor, is challenged. It is clear the patient is in a feisty mood, and connections between Greenson and the professor will not be welcome. This is the resistance that seems most closely available to consciousness. Greenson raises it, but takes the further step of telling the patient that it is his anger toward the analyst that he is avoiding. Greenson clearly has something in mind, which he finally gets to when he tells the patient he is angry about the analyst's upcoming vacation. However, there is nothing in the data to suggest that the patient might have any awareness that one might work with, except in the resistance, that he is really angry at Greenson, or that the reason has to do with Greenson's vacation. In bypassing the resistance, the patient's conscious participation is left out of the analysis, except to passively accept the interpretation. Greenson's explanation for his remarks is that he saw the slip as an indication of the patient's anger, "but he refuses to accept this consciously" (p. 300). This is just the point. *Where* a patient is consciously and *why* he is there are a crucial part of the analytic task. Consciousness is not something to be run roughshod over. Greenson's explanation is, "I believe it is necessary to pursue the resistances until one mobilizes a reasonable ego in the patient" (p. 300). In this one sees Greenson's tendency to confuse the resistance with the feelings behind the resistance. What he pursued were the patient's feelings of anger. What he did not pursue was the patient's reluctance to make a connection between Greenson and the professor (i.e., the most observable component of the resistance at that time). Furthermore, for patients, their conscious ego is always the most reasonable one.

If we believe a patient is warding off something from consciousness, it is not our task to only bring this to their awareness. From the side of the ego, there is a perfectly good reason why it is being warded off; understanding this reason is a first step toward conscious acceptance of that which is being warded off.

This paper will be about the importance of paying attention to what Myerson (1981) aptly describes as the analysand's ability to hear our interpretations. It does not appear that this component of the analytic enterprise has been fully integrated into consistent usable techniques. Herzog (1991) notes that throughout Freud's work there is no systematic elaboration of consciousness, while Joseph (1987) concludes that Freud did not consider consciousness as particularly worthy of study. Possibly this situation might have been righted if we had access to Freud's missing metapsychological paper on consciousness. However, what we have been left with is a situation where, at best, we have taken as given the complex, detailed conscious processing that goes on in psychoanalytic work. At worst, the importance of analysands' conscious readiness to accept and use our interventions remains relatively ignored. I suggest that this developmental lag in integrating a central component of the interpretive process into clinical technique is, in part, a response to Freud's struggle with the integration of his clinical observations with theory, and the relative neglect of the clinical ego in the development of ego psychology. I shall elaborate on the importance of being "in the neighborhood" in the hope that this contribution might prove to be a step in conceptualizing an important but unfinished task in psychoanalysis—the illumination of the role of the ego in the psychoanalytic process.

FREUD, HIS AMBIVALENCE, AND SOME THAT FOLLOWED

In his paper on "wild" psychoanalysis, Freud (1910) gently chides the young physician for his intemperate interpretation. The primary technical error Freud cites is the belief that the patient suffers from a type of ignorance, and that by informing the patient one will have cured the neurosis. Freud then highlights the significance of combating the resistances for the success of the analysis. However, toward the end of this article, Freud offers the following surprising caveat:

> "wild" analysts of this kind do more harm to the cause of psycho-analysis than to individual patients. I have often found that a clumsy procedure like this, even if at first it produced an exacerbation of the patient's condition, led to a recovery in the end. Not always but still often. (p. 227)

In this one passage Freud seems to renounce everything he has said heretofore. He now comes down on the side of the usefulness of even "clumsy" efforts to bring the unconscious wishes to consciousness, even if the initial effect is deleterious. The importance of being "in the neighborhood" now seems insignificant as an interpretive guideline. The emphasis on the patient's readiness to consciously accept an interpretation and all that it implies seems now to be disavowed. This is done even though most of what he said previously cautions against taking such an approach, and expresses doubt about the usefulness of such a technique. The reason Freud gives for this turnaround is that he believes the young physician's remarks "forced her attention to the real cause of her trouble, or in that direction, and in spite of all her opposition this intervention of his cannot be without some favorable results" (p. 227). Freud's view now is that bringing the unconscious wishes into awareness has a generally positive, long-term effect on the patient, no matter how the wishes might be brought to the patient's attention. The beneficial outcome is seen as due to the conscious attention of the patient being directed toward the unconscious, even in the face of the resistances. The resistances are reduced to factors that "intensify the prejudices… against the methods of psycho-analysis" (p. 227).

How do we understand these contradictory views? One useful way is described by Lear (1990) as the contradiction between Freud the clinician, "who helped himself to empathic understanding," and Freud the theorist who "tried to fit psychoanalysis into the scientific image of his day" (p. 5). Freud the clinician understood early on that thoughts were kept out of awareness because of their being associated with frightening and overwhelming feelings. Therefore his clinician side understood that analysands might be upset with the approaching awareness of unconscious thoughts, because of the unpleasurable affects associated with them. Thus Freud's earliest clinical description of the ideas that fell prey to censorship is a complex amalgam of feelings and dangers. He states of thoughts that are censored, "they were all of a distressing nature, calculated to arouse the affects of shame and self-reproach and of psychical pain, and the feeling of being harmed; they were all of a kind one would prefer to have not experienced, that one would rather forget" (Freud 1895, p. 269). This is the Freud who would understand the uselessness of attempting to bring an idea to consciousness until the intense negative feelings surrounding the idea had been ameliorated in some way. This is the Freud who instantly understood the folly of the "young physician's" remarks. This is the Freud who empathically understood the nature of resistances, and kept them at the center of his clinical theory throughout his work.

Freud the theorist held three views in 1910 that are germane to our discussion. The first of these was that anxiety was the result of dammed-up libido. The psychic corollary to this was that only if a wish remained unconscious could it become pathogenic. The final view was that consciousness and unconsciousness existed at two different levels of representation, and only by joining these two levels could an unconscious idea become conscious. The characteristic of consciousness specific to our discussion is that it is represented by "word presentation." This is in contrast to the unconscious represented by "thing presentations." In this model the road to consciousness involves connecting the "thing presentations" to "word presentations." Thus Freud the theorist could see how the "young physician" could reduce anxiety by putting into words, and thus making conscious, unfulfilled unconscious wishes. From this perspective it was the putting ideas into words that would remove them from the unconscious, and ultimately unblock the dammed-up libido. In short, Freud the clinician was drawn one way while Freud the theorist was drawn in the opposite direction. This distinction is one useful way to understand the contradictory advice Freud seems to be giving in this article on the handling of material in relation to being "in the neighborhood."

Throughout the rest of Freud's early technical papers there are references to this same topic, with Freud oscillating between his clinical and theoretical views. In "The Dynamics of the Transference" Freud's (1912) views are dominated by the necessity of bringing the unconscious thoughts to consciousness. He suggests that if the patient falls silent, this stoppage can be eliminated by assuring the patient that he is holding back thoughts about the analyst. "As soon as this explanation is given, the stoppage is removed, or the situation is changed from one in which the associations fail into one in which they are being kept back" (p. 101). In this we can see that the necessity of being in the same neighborhood as the patient is replaced by a more authoritarian stance. A year later Freud (1913) repeats what happened in the paper on "wild" psychoanalysis. At first he repudiates the importance of bringing an idea to consciousness without first taking into account how objectionable it might be to consciousness. He notes (p. 142), "there was no choice but to cease attributing to the fact of knowing, in itself, the importance that had previously been given to it and to place the emphasis on the resistances which had in the past brought about the state of not knowing and which were still ready to defend that state." However, by the end of this same page, Freud states, when referring to bringing repressed material into consciousness, "At first it arouses resistances, but then, when these have been overcome, it sets up a process of thought in the course of which the expected influencing of the unconscious recollection eventually takes place." This same oscillation occurs in later technical papers (Freud 1914, 1916–1917).

While Freud does not specifically return to the topic of being "in the neighborhood" in later papers, the underlying issues are crucial to later theoretical developments. The importance of resistances being unconscious is a central component in the development of the structural theory (Freud 1923). The analysand's readiness to accept interpretations into consciousness, and its relation to the unconscious resistances, become a central factor in the structural theory. Freud's (1926) second theory of anxiety comes much closer to capturing his earliest (Freud 1895) observations on those affects associated with keeping thoughts from awareness. However, it was left to others to continue to work on the clinical significance of this new integration of clinical empathy and psychoanalytic theory.

In Anna Freud's (1936) pioneering investigation of the ego, she notes, "we have realized that large portions of the ego institutions are themselves unconscious and require the help of analysis in order to become conscious. The result is that analysis of the ego has assumed a much greater importance in our eyes" (p. 25). From this perspective the centrality of the ego's ability to become aware of its own thought processes is highlighted, and continues the thrust of Freud's attempts to integrate clinical observations with the theory of the analytic process. Searl's (1936) paper on technique is a clear integration of what was understood to that point on the importance of considering the patient's ability to "hear" interpretations. Her description of the importance of taking into account what the analysand is capable of becoming aware of, while pointing to the dangers of interpreting "absent content," shows a subtle and complex understanding of the implications for technique of the new ego psychology which was not consistent at the time (e.g., Reich 1933).[1] Fenichel (1941) succinctly described the principles under discussion here when he stated:

> Analysis must always go on in the layers accessible to the ego at the moment. When an interpretation has no effect, one often asks oneself: "How could I have interpreted more deeply?" But often the question should more correctly be put: "How could I have interpreted more superficially?" (p. 44)

However, this line of thinking, which started out in such a promising fashion, soon reached a barrier. There are only scattered references to the concepts implied in the interpretive technique of being "in the neighborhood" over the next 30 years. E. Kris (1951) states that in second analyses interpretations that are closer to the surface often lead to significant improvements. Eissler (1965) highlights the importance of interpretations not being isolated from a patient's previous knowledge, while Loewenstein's (1972) concept of identification with the analyst's function is influenced by notions of the importance of autonomous ego functions in the interpretive process.

Similar influences can also be seen in the work of Loewald (1960) and Myerson (1960). Why there was this long barren period seems partly related to Freud's ambivalence, and partly related to issues discussed in the next section. However, it was not until the work of Gray (1973, 1982, 1986, 1987, 1990a, 1990b) that the centrality of the conscious ego in the interpretive process was returned to. No one to that point had approached Gray's meticulous attention to actual techniques in the interpretation of resistances that took into account the conscious ego. Following his work a number of psychoanalysts have recently explored an area that has come to be known as the analytic "surface" (Davison et al. 1986; Levy and Inderbitzin 1990; Paniagua 1985). While the emphasis varies slightly, the "surface" generally refers to behaviors that are observable and demonstrable to the patient. In these investigations the benefits of using the surface, especially in the understanding of resistances, are delved into and elaborated on in a way that gives increasing weight to the significance of the conscious ego. Thus we seem to be on the verge of multiple explorations into the role of the conscious ego in the analytic process.[2] However, before going further into our own in-

---

[1]See Busch 1995b for a fuller exploration of Searl's work.

[2]For a fuller exploration of the earlier struggles to integrate ego psychology with clinical technique see Busch 1999 pp. 111–123; also see the references for a fuller appreciation of the growing contributions to this area. For its application to the work of children, see Sugarman 2003. Also see Paniagua 2001 for a succinct exposition on the salient issues in this approach.

vestigation, it is important to look at another factor that may have inadvertently hampered psychoanalytic inquiry into the role of the ego in the psychoanalytic process—the development of ego psychology.

HARTMANN'S LEGACY

Possibly no one has captured Hartmann's place in psychoanalysis as well as Schafer (1970):

> Heinz Hartmann's contributions to psychoanalytic theory [1939, 1960, 1964] rise up before the student of psychoanalysis as a mountain range whose distant peaks with their immense vistas and rarefied atmosphere it is scarcely possible to reach. And yet the student must not only attempt the arduous climb, he must try to get above that range so that he can include Hartmann's work within his own vision of psychoanalysis, for that work is not the whole of psychoanalysis, nor can it be the last word on psychoanalytic theory; it is and can only be part of the terrain of scientific psychoanalysis and of science generally. (p. 425)

While agreeing with Smith's (1986) view that we still need time to fully evaluate Hartmann's contributions, one is inevitably drawn to his work with regard to the topic at hand. In fact, in this area Hartmann's work has proven to be both an important contribution and an unwelcome diversion. While stimulating studies that added significant depth to our understanding of subtleties in ego functioning, his emphasis on psychoanalysis as a general psychology may have inadvertently contributed to a diversion from in-depth attention to issues of psychoanalytic technique.

Our views of human behavior were radically changed by Hartmann's views of early ego development and his call for research in child development. His view of the ego as an inborn adaptational structure with predetermined strengths and weaknesses interacting with, and affected by an environment which was growth-producing or inhibiting, all since shown to be essentially correct by studies of early development, forever changed our view of the infant/child. This, in turn, opened the potential for a new way of understanding patients, especially in the area of analyzability. Will the patient be able to tolerate the regressive components of the analytic situation? Will he be able to give up enough control to participate in the process of free association? If there are severe, long-term restrictions in ego functioning, is it not more likely these are due to developmental interferences rather than neurotic conflicts? Were there some interferences in his early "average expectable environment" that may have had a profound influence on early ego functions? Such questions come directly from the work of Hartmann and the psychoanalytic investigations into early development he spawned. The importance of the relationship between the infant/child and its caregiver for psychic survival, as well as a sense of self, cohesion, autonomy, individuation, along with tolerance for affects and affect regulation, have all been well documented by now (e.g., Emde 1988; Mahler et al. 1975; Spitz 1945; Stern 1985).

Hartmann's work set the stage for a subtle approach to the understanding of those factors in the ego which affect acceptance into consciousness. The effect on conscious receptivity of thoughts to such things as changes in ego states (e.g., fragmentation), regressions in levels of thinking (e.g., from formal operations to preoperational thought), and the degree to which communication is dominated by action are more easily comprehended because of the work of Hartmann. His inquiries and encouragement of others to map the developmental outline of the ego have had the potential to provide a significant impact on our understanding of what is allowable into consciousness. However, it is not clear this potential has been realized as of yet. As Apfelbaum and Gill (1989) conclude, the technical implications of the structural theory seem not to have been noted and implemented. The heart of the structural theory, that in analyzing the ego resistances one must consider different levels of consciousness, still seems not to be a part of general clinical thinking.[3] To help understand this I think we need to take a look at Hartmann's work from another dimension.

It has been noted that Hartmann's heavy emphasis on metapsychology, which was presented in a way that was removed from clinical data, has had a deleterious effect on clinical theory and technique (Apfelbaum 1962; Schafer 1970; Shaw 1989). The same might be said, in the short run, for his championing the necessity of studies in child development as a way of understanding ego development. The result has been that Hartmann remains a giant in the psychoanalytic pantheon, but as Wyman (1989) notes, his ideas seem to have vanished from the literature. The abstractness of his theorizing, while forsaking clinical examples, has left a generation of analysts in awe of Hartmann's intellectual powers, while shaking their heads when considering its relevance to their last patient. The importance of the clinical ego in ego psychology was pushed aside for a more abstract theorizing. This trend continued

---

[3]For a discussion of how Arlow and Brenner moved from this focus, see Busch 1999, pp. 19–51.

for many years as noted by Arlow (1975) and Joseph (1975). That Hartmann had a sophisticated clinical view of the ego which took note of such issues as levels of conscious ego, and the importance of ego analysis, can be glimpsed in the following:

> Defenses (typically) not only keep thoughts, images, and instinctual drives out of consciousness, but also prevent their assimilation by means of thinking. When defensive processes break down, the mental elements defended against and certain connections of these elements become amenable to recollection and reconstruction. Interpretations not only help to regain the buried material, but must also establish correct causal relations, that is, the causes, range of influence, and effectiveness of these experiences in relation to other elements. I stress this here because the theoretical study of interpretation is often limited to those instances which are concerned with emerging memories or corresponding reconstructions. But even more important for the theory of interpretation are those instances in which the causal connections of elements, and the criteria for these connections, are established. (Hartmann 1939, p. 63)

In this one can see the importance for Hartmann, in the interpretive process, of what is allowable into consciousness. He alerts us to the significance not only of the memories associated with repressed trauma, but also to the importance of elements of ego functioning associated with defenses and connected to these traumas.[4] He underlines the importance of the expanding awareness of the workings of the conscious ego in the interpretive work, and emphasizes the various "mental elements" which are connected to the defenses which become available for entry into consciousness once the defenses become less rigid.[5] We see here the Hartmann that sounds like other voices who have championed expanding awareness of the conscious ego as a primary interpretive goal.

The quandary posed by Hartmann for the psychoanalytic clinician is captured in the following sentence: "Permit me a digression on the nature of thinking in the *psychoanalytic situation,* in which the predominant object of thought is the subject himself" (Hartmann 1939, p. 62). That Hartmann considered thinking about the psychoanalytic situation a "digression" is evident in his theorizing. This approach hampered the translation of ego psychology into a viable component of clinical psychoanalysis. While ego analysis was championed in print, its transla-

---

[4]See Busch 2005.

[5]See Busch 2004.

tion into understandable, workable approaches in the clinical situation lagged behind. Thus the clinical issue of availability to consciousness as one consideration in the analyst's interpretive stance, which began in conflict between Freud the empathic observer and Freud the scientist, once again was obscured behind Hartmann the theoretician. Thus Hartmann's legacy is that while he opened a window to the possibility of subtleties in understanding ego functions, the shade remained drawn on the clinical ego.

IMPORTANCE OF BEING "IN THE NEIGHBORHOOD"

The centrality of being "in the neighborhood" for the analytic process is emphasized in Gray's (1973, 1982, 1986, 1990b) work on resistance analysis, where he champions the importance of the conscious ego in the analytic process. In a twist of Freud's adage, Gray (1990b) points to the usefulness of looking at the goals of the psychoanalytic process in terms of "where unconscious ego was, conscious ego shall be" (p. 1095). He believes that "the therapeutic results of analytic treatment are lasting in proportion to the extent to which, during the analysis, the patient's unbypassed ego functions have become involved in a consciously and increasingly voluntary co-partnership with the analyst" (Gray 1982, p. 624). In a series of articles over the last two decades Gray has given us a clear methodology for analyzing the unconscious ego resistances while helping analysands become aware of their mental activity. His emphasis is on helping patients gain greater access to consciousness of unconscious ego activities that lead to resistances. For Gray a successful interpretation has, as one component, a direction of the patient to something *he can understand* in spite of ongoing resistances. Gray (1990b) asserts that by including the conscious ego in our interpretive stance we encourage and strengthen more mature ego functioning.

The significance of the analysand's conscious awareness of his own thoughts is also seen in the work of A.O. Kris (1982, 1983, 1990). Kris, who considers the conscious ego from a somewhat different perspective, uses the method of free association as the frame of his analytic perspective, and suggests there are inherent satisfactions with freedom of associations. His concept of a pathological process, within the context of the analytic setting, involves inhibition of the pleasure in being able to conceptualize and *become aware of one's thought processes.* Using interferences with the method of free association as a basis of pathology, Kris takes the position that a definition of health needs to take into account the ability to become *consciously* aware of one's thoughts, with a corresponding decrease in unconscious resistances to this process.[6] In the work of both Gray and Kris one sees a view of pathology that is defined within the analytic process as an interference with the ability to become *conscious of one's thought processes.* Both use consciousness as a basis of understanding resistances. A corollary to this from the interpretive side is that the analyst's task is to help make conscious the unconscious resistances in a way that allows analysands to have greater access to their mental life. To do this is to keep in mind at all times that: "The interpretive task is to estimate sensitively the patient's ability to comprehend, in order to make a formulation that is not too superficial, yet does not stimulate more reactive defenses" (Gray 1986, p. 253). In this same vein Gray states: "The effectiveness with which patients can use their capacity for observing ego activities depends primarily on the nature of the burden the analyst's interventions place on them" (p. 253). This burden can be decreased by focusing on the unconscious resistances via the analysand's communications and interferences with the free association method. By directing comments to the "neighborhood" the patient presently occupies, in a way that demystifies the basis of our remarks, we go a long way toward inviting conscious participation in the therapeutic process.

What has not been sufficiently emphasized in the literature to this point are the problems inherent in *not* being "in the neighborhood." Simply put, given the centrality of the unconscious ego resistances in the analytic process, it is futile to be any place else. If one primary purpose of a resistance is to keep thoughts and feelings out of awareness, to fail to take into account what can be allowed into awareness when making an intervention is to risk our comments falling on deaf ears, at best, and potentially arousing more resistances. Since Freud's (1926) elaboration of his second theory of anxiety it has been clear that resistances are, in part, the ego's response to some experienced danger or threat. If a resistance is in operation, it indicates that the analysand is experiencing his thoughts or feelings as a danger. The purpose of the resistance is to keep the dangerous thought or feeling from awareness. The particular type of resistance is an adaptation, from an earlier time, to this threat. Interventions that do not respect the analysand's resistance to certain thoughts and feelings becoming conscious will be either irrelevant or potentially overwhelming. This basic component of the analytic process has been

---

[6]For an elaboration of the method of free association, see Busch (1994, 1999, 2003).

muddled by our "developmental lag" (Gray 1982) in understanding the resistances (see also Busch 1992; Schafer 1983).

A different perspective on the futility of interpreting outside "the neighborhood" is presented in the work of Klein (1976). He shows that the basic purpose of any defensive process is to take the meaning out of behavior that is drive-dominated.[7] Thus the person with exhibitionistic wishes is aware only of feeling self-conscious that people are staring at him, while someone in the throes of an oedipal rivalry knows only about his discomfort around older authority figures. Wishes have an active, ongoing influence on behavior, while the individual has no understanding of the behavior or feeling associated with the wish. The critical accomplishment of defenses is the establishment of a gap between behavior and conscious comprehension of that behavior. The meaning of wishes can be lived out without any conscious understanding. The individual who can "barely" go out in public due to vague feelings of shame and embarrassment when others are looking is living out an ongoing expression of exhibitionistic wishes. The crucial component of the defense is that the individual can live out the wish without any conscious comprehension. One important goal of an interpretation, then, is to *fill out gaps in meaning* (and not necessarily gaps in memory). The bridge must be made between unconscious wishes acted upon in behaviors and their conscious meanings, along with the reasons for their being kept apart (i.e., the resistances). Until such a bridge is made, behaviors remain unresponsive to feedback, and thus not modifiable. The exhibitionist cannot think of leaving the house while fervently believing he is avoiding pain and discomfort by staying home.

The conscious understanding that behaviors have meaning, that there are reasons for our keeping a gap between the behavior and its meaning, and finally what the behaviors mean, become the significant steps in an analysand obtaining understanding of his behavior. By not taking into account the analysand's conscious readiness to grasp the meaning of his behavior, we are missing one of the basic points of the defenses, which is to keep meanings outside awareness. Only by gradually making behaviors consciously meaningful can we hope to modify the basic defensive structure. Defenses are instituted in such a manner

---

[7]Two emendations are needed to this statement. I would now *[2004]* say the basic purpose of a defense is to ward off danger (Busch 2001). That's why meaning is taken out. Also, to relate defenses only to drive determinants simplifies the many others dangers to self and object that motivate defenses (Busch 1999, pp. 139–188).

that wishes can be lived out without comprehension. With our interpretations, we hope to bring meaning to this lack of comprehension, while increasing comprehension. Without participation of the patient's conscious ego, we subvert our own goals.

A more subtle, and potentially more insidious problem, is the enfeebling and undermining of the ego which occur when the analysand's conscious awareness is not taken into account. This can be seen most frequently in what Searl (1936) calls the interpretation of "absent content" (i.e., the interpretation of a fantasy or feeling that the analysand is unaware of), an example of which can be seen in the Greenson vignette cited above. In outlining some of the problems with such interpretations, Searl notes:

> If on the other hand, we say to a patient, "You are thinking so and so," "You have such and such a fantasy," and so on, we give him no help about his inability to know that for himself, and leave him to some extent dependent on the analyst for all such knowledge. If we add "The nature of this thought or fantasy explains your difficulty in knowing it for yourself," we still leave the patient with increased understanding related to a particular type of thought and fantasy only, and imply "one must know the thought or fantasy first before one can understand the difficulty about knowing it." The dynamics about the patient's disability to find his own way have been comparatively untouched if the resistance was more than the thinnest of crusts, and will therefore still be at work to some extent and in some form whatever the change brought about by the absent content. (pp. 478–479)

By including the conscious ego in our interventions we encourage the analysand to take a more active role in his treatment. This is in contrast to those interpretations geared toward absent content which, as Searl demonstrates, enforce a passivity on the patient. Such interpretations encourage a belief in the analyst's omniscience, while stimulating the patient's omnipotent fantasies and reinforcing a belief in magical thinking. Searl's work also suggests that by interpreting content outside of an analysand's awareness we may participate in a bypassing of resistances to independent self-analysis (i.e., the dynamics of the patients' inability to find their own way). This fear and/or distortion of the ability to observe one's own thought processes is a significant resistance in every analysis, but it has been obscured by gaps in our understanding of ego analysis.[8] How frequently have we heard what seem to be rel-

[8] See Busch (1996, 1997) for an elaboration.

atively successful treatments which are in their final stages where the patient "associates," and the analyst "interprets." The patient's participation in the process of analyzing is too infrequently analyzed, partly because we are not paying attention to the nature of what would be most helpful to the analysand in understanding the analytic process. Is it the understanding of his unconscious fantasies, or is it the increasing conscious awareness of his own thought processes and the barriers to this awareness? I do not in any way rule out the centrality of understanding unconscious conflicts and the resulting compromise formations in symptom resolution. Inevitably, all resistances to self-awareness are intertwined with persistent fantasies which dominate unconscious thoughts. It is simply a question of the best way to show these to the patient so that the analytic process is furthered. The analyst's task is a daunting one. Translating the analysand's action thoughts while understanding unconscious components of a communication from the side of the id, ego, and superego is difficult enough. Communicating this to patients so they can hear what they have been talking about, while also being relevant to concerns they are aware of struggling with, is a never-ending test of our cognitive and empathic abilities.

While recently listening to a colleague interpret, for what seemed like the umpteenth time, the patient's passive homosexual wishes as a defense against his active strivings, I thought of our tendency to interpret, and if the patient is not able to use what we say, to interpret again—like trying to give directions to someone who does not speak our language. Invariably in these situations we tend to speak louder and slower, as if by doing this the foreigner will understand better. Our repetitions of the absent unconscious fantasy in its various forms has the same quality. By continuing to focus on absent content, we may be engaging in a process that undermines the ego while, via our empathic disruption with what the analysand is capable of hearing, we may increase the sense of danger and thus intensify resistances.

I have focused on the dangers of not being "in the neighborhood." Yet the question remains as to what the benefits are of including the conscious ego as part of the intervention process. Inviting the analysand's more active participation supports the enlistment of certain ego pleasures which have not been well integrated into psychoanalytic technique. These pleasures are well known to observers of children. Klein (1976) outlined some of these pleasures associated with ego activities as: functioning (i.e., the activity itself is pleasurable); effectance (i.e., changing a course of action through one's behavior); synthesis (i.e., establishing a sense of order and wholeness). These are similar to ego activities noted by Erikson (1959) and White (1963) as well as by many others. In a similar vein, Emde (1988), in reviewing early childhood research, concludes that two of the basic motivations for behavior are activity and self-regulation. It is clear in observational research that from very early on we are driven by, and find pleasure in, a number of ego activities. These have been called by various names over the years (e.g., a drive for competence, a need for mastery); further clarity is still needed. However, what cannot be doubted are the active ego needs and pleasure in them. In our daily analytic work we are much more impressed with how the ego becomes compromised by resistances and unconscious fantasies. Stereotypical, repetitive, restrictions in characteristic ego activities, for much of an analysis, is the observational fare of most analysts. The numbing effect of an ego caught in conflict should not be confused with its potential resilience. We should not, in a countertransference acting out, treat our adult analysands as cognitively impoverished, as they appear when a threatened ego is temporarily restricted. With a respectful eye on the conscious ego and its pleasures, one can point to the way ego functioning becomes compromised by conflict, thus removing pleasure in ego activities. Working with analysands in this way often leads them to a feeling that they have "found a part of themselves" or they consider their thoughts more "their own."

Gray (1982) observed that an important distinguishing element among analysts is their "forms of attention" (p. 621) during the analysis. This can be said both about the type of material listened for and how the analyst communicates his understanding to the patient. In terms of the latter, one hears variations in style from analysts who always seem to "assert" what is going on at any moment in the analysis, to those who seem to believe that it is only the patient who can come to his own understanding and thus say almost nothing. Gray's (1973, 1986, 1990b) method of sharing the data that led to his conclusion invites the analysand's conscious ego to participate in the process. It not only has the advantages associated with including the conscious ego in the analytic process, but also helps to focus in a minute way on resistances to the process. This is essential in analyzing resistances to the self-analytic function which seems crucial for post-termination success.

Weinshel (1984) suggests that a useful way of distinguishing among analysts is that there are those who focus on the goal of analysis, and those who focus on the analytic work. Different ways of interpreting to analysands highlight these differences. Inherent within the position of the analyst who "asserts" his interpretations is the goal of bringing unconscious thoughts to consciousness. Thus this analyst would be working within a topographic model where the therapeutic benefit of analysis is viewed in terms of goals. By sharing with patients the reasons for our inferences, we emphasize the process. We are saying to our patients, "In your use of the method we can learn such and such from what you are saying." It is not that there are no goals with such a method, it is that the goals are reached by focusing on the method. Implicit in one's approach to interventions, there are hidden assumptions about the nature of the analytic process. The approach I have been suggesting is concisely captured in Gill's (1954) felicitous, oft-quoted comment that we still recognize our friends after they have successfully completed an analysis. If one believes that the work of analysis centers on continuing the work of analysis, rather than obliteration of conflict, then including the conscious ego in a variety of ways becomes a necessary component of the process.

In follow-up studies of completed psychoanalyses by Schlessinger and Robbins (1983) there are clear indications that core conflicts are not dissolved. Instead, what one sees post-termination is an emergence of, and then a working on, issues that were central in the analysis. Under periods of stress (i.e., as in the stimulation of the ever-ready transference fantasies arising in a post-termination interview) old conflicts arise, but this time to be handled far more swiftly and with less disruptiveness. Analysis neither obliterates conflict nor the character patterns of resistances and gratifications surrounding conflict. Instead, what analysis accomplishes, from this one perspective, is help in making accessible to consciousness the resistances which are fed by anxiety, and accompanied by an array of unconscious fantasies and traumas. Analysis allows for a greater access to consciousness of these myriad components of conflict, allowing for more rapid resolution of the immediate stresses via self-analysis. This capacity for self-analysis, rather than obliteration of conflict, is one of the prime benefits one sees from successfully completed analyses (Schlessinger and Robbins 1983). As Calef (1982) noted, the outcome of analysis may be most influenced by whether the analysand has been able to identify with its process.

Finally, it is at least important to note there are resistances to including the conscious ego in the interpretive process that lead both analyst and analysand away from the importance of being "in the neighborhood." Gray (1982) and I (Busch 1992) have commented on the magnetism of unconscious fantasies for the analyst in resistances to analyzing the resistances, and the same can be said here. Universal trends from childhood also tend to pull the analysand toward a regressive relationship where the analysand "associates" and the analyst interprets. This can include such wishes as the desire to remain in a dependent position in relation to an omniscient, omnipotent figure; the narcissistic pleasure of being at the center of another's attention, who is observing and attempting to make sense of whatever one is saying; and the pleasure of letting one's mind go without believing there is the need for any structure or control. Furthermore, there are regressions in ego functioning concomitant with development of the transference neurosis which preclude the analysand from observing his own thoughts. For example, a patient functioning under the influence of preoperational thought

> feels neither the compunction to justify his reasoning to others nor to look for possible contradictions in his logic. He is, for example, unable to reconstruct a chain of reasoning which he has just passed through; he thinks but he cannot think about his own thinking. (Flavell 1963, p. 156)

When an analysand is in such a state, his thoughts are closer to actions, and he does not recognize there is a "neighborhood" to be in.[9] Thus, when we observe these resistances to conscious awareness (whether in the form of an ego regression or regression in wish), we need to analyze them as we would any resistance. The danger lies in bypassing an important impediment to self-analysis (i.e., the inability to become aware of one's thought process or the wish not to become aware). This takes on added importance when we consider Loewald's (1971) suggestion that part of the curative process in psychoanalysis rests on experiences coming under the influence of higher-level ego functions which were previously not available to consciousness.

REFERENCES

Apfelbaum B: Some problems in contemporary ego psychology. J Am Psychoanal Assoc 10:526–537, 1962

Apfelbaum B, Gill MM: Ego analysis and the relativity of defense: technical implications of the structural theory. J Am Psychoanal Assoc 37:1071–1096, 1989

Arlow JA: The structural hypothesis: technical considerations. Psychoanal Q 44:509–525, 1975

Busch F: Recurring thoughts on unconscious ego resistances. J Am Psychoanal Assoc 40:1089–1115, 1992

Busch F: Some ambiguities in the method of free association and their implications for technique. J Am Psychoanal Assoc 42:363–384, 1994

---

[9]See Busch 1995a for an elaboration.

Busch F: Do actions speak louder than words? J Am Psychoanal Assoc 43:61–82, 1995a

Busch F: Neglected classics: M.N. Searl's "Some Queries on Principles of Technique." Psychoanal Q 64:306–325, 1995b

Busch F: The ego and its significance in analytic interventions. J Am Psychoanal Assoc 44:1073–1099, 1996

Busch F: Understanding the patient's use of the method of free association: an ego psychological approach. J Am Psychoanal Assoc 45:407–424, 1997

Busch F: Rethinking Clinical Technique. Northvale, NJ, Jason Aronson, 1999

Busch F: Are we losing our mind? J Am Psychoanal Assoc 49:739–751, 2001

Busch F: Telling stories. J Am Psychoanal Assoc 51:25–42, 2003

Busch F: A missing link in psychoanalytic technique: psychoanalytic consciousness. Int J Psychoanal 85:567–571, 575–578, 2004

Busch F: Conflict theory/trauma theory. Psychoanal Q 74:27–46, 2005

Calef V: An introspective on training and nontraining analysis. Annu Psychoanal 10:93–114, 1982

Davison WT, Bristol C, Pray M: Turning aggression on the self: a study of psychoanalytic process. Psychoanal Q 55:273–295, 1986

Eissler KR: Medical Orthodoxy and the Future of Psychoanalysis. New York, International Universities Press, 1965

Emde RN: Development terminable and interminable, II: recent psychoanalytic theory and therapeutic considerations. Int J Psychoanal 69:283–296, 1988

Erikson EH: Identity and the Life Cycle (1959). New York, WW Norton, 1963

Fenichel O: Problems of psychoanalytic technique. Psychoanal Q, 1941

Flavell JH: The Developmental Psychology of Jean Piaget. Princeton, NJ, Van Nostrand, 1963

Freud A: The Ego and the Mechanisms of Defense (1936), in Writings, Vol 2. New York, International Universities Press, 1966, pp 1–176

Freud S: Studies on hysteria (1895), in The Standard Edition of the Complete Psychological Works of Sigmund Freud [SE], Vol 2. Translated and edited by Strachey J. London, Hogarth Press, 1955, pp 1–319

Freud S: "Wild" psycho-analysis (1910). SE, 11:219–227, 1957

Freud S: The dynamics of the transference (1912). SE, 12:97–108, 1958

Freud S: On beginning the treatment (further recommendations on the technique of psycho-analysis I) (1913). SE, 12:121–144, 1958

Freud S: Remembering, repeating, and working through (1914). SE, 12:145–156, 1958

Freud S: Introductory lectures on psycho-analysis (1916–1917). SE, 15,16, 1961, 1963

Freud S: The ego and the id (1923). SE, 19:3–6, 1961

Freud S: Inhibitions, symptoms, and anxiety (1926). SE, 20:77–175, 1959

Gill MM: Psychoanalysis and exploratory psychotherapy. J Am Psychoanal Assoc 2:771–797, 1954

Gray P: Psychoanalytic technique and the ego's capacity for viewing intrapsychic conflict. J Am Psychoanal Assoc 21:474–494, 1973

Gray P: "Developmental lag" in the evolution of technique for psycho-analysis of neurotic conflict. J Am Psychoanal Assoc 30:621–655, 1982

Gray P: On helping analysands observe intrapsychic activity, in Psycho-analysis: The Science of Mental Conflict. Essays in Honor of Charles Brenner. Edited by Richards AD, Willick MS. Hillsdale, NJ, Analytic Press, 1986, pp 245–262

Gray P: On the technique of analysis of the superego—an introduction. Psychoanal Q 56:130–154, 1987

Gray P: A conversation with Paul Gray. Am Psychoanal 24:10–11, 1990a

Gray P: The nature of therapeutic action in psychoanalysis. J Am Psychoanal Assoc 38:1083–1097, 1990b

Greenson RR: The Technique and Practice of Psychoanalysis. New York, International Universities Press, 1967

Hartmann H: Ego Psychology and the Problem of Adaptation (1939). New York, International Universities Press, 1958

Hartmann H: Psychoanalysis and Moral Values. New York, International Universities Press, 1960

Hartmann H: Essays on Ego Psychology. New York, International Universities Press, 1964

Herzog P: Conscious and Unconscious. Psychological Issues, Monogr. 58. New York, International Universities Press, 1991

Joseph ED: Clinical formulations and research. Psychoanal Q 44:526–533, 1975

Joseph ED: The consciousness of being conscious. J Am Psychoanal Assoc 35:5–22, 1987

Klein GS: Psychoanalytic Theory: An Exploration of Essentials. New York, International Universities Press, 1976

Kris AO: Free Association: Method and Process. New Haven, CT, Yale University Press, 1982

Kris AO: The analyst's conceptual freedom in the method of free association. Int J Psychoanal 64:407–411, 1983

Kris AO: Helping patients by analyzing self-criticism. J Am Psychoanal Assoc 38:605–636, 1990

Kris E: Ego psychology and interpretation in psychoanalytic therapy. Psychoanal Q 20:15–30, 1951

Lear J: Love and Its Place in Nature. New York, Farrar, Straus & Giroux, 1990

Levy ST, Inderbitzin CB: The analytic surface and the theory of technique. J Am Psychoanal Assoc 38:371–392, 1990

Loewald HW: On the therapeutic action of psychoanalysis. Int J Psychoanal 41:16–35, 1960

Loewald HW: Some considerations on repetition and repetition compulsion. Int J Psychoanal 52:59–66, 1971

Loewenstein RM: Ego autonomy and psychoanalytic technique. Psychoanal Q 41:1–22, 1972

Mahler MS, Pine F, Bergman A: The Psychological Birth of the Human Infant. New York, Basic Books, 1975

Myerson PG: Awareness and stress: post-psychoanalytic utilization of insight. Int J Psychoanal 41:147–155, 1960

Myerson PG: The nature of transactions that enhance the progressive phase of a psychoanalysis. Int J Psychoanal 62:91–105, 1981

Paniagua C: A methodological approach to surface material. Int Rev Psychoanal 12:311–325, 1985

Paniagua C: The attraction of topographic technique. Int J Psychoanal 82:671–684, 2001

Reich W: Character Analysis (1933). New York, Farrar, Straus & Cudahy, 1949

Schafer R: An overview of Heinz Hartmann's contributions to psychoanalysis. Int J Psychoanal 51:425–446, 1970

Schafer R: The Analytic Attitude. New York, Basic Books, 1983

Schlessinger N, Robbins FP: A Developmental View of the Psychoanalytic Process: Followup Studies and Their Consequences. New York, International Universities Press, 1983

Searl MN: Some queries on principles of technique. Int J Psychoanal 17:471–493, 1936

Shaw RR: Hartmann on adaptation: an incomparable or incomprehensible legacy. Psychoanal Q 58:592–611, 1989

Smith JH: Dualism revisited: Schafer, Hartmann, and Freud. Psychoanalytic Inquiry 6:543–574, 1986

Spitz RA: Hospitalism: an inquiry into the genesis of psychiatric conditions in early childhood. Psychoanal Study Child 1:53–74, 1945

Stern DN: The Interpersonal World of the Infant. New York, Basic Books, 1985

Sugarman A: A new model for conceptualizing insightfulness in the psychoanalysis of young children. Psychoanal Q 72:325–356, 2003

Weinshel EM: Some observations on the psychoanalytic process. Psychoanal Q 53:63–92, 1984

White RW: Ego and Reality in Psychoanalytic Theory. Psychol Issues, Monogr 11. New York, International Universities Press, 1963

Wyman HM: Hartmann, health, and homosexuality: some clinical aspects of "Ego Psychology and the Problem of Adaptation." Psychoanal Q 58:612–639, 1989

4

NANCY J. CHODOROW, PH.D.

INTRODUCTION

Nancy J. Chodorow received her A.B. in social relations/social anthropology from Radcliffe-Harvard in Cambridge, Massachusetts, her Ph.D. in sociology from Brandeis University in Waltham, Massachusetts, and her psychoanalytic training at the San Francisco Psychoanalytic Institute. She is Professor Emerita of Sociology and was Clinical Faculty in Psychology at the University of California, Berkeley. She is in private practice in Boston, Massachusetts, where she is a faculty member of the Psychoanalytic Institute of New England, East, Boston Psychoanalytic Institute, and Massachusetts Institute of Psychoanalysis, and Visiting Professor of Psychiatry at Harvard Medical School.

In addition to being the author of more than 50 published papers, Chodorow has authored four books: *The Power of Feelings: Personal Meaning in Psychoanalysis, Gender, and Culture; Femininities, Masculinities, Sexualities: Freud and Beyond; Feminism and Psychoanalytic Theory;* and *The Reproduction of Mothering.* She has lectured throughout the world. She currently serves as Book Review Editor for North America of *The International Journal of Psychoanalysis* and Associate Editor of *Studies in Gender and Sexuality.*

Chodorow's honors include the Liebert Lecture of the Columbia Psychoanalytic Society, the L. Bryce Boyer Prize of the Society for Psychoanalytic Anthropology, an Award for Distinguished Contribution to Women and Psychoanalysis from the Division 39 Section on Gender, and the Robert Stoller Memorial Lecture. She has been a Fellow of the

Radcliffe Institute for Advanced Study, the Guggenheim Foundation, the American Council of Learned Societies, the National Endowment for the Humanities, and the Center for Advanced Study in the Behavioral Sciences.

Dr. Chodorow has said of herself:

> I have been contributing to psychoanalytic thinking since 1974, 10 years before I began psychoanalytic training.[1] In the broadest sense, I have always questioned the obvious—women's mothering role, gender difference and gender inequality, normative masculinity, the heterosexual norm—leading readers and colleagues to think in new ways about the familiar. My capacities and desires in this realm stem partly from innate turn of mind, partly from personal identity as somewhat of an outsider, and partly from disciplinary training, where I have called several fields my own, including anthropology, sociology, psychoanalysis, and women's studies (which my work helped to establish). Within these fields, sociological ethnomethodology and clinical listening particularly lead one always to ask, What came before? What is not said? What is taken as not needing explanation here? My strengths as a writer are theoretical, while my clinical work seems to be conducted in an intuitive, emotionally immersed sphere. Thus although my writings often include brief case vignettes, and my conclusions emerge from my clinical work, I tend to argue more from analytic and epistemological principle than from detailed clinical process.
>
> My specific influence in psychoanalysis began with *The Reproduction of Mothering*. Here, I as a nonanalyst joined a small number of analysts like Chasseguet-Smirgel, Kestenberg, and Stoller who had dared, after a long hiatus, to challenge Freud on gender, and a smaller number of feminists who wanted to take psychoanalysis seriously. Because it was an overarching theory of the psychologies of women and men, addressing phenomena that many clinicians as well as academic readers found persuasive—the intrapsychic mother-daughter relationship in the female psyche, the development of maternality—the book became widely noticed and drawn upon by analysts. While relying on classical gender writings, I also put forth an object relations theory based in Fairbairn, Balint, and Winnicott that came to influence the development of American relational psychoanalysis. Thus my position within psychoanalysis began as that of a gender theorist and of a theoretically eclectic, nonmainstream psychoanalyst.
>
> With training and clinical experience, my position shifted. In the early 1980s I turned my attention to the role and impact of early women psychoanalysts, foreshadowing a virtual biographical industry of the next 20 years, and I published a collection, *Feminism and Psychoanalytic Theory*, which included widely cited articles on fantasies of maternal

[1]For further discussion of my role and history, see Chodorow 2004b.

perfection, separation and differentiation as relational processes, and the gender consciousness of early women psychoanalysts. In 1994, *Femininities, Masculinities, Sexualities: Freud and Beyond* developed themes of clinical individuality and theoretical syncretism that have been central to my work over the last 10 years. I have subsequently taken this theme beyond sexuality and gender to argue for theoretical multiplicity and for "listening to" our patients rather than "listening for" instantiations of theory (Chodorow 2003a).

Since the publication of *The Power of Feelings: Personal Meaning in Psychoanalysis, Gender, and Culture*, my contribution has extended to include general theory and clinical epistemology. Arguing for the live activity of transference in the consulting room and in everyday life, the book draws its voice and emotional commitment especially from Loewald, who (along with Klein, Winnicott, and of course Freud) forms its theoretical core. Insisting on the inextricable intrapsychic intertwining of psyche and culture, the book is influenced by Erikson. Thus through clinical experience and these theoretical commitments, I have moved toward a primarily North American psychoanalytic identity, as I consider myself part of the Loewaldian intersubjective ego psychological tradition (see also Chodorow 2003c and 2004c).

A second role I have played within psychoanalysis is in bridging (or trying to bridge) the gap between psychoanalysis and the university and representing each venue and approach to the other. This role has taken multiple forms. First, all of my psychoanalytic writings have been widely read and influential across a number of academic fields. Then, for 30 years at the University of California I taught graduate and undergraduate courses on psychoanalytic theory, psyche and culture, listening for affect and transference in social science interviews, and psychoanalysis and feminism. I worked with graduate students, especially helping those who wanted, against the grain, to incorporate psychoanalysis in sociology and clinical psychology dissertations and bringing clinical thinking and theory beyond Freud to students in the humanities. I sponsored several Fellows of the American Psychoanalytic Association. As a professor at the public University of California, I, along with a few other Committee on Research and Special Training (CORST) colleagues across the U.C. campuses, have probably introduced psychoanalytic thinking to more students from varied ethnic, racial, and immigrant backgrounds than all other analysts combined. I was also a cofounder of the University of California Interdisciplinary Psychoanalytic Consortium.

I have written and spoken on both sides of the divide concerning the mutual ignoring and distrust between psychoanalysis and the social sciences. One goal of *The Power of Feelings* was to argue that social science, postmodernist-poststructuralist, and feminist colleagues need to look beyond sociocultural, political, and discursive determinism to the uniqueness of the individual and to the importance of studying individuality in all its multifaceted interest and importance (see also Chodorow 2004c). At the same time, I have called for analytic colleagues to extend their transclinical interests beyond the humanities, high culture, and the medical and neurosciences toward the social sciences, whose interests and methods, as Freud also points out, make them close cognate disciplines to psychoanalysis (Chodorow 2004d).

WHY I CHOSE THIS PAPER

Nancy J. Chodorow, Ph.D.

Among my published papers, "Heterosexuality as a Compromise Formation," which also appeared as a chapter in *Femininities, Masculinities, Sexualities*, is certainly my most influential, widely cited work. In it, I argue that all sexualities are complex compromise formations and that we cannot automatically distinguish heterosexuality and homosexuality on grounds of pathology. In addition to first enunciating ideas developed in subsequent work, the paper led to further opportunities to observe and critique psychoanalytic thinking about sexuality, including contributing a new foreword to Freud's *Three Essays on the Theory of Sexuality* (Chodorow 2000).

"Heterosexuality as a Compromise Formation" marks a turning point. My first paper written *exclusively* for analysts, it represents a response to my own psychoanalytic training, to clinical and theoretical presentations I had heard at professional meetings, and to the psychoanalytic literature. My writings until then had been directed toward both academic colleagues and psychoanalysts. Now several factors converged. I was inspired by students who had written deeply and intelligently about sexuality. I reacted to the ease with which analysts at the time referred to homosexuality as a disorder and to the fact that my training included one course on the perversions and nothing on ordinary sexuality. I was trying to make sense of the fluctuating sexual transferences and identities (and countertransferences and counteridentities, although these were not so willingly attended to in the 1980s as today) in my clinical work and thinking also, as a sometime feminist sociologist of everyday life, about the sexuality of myself and others. All this led me to wonder: How do we understand (what I at the time characterized ironically as) "garden-variety heterosexuality"? It is historically worth noting, given the paper's broad influence, that the two leading journals to which I first submitted it for publication rejected it on the grounds that it was neither new nor psychoanalytic.

This paper represents my most characteristic form of thinking and the dominant form of my contribution to psychoanalytic thought. Beginning with *The Reproduction of Mothering,* I have tended to start from long-standing, taken-for-granted theoretical or pretheoretical assumptions (there, the universality of women's mothering; here, the taken-for-grantedness of heterosexuality) and to unpack the implications, contradictions, and limitations within these. "Heterosexuality as a Compromise Formation" contains my first claim for all genders and sexualities as compromise formations and for what I later call "clinical individuality" in psychologies of gender. It points toward the multiple constitutive components—developmental, bodily, fantasy, object-relational, cultural—of sexuality and implies that individualized and relational developmental understandings of sexuality and gender serve us better than overgeneralized, universalized, and unreflective culturally normative claims (Chodorow 1996, 1999, 2003b, 2004a).

REFERENCES

Chodorow NJ: Theoretical gender and clinical gender: epistemological reflections on the psychology of women. J Am Psychoanal Assoc 44 (suppl: Female Psychology):215–238, 1996

Chodorow NJ: The Power of Feelings: Personal Meaning in Psychoanalysis, Culture, and Gender. New Haven, CT, Yale University Press, 1999

Chodorow NJ: Foreword to Freud's Three Essays on the Theory of Sexuality. New York, Basic Books, 2000, pp vii–xviii

Chodorow NJ: From behind the couch: uncertainty and indeterminacy in psychoanalytic theory and practice. Common Knowledge 9:463–487, 2003a

Chodorow NJ: [Homosexualities as compromise formations: theoretical and clinical complexity in portraying and understanding homosexualities] (French). Revue Française de Psychanalyse 1:41–64, 2003b

Chodorow NJ: The psychoanalytic vision of Hans Loewald. Int J Psychoanal 84:897–913, 2003c

Chodorow NJ: Beyond sexual difference: clinical individuality and same-sex cross-generation relations in the creation of feminine and masculine, in Dialogues on Sexuality, Gender, and Psychoanalysis. Edited by Matthis I. London, Karnac, 2004a, pp 181–203

Chodorow NJ: Psychoanalysis and women: a personal thirty-five-year retrospect, in The Annals of Psychoanalysis XXXII: Psychoanalysis and Women, 2004b, pp 101–129

Chodorow NJ: The American independent tradition: Loewald, Erikson, and the (possible) rise of intersubjective ego psychology. Psychoanalytic Dialogues 14:207–232, 2004c

Chodorow NJ: The question of a *Weltanschauung*: ethnographic observations 70 years later. Unpublished Liebert Lecture, Columbia Psychoanalytic Society and Association for Psychoanalytic Medicine, 2004d

HETEROSEXUALITY AS A COMPROMISE FORMATION

Reflections on the Psychoanalytic Theory of Sexual Development

NANCY J. CHODOROW, PH.D.

THIS PAPER UNPACKS WHAT seem to be psychoanalytic assumptions that take as given a psychosexuality of normal heterosexual development, in which deviation from this norm needs explanation or accounting for but norm-following does not.[1] I make two intertwined arguments. First, because heterosexuality is assumed, its origin and vicissitudes are not described: psychoanalysis does not have a developmental account of what we think of as "normal" heterosexuality (which is, of course, a wide variety of heterosexualities) that compares in richness and specificity to accounts we have of the development of the various homosexualities and what are called perversions.[2] Psychoanalytic writers have

[1]I am very grateful to Janet Adelman and Arlie Hochschild for long discussions about this paper. I thank Adrienne Applegarth, Steven Epstein, Ethel Person, and the Seminar for Semi-Baked Ideas for comments and suggestions, and Karin Martin for valuable research assistance.

"Heterosexuality as a Compromise Formation: Reflections on the Psychoanalytic Theory of Sexual Development," by Nancy J. Chodorow, Ph.D., was first published in *Psychoanalysis and Contemporary Thought*, 15:267–304, 1992.

not paid the kind of attention to heterosexuality that they have to these latter identities and practices. After Freud, most of what one can tease out about the psychoanalytic theory of "normal" heterosexuality comes by reading between the lines of writing about perversion and homosexuality.[3]

Second, insofar as we have a developmental or clinical account of heterosexuality, either it seems to be relatively empty and general, or it implies that heterosexuality is not different in kind from whatever we want to say homosexuality, perversion, or *any* sexual outcome or practice is; that is, a compromise formation, a symptom, a defense, a neurosis, a disorder, a meshing of self development, narcissistic restitutions, object relations, unconscious fantasy, and drive derivatives, and so forth. Thus, within psychoanalytic theory, it is difficult to find persuasive grounds for distinguishing heterosexuality from homosexuality according to criteria of "health," "maturity," "neurosis," "symptom" or any other evaluative terms, or "normal versus abnormal" in other than the statistical or normative sense. At most, we may be able to distinguish according to these terms perverse from nonperverse within the categories of both homosexuality and heterosexuality.

Two preliminaries must preface my discussion. First, I will of necessity skirt a problem of connotation in the literature: when we refer to homosexuality, homosexuals, homosexual object choice, or a variety of

---

[2]Terminological problems are unavoidable in an account of this kind. By "normal" or "ordinary" heterosexuality, I have in mind a socially and culturally taken-for-granted assumption. Within psychoanalysis, normal heterosexuality is represented by Freud's (1924, 1925, 1931, 1933), descriptions of the path to normal femininity in girls and the positive oedipal resolution in boys. We can also define it negatively, as that which tends not to come to psychoanalytic attention as requiring especial notice, as has been the case with homosexuality and the perversions. To say "normal" is not to imply that there is no variety nor that such sexuality might not be intensely meaningful to participants.

[3]This paper is not a review of the literature, but as a quick check on these claims, Karin Martin surveyed eight major psychoanalytic journals for the past 10 years, finding only a couple of articles on love, and a few that address heterosexuality tangentially (Hershey [1989] in particular stands out in taking heterosexuality as problematic). Her conclusion after performing this survey (personal communication): "It struck me that it is not just normal heterosexuality that is neglected by psychoanalysis but more specifically normal male heterosexuality. Female sexuality, heterosexual or not, has been continuously understood as problematic if not deviant by psychoanalysis, and there are accounts of how and why it is so problematic."

perversions, we seem to be referring specifically to sexuality, sexual object choice, lust, erotization, or desire, and in the case of homosexuals and lesbians to someone with a conscious sexual identity.[4] By contrast, when we look for accounts of the development of experience of normal heterosexuality (e.g., Person [1988], or until recently Kernberg [1976a, 1976b, 1980]; in an earlier period, M. Balint [1936, 1947]), it seems that something more than, or "larger than," sex is meant: we are in the realm of "falling in love," "mature love," "romantic passion," "true object love," or "genital love." It is as though heterosexuality is more than a matter of erotic or orgasmic satisfaction, whereas other sexualities are not.[5]

Second, I will indicate but not be able to address satisfactorily the relations between sexuality and gender. Given what we know about men and women, their sexuality and its development, there is some question whether we can talk generically of either homosexuality or heterosexuality. This has been a major issue in nonpsychoanalytic writings on sexuality and in contemporary sexual politics, and most psychoanalytic writing as well tends to differentiate male homosexuals from lesbians, to focus in writing about homosexuality on either men or women.[6] Similar considerations would also seem to apply in the heterosexual case: a woman's choice of a male sexual object or lover is so different developmentally, experientially, dynamically, and in its meaning for her womanliness or femininity, than a man's choice of a female sexual object or lover, that it is not at all clear that we should conceptualize these by the

---

[4]A large contemporary historical and theoretical literature documents persuasively the relatively recent construction of notions of sexual identity or of sexuality. Formerly, Western culture conceptualized sexuality in terms of individual prescribed and proscribed acts: the terms and conceptions of *homosexual* and *heterosexual* as unitary stances, kinds of persons, or object choices were unknown (Foucault 1978; Katz 1983, 1990; Stein 1989; Weeks 1986).

[5]This love may *include* sexual pleasures and meanings but it goes beyond them (Balint 1936, 1956; Kernberg 1976a, 1976b, 1980, 1988, 1991).

[6]Katz (1990, pp. 10–14) provides useful historical insight into this problem, pointing out that the first medical writer to use the term *homosexual* referred exclusively to gender conceptions ("persons whose 'general mental state is that of the opposite sex'"). He also suggests that the turn-of-the-century term, *invert,* allows gender-crossing, deviation from True Womanhood and True Manhood, to stand for homoerotic desire. It is only recently that some psychoanalysts have moved beyond seeing gender identity and personality, as Freud did, exclusively as an issue of sexual orientation and mode (Chodorow 1989a).

same term. We can do so behaviorally and definitionally—a hetero-object is other than or different from the self, whereas a homo-object is like the self, but we may thereby confuse our psychological understanding.[7]

In what follows, I try to consider specific theorists, but I also indicate what I believe to be sometimes unelaborated paradigmatic accounts and assumptions. I do not wish to universalize; I am pointing to trends in thinking that I think bear reflection on our part. I point to the need for more explicit attention to the development of heterosexuality in both men and women (as well as to the need for more explicit attention to the development of love and passion in homosexuals).

BIOEVOLUTIONARY ASSUMPTIONS ABOUT HETEROSEXUALITY

A variety of biological assumptions or understandings, I believe, underlie the striking lack of interest in detailed investigation of the developmental genesis of heterosexuality. The simplest version here, what many psychoanalysts probably think, assumes that heterosexuality is innate or natural—how humans "naturally" develop as we follow our evolutionary heritage and that of other animal species, especially our primate ancestors. Such a position seems obvious and not in need of defense or argument.[8]

There are a number of problems with this kind of psychoanalytic account.[9] First, on the level of logical consistency, it implies that we need an explanation for the development of homosexuality or perversion in the individual but that heterosexuality needs no explanation.

Second, a more complex empirical problem with the claim that peo-

---

[7]Lewes (1988, p. 232) argues that modern psychoanalysis uncharacteristically defines homosexuality in terms of its characteristic behavior rather than its dynamics or phenomenology.

[8]For example, "The problem of the social and psychological reproduction of heterosexuality for the propagation of the species comes after that...for reasons of heterosexuality, all societies have made some, however, different, distinction between the sexes which has, so far, been universal and necessary" (Mitchell 1989).

[9]Stoller (1985), discussing problems with the assumption of a biologically "natural" heterosexuality, asks," Are there really psychoanalysts who believe that human psychic development proceeds 'naturally' with preprogrammed facility?" (p. 101).

ple are biologically programmed to be heterosexual is that normal heterosexuality, like any sexual desire, is always more specified in its object. If it were not, *any* man would suit a heterosexual woman's sexual or relational object need, and the reverse for men. In fact, however, there is great cultural and individual psychological specificity to sexual object choice, erotic attraction, and fantasy. Any *particular* heterosexual man or woman chooses particular objects of desire, or types of object, and in each case we need to give, probably, a cultural and individual developmental story to account for these choices.

By cultural story, I have in mind the fairy tales, myths, tales of love, loss, and betrayal, movies and books that members of a culture grow up with and thus share with others. Since fantasy must be constituted at least partially through language, we are not surprised to find that sexual fantasy has partial resonance with these stories; as they are individually appropriated, we might liken them to what Kris (1956) has called a "personal myth." As we would expect from this cultural component, notions of sexual attraction and attractiveness vary historically and cross-culturally. In our culture, these stories are almost exclusively heterosexual (Greek myths and tales of male friendship are a notable exception here, and, of course, homosexual love was sanctioned in classic Greek culture, while it has been largely proscribed in ours). In a sense, it is easier to construct heterosexual fantasies, because the ingredients are nearer to hand.

Heterosexual fantasy and desire also always have an individual component, a private heterosexual erotism that contrasts with or specifies further the cultural norm. To take an everyday example, different ethnicities are likely to have different norms of attractiveness. People who grow up in these ethnicities, for both cultural and oedipal reasons, are likely to build such norms (directly or indirectly, positively or negatively) into their sexual orientation and object choice. Those called, or who consider themselves, heterosexual, are, in all likelihood, tall blond Wasposexual, short, curly-haired zaftig/Jewishosexual, African American with a Southern accentosexual, erotically excited only by members of their own ethnic group or by those outside that group. Some women find themselves repeatedly attracted to men who turn out to be depressed, others to men who are aggressive or violent, still others to narcissists. Some men are attracted to women who are chattery and flirtatious, others to those who are quiet and distant. Some choose lovers or spouses like a parent (and it can be either parent for either gender or a mixture of the two); others choose lovers or spouses as much unlike their parents as possible (often to find that these mates recapitulate parental characteristics or to find themselves discontented when they don't). These choices have both cultural and individual psychological resonance.

My point is that biology cannot explain the content either of cultural fantasy or private erotism. We need a story to account for the development of any particular person's particular heterosexuality, and it is very hard to know where to draw the line on what needs accounting for in anyone's sexual development or object choice. Any clinician knows this, but we tend for pre-theoretical reasons to assume that such variety is less important. We privilege the overarching division of sexual orientation that our culture has made primary since the nineteenth century.

A third lacuna, or contradiction, in the assumption of innate heterosexuality concerns that assumption's relation to our developmental theories: how do we reconcile a theory that heterosexual preference is innate with our observations and theory concerning the pansexuality of infants and children and their lack of focus on one zone or mode of gratification, or with our knowledge that virtually *everyone's* initial bodily erotic involvement is with their mother? We could argue that the mother-relation (nursing, body contact, and clinging) is not sexual, but this would be a high price to pay in terms of the psychoanalytic theory of sexuality and Freud's argument that sexuality is more than genital and reproductive. Moreover, the little evidence we have suggests that gender labeling typically overrides biology in determining sexual orientation, so that for most cases of "mislabeling" or hormonal abnormality, sexual orientation is heterosexual in complementary relation to the labeled gender (see on this the classic studies of Money and Ehrhardt [1972]).[10]

There is an alternative innatist position, a claim that seems to refer implicitly only to the case of male homosexuality, that most people are programmed to be heterosexual, but some are programmed to be homosexual (see Isay [1989], who takes this position but also claims [p. 21] that "the manner in which [this immutable from birth sexual orientation] is expressed appears to have multiple and diverse roots that may

---

[10]I cannot consider here the whole question of hormonal and genetic impact on gender-typed behavior, a topic that deserves many papers in itself. I am simply pointing out that people labeled as girls tend to desire males, and the reverse is true for people labeled as boys, in both cases regardless of chromosomal or hormonal makeup. The evidence at the same time supports biological influence in particular cases. For example, certain boyhood gender disorders may have an endocrinologic component and sometimes correlate with later homosexuality (see on this Friedman [1988]).

be profoundly influenced by a variety of early experience"; see also Friedman [1988], who thinks some aspects of homosexual object choice for some people are constitutional).[11]

This position raises similar problems to the claim for universally programmed heterosexuality. It does not allow specificity of object choice beyond homo- or heterosexual; it contradicts the gender labeling evidence; and it removes the question of sexuality from psychodynamic concern, since it implies that our developmental stories, transference recapitulations, and understandings about intrapsychic, object-relational, self, and defensive organization are not so important. Here too, everyone lives out their biological tendencies, most of us as heterosexuals.

As clinicians and developmental theorists, then, we are challenge: if everyone's programmed biology is heterosexual, and this goes awry for some who end up homosexual, then homosexuals have developmental stories, and heterosexuals do not. Biology, or evolutionary biology, explains how one kind of sexuality develops, but not others. Even if we want to retain a modified biological story, as in Freud's view that development is a "complemental series" of interactions between constitution and experience (much of modern biology extends this, insisting that experience always affects biological structure and function as much as the reverse), we must then conclude that the *kind* of complemental story of homosexual and heterosexual development will be the same. Since each account and each story will be developmentally and clinically specific, there will be no reason normatively to privilege heterosexuality.

A biological explanation of heterosexuality leads us to deny what

---

[11] Innatist theory is echoed by some nonpsychoanalytic gay theorists as well. These views, while probably a minority position, respond to how insistent, innate, and unchangeable sexual preference feels. By arguing that sexuality, or sexual object choice, is biological and insistent, gay theorists challenge claims that homosexuality can be changed (through choice or therapy), or that it is to be morally condemned. Such an argument implies that one's sexuality is given, what one is born with: it is outside the moral (and therapeutic) realm. Gay and lesbian writings diverge here. Against Rich's (1980) claim that all women would be naturally lesbian if it were not for "compulsory heterosexuality," psychologist Golden (1987) reports research demonstrating that some lesbians see themselves as "primary lesbians," those for whom lesbianism is not a choice but a felt desire and sense of "difference" from an early age. Others, however, see their lesbianism as "elective," consciously chosen for political or erotic reasons. (Golden does not address whether primary lesbianism is biological. What her subjects report is that it is early developed and feels immutable.)

we know clinically, experientially, culturally, and cross culturally, that sexual feelings are psychological, charged, and subjectively meaningful, and that their particularity can always be explained in terms of an individual's life history and cultural-linguistic location. In order to retain our biological assumptions, we lose our psychology. To retain a psychological approach, recognizing that biology and drives always get embroiled in conflict, fantasy, identity, narcissism, passionate object relating, reparation (the particular psychological theory here is irrelevant), we cannot rely on sexual dimorphism to explain heterosexuality.

FREUD AND HIS FOLLOWERS

I am aware that by this point many readers will, quite naturally, raise the objection that Freud's view was much more complex, that he never thought heterosexuality was biological. Freud believed that everyone was constitutionally bisexual and that sexual object choice always needed explaining. In the *Three Essays on the Theory of Sexuality* (Freud 1905) and in "The Psychogenesis of a Case of Homosexuality in a Woman" (Freud 1920), Freud protests that there are upstanding homosexuals and that homosexuality is simply one sexuality among many; in "Analysis Terminable and Interminable" (Freud 1937), he claims that bisexuality is biological and psychological bedrock. The theory of constitutional bisexuality and Freud's clinical cases indeed sustain the view that any sexuality is partly constructed through the repression of its opposite: heterosexual orientation includes repressed homosexuality and vice versa.[12] Freud thought that there were continuities between child and adult sexuality, between homosexuality and heterosexuality, between normal genitality and perversion.

But Freud also thought, probably for teleological reasons about species reproduction, the opposite, that heterosexuality is natural (on Freud's teleology, see Chodorow [1978]; Schafer [1974]). Yet his own theoretical and clinical accounts of the development of heterosexual ori-

[12]Connell (1987, p. 209) points to the systematic layering of masculinity and femininity in the personality, such that normally the surface personality that is compatible with social role is constructed by the repression of its opposite. I adapt his point here. I do not even begin to consider here the fact that there are many homosexualities and many heterosexualities, all of which include and repress each other.

entation in both males and females can be read only as accounts of compromise formations and defense: the boy's terror of castration, based on a fear of and disgust at the female genitals, leads him to give up his mother and fuels his final heterosexual object choice; it is a rare case history that does not recognize castration anxiety and conflict about women in a male patient. A girl's heterosexuality is also fueled by horror at her own genital mutilation, penis envy, and rage and hatred at her mother. Her erotic desire never seems to enter the picture, as she turns to her father not out of libidinal desire but out of narcissistic mortification and a wish to possess his penis as her own organ. When she finds out that she cannot have it, she still doesn't want him. She wants a baby that will substitute for the penis she cannot have.

There are many inconsistencies here, and Lewes's *The Psychoanalytic Theory of Male Homosexuality* (Lewes 1988) brilliantly deconstructs this classical theory, especially for boys. Lewes points out, for instance, that according to the theory, it is the mother who should be identified with rather than the father, since Freud has told us in "Mourning and Melancholia" that it is the lost *object* that casts a shadow on the ego. A proper response to fear, by contrast, is flight. If the boy identifies with his *father* in resolving his Oedipus complex, it can only be to the extent that the boy was homoerotic as well as heteroerotic, to the extent that his *father* was his love object as well as, or rather than, his mother. Lewes also points to Freud's confusion between behavior and psychology. On the level of psychological meaning, the boy's preoedipal love for his mother must be understood as narcissistic and homosexual: it is the phallic mother whom the phallic boy (as well as the phallic girl) loves.

Lewes makes clear that the origins of normal heterosexuality in the Oedipus complex are much more complicated than Freud and those that follow him thought. Indeed, he describes 12 different possible oedipal constellations for the boy, depending on whether his attachment is anaclitic or narcissistic, whether he takes himself, his father, or his mother as object, whether this mother is phallic or castrated, whether he identifies with father or (phallic or castrated) mother, and whether his own sexual stance is passive or active. Six of these are heterosexual, but only one—active, employing an anaclitic mode of object choice, based on identification with his father, and taking as object a castrated mother—is "normal." Lewes points to the problematic nature of his discovery for our ability to accord normality to a single sexuality:

> [T]he mechanisms of the Oedipus complex are really a series of psychic traumas, and all results of it are neurotic compromise formations…even optimal development is the result of a trauma, [so] the fact that a certain

> development results from a "stunting" or "blocking" or "inhibition" of another possibility does not distinguish it from other developments. So all results of the Oedipus complex are traumatic, and, for similar reasons, all are "normal"...the Oedipus complex operates by trauma and necessarily results in neurotic conditions. (pp. 82, 86).

Many psychoanalytic theorists, I believe, have more or less recognized, though they have not forcefully acknowledged, this problem. They do not offer final conclusions on the issue of normality and neurosis. Some, like Stoller (1975, 1979, 1985) and Person (1988), describe the "neurotic" core of passion or heterosexuality, or, like McDougall (1986), think that some handlings of the castration trauma, while traumatic, are normal and others not.

Another solution to the Freudian paradox seems to be more or less to bypass or minimize the castration complex and to see the development of heterosexuality in less dynamic, more interpersonal terms. In what is again a widely assumed though not necessarily explicitly described view that finds origin in Freud, the boy is thought to bounce from his natural preoedipal love for his mother, to oedipal love, to adult sexual desire for women. Complementarily, the girl's desire for autonomy from her mother meets with "mild seduction"—a sort of seduction that is not a seduction—by her father and she becomes heterosexual (Leonard 1966; Chasseguet-Smirgel 1976).

While I do not think that the castration complex is the nodal complex of sexual orientation and desire, its virtue as a theoretical center remains, as Lewes indicates, that it requires consistency in our accounts of all forms of sexual development. Insofar as Freud's story of the castration complex sees sexuality in developmental, dynamic, and conflictual terms, and recognizes that conscious and unconscious fantasy go into sexuality, it also accords with our clinical experience.

By contrast, the interpersonal alternative has tremendous problems. We find here a generality and lack of detail that contrasts with the extremely fine-tuned specificity and the richness of psychoanalytic accounts of homosexuality and the perversions (for example, Freud's [1905], Greenacre's [1968], Chasseguet-Smirgel's [1985], and others' descriptions of the primitive denials and splits in the ego that enable a man to deny sexual difference; Stoller's [1975, 1979, 1985] accounts of the transcending and reversal of humiliation that is at the core of all perversion; Stoller's [1975, 1979, 1985] and McDougall's [1986] descriptions of the driven compulsiveness in perversion; Stolorow and Lachman's [1980], and Socarides' [1978, 1979, 1988] accounts of self–other problems and gender identity confusion; McDougall's [1970], Stoller's [1975,

1979, 1985], and others' descriptions of extremely problematic maternal and paternal behavior and parental appropriation or punishment of the child's erotism, gender, and pleasure). Normal heterosexuals in this account look more or less alike; their sexuality does not seem experientially to attain great importance or meaning for them.

The interpersonal account, moreover, does not stand up to close examination. Psychoanalysts repeatedly document the defensiveness and fear of women and things feminine that characterize many of the most normal heterosexual men in our society (Kernberg [1976] reviews this literature, which begins with Horney [1932]; see also Slater [1968]). Male love and erotic desire for women are not so simple or straightforward. With the girl's story, we confront a different set of problems in the way that the account glosses over a rather problematic content. Culturally, we might ask, what is the "femininity" that a father should appreciate in his preschool-aged daughter? Where does it come from? Psychologically, we wonder, why does she engage in what we can only assume are demure, flirtatious, idealizing behaviors, and why does she have to engage in such behavior to win her father's attention? We know that such behavior is not biologically determined nor even prevalent transhistorically or cross-culturally; it is historically and culturally specific.

Reciprocally, why do fathers in our society, as many developmental psychology studies demonstrate, seem to need to reinforce and instill gender-typed behavior in their sons and daughters, whereas mothers do not (indeed, we take any sexualization of a mother's relationship toward her son to be problematic) (see on this point Maccoby and Jacklin [1974]; Johnson [1988])? What is appropriate paternal "seductiveness" and heterosexual behavior from father to young daughter, and what do we make of such a prescriptive model of father–daughter relations in the context of our growing awareness of the prevalence of incest, child sexual abuse, and sexual objectification of little girls in our society?

NORMALITY AND NEUROSIS IN MODERN PSYCHOANALYTIC ACCOUNTS

Since Freud, then, dominant psychoanalytic understandings have moved from some recognition of continuity and commonality among sexualities, and of the problematic nature of everyone's sexuality, to assumptions more in accord with a popular culture that treats only deviant sexualities as problematic. But those few modern psychoanalysts who do discuss heterosexuality, like Kernberg and Person, or the German psychoanalyst and ethnographer Morgenthaler (1988), as well as some, like McDougall and Stoller, who discuss perversion, point in the directions that I am suggesting. They all give us reason to conclude either that heterosexuality is, like homosexuality and perversion, a defensive structure or compromise formation, in some sense, "symptomatic" or a "disorder," or that it has symptomatic or defensive features. A few papers address the disorders or problematic features of "normal" sexuality (see Hershey [1989] and Person [1986], or, in an earlier era, A. Reich [1953]).[13] When we cannot reach such a conclusion, it is in regard to distinguishing elements in heterosexuality that seem to have a deus ex machina quality inconsistent with the rest of the account.

Like Freud, modern theorists tend toward what could be taken as a contradictory position, claiming or implying, that homosexuality is less healthy or normal but also indicating that it is not or need not be. M. Balint (1956), for example, argues for the unique primacy of heterosexual true object love and genitality, and he classes homosexuality as a perversion. At the same time, he claims: "anybody who has had any experience with homosexuals knows that, in them, we may find practically the whole scale of love and hatred that is exemplified in heterosexuality" and that "one quite often finds in homosexuals an object-love as rich and as diversified as among heterosexuals" (M. Balint 1956, pp. 136, 142).[14] Similarly, McDougall (1986) refers to "the different homosexualities, some of which do not qualify as neosexualities [McDougall's term for perversions]" (p. 256) and claims that "nondeviant sexuality may also display addictive and compulsive qualities" (p. 280).

Among analysts, Stoller has taken on the issue of normality and

---

[13]Wolfson (Panel 1987) cites Kirkpatrick, "Many assertions about homosexuals—hatred of the opposite sex, regression from oedipal disappointments, inability to tolerate the discovery of sexual differences—can be applied equally to many heterosexuals" (p. 169). We also find such accounts outside of the psychoanalytic mainstream: Contratto (1987) provides clinical examples and theory concerning problems in "normal" heterosexual love in women.

[14]Balint (1956) seems to classify homosexuality as a perversion because of what he takes to be "an atmosphere of overpretence and denial" that characterizes perversions more generally. According to Balint, homosexuals insist that their sexuality and its pleasures are far superior to that of heterosexuals. Their overemphasis is "in order to deny—what they all know—that without normal intercourse, there is no real contentment" (p. 142). Lewes points out that it seems to be heterosexuals, among psychoanalysts at least, who assert the superiority of their own sexuality, but in the case of Balint, I think such a critique may read contemporary discourse and politics into an earlier era.

neurosis most directly. In some sense putting "perversion" in the center of normal sexuality (Kernberg [1991] more recently takes a similar position), he argues that "the overall structure of erotic excitement... is similar in most everyone, [that] it is not [hostile] dynamics that differentiate perversions from the lesser perversions—those states that others call normal or normative behavior—but whether the erotic excitement brings one toward or away from sustained intimacy with another person" (Stoller 1985, pp. vii–viii). Stoller describes how his early work demonstrated that hatred, and the desire to humiliate the other and thereby to revenge oneself and triumph over childhood trauma, formed the basic fantasy script in perversion and pornography. He came subsequently to conclude that "what makes excitement out of boredom for most people is the introducing of hostility into the fantasy" (p. vii). For him, the differentiating criteria in perversion is the "desire to sin... to hurt, harm, be cruel to, degrade, *humiliate* someone" (Stoller 1985, p. 7). But this leads circularly back to the conclusion that there is a perverse element in all sexuality, since the desire to sin is itself the hostility that is at the core of sexual excitement for all people. Stoller indicates a continuum, as he does seem to want to differentiate what we might consider extremes of perversion and nonperversion without specifying exactly where the dividing line between perverse and nonperverse lies.

The extent of desire to harm allows us to begin to differentiate "perverse" from "nonperverse" sexuality, but not according to the gender of the object in relation to the self. In both heterosexuality and homosexuality, one could "search for the circumstances in which affection, tenderness, and other nonhostile components of love participate in, perhaps even dominate, the excitement" (Stoller 1985, p. vii). Echoing McDougall, Stoller claims that "it is better to talk of the homosexualities rather than of homosexuality... there are as many different homosexualities as there are heterosexualities" (p. 97).

Person, whose book is about love more than sex, takes a similar position. She writes:

> [L]ove between homosexuals—is experienced in exactly the same way as it is experienced between heterosexuals.... Homosexual love draws fire for much the same reason as adulterous love, it appears to be a threat to the social order. Homosexual love is disapproved of for its unconventionality, its threat to social role, and, perhaps, its threat to people's own security about their sexual identities. However, none of these fears ought to blind others to the experience of the participants themselves, which seems identical to the experience of heterosexuals in love. (Stoller 1988, p. 347)

The solution to this inconsistent and equivocal treatment would seem to be either to see both homosexuality and heterosexuality as symptomatic and perverse or neither. Stoller affirms, on the one hand, that "everyone is erotically aberrant and most people most of the time are at least a bit perverse"; on the other that "homosexuality, like heterosexuality, is a mix of desires, not a symptom, not a diagnosis" (Stoller 1985, pp. 9, 184). Person (referring implicitly to heterosexual love) claims, "The customary mental health prescription for love relies too much on psychic maturity, but maturity is hardly a guarantor of passion. Intensity is just as likely to come out of a good neurotic fit, perhaps with one person needing to be subordinate, the other dominant" (Stoller 1988, p. 339).

Of modern writers, Kernberg has most consistently addressed himself to normal heterosexuality. According to one possible reading, his writing seems to speak to any intense, passionate, sexual love. He describes a "continuum of character constellations" in the capacity to fall and remain in love, with the "capacity to integrate genitality with tenderness and a stable, mature object relation" at its apogee (Kernberg 1980, pp. 278–279). Definitions of mature love require not heterosexual object choice but instead a coming to terms with and sublimating both homosexual and heterosexual, preoedipal and oedipal, identifications (Kernberg 1976a). Kernberg claims:

> [S]exual passion is a basic experience of simultaneous forms of transcendence beyond the boundaries of the self. [It] reactivates and normally contains the entire sequence of emotional states which assure the individual of his own, his parents', the entire world of objects' "goodness" and the hope of fulfillment of love in the face of frustration, hostility, and normal ambivalence. (Kernberg 1980, p. 293)

He describes further "the couple's intuitive capacity to weave changing personal needs and experiences into the complex net of heterosexual and homosexual, loving and aggressive, aspects of the total relationship expressed in unconscious and conscious fantasies and their enactment in sexual relations" (Kernberg 1980, p. 297). Like Balint, Kernberg writes movingly of the transcendent potential of love:

> [T]he "coming alive" of inanimate objects—the background figures of human experience—illuminated by a love relation. This reaction to inanimate objects, as well as to nature and art, is intimately connected with the transcending aspect of a full love relation… the capacity to experience in depth the nonhuman environment, to appreciate nature and art, and to experience one's self within a historical and cultural continuum are intimately linked with the capacity for being in love… falling

> in love represents a developmental crisis powerfully favoring the deepening of these other potentials. (Kernberg 1976b, pp. 227–228)

Kernberg is careful to insist that heterosexuality itself does not necessarily accompany or result from psychological health; in fact, sexual *inhibition* is often a progressive *result* of reaching the triangular oedipal level of development, when genital prohibitions become meaningful. Those with borderline pathology may by contrast achieve enjoyment as a flight from orality, precisely because their pathology goes along with splitting and idealization:

> [T]he capacity for sexual intercourse and orgasm does not guarantee sexual maturity, or even necessarily represent a relatively higher level of psychosexual development.... Clinically one finds that the full capacity for orgasm in sexual intercourse is present both in severe narcissistic personalities and in mature people and that sexual inhibition is present both in the most severe type of narcissistic isolation and in relatively mild neuroses and character pathology. (Kernberg 1976b, p. 217)

At the same time as his characterization of mature love does not specify or seem to require a specific form of object choice, Kernberg assumes that mature love will be heterosexual. He does not say why such gender complementarity is necessary; he only asserts that it is.[15] He refers to "the capacity for tenderness and a stable, deep object relation with a person of the other sex," to a total object relation "including a complementary sexual identification," and to the fact that mature love requires "resolution of oedipal conflicts"—explicitly in the first two cases, implicitly in the third, privileging heterosexual object choice (Kernberg 1980, pp. 279, 278; Kernberg 1976a, p. 212).

GENDER, POWER, AND HETEROSEXUALITY

As my discussion of Kernberg implies, it is by tying the developmental story of heterosexuality to the psychology and culture of gender that accounts differentiate homosexuality and heterosexuality. One tendency here ties sexual object choice to gender identification, without explaining erotization; the second explains erotization, but makes sexual inequality and male dominance its necessary complement or prerequisites. In

[15]As I indicate below, he seems to be influenced here by French theorists like Chasseguet-Smirgel and McDougall.

both, accounts are formulated differently for the two cases. In the case of homosexuality (or perversion), the story is of what went wrong to produce the deviation; in the case of heterosexuality, it is a less explicit account of what needs to go right. As in Freud's original theories, then, gender identity and sexual orientation here are conflated, and biology has self-evident psychological meaning. For all these theorists, this aspect of the account shows little intrinsic relation to other aspects of its characterization of sexual object choice.

According to Kernberg, identification with the same sex parent is an oedipal task: "women ... are to cross the final boundary of an identification with the oedipal mother,... Men have to cross the final boundary of the identification with the oedipal father" (Kernberg 1980, p. 299). Kernberg is explicit about the relation between this "achievement" and normative social conformity, as he ties a "full sexual identify" or "normal sexual identity" (meaning gender identity and heterosexual object choice) to "reciprocal sexual roles and... full awareness of social and cultural values." He argues that a "stable sexual identity and a realistic awareness of the love object... includes social and cultural in addition to personal and sexual ideals" (Kernberg 1976b, pp. 200–221). Gender identity and identification thus build into heterosexual development.

Like Kernberg, Person has developed her account in the first instance without explicit normative claims. Love is characterized by a:

> leap out of objectivity and into subjectivity,... sharing in each other's subjective realities.... [Love] denies the barriers separating us, offering hope for a concordance of two souls... "emotional telepathy"... an emotion of extraordinary intensity.... The experience of love can make time stop... may confer a sense of inner rightness, peace, and richness; or it may be a mode of transforming the self,... a mode of transcendence,... a religion of two. (Person 1988, p. 14)

She has acknowledged that the longing for love usually crosses perceived difference—"otherwise the lover has essentially chosen a narcissistic love object and the enormous transcendent power of love is lost" (Person 1998, p. 286)—but she points out that humans can vary in ways other than in their biological sex (e.g., in age, background, culture, interests, abilities, character—we could add, in terms of many other aspects of appearance and physiology as well).[16]

At the same time, Person assumes heterosexual love and follows the dominant psychoanalytic model in accounting for its development.[17] Each person experiences "a developmental series of 'love dialogues'" (p. 93), beginning with idealization of the mother, following through a family romance to idealization of and identification with outsiders. In the "normal" course of development, the child consolidates her or his identification with the same gender parent, and this identification enables and fuels desire for the opposite sex. Gender identification here leads to opposite sex object choice, as a "complementary" relationship replaces an identificatory relationship. Adolescents, in transition, may desire the heterosexual love object of their best friend, because their identification, rather than sense of complementarity, shapes desire, but "[i]n the normal course of development,... the yearning that attaches to idealization is transformed from the wish *to be like* (or to replace) to the wish *to be with*... desire shifts toward complementariness" (Person 1988, p. 100).

There are two major problems with such accounts. First, one is left without a sense of the *motivation* for such shifts in identificatory choices. More important, the account does not tell us how *identification*—an ego choice which might well tell the developing child whom he or she *ought* to love in order to be like the identificatory object—relates to erotization. If appropriate sexual object choice comes from identification with the same-gender parent, it is almost an aspect of role-modeling. But erotization here seems to run counter to object choice, as attachment to the identificatory object, a homoerotic object, is foremost in the psyche: in the boy's case, love for the father and attachment to him leads the boy to take the mother or women as object.

French theory provides another perspective on the tie between gender and heterosexual development. This theory ties heterosexuality more to passion, conflict, and erotism that American identification theories, but it relates this heterosexuality not only to gender difference but also to sexual inequality and power, so that gender inequality and

---

[16]I cannot do justice to this complex topic here. Let me simply point out that if people indeed choose opposite gender partners because erotic passion, or love, thrives on difference, we should then be surprised by the extensive age, class, race, and religious endogamy still present in our society. We should also note that although homosexual object choice often crosses these other categories of difference—perhaps to enhance the excitement that comes from difference in a case of same-gender choice—accounts of problems in lesbian object choice point rather to similarity bordering on merging (Krieger 1983; Lindenbaum 1985).

[17]It seems appropriate to center an account of romantic passion in our culture on heterosexual passion, since that is the passion that most people experience or dream about, and what our cultural categories offer us. It is Person's normative development theory that I address here.

power difference become the sine qua non of heterosexual desire. Chasseguet-Smirgel (1985), for example, claims an identity between "the universe of differences" and "the genital universe" and considers that the pervert refuses the "(genital) universe of difference" (pp. 4, 6). Echoing Lacan, for whom genital difference is implicitly unequal, constituted as law exclusively by the father, she claims that the genital universe is also the "paternal universe [of] constraints of the law" and that the pervert wants to "dethrone God the Father" (p. 12). McDougall (1986) asserts that normal heterosexuality requires acknowledgment of the bipolarity of the sexes, of the primal scene, of castration, and of genital difference as the basis of sexual arousal: "The belief that the difference between the sexes plays no role in the arousal of sexual desire underlies every neosexual scenario" (p. 249). Like other writers, she recognizes the universal prevalence of bisexuality and a desire to possess the genital organs of both sexes, but such bisexuality must rest on recognition of a sexual difference privileging heterosexual phallocentrism: "the phallus, symbol of power, fertility, and life, must...come to represent, for both sexes, the image of narcissistic completion and sexual desire...should a symbolic phallic image be entirely missing, psychotic confusion about sexual relationships would ensue" (pp. 267–268). Thus, "neosexual inventions...attempt to short-circuit the multiple effects of castration anxiety" (p. 248). In implicit linguistic support for her asymmetrical view, McDougall refers to the relation of the [named] "father's penis" and the [unnamed] "mother's sexual organ" (p. 268). Thus, as with Lacan (1966, 1968, 1975), "inscription" in the gender system is the same thing as inscription in a (hetero)sexual subjectivity that privileges the phallus.

Kernberg, who at the same time warns analysts against identifying "with a traditional cultural outlook" toward sexual roles and inequality (Kernberg 1976b, p. 268), nonetheless follows French theory. According to him, a boy's oedipal complex can be impeded by a mother who has rebelled against the "'dominance' of the paternal penis and the 'paternal law' in general" (Kernberg 1980, p. 284), and a girl's progress toward heterosexuality can develop only as she accepts the inferiority of her own genitals and recognizes her mother's own conflicts about female genitals and genital functions. This acceptance and recognition propel her to turn to her father to get an affirmation of her female sexuality.

Person, a leading feminist analyst who is critical of male dominance in her other writings, nonetheless implies in *Dreams of Love* (Person 1988) an acceptance of an almost necessary inequality in heterosexual relations. She suggests that a power differential in love may be ineradicable, and that insofar as women long for love and men fear it, normal heterosexuality will tend to include female submission and male domination, or, more tentatively, that women will distort love in the direction of the former and men in the direction of the latter. Such a tendency originates in cultural imperatives, early object relations, and the asymmetric structures of the Oedipus complex, and it finds reflection in transference patterns, in which women eroticize relationships with men in authority and seek the shelter of power, and men split sex and dependency and need the safety of a power advantage. As a developmental outcome, "women are more at ease with the mutuality implicit in love, as well as the surrender, while men tend to interpret mutuality as dependency and defend against it by separating sex from love, or alternatively, by attempting to dominate the beloved" (Person 1988, p. 265).

Person here points to congruence with our society's dominant romantic fantasies, suggesting that culture both embeds itself in and grows out of defensive structures and intrapsychic patterns.[18] She also implies that these modes of relationship are themselves defensive structures, based on felt need and attempts at resolution of anxieties, fears, and conflicts.

The *asymmetry* in heterosexual desire, its intertwining with patterns of dominance and submission, begin to indicate its defensive features and symptomatic nature. Contratto (1987) and Benjamin (1988) provide its developmental story. Reformulating Chodorow (1978, 1979), Benjamin shows us how, developmentally, males develop a "false differentiation" from their mother, resting on denial of the mother's subjectivity and objectification of her. Objectification, and the difficulties faced by the boy who wants recognition and response from his mother, on whom he at the same time does not want to be dependent, twist into a need to dominate women, into the eroticization of domination in the normal case and into erotic violence in the abnormal.[19]

Contratto and Benjamin suggest that "woman's desire" (Benjamin's

---

[18]I am indebted to Connell (1987) for this double conceptualization. Connell points out that psychoanalytic sociologies and culture and personality studies have tended to see culture and society as in some sense *resultants* of prevalent psychological tendencies and conflicts. In the case of gender and sexuality, he suggests, the reverse is also true: "the power relations of the society become a constitutive principle of personality dynamics through being adopted as a personal project" (p. 215). Institutions, practices, cultural productions, and inegalitarian social relations inform and help to constitute masculinities and femininities and the forms of sexuality.

term) is formed through idealization, alienation and submission. According to Benjamin, difficulties in the girl's heterosexuality begin during the rapprochement subphase. Because this coincides with an early genital phase (Roiphe and Galenson 1981), classic rapprochement preoccupations with agency and independence become tied to sexuality. Mahler has noted that girls tend to respond during this phase with depressive affect and a sense of helplessness, and Benjamin argues against Roiphe and Galenson that this is not a direct response to the discovery of genital difference. Rather, their common gender with their mother does not allow girls to use their father (as boys do) to represent and mediate independence and separateness.

Fathers collude here: they prefer boy babies and develop a more intense bond with them.[20] As the boy resolves the rapprochement crisis, his father acts as a vehicle for separation and as a model of activity and desire: "In rapprochement, the little boy's 'love affair with the world' turns into a homoerotic love affair with the father, who *represents* the world" (Benjamin 1988, p. 106). For both boy and girl during the rapprochement phase and later, the father represents active desire, the mother a more desexualized regression. The girl (as McDougall also suggests) must represent her own desire by something that is not hers and not feminine. Her desire is alienated, because male sexuality and the male genitals, with their symbolic intertwining of agency and separation, represent excitement and erotism. Contratto suggests that such a pattern continues throughout childhood. She describes the working fathers of her patients, to all intents and purposes "good" fathers, who energetically returned to the household evenings and weekends, bringing treats, engaging in exciting adventures and interactions, who needed to be carefully catered to when short-tempered or preoccupied

---

[19]Johnson (1988) contrasts the girl's gendered oedipal change of object, from mother to father, with what is symbolically a generational change on the part of the boy—from passive, less powerful son in relation to mother, to active, more powerful man in relation to less powerful women.

[20]There is a large literature on father preference for boys, differential treatment of boys and girls, and greater concern than mothers with gender difference and gender-appropriate behavior. This differentiation is often normatively approved. I cannot cite this literature here, but adapt my points from Kerig (1989, pp. 23–27), who reviews it. I note also that in this part of my account I have had to look beyond the psychoanalytic mainstream for clinical and developmental treatments (like Contratto and Benjamin) that take sexual inequality and its sexual and relational sequelae to be problematic.

and who contrasted with taken-for-granted, everyday mothers. Such accounts accord with the traditional theory, in which female sexuality is not active or autonomous but passive in relation to the father and men.

Contratto and Benjamin suggest that such a solution undermines female sexuality. Women find it difficult to integrate agency and love and often accept whatever love they can get in exchange for identification with and love from a heterosexual lover. The unavailability of the father (less available to her than to his son, less available to her than a mother to her son) coupled with his specialness leads girls, in the normal case, to develop tendencies toward "ideal love" for their fathers that forms the basis of their heterosexuality. Such love pulls toward submission, one-sided accommodation, idealization, masochism, and the borrowing of subjectivity from the lover (on this see also A. Reich [1953]).

Identification with the same-sex parent, then, differs for the girl and the boy. For the girl, mother identification is likely to be with her mother's maternality rather than with her mother as an active sexual being. The mother is not seen psychologically or portrayed culturally as a sexual subject; she is there to serve the child's interests, and her sexual power is frightening and denied.[21] She is not exciting. Moreover, the mother may have made a similar bargain in her own development and may therefore experience her own sexuality as more passive and submissive. If the daughter identifies with her mother's sexuality in this situation, she identifies with submission and accommodation. By contrast, it is through ideal love for a father who makes himself available that a boy can come to his own heterosexual position (paradoxically pointing us to a link between homoerotic identification and heterosexual object choice). The boy's oedipal and preoedipal relations with his mother ensure that such sexuality will require objectification and power, that is, will undermine true object love.

In looking at these accounts of gender and heterosexuality, one has the sense that with the exception of Contratto and Benjamin, they are undermined by the taken for granted. How does identification with one sex parent lead to erotic desire for the other? How do we reconcile a complex and varied view of the multiplicity of sexualities and of the problematic nature of conceptions of normality and abnormality with a dichotomous, unreflected upon, traditional view of gender and gender role or an appeal to an undefined "masculinity" and "femininity"? As-

---

[21]This theme is found in psychoanalytic writings since Horney (1932); see also A. Balint (1939), Chasseguet-Smirgel (1976), and Chodorow (1978, 1989a).

sumptions about cultural normality, conformity, and biological function and cause are allowed to stand in a way that would rarely happen in regard to other features of psychic functioning or development.[22] A psychic wish, "need," or tendency to be dominant or submissive is not problematized, inherent inequality and hierarchy of role and valuation between two kinds of people and their genital constitution is taken for granted. Those who do not accept such inequality and hierarchy are seen as neurotic or perverse, engaged in special pleading or a refusal to accept nature. One's own psychology is taken as a model of normality and desirability.

Even the language of description of homosexual development often presumes heterosexual structures of attraction. Developing homosexual boys are "feminized," as if it is only by being feminine that someone could desire a male, and developing lesbians are "tomboys"—a homosexual woman must be masculine, since one has to be masculine to desire women. Even as the evidence of fantasy and behavior disentangles gender and sexuality, psychoanalytic theory often assumes it.[23]

HETEROSEXUALITY AND HOMOSEXUALITY: SEXUALITY AS A COMPROMISE FORMATION

I have suggested that we know, or conceptualize theoretically, much more about the homosexualities and perversions than we do about what we take for granted to be most people's sexuality, and that what we do know about this normal sexuality indicates that it is difficult to privilege it in evaluative psychological terms. On the "healthy," or "mature," end of the spectrum, we can conceptualize forms of homosexuality in which the quality of object-relationship (in terms of wholeness, respect for the other, and so forth) is equivalent to our conceptions of

---

[22]As a social scientist trained to assume the basic cultural and social constructedness of all gendered and sexual experience and categories, including the social and cultural construction of our understandings of biology, I have wondered at the ease with which psychoanalysts turn to "real" biological function and anatomy in the case of gender and sexuality. It has occurred to me that training has a role in this case as well, in addition to Freud's similar inclinations. Such functions and anatomy were first introduced in the medical context, whereas notions about conflict, psychic structure, unconscious mental functioning, and so forth are introduced only in the more exclusively psychoanalytic-psychodynamic context.

mature heterosexuality, and homosexuals who can fully differentiate their gender identity (unless this by definition includes heterosexual object choice) and have a firm and relatively unproblematic sense of gendered self (I use the word *relatively* here only to stress that no one's sense of gendered self is entirely unproblematic). On the more problematic end, we have accounts such as those of Hershey, Person, Contratto, Benjamin, McDougall, and others that demonstrate the inherent conflict, domination, and "perversion" in normal heterosexuality. Both of these perspectives converge in suggesting that normal heterosexuality has the same *kind* of dynamic and developmental ingredients as all sexuality.

Such a conclusion accords with our clinical experience, which demonstrates, whatever our cultural and biological assumptions might be, that the sexual stories and transference processes of heterosexuals are as complex and individualized as those of homosexuals. We give up a lot theoretically and methodologically if we do not hold such a position. Erotic feelings, conflicts, defenses, accounts of relationships with parents, attempts to sort out a self, accountings for what gives pleasure and why, or what is desired and what fantasied, and the developmental and transferential history of all these, are the bread and butter of clinical work. We find clinical stories that are wild and tame, people focused on

---

[23]I am grateful to Frann Michel for first pointing out this inconsistency to me, in an early version of her dissertation chapter "William Faulkner as a Lesbian Author" (Michel 1990).

Lewes (1988, pp. 236–238) points out that a pejorative psychoanalytic theory and discriminatory organizational practice have themselves prevented homosexuals from having the possibility, as practitioners, of contributing to the creation of a theory of their own functioning. Historically, women's entrance into the field was essential to allowing a view of women as different rather than inferior, as well as a view of a differentiated and complex femininity with both advantages and problems. Lewes links these two discourses, pointing out that the traditional psychoanalytic theory of homosexuality parallels the theory of female psychology: homosexuals identify with their mother, make narcissistic object choices, are convinced of their own castration, choose sexual objects in order to gain a penis, attempt to be loved instead of to love, and have flawed superegos and other ego deficits: the "gynecophobia" of the early theory of female development that was challenged especially by female analysts now characterizes the view of homosexuality. As analysts saw disturbed homosexuals who came for treatment, they concluded that all homosexuals were disturbed, whereas their treatment of neurotic heterosexuals did not lead to the presumption that heterosexuality was a disorder (Lewes 1988, pp. 231–239).

or obsessed with sexuality and those who are not (these latter are more likely to be "normal" heterosexuals, who culturally can take their sexuality for granted), but we *always* find a story. Clinically, there is no normal heterosexuality: any heterosexuality is a developmental *outcome* reflected in transference, whatever the admixture of biology or culture (and whether we define "culture" as gender identity, sexual rules, dominant cultural fantasies, or mother's and father's gender identifications) that may contribute to it. This developmental and transferential outcome results from fantasy, conflict, defenses, regressions, making and breaking relationships internally and externally, and trying to constitute a stable self and maintain self-esteem. Whatever our theoretical approach, whether classical, structural, object relational, Kleinian, or Kohutian, sexual development and orientation, fantasy and erotism, need explaining and describing in the individual clinical case.

We return to the two elements in my argument. First, we have been able to elicit in the literature some accounts of normal heterosexuality. However, compared to the luxuriant richness of clinical accounts, let alone general theories, of deviant sexualities of many sorts, we must be struck by the relative paucity of case studies and clinical observations, let alone by the underdevelopment of general theory, about "normal" heterosexuality. Second, in the sphere of transference and developmental understandings that emerge from the clinical situation, we cannot find a reason to differentiate out heterosexuality or to see homosexuality as more of a defense or compromise formation. Logically and experientially, insofar as we have a clinical or developmental account of heterosexuality, it is either relatively empty and uninteresting or it makes heterosexuality as an object of inquiry and understanding and as an experience into whatever we want to say any sexuality in general is.

A final objection to my argument could still be raised: Is there not a difference between a normal everyday defense or compromise formation and a disorder or symptom, since, as we know, all psychic products and processes involve defense and compromise formation? There probably is, and we can probably differentiate out what we might want to call "perversion" of the homosexual and heterosexual (and even autoerotic) variety from what we might want to call "normal" homosexuality and heterosexuality. At least, following Stoller, we can delineate the extremes.

Following out some lines of delineation demonstrates the limitations and difficulties with such a strategy. McDougall (1986) singles out the compulsive and addictive qualities of the neosexualities, as they fulfill multiple needs of a "complex psychic state in which anxiety, depression, inhibitions, and narcissistic perturbation all play a role" (p. 247).

Many accounts of perversion stress the driven intensity, the insistent, narrowly specific object choice and sexual aim, and the necessity to repeat. What follows from this view is that normal heterosexuality is less intense, more diffuse, and affectively flatter. Many heterosexuals would not agree with this view, nor does that which we learn from clinical experience, literature, or our own or our acquaintances' lives support it. What would we make, in this view, of the compelled lovers of literature, of Tristan and Isolde, of Romeo and Juliet, of Anna and Vronsky, of Heathcliff and Cathy, of Florentino Ariza in Garcia Marquez's (1988) *Love in the Time of Cholera*? As clinicians, we can easily demonstrate their "neurosis," their compulsive drivenness, narrowly specific object choice, and perversity (the main point of Garcia Marquez's book is that love is a disease, though in his case, a cholera). But this leaves us explaining the passion, intensity, addiction, and obsession of their desire in terms of perversion.

What is left after we factor out the "perverse" elements in these examples of obsessive, intense, erotic heterosexual passion seems, to be blunt, boring. We are left either implying that the subjectively important and intense parts of all sexual experience and fantasy are perverse or symptomatic, or recognizing that addiction and compulsion may be ingredients in all intense sexual experience and fantasy. If we take the former point of view, arguing that only the noncompulsive, nonaddictive parts of sex constitute normal heterosexuality and that the rest is "perversion," we still need individual, detailed complex accounts to explain the mix that is both intense and flat. The traditional psychoanalytic account that distinguishes "perverse" from "normal" sexuality does not do that. We will still be hard pressed to distinguish passionate homoerotic true object love (with whatever true object love should include, as indicated by Balint, Kernberg, Person, and others) and passionate heteroerotic true object love. Alternately, many accounts imply that distinctions about compulsion, addiction, narrowness of aim and object, intensity, and so forth do better in differentiating male sexuality in general, whether homosexual or heterosexual, from female sexuality in general. In this case, it is women, both heterosexual and lesbian, who find themselves on the noncompulsive, nondriven, nonintense (verging on sexless) end of the spectrum of sexual desire.

Similar considerations hold true, I believe, for the issue of humiliation. Stoller puts humiliation at the core of perversion and also at the core of sexual excitement in general. We might, at Stoller suggests, turn to the outcome of the sexual excitement—does it lead to sustained intimacy or not?—but this will not distinguish for us all homosexualities from heterosexuality, and it certainly differentiates among heterosexualities as well. (We might also wonder—at the risk of idealizing and desexualizing women—about the extent to which hostility and the desire to harm are more characteristic of the sexual fantasies and practices of men than of women, since "perversion" as well as actual and fantasied sexual violence, abuse, and rape, seem more widespread among men than among women (see on this Person [1986], p. 74).

A variety of other pathological, symptomatic elements like weak self–other differentiation, narcissistic object choice, severe reaction to narcissistic injury, conflictual or not firmly established gender identity, problematic body image, and borderline, narcissistic, or even psychotic ideation and character, are thought to distinguish homosexuality and perversion from heterosexuality (McDougall 1970; Socarides 1978, 1979, 1988; Stolorow and Lachman 1980). This focus on the early origins of deviant sexualities has enabled a pathologization of these sexualities, since, in psychoanalytic developmental theory, we have tended to correlate the degree of pathology in a trait with the earliness of its origins.[24] Such a focus may also have been fostered by greater access to a clinical population as well as by lack of scrutiny of the origins of apparently normal because behaviorally typical heterosexualities.

In any case, the problem here is, as Kernberg (1976a, 1980) points out, that heterosexual object choice and heterosexual behavior can characterize the most disturbed individual (indeed, he has more hope regarding love relations for what we think of as the more disturbed borderline personality than for the narcissist). Lewes, following Freud, further reminds us that homosexual object choice, or many homosexualities, are oedipal (thereby later developmental) products. There is no inherent incompatibility between postoedipal "true object love," concern for the wishes of the other, capacity for whole object relations, or an established gender identity (unless we *define* this gender identity as needing to include heterosexual object choice) and homosexual object choice, even if there are many homosexuals, like heterosexuals, who do not have these capacities.

Whether we take Freud's bifurcate model of the complete Oedipus complex or Lewes's twelvefold model, we have only a variety of ad hoc criteria for privileging one postoedipal outcome over the other or over 11 others. I have reviewed these above. They are, first, a presumed bio-

---

[24]This point is made by Steven Epstein (1991). Such an account also tends to locate the origins of the pathology in disturbances in the relation to the mother, since the father is traditionally not seen as important until the oedipal period.

logical normality; second, what we have seen to be the relatively weak criterion of identification with the right parent in the right way, in which case erotic desire and passion somehow emerge out of identification, or sexual orientation is simply role acceptance; third, acceptance of cultural values; fourth, acceptance of a pregiven reality that gender difference *means* sexual orientation; fifth, acceptance of pregiven valuation of the phallus as a sign of sexual difference and gender hierarchy, in which view there is one right outcome to castration anxiety and sexual desire must incorporate and reproduce sexual inequality (if one argues in this last case that such acceptance is ego-syntonic, one then confronts the argument for ego-syntonicity in various alternative sexualities). I have suggested problems with each of these five assumptions.

It seems, finally, and analytic writers occasionally imply as much, that there is a spectrum of qualities of object relatedness, erotization, compulsiveness, drivenness, castration anxiety or penis envy, imaging of gender, specificity versus broadness of object choice and sexual aim, denial or defense, character pathology or neurosis, conjoinings of fantasy and reparative goals, in those who make heterosexual and those who make homosexual object choices. Any evaluation according to criteria like compulsiveness, addictiveness, humiliation, or the presence or absence of a "true object relationship," will apply to both sexual orientations.

The second part of my argument simply noted the paucity of clinical accounts that focus on heterosexuality and of theory about heterosexuality. We cannot claim that homosexuality is more symptomatic than heterosexuality without better accounts of heterosexuality, and the accounts we have suggest that we will not find that it is. But I am also suggesting that we should investigate heterosexuality for its own sake. There are very good reasons, which have nothing to do with what is or is not normal, for translating our complex clinical understandings of individual cases toward a more general theory; for challenging our simple normative model of one modal boy and one modal girl who develop into "normal" heterosexuals; for assuming rather that we will find a wide variety of "normal" heterosexualities just as we know there are many homosexualities and many heterosexual perversions.

In response to occasional analytic reference to homosexuality as a symptom, I had previously titled this paper "Heterosexuality as a Symptom." I believe we must reserve judgment about the symptomatic nature of heterosexuality and the normality of some homosexualities; this paper argues that such differentiation, given our current clinical and developmental knowledge, is not possible. I also reserve judgment on final causes in any individual case: there may well be variations in how any person's sexual orientation, organization, fantasy, and practices result from biology, from cultural valuation and construction, from intrapsychic solutions to conflict, from family experience, and from gender identity.

Some people might want to make a moral or political argument in either direction, either that heterosexuality is morally superior or better for society (that some people must behave heterosexually some of the time for species reproduction is self-evident but does not explain the individual and cultural variety and specificity I allude to earlier), or that we must, for moral or political reasons, defend any sexuality. But I think we must be quite clear about the nature of this kind of argument. Psychoanalytic theory, as we have it, does not give us a basis for answering such moral and political questions.

Someone may eventually find grounds from a psychoanalytic point of view for evaluating the relative healthiness (symptom freedom, lack of pathology, secondary autonomy) of homosexuality and heterosexuality. I do not argue for a total relativism: as McDougall, Stoller, and others make clear, there are probably good grounds within the theory for making comparative evaluations among sexualities. But at this stage in our knowledge, these do not differentiate homosexuality and heterosexuality. Currently, when we make evaluative claims, we do so in the context of a normative cultural system that includes a set of biological assumptions, probably one in which normal sexuality means not only reifying gender and sexual difference but also sustaining gender inequality. If we retain passion and intensity for heterosexuality, we are in the arena of symptom, neurosis, and disorder; if we deperversionize heterosexuality, giving up its claim to intensity and passion, we make it less interesting to us and to its practitioners. This paper suggests that we treat all sexuality as problematic and to be accounted for. Psychoanalysts have nearly unique access to many people's sexual fantasies, identities, and practices. We should use this access to help us fully to understand sexuality in all its forms.

REFERENCES

Balint A: Love for the mother and mother-love (1939), in Primary Love and Psycho-Analytic Technique, by M. Balint. New York, Liveright, 1965, pp 91–108

Balint M: Eros and Aphrodite (1936), in Primary Love and Psycho-Analytic Technique. New York, Liveright, 1965, pp 59–73

Balint M: On genital love (1947), in Primary Love and Psycho-Analytic Technique. New York, Liveright, 1965, pp 109–120

Balint M: Perversions and genitality (1956), in Primary Love and Psycho-Analytic Technique. New York, Liveright, 1965, pp 136–147

Benjamin J: The Bonds of Love: Psychoanalysis, Feminism, and the Problem of Domination. New York, Pantheon, 1988

Chasseguet-Smirgel J: Freud and female sexuality: the consideration of some blind spots in the exploration of the "Dark Continent" (1976), in Sexuality and Mind. New York, New York University Press, 1986, pp 9–28

Chasseguet-Smirgel J: Creativity and Perversion. London, Free Association Books, 1985

Chodorow NJ: The Reproduction of Mothering. Berkeley and Los Angeles, University of California Press, 1978

Chodorow NJ: Gender, relation and difference in psychoanalytic perspective (1979), in Feminism and Psychoanalytic Theory. New Haven, CT, Yale University Press, and Cambridge, UK, Polity Press, 1989, pp 99–113

Chodorow NJ: Feminism and Psychoanalytic Theory. New Haven. CT, Yale University Press, and Cambridge, UK, Polity Press, 1989a

Chodorow NJ: Psychoanalytic feminism and the psychoanalytic psychology of women, in Feminism and Psychoanalytic Theory. New Haven, CT, Yale University Press, and Cambridge, UK, Polity Press, 1989b, pp 178–198

Connell RW: Gender and Power. Stanford, CA, Stanford University Press, 1987

Contratto S: Father presence in women's psychological development, in Advances in Psychoanalytic Sociology. Edited by Rabow J, Platt GM, Goldman M. Malabar, FL, Krieger, 1987, pp 138–157

Epstein S: Sexuality and identity: the contribution of object-relations theory to a constructionist sociology. Theory and Society 20:825–873, 1991

Foucault M: The History of Sexuality, Vol I. New York, Pantheon, 1978

Friedman R: Male Homosexuality: A Contemporary Psychoanalytic Perspective. New Haven, CT, Yale University Press, 1988

Freud S: Three essays on the theory of sexuality (1905), in The Standard Edition of the Complete Psychological Works of Sigmund Freud [SE], Vol 7. Translated and edited by Strachey J. London, Hogarth Press, 1953, pp 125–243

Freud S: The psychogenesis of a case of homosexuality in a woman (1920). SE, 18:145–172, 1955

Freud S: The dissolution of the Oedipus complex (1924). SE, 19:173–179, 1961

Freud S: Some psychical consequences of the anatomical distinction between the sexes (1925). SE, 19:248–258, 1961

Freud S: Female sexuality (1931). SE, 21:225–243, 1961

Freud S: New introductory lectures on psycho-analysis (1933). SE, 22:112–135, 1964

Freud S: Analysis terminable and interminable (1937). SE, 23:216–253, 1964

Garcia Marquez G: Love in the Time of Cholera. New York, Alfred A Knopf, 1988

Gaylin W, Person E (eds): Passionate Attachments: Thinking About Love. New York, Free Press, 1988

Golden C: Diversity and variability in women's sexual identities, in Lesbian Psychologies. Edited by Boston Lesbian Psychologies Collective. Urbana and Chicago, University of Illinois Press, 1987, pp 19–34

Greenacre P: Perversions: general considerations regarding their genetic and dynamic background. Psychoanal Study Child 23:47–62, 1968

Hershey DW: On a type of heterosexuality, and the fluidity of object relations. J Am Psychoanal Assoc 37:147–171, 1989

Horney K: The dread of women (1932), in Feminine Psychology. New York, WW Norton, 1967, pp 43–67

Isay R: Being Homosexual: Gay Men and Their Development. New York, Farrar, Straus, & Giroux, 1989

Johnson M: Strong Mothers, Weak Wives. Berkeley and Los Angeles, University of California Press, 1988

Katz JN: The invention of the homosexual, 1880–1950, in The Gay/Lesbian Almanac: A New Documentary. Edited by Katz JN. New York, Harper and Row, 1983, pp 137–174

Katz JN: The invention of heterosexuality. Socialist Review 20:7–34, 1990

Kerig P: The Engendered Family: The Influence of Marital Satisfaction on Gender Differences in Parent-Child Interaction. Unpublished Ph.D. dissertation. University of California, Berkeley, Department of Psychology, 1989

Kernberg O: Barriers to falling and remaining in love, in Object Relations Theory and Clinical Psycho-Analysis. New York, Jason Aronson, 1976a, pp 185–213

Kernberg O: Mature love: prerequisites and characteristics, in Object Relations Theory and Clinical Psycho-Analysis. New York, Jason Aronson, 1976b, pp 215–239

Kernberg O: Boundaries and structures in love relations, in Internal World and External Reality. New York, Jason Aronson, 1980, pp 277–305

Kernberg O: Between conventionality and aggression: the boundaries of passion, in Passionate Attachments: Thinking About Love. Edited by Gaylin WE, Person E. New York, Free Press, 1988, pp 63–83

Kernberg O: Aggression and love in the relationship of the couple. J Am Psychoanal Assoc 39:45–70, 1991

Krieger S: The Mirror Dance. Philadelphia, PA, Temple University Press, 1983

Kris E: The personal myth. J Am Psychoanal Assoc 4:653–681, 1956

Lacan J: [Selections] (1966, 1968, 1975), in Feminine Sexuality: Jacques Lacan and the école freudienne. Translated by Rose J. Edited by Mitchell J, Rose J. New York, WW Norton, 1982

Leonard MR: Fathers and daughters: the significance of "fathering" in the psychosexual development of the girl. Int J Psychoanal 47:325–334, 1966

Lewes K: The Psychoanalytic Theory of Male Homosexuality. New York, Simon & Schuster, 1988

Lindenbaum JP: The shattering of an illusion: the problem of competition in lesbian relationships. Feminist Studies 11:85–103, 1985

Maccoby E, Jacklin C: The Psychology of Sex Differences. Stanford, CA, Stanford University Press, 1974

McDougall J: Homosexuality in women, in Female Sexuality: New Psychoanalytic Views. Edited by Chasseguet-Smirgel J. Ann Arbor, University of Michigan Press, 1970

McDougall J: Theatres of the Mind: Illusion and Truth on the Psychoanalytic Stage. London, Free Association Books, 1986

Michel F: After the World Broke: Cross-Gender Representation in Works by Willa Cather, William Faulkner, and Djuna Barnes. Unpublished Ph.D. dissertation. University of California, Berkeley, Department of English, 1990

Mitchell J: Eternal divide. Times Higher Education Supplement, 17 Nov 1989

Money J, Ehrhardt A: Man and Woman, Boy and Girl. Baltimore, MD, Johns Hopkins University Press, 1972

Morgenthaler F: Homosexuality, Heterosexuality, Perversion. Hillside, NJ, Analytic Press, 1988

Panel: Toward the further understanding of homosexual women. Wolfson A, reporter. J Am Psychoanal Assoc 35:165–173, 1987

Person ES: The omni-available woman and lesbian sex: two fantasy themes and their relationship to the male developmental experience, in The Psychology of Men. Edited by Fogel GI, Lane FM, Liebert RS. New York, Basic Books, 1986, pp 71–94

Person ES: Dreams of Love and Fateful Encounters: The Power of Romantic Passion. New York, WW Norton, 1988

Reich A: Narcissistic object choice in women J Am Psychoanal Assoc 1:22–44, 1953

Rich A: Compulsory heterosexuality and lesbian existence. Signs 5:631–660, 1980

Roiphe H, Galenson E: Infantile Origins of Sexual Identity. New York, International Universities Press, 1981

Schafer R: Problems in Freud's psychology of women. J Am Psychoanal Assoc 22:459–485, 1974

Slater P: The Glory of Hera: Greek Mythology and the Greek Family. Boston, MA, Beacon Press, 1968

Socarides C: Homosexuality. New York, Jason Aronson, 1978

Socarides C: A unitary theory of sexual perversions, in On Sexuality. Edited by Karasu T, Socarides C. New York, International Universities Press, 1979, pp 161–188

Socarides C: The Preoedipal Origin and Psychoanalytic Therapy of Sexual Perversions. Madison, CT, International Universities Press, 1988

Stein A: Three models of sexuality: drives, identities and practices. Sociological Theory 7:1–13, 1989

Stoller R: Perversion: The Erotic Form of Hatred. New York, Pantheon, 1975

Stoller R: Sexual Excitement. New York, Pantheon, 1979

Stoller R: Observing the Erotic Imagination. New Haven, CT, Yale University Press, 1985

Stolorow RD, Lachman F: Psychoanalysis of Developmental Arrests. New York, International Universities Press, 1980

Weeks J: Sexuality. London, Tavistock, 1986

5

ARNOLD M. COOPER, M.D.

INTRODUCTION

Arnold Cooper is a graduate of Columbia College, the University of Utah School of Medicine, and the Columbia University Psychoanalytic Center for Training and Research, where he is a Training and Supervising Analyst. After graduating from medical school, he held a Research Fellowship in Physiology at the Thorndike Laboratory of Harvard University, spent 2 years in Medicine at Presbyterian Hospital in New York, and did his psychiatric residency at Bellevue Hospital in New York. He is the Stephen P. Tobin and Dr. Arnold M. Cooper Professor Emeritus in Consultation-Liaison Psychiatry at Weill Cornell Medical College and has been Professor of Psychiatry at Columbia College of Physicians and Surgeons and Adjunct Professor of Literature at Columbia University.

Teaching has been a central focus of his career. From 1965 to 1974, he was the Director of the Program in Psychoanalytic Studies at Columbia College, a program in psychoanalysis and related academic disciplines for college undergraduates, and he served as Associate Chairman of the Department of Psychiatry at Weill-Cornell Medical College, responsible for medical student and resident education. He has at various times been Chair of the Curriculum Committee and Associate Director of the Columbia Psychoanalytic Center, Chair of the Program Committee and President of the American Psychoanalytic Association, Vice President, Councilor and North American Secretary of the International Psychoanalytic Association, North American Editor of *The International Journal of Psychoanalysis*, and Deputy Editor of the *American Journal of Psychiatry*.

He is the author of over 100 papers and most recently of *The Quiet Revolution in American Psychoanalysis: Selected Papers of Arnold M. Cooper,* edited by Elizabeth L. Auchincloss.

Dr. Cooper has, from early in his analytic career, been interested in the struggle within psychoanalysis between the orthodoxy of American ego psychology and the variety of alternative or complementary theories struggling for their place in the analytic sun. He was influenced early by the work of Edmund Bergler, and he attempted to explore the narcissistic, preoedipal, clinically observable roots of varieties of neurotic disturbances. He has written on masochism, perversion, castration anxiety, the relationship of psychoanalysis to psychotherapy, psychoanalytic education, noninterpretive measures in psychoanalysis, and organizational resistance to change, among other topics. He has been a leader in opening psychoanalysis to related disciplines, such as literature, anthropology, and art history, and in stressing the urgent need for empirical research studies in psychoanalysis.

WHY I CHOSE THIS PAPER

Arnold M. Cooper, M.D.

"The Narcissistic-Masochistic Character," one of the earliest of my works, has provided a basic grounding for much of my later work in psychoanalysis. The paper attempts to bring together an understanding of the centrality of early narcissistic conflict and the attempted resolution of anxieties and conflicts at preoedipal stages and to suggest a solution to the riddle of the pervasive pathology of psychic masochism and resistance to change. Over several generations, and continuing to the present, students have told me that this paper was one of the great influences that helped guide them to a more successful and gratifying clinical outcome in their analytic work.

THE NARCISSISTIC-MASOCHISTIC CHARACTER

ARNOLD M. COOPER, M.D.

THERE IS AN OLD Chinese curse: "May you live in interesting times." These are analytically interesting times, in which, more than ever before in the history of psychoanalysis, accepted paradigms have been called into question, and a congeries of new and old ideas compete for attention and allegiance. In intellectual history, such periods of enthusiastic creative ferment have led to the development of new ideas. Sciences make their great advances when new techniques lead to new experiments, when new data contradict old theories, and when new ideas lead to new theories. Since the early 1970s, much of the interesting creative tension in psychoanalysis has focused on the crucial role of preoedipal experiences and the centrality of issues of self or narcissism in character development. I propose that masochistic defenses are ubiquitous in preoedipal narcissistic development and that a deeper understanding of the development of masochism may help to clarify a number of clinical problems. I suggest that a full appreciation of the roles of narcissism and masochism in development and in pathology requires that we relinquish whatever remains of what Freud referred to as the "shibboleth" of the centrality of the Oedipus complex in neurosogenesis. I further suggest that masochism and narcissism are so entwined, both in development and in clinical presentation, that we clarify our clinical work by considering that there is a narcissistic-masochistic character and that neither appears alone.

"The Narcissistic-Masochistic Character," by Arnold M. Cooper, M.D., was first published in *Masochism: Current Psychological Perspectives,* edited by Robert A. Glick and Donald I. Meyers, pp. 117–139.

The problem of reformulating our ideas was foreshadowed over half a century ago, when Freud (1931), in speaking of the intensity and duration of the little girl's attachment to her mother, wrote:

> The pre-Oedipus phase in women gains an importance which we have not attributed to it hitherto. Since this phase allows room for all the fixations and repressions from which we must trace the origin of the neuroses, it would seem as though we must retract the universality of the thesis that the Oedipus complex is the nucleus of neurosis. But if anyone feels reluctant about making this correction, there is no need for him to do so. (p. 225)

Freud then went on to reveal some of his own difficulties in accepting his new findings by stating that those who are reluctant to make this clearly necessary revision need not do so, if they are willing to accept a redefinition of the Oedipus complex to include earlier events. He said:

> Our insights into this early pre-Oedipus phase in girls comes to us as a surprise like the discovery, in another field, of the Minoan-Mycenean civilization behind the civilization of Greece. Everything in the sphere of the first attachment to the mother seems to be so difficult to grasp in analysis—so gray with age and shadowy, and almost impossible to revivify, that it was as if it has succumbed to an especially inexorable repression. (p. 226)

Perhaps this is an indication of Freud's and our own difficulty in accepting the breadth of theoretical revision that our data may require. The fact is that in his posthumous work, "The Outline of Psychoanalysis" (Freud 1938), he again stated without reservation that the Oedipus complex is the nucleus of neurosis.

It is questionable whether it was ever the case that most analytic patients presented with primary oedipal pathology. Edward Glover in his "Technique of Psychoanalysis" published in 1955, was already lamenting the scarcity of cases of classical transference neurosis. He referred to "those mild and mostly favorable cases which incidentally *appear all too infrequently* in the average analyst's case list" (p. 205). I suspect that few of us have ever seen many cases of "classical transference neurosis" and yet it has been difficult for us to give up the accompanying clinical idea, so dear to Freud, that the nucleus of neurosis is the Oedipus complex. I in no way depreciate the immensity of the discovery of the Oedipus complex and its vital role in human affairs. But we need not share Freud's reluctance to place the Oedipus complex in perspective as one of a number of crucial developmental epochs, and not necessarily the one most significant for our understanding of narcissistic and masochistic pathology, and perhaps not even for understanding neurosis generally.

Kohut's (1971) self psychology represented the most radical attempt to date to address, and resolve, the various dissonant elements in psychoanalytic developmental research, clinical experience and general theory. As I have written elsewhere (Cooper 1983), I believe it is this exposure of some of the major unresolved problems of psychoanalytic work that accounts for much of the passion—positive and negative—that was generated by self psychology. For more than a decade, psychoanalysis has been productively preoccupied with developing a new understanding of narcissism in the light of our newer emphasis on preoedipal events. The scientific and clinical yield of this investigation has been high, and it should prompt us to apply these methods to other of our metapsychological and clinical formulations that are a bit fuzzy. Prominent among these are the concepts of masochism and the masochistic character.

Our major ideas concerning masochism date to an earlier period of psychoanalytic thinking, when the focus was on the Oedipus complex. The cultural climate of psychoanalysis was different then. A reexamination of masochism at this time, using our newer ideas of separation-individuation, self-esteem regulation, the nature of early object relations, and so on, might help clarify our understanding of masochistic phenomena.

REVIEW OF THEORIES AND DEFINITIONS

The literature is vast, and I will mention only a few salient points. The term *masochism* was coined by Krafft-Ebing in 1895 with reference to Leopold von Sacher-Masoch's (1870) novel *Venus in Furs.* The novel described, and Krafft-Ebing referred to, a situation of seeking physical and mental torture at the hands of another person through willing submission to experiences of enslavement, passivity, and humiliation. Freud (1920) used Krafft-Ebing's terminology, although in his early writings on masochism he was concerned with perversion masochism with clear sexual pleasure attached to pain, and only later was he concerned with the problems of moral masochism in which humiliation and suffering are sought as part of the character formation and without evident sexual satisfactions. Freud postulated several explanations for these puzzling phenomena:

1. It is the nature of physiology that an excess of stimulation in the nervous system automatically leads to experiences of both pain and pleasure.

2. Masochism is a vicissitude of instinct; sadism or aggression, a primary instinct, turns against the self as masochism, a secondary instinctual phenomenon.
3. Masochism is defined as "beyond the pleasure principle," a primary instinct, a component of the death instinct, a consequence of the repetition compulsion, and thus an independent, automatically operating regulatory principle. Masochism as a primary instinct is, in the course of development, directed outward, and as a tertiary phenomenon, is redirected inward, as clinical masochism.
4. Moral masochism is the need for punishment, consequent to the excessive harshness of the superego. Persons feeling guilty for sexual, generally oedipal, forbidden wishes seek punishment as a means of expiation.
5. Masochistic suffering is a condition for pleasure, not a source of pleasure. That is, masochists do not enjoy the suffering per se; rather they willingly endure the pain as an unavoidable guilty ransom for access to forbidden or undeserved pleasures.
6. Masochism is related to feminine characteristics and passivity.

I think it is fair to say that Freud struggled throughout his lifetime for a satisfactory explanation of the paradox of pleasure-in-unpleasure. In "Analysis Terminable and Interminable" (Freud 1937), he wrote:

> No stronger impression arises from resistances during the work of analysis than of there being a force which is defending itself by every possible means against recovery and which is absolutely resolved to hold on to illness and suffering. One portion of this force has been recognized by us, undoubtedly with justice, as a sense of guilt and need for punishment, and has been localized by us in the ego's relation to the super-ego. But this is only the portion of it which is, as it were, psychically bound by the super-ego and thus becomes recognizable; other quotas of the same force, whether bound or free, may be at work in other, unspecified places. If we take into consideration the total picture made up by the phenomena of masochism immanent in so many people, the negative therapeutic reaction and sense of guilt found in so many neurotics, we shall no longer be able to adhere to the belief that mental events are exclusively governed by the desire for pleasure. These phenomena are unmistakable indications of the presence of a power in mental life which we call the instinct of aggression or of destruction according to its aims, and which we trace back to the original death instinct of living matter. It is not a question of an antithesis between an optimistic and pessimistic theory of life. Only by the concurrent or mutually opposing action of the two primal instincts—Eros and the death-instinct—never by one or the other alone, can we explain the rich multiplicity of the phenomena of life. (p. 242)

The death instinct, as we all know, is an idea that never caught on.

The vast subsequent literature on masochism was well summarized by Brenner (1959), Stolorow (1975), Maleson (1984), and Grossman (1986), and a panel of the American Psychoanalytic Association, in which I participated (Fischer 1981). I will not repeat these summaries, which succinctly convey the large array of functions and etiologies ascribed to masochism. Stolorow's paper deserves special note because he also concerned himself with the narcissistic functions of masochism, pointing out that sadomasochistic development can aid in maintaining a satisfactory self-image. I will, through the remainder of this paper, confine my discussion to so-called moral masochism, or, as some have referred to it, "psychic" masochism. I will not discuss perversion masochism, which I believe to be a developmentally different phenomenon.... Perverse fantasies, however, are common in persons of very varied personalities.

While many definitions of masochism have been attempted, Brenner's (1959) definition has remained authoritative. He defined masochism as "the seeking of unpleasure, by which is meant physical or mental pain, discomfort or wretchedness, for the sake of *sexual* pleasure, with the qualification that either the seeking or the pleasure or both may often be unconscious rather than conscious" (p. 197). Brenner emphasized that masochism represented an acceptance of a painful penalty for forbidden sexual pleasures associated with the Oedipus complex. He agreed that masochistic phenomena are ubiquitous in both normality and pathology, serving multiple psychic functions including such aims as seduction of the aggressor, maintenance of object-control, and the like. Brenner believed that the genesis of the masochistic character seemed related to excessively frustrating or rejecting parents.

A somewhat different, highly organized view of masochism was put forth in the voluminous writings of the late Edmund Bergler (1949, 1961). Because his theories seem to me relevant to topics that are currently of great interest, because they have influenced my own thinking, and because they are so little referred to in the literature, having been premature in their emphasis on the preoedipal period and narcissism, I will present a brief summary of his work. As long ago as 1949, Bergler stated that masochism was a fundamental aspect of all neurotic behavior, and he linked masochistic phenomena with issues of narcissistic development, or development of self-esteem systems. Bergler described in detail a proposed genetic schema out of which psychic masochism develops as an unavoidable aspect of human development. I will mention only a few elements that are particularly germane to the thesis of this paper.

1. Bergler assumed that the preservation of infantile megalomania or infantile omnipotence (we today would say narcissism) is of prime importance for the reduction of anxiety and as a source of satisfaction—on a par with the maintenance of libidinal satisfactions. This formulation is not dissimilar to Kohut's many years later.
2. Every infant is, by its own standards, excessively frustrated, disappointed, refused. These disappointments always have the effect of a narcissistic humiliation because they are an offense to the infant's omnipotent fantasy.
3. The infant responds with fury to this offense to his omnipotent self, but in his helplessness to vent fury on an outer object, the fury is deflected against the self (what Rado [1969] termed retroflexed rage) and eventually contributes to the harshness of the superego.
4. Faced with unavoidable frustration, the danger of aggression against parents, who are also needed and loved, and the pain of self-directed aggression, the infant nonetheless attempts to maintain essential feelings of omnipotence and self-esteem, and in Bergler's terms, he "libidinizes" or "sugarcoats" his disappointments. He learns to extract pleasure from displeasure for the sake of the illusion of continuing, total, omnipotent control, both of himself and of the differentiating object. "No one frustrated me against my wishes; I frustrated myself because I like it." It was Bergler's belief that some inborn tendency made it easy and inevitable that a pleasure-in-displeasure pattern would develop. He insisted that this develops at the very earliest stages of object differentiation and perhaps, I would add, becomes consolidated during the disappointing realization of helplessness that occurs during the rapprochement phase of the separation-individuation process as described by Mahler (1972).

According to Bergler, these hypothesized early events of psychic development resulted in the "clinical picture" of psychic masochism, which was characterized by the "oral triad." The oral triad, a phrase he used many years before Lewin (1950) used the term for a different purpose, consists of a three-step behavioral sequence that is paradigmatic for masochistic behavior.

- *Step 1.* Through his own behavior or through the misuse of an available external situation, the masochist unconsciously provokes disappointment, refusal, and humiliation. He identifies the outer world with a disappointing, refusing, preoedipal mother. *Unconsciously,* the rejection provides satisfaction.
- *Step 2.* Consciously, the masochist has repressed his knowledge of his

own provocation and reacts with righteous indignation and *seeming* self-defense to the rejection, which he consciously perceives as externally delivered. He responds, thus, with "pseudoaggression," that is, defensive aggression designed to disclaim his responsibility for, and unconscious pleasure in, the defeat he has experienced. Step 2 represents an attempt to appease inner guilt for forbidden unconscious masochistic pleasure.

- *Step 3.* After the subsidence of pseudoaggression, which, because often ill-dosed or ill-timed, and not intended for genuine self-defense, may provoke additional unconsciously wished-for defeats, the masochist indulges in conscious self-pity, feelings of "this only happens to me." Unconsciously he enjoys the masochistic rebuff.

This clinical oral triad, or, as Bergler calls it, the mechanism of "injustice collecting," is, I think, an excellent description of a repetitive sequence of events observable in almost all neurotic behavior. The term "injustice collector" was coined by Bergler, and later used by Louis Auchincloss (1950) as the title of a collection of stories. In Bergler's view, all human beings have more or less masochistic propensities. The issue of pathology is one of quantity.

THEORETICAL ISSUES

I would like now to explore some of the theoretical issues that have been raised in previous discussions of masochism.

Today there is little disagreement that we can explain masochism in terms of its defensive and adaptive functions without recourse to a primary drive. The extraordinary ease with which pleasure-in-displeasure phenomena develop, and their stickiness, suggests a psychic apparatus that is well prepared for the use of such defensive structures, and there is no theoretical need to call on a primary instinctive masochism.

What is the nature of the pleasure in masochism? The generally accepted formulation, that the pleasure is the same as any other pleasure and that the pain is the necessary guilty price, has the great merit of preserving the pleasure principle intact. There has always been a group of analysts, however, including Loewenstein and Bergler, who insisted, to quote Loewenstein, that "in the masochistic behavior we observe an unconscious libidinization of suffering caused by aggression from without and within" (Loewenstein 1957, p. 230). The operating principle seems to be, "If you can't lick 'em, join 'em." Perhaps, more simply, one may speculate that the infant claims as his own, and endows with as much pleasure as possible, whatever is familiar, whether painful experiences or unempathic mothers. The defensive capacity to alter the meaning of painful experience so that it is experienced as ego-syntonic has also been described in certain circumstances in infancy by Greenacre (1960) and Jacobson (1964). Greenacre reported that babies under conditions of extreme distress will have genital, orgasticlike responses, as early as the second half of the first year, and that these early events may result in ego distortions creating sexual excitation arising from self-directed aggression. This is similar to Freud's original formulation, and I think we must leave open the possibility that there is a dialectic here of excessive quantity changing quality.

From a different point of view, we may ask, What are the gratifying and constructive aspects of pain? We do not dispute every mother's observation that painful frustration, disappointment, and injury are inevitable concomitants of infancy. It is rare that any infant goes through a 24-hour period without exhibiting what we adults interpret to be cries of discomfort, frustration, and need. Even the most loving and competent mother cannot spare the infant these experiences, and, indeed, there is good reason to believe that no infant should be spared these experiences in proper dosage. It seems likely that painful bodily, particularly skin, experiences are important proprioceptive mechanisms that serve not only to avoid damage, but also, developmentally, to provide important components of the forming body image and self-image. There are many cases in the literature, summarized by Stolorow (1975), of persons who experience a relief from identity diffusion by inflicting pain upon their skin.

A typical pattern for borderline self-mutilators is to cut or otherwise injure themselves in privacy, experiencing little pain in the process. They later exhibit the injury to the usually surprised caretaking person, be it parent or physician, with evident satisfaction in the demonstration that they are suffering, in danger, and beyond the control of the caretaking person. A prominent motivation for this behavior is the need to demonstrate autonomy via the capacity for self-mutilation.

Head banging in infants, a far more common phenomenon than is usually acknowledged and quite compatible with normal development is also, I suggest, one of the normal, painful ways of achieving necessary and gratifying self-definition. Skin sensations of all kinds, and perhaps moderately painful sensations particularly, are a regular mode of establishing self-boundaries.

Hermann (1976) stated:

> In order to understand masochistic pleasure, one has to recognize that it is quite closely interwoven with the castration complex but behind

> this link is the reaction-formation to the urge to cling—namely the drive to separate oneself. At this point, we have to go far back to early development. Our guess is that the emergence of the process of separation of the mother and child dual unit constitutes a pre-stage of narcissism and painful masochism; normal separation goes along with "healthy" narcissism. (p. 30)

Hermann then went on to describe that pain is a necessary concomitant of separation but is a lesser evil than the damage and decay of the self, which would result from failure of separation in infancy. He referred to a healing tendency within the psyche and the erotization of pain, which facilitates healing of a damaged psychic area. Hermann viewed all later self-mutilations, such as self-biting, tearing one's cuticles, pulling hair, tearing scabs, and the like as attempts to reinforce a sense of freedom from the need to cling: "pain arises in connection with the *separation that is striven for,* while its *successful accomplishment* brings pleasure" (p. 30). Hermann viewed masochistic character traits as a consequence of failure of successful separation with reactive repetition of separation traumas.

Pain, it is suggested, serves the person's need for self-definition and separation-individuation and is part of a gratifying accomplishment. Mastery—not avoidance—of pain is a major achievement in the course of self-development; mastery may imply the capacity to derive satisfaction and accomplishment from self-induced, self-dosed pain. The tendency for such an achievement to miscarry is self-evident. The pleasurable fatigue after a day's work, the ecstasy of an athlete's exhaustion, the dogged pursuit of distant goals, the willingness to cling to a seemingly absurd ideal—all of these represent constructive uses of pleasure in pain and a source of creative energies.

All cultures at all times have idealized heroes whose achievement involves painful and dangerous feats, if not actual martyrdom. The achievement is not valued unless it is fired in pain. No culture chooses to live without inflicting pain on itself; even cultures seemingly devoted to nirvana-type ideals have painful rituals. Rites of passage and experiences of mortification, "baptism by fire," are means of assuring essential aspects of cultural and individual identity , and their effectiveness may be proportional to their painfulness and sharpness of definition. A circumcision ceremony at puberty is obviously a clearer marker of a stage in self-development and onset of manhood than is a Bar Mitzvah ceremony.

The question of aggression in the induction of masochism is interesting but, I think, not satisfactorily answerable at this time. Regularly in the course of development, aggression is distributed in at least five directions: 1) in legitimate self-assertion; 2) in projection; 3) turned against the self; 4) toward the formation of the superego; and 5) used defensively as "pseudoaggression." The proportions vary, but in the narcissistic-masochistic character legitimate self-assertion is in short supply. I will not discuss here the many issues of the relationship of sadism to masochism, double identifications with both aggressor and victim, and so forth. It seems clear that experiences of frustration and the absence of loving care, whether in infant children or infant monkeys, induce self-directed aggression and mutilation. The usual explanations involve ideas of retroflexed rage or failure of instinct fusion. These concepts are convenient, but not entirely adequate. Stoller (1979) states that hostility, in retaliation for and in disavowal of early experiences of passivity and humiliation at the hands of a woman, is the crucial motivation in *all* perversions, not only masochistic perversion. (Hostility, in his view, is an important aspect of all sexuality.) Referring to the risks that perverts take, he says, "Masochism is a technique of control, first discovered in childhood following trauma, the onslaught of the unexpected. The child believes it can prevent further trauma by reenacting the original trauma. Then, as master of the script, he is no longer victim; he can decide for himself when to suffer pain rather than having it strike without warning" (p. 125). Dizmang and Cheatham (1970), discussing the Lesch-Nyhan syndrome, have suggested a psychobiological basis for masochistic behavior in the postulate of a low threshold for activation of a mechanism that ordinarily controls tendencies toward repetitive compulsive behaviors and self-inflicted aggression.

At what stage of development do the decisive events leading to masochistic character disorder occur? It is clear from what I have been describing that I feel it is now evident that the masochistic conflicts of the Oedipus complex are reworkings of much earlier established masochistic functions. In the later character development, these defenses, by means of the mechanism of secondary autonomy (Hartmann and Loewenstein 1962) function as if they were wishes.

AN ATTEMPT AT CLARIFICATION

If even part of what I have been suggesting is correct, then masochistic tendencies are a necessary and ubiquitous aspect of narcissistic development. I think there is convincing evidence that Freud was right: the pleasure principle alone is inadequate to explain masochism, nor does the dual-instinct theory add sufficient heuristic power. If we add an instinct or tendency toward aggression, we still lack heuristic power. Our knowledge of early development and our knowledge derived from the studies of borderline and psychotic disorders make it abundantly clear that a newer theoretical perspective requires that issues of self-development and object relations be accorded their proper weight as crucial factors in early psychological development. Libidinal pleasures and aggressive satisfactions will be sacrificed or distorted if necessary to help prevent the shattering disorganizing anxieties that arise when the self-system is disturbed or the ties to the object disrupted. Whether one refers to Kohut's (1972) narcissistic libido, or Erikson's (1963) basic trust, or Sullivan's (1953) sense of security, or Rado's (1969) basic pride and dependency needs, or Sandler and Joffee's (1969) feelings of safety, or Bergler's (1949) omnipotent fantasy, or Winnicott's (1971) true self—all are ways of addressing the crucial issues of the organism's primary needs for self-definition out of an original symbiotic bond. In fact, Freud, under the unfortunately termed "death instinct," was making the same point. The organism will give up libidinal pleasure for the safety, satisfaction, or pleasure of maintaining a coherent self.

Let me summarize my view of the relevant issues:

1. Pain is a necessary and unavoidable concomitant of separation-individuation and the achievement of selfhood. Perhaps "Doleo ergo sum" (I suffer, therefore I am) is a precursor of "Sentio ergo sum" (I feel, therefore I am), and "Cogito ergo sum" (I think, therefore I am).
2. The frustrations and discomforts of separation-individuation, necessary events in turning us toward the world, are perceived as narcissistic injuries—that is, they damage the sense of magical omnipotent control and threaten intolerable passivity and helplessness in the face of a perceived external danger. This is the prototype of narcissistic humiliation.
3. The infant attempts defensively to restore threatened self-esteem by distorting the nature of his experience. Rather than accept the fact of helplessness, the infant reasserts control by making suffering ego-syntonic. "I am frustrated because I want to be. I force my mother to be cruel." Freud (1937), of course, often discussed the general human intolerance of passivity and the tendency to assert mastery by converting passively endured experiences into actively sought ones. The mastery of pain is part of normal development, and this always implies a capacity to derive satisfaction from pain.
4. Alternatively, one may consider that the infant, out of the need to maintain some vestiges of self-esteem in situations of more than ordinary pain, displeasure, failure of reward, and diminished self-esteem, will still attempt to salvage pleasure by equating the familiar with the

pleasurable. Survival in infancy undoubtedly depends on retaining some capacity for receiving pleasurable impressions from the self and object. We may theorize that the infant makes the best adaptation he can, and familiar pains may be the best available pleasure.

5. What I am terming narcissistic-masochistic tendencies are compatible with normal development and with loving, although never unambivalent, ties to objects.
6. Where the experience of early narcissistic humiliation is excessive for external or internal reasons, these mechanisms of repair miscarry. The object is perceived as excessively cruel and refusing; the self is perceived as incapable of genuine self-assertion in the pursuit of gratification; the gratifications obtained from disappointment take precedence over genuine but unavailable and unfamiliar libidinal, assertive, or ego-functional satisfactions. Being disappointed, or refused, becomes the *preferred* mode of narcissistic assertion to the extent that narcissistic and masochistic distortions dominate the character. Nietzsche, quoted by Hartmann and Loewenstein (1962), said, "He who despises himself, nevertheless esteems himself thereby as despisor" (p. 59). One can always omnipotently guarantee rejection—love is much chancier. If one can securely enjoy disappointment, it is no longer possible to be disappointed. To the extent that narcissistic-masochistic defenses are used, the aim is not a fantasied reunion with a loving and caring mother; rather it is fantasied control over a cruel and damaging mother. Original sources of gratification have been degraded, and gratification is secondarily derived from the special sense of suffering.
7. It seems clear that the pleasure sought is not genital-sexual in origin, is preoedipal, and is the satisfaction and pride of a more satisfying self-representation, a pleasure in an ego function, the regulation of self-esteem. Psychic masochism is not a derivative of perversion masochism, although the two are often related. Exhibitionistic drives, pleasures of self-pity , and many other gratifications play a role secondarily.
8. Inevitably, when narcissistic-masochistic pathology predominates, superego distortions also occur. The excessive harshness of the superego is, in my view, a feature of all narcissistic and masochistic pathology and often dominates the *clinical* picture.
9. In any particular instance, the presenting clinical picture may seem more narcissistic or more masochistic. The surface may be full of charm, preening, dazzling accomplishment, or ambition. Or the surface may present obvious depression, invitations to humiliation, and feelings of failure. However, only a short period of analysis will

reveal that both types share the sense of deadened capacity to feel, muted pleasure, a hypersensitive self-esteem alternating between grandiosity and humiliation, an inability to sustain or derive satisfaction from their relationships or their work, a constant sense of envy, an unshakable conviction of being wronged and deprived by those who are supposed to care for them, and an infinite capacity for provocation.

Trilling (1963), in his brilliant essay "The Fate of Pleasure," based on Freud's "Beyond the Pleasure Principle," spoke of the change in cultural attitude from the time of Wordsworth, who wrote of "the grand elementary principle of pleasure," which he said constituted "the named and native dignity of man," and which was "the principle by which man knows and feels, and lives, and moves." Trilling referred to a

> change in quantity. It has always been true of some men that to pleasure they have preferred unpleasure. They imposed upon themselves difficult and painful tasks, they committed themselves to strange "unnatural" modes of life, they sought after stressing emotions, in order to know psychic energies which are not to be summoned up in felicity. These psychic energies, even when they are experienced in self-destruction, are a means of self-definition and self-affirmation. As such, they have a social reference—the election of unpleasure, however isolated and private the act may be, must refer to society if only because the choice denies the valuation which society in general puts upon pleasure; of course it often receives social approbation of the highest degree, even if at a remove of time: it is the choice of the hero, the saint and martyr, and, in some cultures, the artist. The quantitative change which we have to take account of is: what was once a mode of experience of a few has now become an ideal of experience of many. For reasons which, at least here, must defy speculation, the ideal of pleasure has exhausted itself, almost as if it had been actually realized and had issued in satiety and ennui. In its place or, at least, beside it, there is developing—conceivably at the behest of literature! —an ideal of the experience of those psychic energies which are linked with unpleasure and which are directed towards self-definition and self-affirmation. (p. 85)

The model for Trilling here is Dostoevsky's "Underground Man," the provocateur without peer. One could add Melville's "Bartleby" as the other pole of the masochistic-narcissistic character who dominates through his seeming passivity. I believe that Trilling was, with his usual extraordinary perspicacity, describing at the level of culture the same shift we have experienced in psychoanalysis at the level of clinical practice. This new type that he described was the same new type with which psychoanalysis has been struggling now for years, the so-called narcissistic-masochistic character. Trilling clearly perceived that this character type struggles to achieve self-definition through the experience of unpleasure. When this occurs within socially acceptable limits we have "normal" narcissistic-masochistic character development. The narcissistic-masochistic character as a pathological type, of varying severity, is marked by the preferential pursuit of suffering and rejection with little positive achievement. Every quantitative gradation occurs between normal and severely pathological or borderline. The mildly neurotic "plays" with self-torture, while the borderline or psychotic may cause irreparable self-damage.

CLINICAL EXAMPLES

I would like now to illustrate this thesis with a clinical vignette and a condensed account of an analysis. Once again, I emphasize that I will not in this brief presentation elaborate a great many significant elements but will focus on a few of these relevant to the view I am suggesting.

Clinical Vignette 1

Miss A, a 26-year-old student, entered treatment with complaints of chronic anxiety and depression, feelings of social isolation, and a series of unfortunate relationships with men. She was the younger by 3 years of two sisters, who were the children of an aloof, taciturn, successful businessman father and a mother who was widely admired for her beauty and who devoted herself almost full time to the preservation of her beauty. Miss A recalled having had severe temper tantrums in childhood that would intimidate the family, but in between tantrums she was an obedient child and an excellent student. Although she always felt cold and distant in her relationships, she recalled that almost up to puberty she had continued to make a huge fuss whenever the parents were going out for an evening. She couldn't bear their leaving her alone. When she began to date at age 14, this middle-class Jewish girl chose lower-class black boys for her companions and insisted on bringing them home to meet her parents. As a consequence, she and the father fought and literally did not speak to each other from that time until the father died when she was 16. By the time that she entered treatment, she had repeated several times the following pattern with men: she would become intensely involved with a man who she knew from the start was unsuitable. He might be married, or someone who was intellectually her inferior, or someone she really didn't like. From the beginning of the relationship, she would be aware that this could not last. She would project this feeling and become intensely angry at the man because he, in her view, was unreliable and threatened to leave her. She would in her fury become increasingly provocative, finally bringing about the separation she both desired and feared. She would then become depressed and feel abandoned.

The repetition of this pattern was a major element in the transference. She was never late for an appointment, paid her bills on time, tried hard to be a "good patient," although she found it difficult to talk. She was convinced that I eagerly awaited the end of every session, the break for the weekend, or the start of a holiday because I was delighted to be rid of her, and she felt that she could not survive without me. (She had dreams of floating in space, isolated, and dreams of accidents.) On the surface, her idealization of me was complete, but dreams and other data revealed the anger and devaluation which permeated that seeming idealization. Idealization in the adult transference is, in fact, never pure idealization but is always merged with the hidden rage that the child experienced in the course of separation-individuation. She would never allow herself to take a holiday or miss an appointment, obviously to maintain the clear record that I was the one who did all the abandoning. This was analyzed at length. Midway in the analysis, in the spring of the year, she planned her summer holiday before knowing precisely what my holiday dates would be. We discussed her plan at length, and for the first time she felt confident and pleased about being able to go away on a self-initiated separation. Several weeks later, I mentioned in the course of a session that the vacation dates had worked out well because, in fact, my holiday would coincide with hers. She immediately was enraged and self-pitying that I would go away and leave her, and it became utterly unimportant that she had previously made her own arrangements to go away.

Several things became apparent in the analysis of this episode.

1. A major portion of her self-esteem and self-knowledge consisted of her representation to herself of herself as an innocent abandoned martyr.
2. She felt a comfortable familiarity and control of her intimate objects only in the context of her ability to create a feeling of abandonment or to provoke an actual abandonment by the object. This was at its basic level preoedipal in nature and clearly reflected her sense of being uncared for by her narcissistic mother.
3. Additionally, this constellation represented the repetition of oedipal issues, and in the transference she was also reliving aspects of her oedipal relationship to her father. All preoedipal constellations have another reworking during the oedipal phase, but that latter does not constitute all the recoverable content of the genetic constellation.
4. The intolerable frustration of the original infantile demands for love and union had led to narcissistic-masochistic defenses. What she *now* sought in her relationships, disguised as an insatiable demand for attention, was the repetition of the painful abandonment, but

> with the hidden gratification of narcissistic control and masochistic satisfaction. The demand for love had been given up in favor of the pleasure of rejection.

This is the paradigmatic sequence for narcissistic-masochistic pathology.

Clinical Vignette 2

A 40-year-old successful corporate executive entered analysis because he had plunged into a deep depression following an accusation of minor wrongdoing in some financial maneuvers. In fact he was innocent of the charge, which had arisen out of an equally innocent error of one of his assistants, whom he had inadequately supervised. He had been officially cleared of any taint, and the whole matter was minor to begin with. However, this was one in a lifelong series of actually, or potentially, self-damaging provocations in important situations, which were further characterized by his inappropriate failure to defend himself with sufficient vigor in the face of the attack that followed his provocation. These incidents had regularly been followed by feelings of depression and self-pity, but this time the feelings were severe. He could not rid himself of the feelings that he had shamefully exposed himself to his colleagues, that his entire career would collapse, and that he would turn out to be a laughingstock with fraudulent pretensions to greatness. The presenting symptom thus combined masochistic, provocative self-damage and self-pity, with a sense of narcissistic collapse. I will present only a few relevant aspects of the history and treatment course. I will deliberately neglect much of the oedipal material that arose during the course of the four session a week analysis and that was interpreted; instead I will concentrate on earlier aspects of development. This will be a sketch, and many significant issues will not be elaborated.

He was the youngest of three children, the only boy and, as he acknowledged only later, the favorite child. He viewed his own childhood with great bitterness. He felt he had received nothing of value from his parents and that they had played no positive role in his life. He regarded himself as a phoenix—born out of himself, his own father and mother. These feelings of bitter deprivation—nobody ever gave me anything—had formed a masochistic current throughout his life. His mother had been a powerfully narcissistic woman, who saw in her son the opportunity for realizing her ambitions for wealth and status, cravings she unceasingly berated the father for not satisfying. The patient recalled little affection from his mother and felt she had used him only for her own satisfaction and as an ally against his weak, passive father. His father had been a modest success until the depression hit, when the patient was 4, and both the father and his business collapsed, never to recover. This probably provided a serious blow to whatever attempts at idealization may have been underway. The parents fought constantly, mother reminding father daily of his failure, and the boy remembered great anxiety that they would separate and he would be abandoned.

The sharp edge of his depression lifted shortly after analysis began, revealing a level of chronic depression and a character of endless injustice collecting and self-pity, covered by a socially successful facade of charm and joviality. He felt that although many people regarded him as a friend and sought him out, he had no friends and felt no warmth toward anyone. Perhaps he loved his wife and children, but he arranged his work schedule so that he would never have to be near them for any length of time. He felt isolated and lived with a constant dread that some disaster would befall him. The incident that precipitated his depression bothered him partly because he felt he was being hauled down by something trivial rather than by an episode fittingly grandiose. He battled endlessly with his associates in business, making wildly unreasonable demands and feeling unjustly treated when they were not yielded to. At the same time, he maintained a killing work pace and never asked for the readily available help that might have reduced his work load. He had a mechanically adequate sex life with his wife and fantasied endlessly about the beautiful women he wanted to sleep with. In fact, he was convinced that he would be impotent with anyone except his wife, and he never dared to attempt an affair.

Early in the treatment, he expressed two major concerns with regard to me. First, that it was my goal to make him "like everyone else." "I couldn't bear to live if I thought I was like everyone else. I'd rather be bad or dead than not be a somebody. Before I give up the feeling of awful things happening to me, I want to be sure I won't be giving up my sense of being special." Second, he was convinced that I had no interest in him, that I saw him only because I wanted the fee. That suited him fine because he had no interest in me, but it worried him that I might not need the fee badly enough so that he could count on my availability for as long as he might want me. Interestingly, convinced that I only saw him for the money, he was regularly late in paying his bills and would worry about the consequences, but not mention it himself. When I would bring up his tardiness, he would feel a combination of terror that I was now going to be angry with him and throw him out and fury that I had the nerve to dun him for money, when everyone knew he was an honest man. Quickly, then, the transference, like his life, developed a variety of narcissistic and masochistic themes.

The early transference combined both idealizing and mirror forms. These narcissistic transferences are, in my view, always equally masochistic, since they are regularly suffused with rage and the expectation of disappointment. The idealization often is the façade for constructing larger, later disappointments. As adults, narcissistic-masochistic characters no longer have genuine expectations of their grandiose fantasies being met. Rather, grandiose fantasies are the occasion for reenactment of unconsciously gratifying disappointments. The seeming insatiability of so many of these patients is not due to excessive need; instead, it represents their raising the demand for love, time, attention, or whatever to the level necessary to be sure it cannot be met. This man, for example, seemed to look forward to sessions, was friendly, felt that my most obvious remarks were brilliant, seemed happy to attribute to me all of the intelligent ideas that he had in the analysis. The other side of this coin, however, was his angry conviction that I used my intelligence totally in my own behalf and had no interest in helping him. He felt that all the work in analysis was being done by himself. A typical dream was of him and a guide scaling a high mountain, making remarkable progress but never speaking, and with him in the lead. In discussing this dream, he said, "All you do here is nudge me along. Why don't you help me more? The work is all mine. I can't bear the thought that anyone else has a part in anything I do." Fantasies of this sort have the double purpose of maintaining a grandiose, omnipotent image of himself and of maintaining an image of the totally refusing mother. The narcissistic portion of the fantasy requires the masochistic portion. "I give myself everything; my mother gives me nothing." A sense of grandiosity and a sense of self-pitying deprivation paradoxically are sides of the same coin, and neither can exist without the other. The narcissistic grandiose self as seen in the adult can never be the original germ of narcissism but is always tempered by the experiences of frustration, which then become part and parcel of the narcissistic fantasy. "I am a great person because I overcome the malice of my refusing mother."

At a later stage of treatment, when I insistently brought up the issue of his feelings about me, he reacted fiercely, saying, "This is a process, not a human relationship. You are not here. You are not. There is just a disembodied voice sitting behind me." As I persisted and discussed how difficult it was for him to acknowledge that he received something from me and felt something for me, he reported, "I feel creepy. I have a physical reaction to this discussion." He was experiencing mild depersonalization, related to the disturbance of self and narcissistic stability, which resulted from the revival of remnants of the repressed affectionate bond toward his mother. The acknowledgment of this bond immediately induced feelings of terrifying weakness, of being passively at the mercy of a malicious giant. On the other hand, this masochistic, passive, victimized relationship to a maliciously perceived mother was an unconscious source of narcissistic gratification (I never yield to her) and masochistic gratification (I enjoy suffering at the hands of a monster). One could see much of this man's life as an attempt at narcissistic denial of underlying, passive masochistic wishes.

As further memories of affectionate interactions with his mother were recovered, he began to weep, was depressed, and dreamed that I was pulling a big black thing out of the middle of him, a cancer that wouldn't come out but that would kill him if it did come out. The analysis, which had been pleasant for him before, now became extremely painful, and he insisted that I was deliberately humiliating him by forcing him to reveal his stupidity, because I knew the answers to all the questions that I was raising with him and he did not. I enjoyed making a helpless fool out of him. He dreamed he was in a psychiatrist's office in Brooklyn, which for him was a term of derogation, and receiving a special form of treatment. "I was hypnotized and totally helpless. People are ridiculing me, screaming guffaws like a fun house. Then I run down a hill through a big garage antique shop." In another dream at this time he was driving a huge shiny antique 1928 Cadillac in perfect condition. "As I am driving, the steering wheel comes apart, the right half of it comes off in my hand, then the big black shiny hood is gone, then the radiator cap is gone." He was born in 1928. At this time he also developed a transitory symptom of retarded ejaculation, which was a form of actively withholding the milk he insisted was being withheld from him.

The revival of repressed positive ties to his mother threatened his major masochistic and narcissistic characterological defenses. His entire sense of being exceptional depended on his pride in having suffered unusual deprivation at the hands of mother, and his entire experience of being loved and favored by his mother had been perceived by him as a threat of passive submission to a superior malicious force. He perceived this turn in the treatment as endangering his life of narcissistic and masochistic satisfactions and exposing him to the hazards of intimacy, mutual dependence, and a genuine recognition of the extent of his unconsciously sought-for bittersweet pleasure in self-damage and self-deprivation. The increasing recognition of a bond to me was accompanied by an exacerbation of the fantasy that I was the all-powerful, withholding mother and he was the victimized child. Loewenstein (1957) has remarked, "Masochism is the weapon of the weak—of every child—faced with the danger of human aggression." I would only emphasize that, indeed, every child, in his own perception, faces the danger of human aggression.

At this stage in treatment his injustice collecting surged to new refinements. Frequent requests for appointment changes, complicated dreams to which I did not have magical, brilliant interpretations, the fact that he was not already cured, my insistence that sessions had to be paid for—all of these were proof of my malicious withholding and of his innocent victimization. The injustice collecting, partly a result of fragile and fragmented self- and object representation, is also a guilt-relieving, rage-empowering reinforcement of masochistic and narcissistic defenses. These patients are indeed singled out for mistreatment by especially powerful figures to whom they have a special painful attachment.

After a great deal of working through, two incidents occurred that signaled a change in the transference. The first was that I had made an error in noting the date of an appointment he had cancelled. Instead of his usual reaction of outrage and indignation, he sat bolt upright on the couch, looking at me as if this were the first mistake I had ever made and said, "You mean, you make mistakes too?" The second incident occurred a few weeks later. After a particularly resistant session, I said, "I wish we could better understand your relationship to your mother." He was again startled and said, "You mean you really don't know the answer?" I assured him that I did not and that we would have to work it out together. He now began to acknowledge my reality as a human being, fallible and yet concerned for his welfare. Increasingly from this point the case tended to resemble that of a classical neurosis, although with many, many detours to deep masochistic and narcissistic issues.

One could further discuss the nature of the Oedipus complex in this type of patient, from this point of view, but that is beyond the scope of this paper.

SUMMARY

I have attempted to suggest, on the basis of genetic hypotheses and clinical data, that the themes of narcissism and masochism, crucial in all human psychic development, achieve their particular individual character at preoedipal stages of development. Furthermore, narcissistic tendencies and masochistic defenses are intimately and inevitably interwoven in the course of development; so interwoven, in fact, that I further suggest that the narcissistic character and the masochistic character are one and the same. I think the vast literature on these entities may become more coherent when considered from the point of view of a single nosological entity—the narcissistic-masochistic character.

In any particular person either the narcissistic or masochistic qualities may be more apparent in the lifestyle, as a result of internal and external contingencies that may be traced and clarified in the course of an analysis. A closer examination, however, will reveal the structural unity and mutual support of the two characterologic modes, despite the surface distinctions. Neither can exist without the other. Interpreting masochistic behavior produces narcissistic mortification, and interpreting narcissistic defenses produces feelings of masochistic victimization, self-pity, and humiliation.

The analysis of the narcissistic-masochistic character is always a difficult task. I hope that our changing frame of reference and the beginning elucidation of the genetic and clinical unity of the seemingly disparate pathologies may help to make our efforts more consistent, coherent, and successful.

REFERENCES

Auchincloss L: The Injustice Collectors, Boston, MA, Houghton Mifflin, 1950

Bergler E: The Basic Neurosis, Oral Regression and Psychic Masochism. New York, Grune & Stratton, 1949

Bergler E: Curable and Incurable Neurotics. New York, Liveright, 1961

Brenner C: The masochistic character: genesis and treatment. J Am Psychoanal Assoc 7:197–226, 1959

Cooper A: Psychoanalytic inquiry and new knowledge, in Reflections on Self Psychology. Edited by Lichtenberg J, Kaplan S. Hillsdale, NJ, Analytic Press, 1983

Dizmang L, Cheatham C: The Lesch-Nyhan Syndrome. Am J Psychiatry 127:131–137, 1970

Erikson E: Childhood and Society. New York, WW Norton, 1963

Fischer N: Masochism: Current concepts. J Am Psychoanal Assoc 29:673–688, 1981

Freud S: On the history of psycho-analytic movement (1914), in The Standard Edition of the Complete Psychological Works of Sigmund Freud [SE], Vol 14. Translated and edited by Strachey J. London, Hogarth Press, 1957, pp 7–66

Freud S: Beyond the pleasure principle (1920). SE, 18:3–66, 1955

Freud S: Female sexuality (1931). SE, 21:223–246, 1961

Freud S: Analysis, terminable and interminable (1937). SE, 23:250–251, 1964

Freud S: An outline of psychoanalysis (1938). SE, 23:141–208, 1964

Glover E: Technique of Psychoanalysis. New York, International Universities Press, 1955

Greenacre P: Regression and fixation: considerations concerning the development of the ego. J Am Psychoanal Assoc 8:703–723, 1960

Grossman WI: Notes on masochism: a discussion of the history and development of a psychoanalysis concept. Psychoanal Q 54:379–413, 1986

Hartmann H, Loewenstein RM: Notes on the superego. Psychoanal Study Child 17:42–81, 1962

Hermann I: Clinging-going-in-search: a contrasting pair of instincts and their relation to sadism and masochism. Psychoanal Q 44:5–36, 1976

Jacobson E: The Self and The Object World. New York, International Universities Press, 1964

Kohut H: The Analysis of the Self. New York, International Universities Press, 1971

Kohut H: Thoughts on narcissism and narcissistic rage. Psychoanal Study Child 27:360–400, 1972

Krafft-Ebing RF von: Psychopathia Sexualis. London, FA Davis, 1895

Lewin B: Psychoanalysis of Elation. New York, WW Norton, 1950

Loewenstein R: A contribution to the psychoanalytic theory of masochism. J Am Psychoanal Assoc 5:197–234, 1957

Mahler M: Rapprochement subphase of the separation-individuation process. Psychoanal Q 44:487–506, 1972

Maleson F: The multiple meanings of masochism in psychoanalytic discourse. J Am Psychoanal Assoc 32:325–356, 1984

Rado S: Adaptational Psychodynamics. New York, Science House, 1969

Sacher-Masoch L von: Sacher-Masoch: An Interpretation by Gilles Deleuze, together with the entire text of "Venus in Furs" [1870]. Translated by McNeil JM. London, Faber and Faber, 1971

Sandler J, Joffee WG: Towards a basic psychoanalytic model. Int J Psychoanal 50:79–90, 1969

Stoller RJ: The Sexual Excitement: Dynamics of Erotic Life. New York, Pantheon, 1979

Stolorow RD: The narcissistic function of masochism and sadism. Int J Psychoanal 56:441–448, 1975

Sullivan HS: The Interpersonal Theory of Psychiatry. New York, WW Norton, 1953

Trilling L: Beyond Culture. New York, Viking Press, 1963

Winnicott DW: Playing and Reality. New York, Basic Books, 1971

6

ROBERT N. EMDE, M.D.

INTRODUCTION

Robert Emde received his A.B. from Dartmouth College in Hanover, New Hampshire, and his M.D. from the Columbia University College of Physicians and Surgeons in New York. He did his psychiatric residency at the University of Colorado School of Medicine and analytic training at the Denver Institute of Psychoanalysis, where he is currently Emeritus Professor of Psychiatry at the University of Colorado Health Sciences Center. His first paper, in 1961, was "Sarcoptic Mange in the Human: A Report of an Epidemic of 10 Cases of Infection by *Sarcoptes scabiei,* Variety Canis," published in *Archives of Dermatology.* His second paper, in 1963, was "The Use of Intravenous Sodium Amytal to Overcome Resistance to Hypnotic Suggestion," in *The American Journal of Clinical Hypnosis,* and his third paper, in 1964 (in collaboration with P. Polak and R.A. Spitz), was "The Smiling Response I. Methodology, Quantification, and Natural History," published in *The Journal of Nervous and Mental Disease.* These three early papers are clues to the course of Dr. Emde's career. He is a careful observer of the external. He is interested in unconscious psychoanalytic processes and how they develop and are influenced, and he brings to his interest sophisticated quantitative and naturalistic research techniques. Dr. Emde is the author of almost 200 papers, which have brought rigorous methodology to the study of infant and child development. His interests are broad, ranging from the study of innate processes and their social influences to the study of almost every aspect of emotional and cognitive development and its social surround.

Dr. Emde has been a generative teacher for several generations of developmental clinical scientists and psychoanalysts. He is the author of 12 books in collaboration with others. His most recent titles are *Infancy to Early Childhood: Genetic and Environmental Influences on Developmental Change* and *Revealing the Inner Worlds of Young Children: The MacArthur Story Stem Battery and Parent-Child Narratives.*

Emde has said of himself:

> I am devoted to furthering several aspects of psychoanalysis in today's world. They include 1) a developmental orientation for psychoanalytic thinking and practice, 2) the growth of empirical research in psychoanalysis, 3) the incorporation of psychobiological and systems thinking in psychoanalysis, and 4) the infusion of critical thinking within psychoanalytic education. I have, with Peter Fonagy, been a founding faculty member of the Research Training Program and the International College of Research Fellows of the International Psychoanalytic Association (IPA) (see Emde and Fonagy 1997), and with Stuart Hauser I have been a founding co-chair of the Committee on Research in Education (CORE) of the Board of Professional Standards of the American Psychoanalytic Association as well as a Scientific Advisor to the Board.

Dr. Emde's work on early mother-infant communication and the mother's emotional responses to the infant's visual cliff behavior has been of enormous importance in alerting psychoanalysts to the affective core of mental life and to the relational roots of early affective and cognitive dispositions.

Dr. Emde has won multiple awards, has given plenary addresses to scientific organizations, and has delivered invited lectures in 22 countries outside the United States. He has served as Editor for the *Monographs of the Society for Research in Child Development* and Associate Editor for *The Journal of the American Psychoanalytic Association* and *Psychiatry.* He has also served in leadership roles for the Society for Research in Child Development, the World Association of Infant Mental Health, and many other interdisciplinary and clinical organizations. It would be difficult to overestimate his role in developmental psychiatry, the mental health community, and psychoanalysis. He has brought knowledge, information, and a research outlook to help change the way psychoanalysts see the world and conduct clinical practice.

WHY I CHOSE THIS PAPER

Robert N. Emde, M.D.

I am a thoroughgoing developmentalist. Developmental processes are biologically based and intrinsically social. Because we participate in development with others, and continue to do so throughout the life span, participating in development is an important consideration for the developmental orientation of psychoanalysis. Psychoanalytic therapeutic encounters rely on such processes for moving to new understandings and possibilities. In this essay, "Mobilizing Fundamental Modes of Development," I find it useful to specify a number of powerful developmental influences (or general motives) that we mobilize over time in meaningful psychoanalytic work with our patients. For my thinking, I draw not only on my clinical experience but also on my research experience with infants and young children. Observations of early development tend to highlight motivational processes that are biologically based, organizing, and universal. I chose this theoretical paper for inclusion in this volume because its principles underlie many of the other papers (empirical and theoretical) that I have written for the psychoanalytic literature as well as my two invited plenary addresses to IPA World Congresses.

REFERENCE

Emde RN, Fonagy P. An emerging culture for psychoanalytic research? Int J Psychoanal 78:643–651, 1997

MOBILIZING FUNDAMENTAL MODES OF DEVELOPMENT

Empathic Availability and Therapeutic Action

ROBERT N. EMDE, M.D.

THIS ESSAY WILL CONSIDER some new views of early developmental processes in terms of their contributions to a theory of therapy.

We begin with a major dilemma. Psychoanalytic theoreticians in recent decades have expressed insights about therapeutic action being connected to the early caregiving process. But formulations linking these two domains have not received wide acceptance in clinical work. Why? Upon reflection, several explanations seem possible. First, formulations have often been appealing metaphorically but have carried awkward implications about violating technical rules of analytic procedure. Second, formulations have often stood alone without integration with a larger body of clinical theory. The emotional aspect of the therapeutic experience received primary emphasis without connection to its better-known cognitive or interpretive aspects. Third, such formulations have not been integrated with knowledge from child observation or research; even more problematic

---

This work was supported by National Institute of Mental Health project grant MH22803, Research Scientist Award 5 K02 MH36808, and the John D. and Catherine T. MacArthur Foundation Network on Early Childhood Transitions.

"Mobilizing Fundamental Modes of Development: Empathic Availability and Therapeutic Action," by Robert N. Emde, M.D., was first published in *The Journal of the American Psychoanalytic Association*, 38:881–913, 1990.

when integrations have been attempted, little evidence of continuity has been found from early development to later development (see Emde 1981). Fourth, there has been a "leapfrogging" problem. Formulations bridging infancy experience to adult transference experiences in therapy or analysis have tended to be applied directly; there has been little regard for developmental processes operating in the years in between.

Controversies about Alexander's formulation of a "corrective emotional experience" in psychotherapy can be understood in this light (see original statement by Alexander [Alexander and French 1946], the challenge by Eissler [1950, 1953] and the later perspective by Lipton [1977]). So can more recent controversies about Kohut's (1971, 1977) formulation of what can be regarded as a "corrective empathic experience" (i.e., that empathic failures of primary caregivers during earliest childhood are causes of psychopathology that require later corrective empathic experiences during analysis).

I believe our views about these matters are enlarging. Clinicians have come to recognize that empathy occupies an important role in psychoanalytic work alongside that of interpretation (see Beres and Arlow 1974; Friedman 1978; Kohut 1959; Schafer 1959; Shapiro 1981; and Stolorow et al. 1987). Partly due to such recognition, Kohut's formulation, in spite of its problems, has received more clinical attention than was the case for Alexander's. Developmentalists, correspondingly, have come to recognize new aspects of continuity as well as change.

An earlier paper (Emde 1988) reviewed how current infancy research points to the centrality of the infant-caregiving relationship experience and of emotional availability in the context of that experience for establishing both continuity and the potential for later adaptive change. Moreover, linking infancy research with psychoanalytic clinical theory generated a proposal about motivational structures. The proposal is as follows. Early appearing motivational structures are strongly biologically prepared in our species, develop in the specific context of the infant-caregiver relationship, and persist throughout life. I have since realized that more can be said. These motivational structures can also be regarded as fundamental modes of development. As such, they are life-span processes that can be mobilized through empathy in the course of therapeutic action with adults.

DEVELOPMENTAL ASPECTS OF EMPATHY

Thinking about life-span developmental processes has been recognized as important by some (e.g., Benedek 1970; Bowlby 1988; Emde 1980;

Erikson 1950; Fleming 1975; Loewald 1960; Sander 1985; Settlage 1980) but has not been integrated into the mainstream of psychoanalysis. The following principles are ones that I believe are in need of emphasis as we consider the enabling role of empathy.

The first set of principles has to do with development in the individual. Development is a continuous process. It is ongoing, not only in childhood and adolescence, but through adulthood. Developmental influences, throughout life, are bidirectional with respect to the individual and others in the social environment. Moreover, development is an integrative process that is continuously organizing. With the symbolic capacities of the human, development makes use of the past so as to have a future orientation in the present.

The second set of principles has to do with development in context. Development occurs in the context of social relationships. Early caregiving relationships are formative because of the internalization of relationship experiences at the same time as representations of self and others are first taking place. Later relationships also "shape" or influence development in childhood and throughout life. Furthermore, later relationships can induce profound salutary influences on early internalized relationships that are problematic. This can occur when such relationships are intimate (i.e., when there is an atmosphere of commitment, trust, and emotional availability) and when the conditions exist for new dialogues and explorations to occur. Thus development is always to some extent mutual and shared.

The first set of principles puts us in mind of some general features in the *therapist* that are seldom discussed but seem important for empathy. The second set of principles puts us in mind of some general features of the *therapeutic process.*

THERAPIST FEATURES OF EMPATHY

The caregiving role is the first feature to be highlighted. Many psychoanalytic authors have pointed to the roots of the psychotherapist's empathy in the mutuality experiences provided within the early mother-child relationship (e.g., Deutsch 1926; Ferreira 1961; Gitelson 1962; Loewald 1960). Indeed, there is now substantial research evidence that the formative experience of caregiving in early childhood influences the later caregiving role of the child who becomes parent (Fraiberg et al. 1975; Main et al. 1985; Ricks 1985). Still, in psychoanalytic discussions about caregiving a key point is often neglected. The empathic response of the therapist models the role of the caregiver's response, not the infant's response. While it is true that those who have been given to are more likely to give in return, it seems unnecessarily complex for theoreticians to postulate that in order to care one must regress to the infantile experience and somehow then reverse that role. Therapeutic care makes use of adult caregiving functions.

Winnicott (1960) provided a basis for this realization when he asserted that psychoanalytic thinking about the parent-infant relationship requires thinking not only about the infant's side of the experience but also about mother's side of the experience. In particular, we need to think about the qualities and the changes in the mother that allow her to meet the developing needs of her infant. As Winnicott put it, there are two halves of a relationship theory, and this has often been neglected in our therapeutic applications. Spitz (1956) and later Gitelson (1962) wrote compellingly about the "diatrophic function of the analyst." This function involves the analyst's healing intention and, we might say, it involves countertransference in an affirmative sense. The assumption was that the diatrophic function derived from infancy, but we now know that it undoubtedly has independent, biological, and maturational contributions with respect to adult caregiving. As Papousek and Papousek (1979) have reviewed, there is clear evidence for a biological preparation for caregiving. From the standpoint of the knowledge of animal behavior and of Darwinian evolution, we might well ask: "How could it be otherwise?" How could the species survive without a strong biological preparedness for caregiving?

Since the psychology of caregiving includes a strong universal biological preparedness, we might well wonder if this preparedness is not activated by the therapist in the course of the psychotherapeutic-psychoanalytic relationship. If so, it deserves more of our attention. Will some therapists have more of this preparedness than others? Will some have more needs than others for attunement of this aspect of adult development?

A related aspect of adult development and the caregiving role has to do with the therapist's capacity for what I refer to as "developmental empathy." Empathy in therapeutic work is developmentally based. This kind of empathy requires considerable ego development, and it usually increases with age and experience. Transient identifications occurring in the midst of empathy require a temporary sense of oneness with the other, followed by a sense of separateness in order to be helpful. Also required is a sense of what is developmentally appropriate for the patient. This process is analogous to another aspect of early caregiving, namely, what has been referred to as operating in the zone of "proximal development." In this, a mother is affectively intimate and shares, but provides her child with the kind of environment needed to pull the child forward to a higher level of development—just enough but not too much. This aspect of adaptive caregiving, originally described by Vygotsky (1934, 1978), has since been documented and studied in the mainstream of developmental psychology by Bruner (1983), Kaye (1982), Rogoff (1987), and Wertsch (1985), among others.

In psychoanalysis, this feature of the therapist's activity has been noted by many. Beres and Arlow (1974) point out quite aptly that narcissistic individuals have difficulty being empathic because of their tendency to merge with another for the purpose of gratification, without ability to maintain a sense of separateness. Greenson (1960), Loewald (1960), and Schafer (1959) all discuss an empathic availability of the therapist that involves a dynamic and shifting view of the patient's potential. Schafer, in his notion of "generative empathy," indicates that this process is a "sublimated parental response" (p. 354), one that comes from a high level of psychic organization in the adult and promotes growth. Moreover, signal affects of the therapist are involved in empathy and, in addition to conflictual influences, one must consider preconscious and autonomous influences (Emde 1980; Engel 1962).

Greenson emphasizes that there can be two problematic extremes with respect to this process, one involving the inhibited empathizer and the other involving the uncontrolled empathizer. Thus empathy, like emotional availability in the caregiver, is a regulatory affective process. As such, just as in caregiving, there can be regulatory disturbances—of under-regulation and of over-regulation or of irregular/inconsistent regulation. Greenson's two types consist of the inhibited empathizer who is afraid to become involved with the patient and the uncontrolled empathizer who becomes too intensely involved, so that there is a loss of the position of observer and analyzer. As Greenson puts it, the therapist must become both detached and involved and allow for transitions between these two states. Others have noted similar features to be as important for empathy in the nonconflictual or broader sense (Ferenczi 1928; Fliess 1953; Kohut 1971; Reik 1936; Schafer 1959; Sharpe 1930). More recently, Shapiro (1981) has discussed the "misfirings" of empathic responsiveness having to do with countertransference or the current stresses or preoccupations of the analyst. Schafer (1959) emphasizes the "free availability of affect signals" (p. 348) in a regulatory process, such that the therapist moves between optimal states of involvement and of observation. Fleming (1975) includes a similar capacity in what she refers to as "systems sensitivity and responsiveness"—a cardinal skill of the analyst in which signal affects are sensed, available, and applied.

Creativity is another feature of the therapist that our developmental perspective brings into focus. Like caregiving, it is an aspect of adult development and probably shares some of its biological preparedness qualities. Empathic communication, for example, can be viewed as a creative act within the therapeutic relationship; it condenses multiple meanings, exercises tact and therefore, like the esthetic experience, has evocative ambiguity. It is also likely to give permission for expressing affects in a special protected context. As Schafer has pointed out, this therapeutic activity has a parallel with Kris's (1952) portrayal of the esthetic experience. In viewing a work of art, one seeks to achieve a balance between optimal distance and the esthetic illusion. All of this reminds us of a major caregiving function, one described so compellingly by Winnicott (1953) in terms of the "intermediate area of experience": a mother repeatedly fosters a special shared time with her child; judgments about logic and judgments about reality are suspended in order to enhance exploration and playfulness.

This brings us to a related aspect of the creative empathic attitude. It is playful. Not only does it encourage exploration in the midst of negative affects and what is painful, but it also encourages and makes use of the potential for surprise and other positive affects. The therapist's capacity for pleasurable surprise, in fact, seems basic for exploration and for the discovery of the unexpected (Reik 1936; Schafer 1959). Curiously, positive affects are seldom acknowledged in psychoanalytic literature on therapeutic activity. With the use of positive affects, however, there is not only an atmosphere of tolerance for errors but, in addition, an interest in them. Major errors are of course introduced by transference distortions. But, as several theorists have emphasized (Kohut 1977; Loewald 1980; Rothenberg 1987; see also discussion, below), transference has its positive affirmative aspects in addition to its self-defeating aspects.

Rothenberg (1987) has contributed a substantial psychoanalytically oriented treatise on the role of creativity in psychotherapy. Creativity is a valued, higher-order aspect of adult functioning. The therapist's creativity may manifest itself in the use of paradox, metaphor, and occasional humor, often with a sense of irony (with the therapist taking pleasure in that process). Rothenberg also emphasizes that empathy is a mutual creative process involving a "highly unstable sense of dynamic interactive sharing" (p. 64). As such, it is apt to be arousing, cognitively conflictual, and lead to new images and formulations. The creative therapist engages what Rothenberg describes as Janusian and homospatial processes in order to apprehend and grasp levels of experience across time and space. These are not reflections of primary process (condensation and displacement), but instead reflect complex abilities to mix levels of experience with both affective and cognitive components in order to achieve a creative outcome. Like the artist, the creative therapist, as Rothenberg points out, has a love for "the material" whether it be a puzzling dream report, a pattern of resistance or symptom formation, a personal fantasy, or a feeling of being blocked. I believe the creative therapist also has a love for the developmental process. There is an expectation that exploration will lead to both differentiation and integration. There is a persistent attitude of cautious optimism. Like the good mother, the therapist expresses a willingness to court uncertainty and tolerate anxiety in the interest of promoting exploration and growth.

A clinical vignette from Aichhorn's *Wayward Youth* (1951), cited in Schafer's (1959) paper on "generative empathy," illustrates how a paradoxical intervention can be a creative form of emotional responsiveness. The intervention moves the patient to the next step, explicitly recognizes autonomy, and allows for multiple options. In this vignette, Aichhorn tells a mistrustful defiant boy, "I'll make you a proposition... don't answer any question you don't like." The youth asks why. Aichhorn responds, "You wouldn't tell me the truth if I asked questions you didn't like." The youth then asks, "How did you know that?" Aichhorn responds, "Because that is what everybody does and you are no exception. I wouldn't tell everything either to someone whom I'd met for the first time."

We have emphasized the therapist features of empathy as those of adult development. Before leaving this topic, it is probably important to add one more point. Empathy, although based on emotional sensitivity and responsiveness, is exercised from a prepared mind. It involves more than emotion. As Kohut put it, empathy involves "vicarious introspection" (Kohut 1959). It depends on cognition, on perspective-taking, and on a knowledge base about the other person and the situation. The knowledge base that provides a background for empathy in therapeutic work is quite complex. It can be thought of as a set of schemas or as a "working model" of the patient (including past, current, and transference aspects) that undergoes continual updating over the course of treatment (Basch 1983; Greenson 1960).

PROCESS FEATURES OF EMPATHY

Most would agree that a goal of intensive psychotherapy and analysis is to obtain freedom from repeating the painful self-defeating patterns of the past. But there is also another important goal. This involves an affirmation of connections between past and current experience. It might be said that while we seek to establish a sense of discontinuity (putting the past in its place), we also seek to establish a sense of continuity (gaining a sense of ownership and connectedness with one's past, including both its positive aspects and the struggles that one has overcome). We might refer to this feature of the therapeutic process as *affirmative empathy*. With successful treatment the patient gains an affirmative sense of life continuity—both in terms of self- and other representations. As stated by Beres and Arlow (1974), a goal of psychoanalytic work is to enable the patient to develop an empathy for his self of the past, to see himself on a continuum from his early life to his current life, along with an acceptance of formerly repudiated aspects of himself. As Erikson (1950) put it, the goal is one of helping the patient to make his own biography. This has to do with affirming individuality and basic values rooted in biology, family, and culture. Kohut (1971) placed an affirmative empathic attitude at the center of the therapeutic process in his self psychology. Whatever else, most psychoanalytic clinicians undoubtedly convey a deep and abiding respect for a patient's individuality. What could be more affirming?

Another important feature of the process of empathy is that it involves *nonconscious as well as conscious* aspects. That empathy involves unconscious communication is a view that has a long history in psychoanalysis, at first given explicit statement by Deutsch (1926) and recently reviewed by Basch (1983). In addition to dynamic unconscious processes of the therapist, there are those processes that are preconscious and nonconscious in another sense. These are multiple, parallel information-processing capacities which involve sensing, selecting, filtering, integrating, and constructing. Some involve knowledge stores that are schematic and general while others involve knowledge stores that are episodic and particular. The cognitive sciences, including artificial intelligence, are making advances which will likely find direct application in our work (for psychoanalytically oriented integrations see Erdelyi 1984; Horowitz 1988; and Kihlstrom 1987). Similarly, the developmental sciences are likely to add important information that can be applied to the area of therapeutic functioning (Mandler 1983; Nelson 1986).

The mechanisms underlying unconscious communication have been addressed by psychoanalytic clinicians in limited fashion only. Beres and Arlow (1974) emphasize that empathy is mediated by nonverbal as well as verbal cues in a process analogous to the shared esthetic experience of the artist and his audience. Jacobs (1973) emphasizes the role of motor activity of the analyst (e.g., gestures engaged in unconsciously) in empathy, and Arlow (1969), in related fashion, discusses the role of motor metaphors in empathy.

Psychoanalytic clinicians have considered nonconscious aspects of empathy mainly from the viewpoint of shared experience between analyst and patient. This brings us to our third point about the process of empathic action: it involves *both shared and nonshared meaning.* Empathy involves signal affects connected with preconscious and unconscious fantasies; hence the dynamics of countertransference, as well as transference, must be considered. Many have emphasized the role of affective sharing in psychotherapeutic work (Beres and Arlow 1974; Greenson 1960; Little 1951; Racker 1958; Schafer 1959). Beres and Arlow (1974) emphasize the alerting role of the analyst's signal affect in understanding the patient's motivation and fantasy that is being shared. Moreover, the analyst comes to know the shared experience as involving a reexperiencing of the patient's past, whereas the patient experiences it totally in the present relationship (Little 1951).

A developmental perspective reveals a further fact: the shared affective experience between analyst and patient is one in which a new dyadic organizational field is created, one that is affirming both of the patient's common humanity and unique participating individuality. In other words, empathy is a mutual creative process wherein the independent validity of the therapeutic relationship experience is acknowledged. This process often involves metaphor that presents truth as manifold; it is a creative act wherein the whole is more than the sum of its parts (Rothenberg 1987). What we might call "transactional empathy" is a process in which the therapist can take multiple roles of self and other at the same time and transform the experience even as this is done. At appropriate times, such creative, generative empathy is shared with the patient with the goal of encouraging exploration.

In psychoanalytic work, the bulk of transactional empathy is probably nonconscious. Indeed, much of its components in terms of shared meaning may operate at the level of the dynamic unconscious. Greenson (1960) states that "for proper empathy, it is necessary to forget and re-repress *almost* as the patient does" (p. 422). But, the more I think about it, another quote from Beres and Arlow is quite extraordinary. I believe it would serve to separate analysts from all other individuals. The former would agree with it on some level, and the latter would think it mysterious. Beres and Arlow (1974) maintain that "a measure of the analyst's empathic capacity lies in his ability to be stimulated by the patient's unconscious fantasy when the analyst himself is not yet aware of the existence or the nature of the patient's unconscious fantasy" (p. 45).

DEVELOPMENTAL ASPECTS OF AVAILABILITY

One cannot have empathy without availability. Analysts agree that the availability of the professional helper is what sets the stage for therapeutic action. Availability is what fosters trust, confidence, and a consistency of expectations; it is therefore a presupposition for the therapeutic alliance. Developmental analogues in infancy and in caregiving have been described, both in terms of the patient's experience—"basic trust" (Erikson 1950), "confidence" (Benedek 1973)—and in terms of the analyst's experience—"diatrophic attitude" (Gitelson 1962; Spitz 1956).

As I see it, availability, both in the early caregiving situation and in the analytic/therapeutic situation, becomes manifest through regulation. Regulation ensures balance, the avoidance of extremes, and the maintenance of individual integrity during the flow of life; from a developmental view, regulation functions to ensure optimal exploration against a background of safety. This view is consistent with that advanced by psychoanalytic and developmental theorists including Sandler (1960), Sandler and Sandler (1978), Sameroff (1983), Sander (1985), and Sameroff and Emde (1989). The view is also consistent with the advice of textbook writers concerning analytic technique: the analyst needs to maintain a balance between affective experiencing and interpretive activity (Fenichel 1941; Thomä and Kächele 1987). Correspondingly, this section will discuss developmental aspects of two forms of therapeutic availability. One occurs through affect regulation. The other occurs through interpretation.

Availability Through Affect Regulation

This is a developmental analogue that begins with uncertainty. Uncertainty and related affective experiences generally signal a state of mind that in the presence of an empathic, responsive other leads to a searching tendency. We might say that the emotional availability of the therapist involves not only a tolerance, but an encouragement for experiencing uncertainty and some anxiety as a shared interactive experience in order to encourage exploration and the possibility of new directions.

That this has a developmental analogue is illustrated by recent research on social referencing in infancy. Social referencing is a process whereby an individual, when confronted with a situation of uncertainty, seeks out emotional information from a significant other in order to resolve the uncertainty and regulate behavior accordingly. In our experimental social referencing paradigms we have constructed situations of uncertainty that involve an unfamiliar toy robot, an unfamiliar person, or a glass-topped crawling surface with an apparent drop-off (the so-called "visual cliff"). When an infant, in the course of exploration, encounters the uncertainty situation (e.g., the apparent drop-off surface) he looks to mother's face. If she signals fear or anger, the infant ceases exploration or withdraws; if she signals pleasure or interest, the infant continues exploration (Emde 1983; Klinnert et al. 1983; Sorce et al. 1985). Social referencing has also been documented in situations of uncertainty involving parental prohibitions and in the more free ranging explorations of toddlers. The social referencing of toddlers reminds one of "checking back" and "emotional re-fueling" as described by Mahler and her colleagues (Mahler et al. 1975) and of using mother as a "secure base" for exploration as described by Ainsworth and her colleagues (Ainsworth et al. 1978).

But in therapy as well as in infancy, total availability would not be helpful. Winnicott (1958) described the important state of "being alone in the presence of the other." There are moments where the patient may be reviewing, thinking through issues, or perhaps having other vital affective experiences. These are moments when the therapist needs only to be silent and indicate a supportive presence. Such moments remind me of some paradoxical times in our infant studies when mothers appear to signal their own emotional unavailability as part of being emotionally available in a larger context. Instead of emotional unavailability, we have come to appreciate this as a different level of emotional availability. This occurs, for example, when mother is busily doing something such as reading, preparing a meal, or talking on the telephone; she signals she is unavailable to the child by subtleties of glance and direction of looking. If the relationship is going well, the child understands these signals and continues with exploration, play, or other activity. It is as if the mother is saying, "I will be available later" or "I will be available if you really need me if you are hurt."

Similarly, the therapist is not always giving or expressing availability. Indeed, this would be intrusive. Emotional availability in the therapeutic sense involves, in a paramount way, respect for the patient's development. If one is too expressive or giving, one may obscure opportunities for development and, in more intensive work, one might obscure the unfolding of repetitive neurotic patterns and their integration.

It has been said that no therapy works unless you become part of the problem, and that psychoanalysis does not work unless you become most of the problem. In addition to the obvious reference to the centrality of the transference neurosis, the saying has reference—on the analyst's side—to such aspects as "role responsiveness," as discussed by Sandler (1976), and immersions in projective identifications and productive countertransferences, as discussed by Ogden (1979) and Fleming and Benedek (1966). Still, all of these developments occur in a contained—or regulated—sense. A special context allows for this kind of experience. The context is one where there is a shared zone of understanding for both patient and analyst. In addition to a shared sense of the openness about what can be expressed, there is a shared sense of safety and restraint about what will not happen. One thinks of child analysis where the latter understanding is sometimes more direct by virtue of words and action. Particularly with the young child, the analyst sometimes prohibits with statements of what is inappropriate and even says "no" on occasion. This is usually seen as the analyst's being emotionally available and participating in a form of special developmental experience with the child.

In the intensive therapeutic process, one attends to current affective states and inferred signal affects, as well as what the patient is attempting to accomplish. One places one's own signal affect processes at the patient's disposal and allows a resonance with what the patient is attempting to communicate. This reminds us of two other developmental analogues of affect regulation. The most obvious is affective mirroring, a confirmatory experience both in therapeutic action and in early caregiving that has been so well articulated by Kohut (1971, 1977). Another is what might be referred to as the provision of affective "scaffolding" by the therapist. As Kohut (1977), and Stolorow et al. (1987) have pointed out, mother's soothing and comforting of negative affects provides a basis for the child's tolerance and for "dosing" of affects (cf. the "holding environment" of Winnicott [1960]). The patient, like the young child, learns from the therapeutic experience about how to "dose" particular affects in certain circumstances. One might carry this a step further and say, following the developmentalist Vygotsky, that this illustrates a process whereby one learns from another by means of "scaffolding" and pulling forward in development—in this case by the therapist (in analogy to mother) demonstrating and making possible the use of affects as internal signals.

Availability Through Interpretation

This is a developmental analogue that emphasizes movement and direction. Such availability includes an appreciation not only of complex affects, but of complex intentions, and of a wider cognitive range that contributes to the patient's feeling of "being understood." But in a fundamental way, the availability of the therapist does more: it anticipates movement and encourages exploration. Spitz (personal communication) used to say that a good psychoanalytic interpretation guides the patient to his next step. I have found this a powerful metaphor from early caregiving. A similar sentiment is expressed by Rothenberg (1987) who discusses creative interventions (metaphor, paradox, and irony) as "enacted types of interpretations" (p. 180) that are geared to stimulating patient response in a new direction.

There is something else that needs to be said about availability through interpretation. Like the caregiver's scaffolding, therapeutic interpretations exert a "pull" to a higher level of integration. In the words of Loewald (1960), such interpretations therefore represent "the mutual recognition involved in the creation of identity of experience in two individuals of different levels of ego-organization. Insight gained in such an interaction is an integrative experience" (p. 25).

Loewald also reminds us with his discussion that this kind of integration is not necessarily a conscious process. Similarly, Blum (1979) points out that Freud (1893), in an early case report, discusses the attainment of insight even though the patient was not conscious of the dynamic connections that led to therapeutic outcome.

Finally, we should note that there are limitations to availability through interpretation. In the course of treatment, there is often a focus on separations and reunions in the context of the therapeutic relationship and its meaning; understanding such events is likely to lead to new capacities and to increasing autonomy. Still, understanding variations in interactive availability is limited by virtue of exploring dyadic representations; there is a need for exploring triadic representations, conflicts, and structuring. There is also a need for exploration beyond the therapeutic encounter, for consolidating and extending integrations by practicing experiences with family, peers, and friends.

MOBILIZING FUNDAMENTAL MODES OF DEVELOPMENT

The role of empathy in therapeutic action has gained increasing recognition alongside that of interpretation in psychoanalytic work. A developmental perspective serves to highlight certain features. Empathy, from the therapist's side, depends on adult functioning rather than on a regressive repetition of infantile experience. Caregiving and creative aspects of empathy are adult competencies. These aspects of empathy have strong connections with fostering development in early childhood, and they are also important for development in psychotherapy. Empathic processes, both in early caregiving and in psychotherapy, tend to be affirmative, nonconscious, and shared experiences. Again, strong analogues to early development are apparent. In infancy there is a fostering of development by communications that are mostly nonverbal, emotional, and nonconscious; moreover, much of shared meaning is implicit, procedural, and expanding in the midst of new explorations. Finally, we have learned that there are important developmental aspects of therapeutic availability. Similar to this process in early caregiving, consistent availability is paramount for fostering the kind of special development we usually refer to as therapeutic action. Such availability involves regulation as its central functional aspect, both in terms of optimizing affective signaling and interpretive activity.

The foregoing discussion has emphasized that psychoanalytic clinicians have described cogent analogues to processes of therapeutic action in the early caregiving situation. Some of these, from the therapist's side, are analogous to the caregiving role and to related features of adult development. Others, from the patient's side, are analogous to infant developmental experiences in the context of the early caregiving relationship. Now we come to a crucial point. These are not just analogues. I believe that what we have been articulating and what three decades of clinicians have been describing are not so much analogues as they are basic developmental principles. The introduction to this essay alluded to a proposal along this line. Certain early-appearing motivational structures are strongly biologically prepared, necessary for development, and persist throughout life. Developing in the specific context of the infant-caregiver relationship, these structures can also be regarded as fundamental modes of development. As such, they can be mobilized through empathy so as to enhance therapeutic action with adults.

What I propose about therapeutic action owes much to Loewald and to others who have conceptualized the psychoanalytic process as a special form of developmental experience. It is fully consistent with a good deal of self psychology, as well as object-relations theory and recent work on projective identification and countertransference. It is also consistent with recent infancy research. What it adds from a theoretical standpoint, however, is an important biological framework—one that might be referred to as an evolving, sometimes "silent" biology that operates throughout life.

I believe there are fundamental motivational aspects of the developmental process that first appear in infancy. Basic motives of activity, self-regulation, social fittedness, and affective monitoring have been identified as species-wide regulatory functions that are preprogrammed by our evolutionary biology. They are universal features of normal development, and perhaps this universality accounts for why they are generally assumed by our theories and are not specified as motivations. Still, when such motives are normatively brought into play by an infant who "exercises" them with an emotionally available parenting figure, they facilitate the development of important psychological structures prior to 3 years of age. The first of these is a consolidation of the affective core of self. The second is the development of a sense of reciprocity, rules, and empathy, as well as some aspects of early moral internalization (for example, the internalization of prohibitions). Social referencing of the parent in the midst of the infant's expanding interest in the world contributes to an enhanced sense of shared meaning and is considered important in this process. A third structure that develops in such circumstances has only recently been appreciated. In an adaptive caregiving environment, and with sufficient positive emotions, these early motivational structures can contribute to the development of an executive sense of "we."

Although much research is needed, there is every reason to believe that important individual differences exist with respect to these early-appearing motivational structures. Although untested, I wonder if the infant-caregiver relationship experience does not have an influence on these early motivational structures of a unique sort, one that is pervasive and resistant to later change with experience. At times I have even wondered whether such an early influence on experience, especially when reactivated in subsequent life relationships, might contain elements of what we have thought of as "constitutional." I believe such a view is consistent with that of psychoanalytic clinical theorists, including Loewald (1971), Kernberg (1976), Kohut (1977), Sander (1985), and Robbins (1983).

The assumption I am making is that psychopathology, to a greater or lesser extent, is developmental psychopathology. One's developmental thrust through life has gotten "off track" or has been blocked in some way. Setting forth therapeutic action involves amelioration through a special form of developmental experience. It is interactive, it rests on empathy, and it mobilizes fundamental modes of development.

A NEW BEGINNING IN THERAPEUTIC ACTION

My formulation owes a special debt to the thinking of Hans Loewald. The phrase "therapeutic action" in my title is taken from Loewald's generative 1960 essay in which he conceptualized the therapeutic process from a developmental orientation. Loewald pointed to the importance of thinking about interaction processes between analyst and patient. In an analysis, one observes and explores primitive as well as more advanced interaction processes, with steps in ego integration and disintegration. In other words, the analyst is a co-actor, especially on the "analytic stage" on which child development and the infantile neurosis are reenacted. Development is set in motion by the fact that the analyst makes himself available for a new internalized relationship. In Loewald's words: "Analysis is thus understood as an intervention designed to set ego-development in motion...not simply by the technical skill of the analyst, but by the fact that the analyst makes himself available for the development of a new 'object-relationship'" (p. 17).

Loewald borrowed the idea of a "new beginning" from Balint (1952) in order to refer to the developmental opportunities provided by the psychoanalytic experience. Balint was apparently using more than a loose metaphor in his phrase for he referred to an impetus toward development that can occur, almost a developmental drive. In a similar vein, others have discussed the dyadic conditions required for the opening phase of analysis. Gitelson (1962) referred to these conditions as setting up a "primitive rapport," and Glover (1955) referred to it as a "readiness for transference." Loewald (1960) referred to a dynamism involving a diffuse potential for loving and hating transference which mobilizes drives and allows them to be deployed for a new developmental beginning. In his view, "curative factors" in the opening phase of psychoanalysis are similar to conditions found in "the early 'more or less' good mother-child situation" (p. 196).

Another theoretician who provides a groundwork for the current formulation is Gitelson (1962). Gitelson, like Loewald, indicated the possibility of strong early developmental forces that could be activated in treatment. He refers to "curative factors" as "a second presentation in the analytic situation of influences that originally operate to favor more or less normal development" (p. 198). Gitelson's idea was that in the analytic situation, there is an induction of an infantile dyadic condition that gathers the impetus for a developmental thrust. Both Gitelson and Loewald indicate that in the fostering of this condition, the analyst has no personal stake. There is no manipulation. Psychoanalysis may best be regarded as a special form of developmental experience. A neurotic system, closed off in early development, can be opened and developmental processes can be reactivated in psychoanalysis. One should add that what begins in psychoanalysis is not infantile or regressive. It is true that what begins reminds us of infancy because we see a setting condition for mobilizing basic motivational processes. But the latter, although salient in infancy, operate throughout life in the context of intimate relationships. It is for this reason that I now refer to these as fundamental modes of development.

Toward an "Executive We" in Therapeutic Action

The middle phase of analysis is when there is a deepening of transference experiences and their resistances. In the course of work, there is an expanding sense of meaning. This phase is usually portrayed as the time when there is the development and the working through of the transference neurosis. In Loewald's terms, there is a resumption of ego development in general because of the analyst's availability as a new object. I prefer to put it slightly differently. The middle phase is one in which the analyst is available to the patient for a dynamic transactional experience in which there is an increasing respect for individuality, defensive struggling, and the quest for truth. Both participants engage in a contrasting of "now" versus "then" experiences in the light of varying transference manifestations. Exploration is jointly valued in the face of conflict.

I believe this process is enabled by virtue of a new shared meaning structure that develops. The sense of mutuality has now progressed within the patient-analyst relationship experience to the point where the patient's "executive we" is affective as well as cognitive. In addition to the analyst's emotional availability providing a "background of safety" for overall analytic work (Sandler 1960), the analyst serves as a "beacon of orientation" (Mahler et al. 1975), providing reassurance for new directions and more specific work. Exploration can go on in the midst of uncertainty and painful emotions. In other words, throughout the middle phase of analysis, the analyst is used as a reference point for exploration. One could use the word "mirroring" from the literature of Kohut and of Lacan—to describe the analyst's responsiveness—but I prefer the Mahlerian metaphor of a "beacon of orientation," since it is less passive and implies guidance for developmental activity.

Moreover, from the vantage point of fundamental modes of development, we can now add some further details to this process. Normative, biologically prepared processes are actualized, and they depend on the interactive, emotional availability of the analyst. Loewald (1960) implied much of this, stating: "We postulate thus internalization of an interaction-process, not simply internalization of 'objects,' as an essential element in ego-development as well as in the resumption of it in analysis" (p. 30).

We are reminded that moments of intense feelings of togetherness and of shared meaning are extremely important for psychoanalytic work. They often precede and surround productive work within interpretive activity and they contribute to the regulation of previously warded-off affects. It is also the case that such moments occur at different levels of organization (and co-organization).

J. Jacobson (1987, unpublished) provides a clinical discussion of such moments. The analyst's responsive empathy is a form of deep mutuality that allows for the patient's security and for further exploration. Jacobson provides a clinical vignette where the therapist's interpretation is seen as an emotionally available response to the patient. A patient's provocative statement reminds Jacobson of our research observations of social referencing. He then understands the patient's comment as

> a questioning glance at the mother to see if this area was going to be acceptable and tolerable to the "caregiver." I think patients often enter new areas in this kind of way, anticipating disapproval or catastrophe in some form, and then scrutinizing us closely for our responses. The concept of referencing behaviors gives us a valid respect for the Darwinian survival dimensions which, in some instances, form the underpinning of these behaviors.

Others have discussed the sense of mutuality and shared meaning as an important background variable for psychoanalytic work. Sandler (1988) equates the sense of "we" in treatment to a "background sense of mutuality" that is present in some patients in their analytic experience. What I refer to is more, however, involving a sense of confidence, even a sense of some power in the midst of uncertainty and painful affects. Over time, this sense incorporates shared meaning from therapeutic experience and gains momentum and dynamic directionality. In its original optimal form, I have referred to it as an "executive we." In its adaptive form during psychoanalysis, it will become part of a mutually endorsed self-analyzing function.

An intriguing incentive for this kind of clinical thinking comes from Eastern psychoanalysis. It can be said that Western thinking and psychoanalysis have been typified by an "I-thou" dialectic and have heretofore been relatively oblivious to ideas of a "we" sense or of an "I-we" dialectic. Not so for Eastern thought. Perhaps it is a welcome irony that in our Western current era, so preoccupied with concerns about narcissism, we may be shifting to a world view that incorporates an Eastern "we" sense. The writings of Takeo Doi, concerning a universal aspect of a culturally embedded Japanese form of passive love, now seems headed for intensive discussion. This form of love, originating in infancy, and known as *amae,* may also be a fundamental process of importance that is influenced by variations in early caregiving. Salient in Japanese culture, it reflects a profound sense of mutuality and a "we" sense that becomes internalized in infancy and guides behavior throughout the life span. Although much of *amae* is implicit, automatic, and beyond awareness—manifesting itself in procedural rather than declarative knowledge—Doi attempts to objectify its structure and decode it. In so doing, he finds universal features applicable to the psychoanalytic treatment relationship (Doi 1987, unpublished). We await his further work.

We return again to interpretation. Empathy does not automatically lead to change. Interpretation of internal conflict in the context of the transference remains the sine qua non for therapeutic action. But the analyst's empathic availability during the middle phase is what fosters interpretation. The thinking of Loewald (1960) is especially instructive in this area. He indicates there is an analytic "pull" toward higher levels of differentiation and integration. An analogy is made to the early parent-child experience wherein the parent exerts such a pull—even though Loewald is apparently not aware of the background for this view in the developmental research of Vygotsky. Loewald speaks of the "positive nature" of the "neutrality" of the analyst which includes

> the capacity for mature object-relations, as manifested in the parent by his or her ability to follow and, at the same time, be ahead of the child's development.... In analysis, a mature object relationship is maintained with a given patient if the analyst relates to the patient in tune with the shifting levels of development manifested by the patient at different times, but always from the viewpoint of potential growth, that is, from the viewpoint of the future. (p. 20)

Thus the sense of "we" that develops in analysis, in analogy to the early caregiving experience, organizes (by interpretation) what was previously less organized. That is, it mediates a higher level of organization, and then a new level of "we" can develop. One therefore wonders: are there not cycles of "we" that occur in development (including in psychoanalysis) that facilitate successive processes of integration? That Loewald sees a basic developmental process at work is indicated by the following:

> the higher organizational stage of the environment is indispensable for the development of the psychic apparatus.... Without such a "differential" between organism and environment, no development takes place... The analyst functions as a representative of a higher stage of organization and mediates this to the patient. (p. 24)

Analytic work is not easy. Disorganization and reorganization are recurring processes within the analytic experience. Loewald uses an example very much like the visual cliff we have used in our infant social referencing studies: "The fear of reliving the past is fear of toppling off a plateau we have reached and fear of that more chaotic past itself... genuine reintegration requires psychic 'work'" (p. 26). Indeed, a social referencing process in analysis may contribute to exploration and integration as Jacobson has suggested.

We have already implied that the special therapeutic atmosphere of shared meaning allows for a reexperiencing of the past such that it is not only less frightening, but becomes a potential source of affirmative continuity. Loewald (1960) speaks of this process as a form of shared meaning in which "ghosts" of the past are liberated in the transference and then converted to ancestors.

One might say that there are three aspects of reexperiencing from the early caregiving experience. There are early *modes* of relating which will be reexperienced; there are early *conflicts* in relating which will be reexperienced; and there are early incorporated images and attitudes of the parent which will be reexperienced as a part of the self (a distorted "mirroring"). In other words, the patient may come to reexperience an early childhood core of himself—"seeing as he was seen"—*then*. He will misinterpret this experience in the transference as applying to the *now*. The analyst's availability is to help the patient clear away transference distortions and see himself as he is seen now.

A Biblical passage offers poetic illustration of this process. It suggests hope about social referencing and the mobilizing of a new sense of "we."

> When I was a child, I spake as a child, I understood as a child, I thought as a child: But when I became a man, I put away childish things. For now we see through a glass, darkly; But then face to face; Now I know in part; But then shall I know even as also I am known. (13 Corinthians, Holy Bible, King James version)

A few words about the termination process. In terminating, there is a necessary reworking not only of conflicts about leaving, but also of what has been experienced throughout treatment. The patient needs to put in place the shared meaning of what has occurred. Correspondingly, the analyst needs to acknowledge the validity of the patient's increasing autonomy. We are reminded again of a basic feature of the development process: in early caregiving secure attachment generates exploration (Bowlby 1969); in like manner, the capacity for intimacy and the capacity for autonomy develop alongside each other—they do not compete.

STEPS BEYOND

In concluding, we return to our opening thoughts about analytic technique in the light of a historical perspective. We again see the need for a balanced perspective. Viewing therapeutic action as a corrective emotional experience and viewing it as a corrective empathic experience portrays the therapeutic relationship as complementary. The patient is portrayed in negative terms (i.e., having an early childhood deficit or distortion needing correction) and the therapist is portrayed in positive terms (i.e., having a mature empathy that can provide for a corrective experience). An expanding clinical literature on countertransference broadens this view—on the negative side (see Emde 1988). The therapist, like the patient, is also seen as having negative aspects (i.e., distortions in empathy); such negative aspects occur commonly and, if taken into account, are used to advantage in therapeutic action. This essay adds balance to the broadened view—on the positive side. There are positive aspects of patient as well as analyst. An important, biologically prepared, positive developmental thrust becomes mobilized in the patient by virtue of therapeutic action. This thrust is specified in terms of a set of fundamental modes of development that have been identified through recent developmental research. These modes begin in infancy, and may or may not get deflected during early experience, but they continue as a developmental potential throughout life. The therapeutic relationship provides the setting conditions that allow for fundamental modes of development to be reactivated. The empathic availability of the therapist is deemed especially important in enabling these modes to operate as powerful background influences in our work.

Our positive, optimistic essay must end with some cautionary points. First, it is important to remember that a sense of mutuality and "we" can be resisted in therapy and may require vigorous interpretive work (Sandler 1988). Second, in spite of the positive forces we have enumerated, the therapeutic process is apt to be a difficult one. There are aspects of early experience that severely limit the capacity for change. Perhaps these aspects are close to what Freud referred to as "constitutional" and stem from early internalized relationship experiences. Perhaps these aspects are what Anna Freud referred to as "ego restrictions" and represent a psychobiological "bedrock" that is especially difficult to change (Sandler 1988). Third, we must not idealize empathy. As Shapiro (1981) has pointed out, there are hazards stemming from errors in the analyst's empathic responsiveness. Similar to what Glover (1931) documented for inexact or premature interpretations, there can be untoward effects of empathic "misfiring" such as intellectualization, a thickening of defenses, or increasing dependence. We are reminded that every therapeutic intervention—whether an interpretation, an empathic affirmation, or a nonresponse to a question—requires sensitivity, tact, and appropriate timing. The analyst must attend both to the patient's immediate needs and to the developmental process of analysis. There are times when the analyst's empathic responsiveness, paradoxically, calls for silence; at such times it is well to remember that, like in early caregiving, not intervening can promote exploration, and not being intrusive can allow development.

Our fourth cautionary point is the most important of all. We need more knowledge. Processes of empathic availability are not outside of natural science as some have feared (Shapiro 1981). Emotional communication is the subject of increasing empirical inquiry (see Campos et al. 1983). Correspondingly, the formulations of this essay regarding the fundamental modes of development and their therapeutic activation will be of value only if they meet an empirical test. They must guide trials of application and lead to research.

REFERENCES

Aichhorn A: Wayward Youth. London, Imago, 1951

Ainsworth MDS, Blehar M, Waters E, Wall S: Patterns of Attachment. Hillsdale, NJ, Lawrence Erlbaum, 1978

Alexander F, French TM: The principle of flexibility, in Psychoanalytic Therapy: Principles and Application. New York, Ronald Press, 1946

Arlow JA: Motor behavior as nonverbal communication. J Am Psychoanal Assoc 17:955–967, 1969

Balint M: New beginning and the paranoid and the depressive syndromes. Int J Psychoanal 33:214–224, 1952

Basch MF: Empathic understanding: a review of the concept and some theoretical considerations. J Am Psychoanal Assoc 31:101–126, 1983

Benedek T: Parenthood during the life cycle, in Parenthood: Its Psychology and Psychopathology. Edited by Anthony EJ, Benedek T. Boston, MA, Little, Brown, 1970, pp 185–206

Benedek T: Adaptation to Reality in Early Infancy: Psychoanalytic Investigations. New York, Quadrangle, 1973

Beres D, Arlow JA: Fantasy and identification in empathy. Psychoanal Q 43:26–50, 1974

Blum HP: The curative and creative aspects of insight. J Am Psychoanal Assoc 27(suppl):41–69, 1979

Bowlby J: Attachment and Loss, Vol 1: Attachment. New York, Basic Books, 1969

Bowlby J: Developmental psychiatry comes of age. Am J Psychiatry 145:1–10, 1988

Bruner J: Child's Talk. New York, WW Norton, 1983

Campos JJ, Barrett, KC, Lamb ME, Goldsmith HH, Stenberg C: Socioemotional development, in Handbook of Child Psychology, Vol 2. Edited by Mussen PH. New York, Wiley, 1983

Deutsch H: Occult processes occurring during psychoanalysis (1926), in Psychoanalysis and the Occult. Edited by Devereux G. New York, International Universities Press, 1953, pp 133–146

Eissler KR: The Chicago Institute of Psychoanalysis and the sixth period of the development of psychoanalytic technique. J Gen Psychol 42:103–157, 1950

Eissler KR: The effect of the structure of the ego on psychoanalytic technique. J Am Psychoanal Assoc 1:104–143, 1953

Emde RN: A developmental orientation in psychoanalysis: ways of thinking about new knowledge and further research. Psychoanal Contemp Thought 3:213–235, 1980

Emde RN: Changing models of infancy and the nature of early development: remodeling the foundation. J Am Psychoanal Assoc 29:179–219, 1981

Emde RN: The prerepresentational self and its affective core. Psychoanal Study Child 38:165–192, 1983

Emde RN: Development terminable and interminable, I: innate and motivational factors from infancy. Int J Psychoanal 69:23–42, 1988

Engel E: Anxiety and depression withdrawal: the primary affects of unpleasure. Int J Psychoanal 43:89–97, 1962

Erdelyi NH: Psychoanalysis: Freud's Cognitive Psychology. San Francisco, CA, WH Freeman, 1984

Erikson EH: Childhood and Society. New York, WW Norton, 1950

Fenichel O: Problems of Psychoanalytic Technique. New York, Psychoanalytic Quarterly, 1941

Ferenczi S: The elasticity of psychoanalytic technique (1928), in Problems and Methods of Psychoanalysis. New York, Basic Books, 1955, pp 7–102

Ferreira AJ: Empathy and the bridge function of the ego. J Am Psychoanal Assoc 9:91–105, 1961

Fleming J: Some observations on object constancy in the psychoanalysis of adults. J Am Psychoanal Assoc 23:743–759, 1975

Fleming J, Benedek T: Psychoanalytic Supervision. New York, Grune & Stratton, 1966

Fliess R: Countertransference and counteridentification. J Am Psychoanal Assoc 1:268–284, 1953

Fraiberg S, Adelson E, Shapiro V: Ghosts in the nursery. J Child Psychiatry 14:387–421, 1975

Freud S: A case of successful treatment by hypnotism (1893), in The Standard Edition of the Complete Psychological Works of Sigmund Freud [SE], Vol 1. Translated and edited by Strachey J. London, Hogarth Press, 1966, pp 115–128

Freud S: Lines of advance in psycho-analytic therapy (1918). SE, 17:157–168, 1955

Friedman L: Trends in the psychoanalytic theory of treatment. Psychoanal Q 47:524–567, 1978

Gitelson M: The curative factors in psycho-analysis, I: the first phase of psychoanalysis. Int J Psychoanal 43:194–204, 1962

Glover E: The therapeutic effect of inexact interpretation: a contribution to the theory of suggestion. Int J Psychoanal 12:397–411, 1931

Glover E: The Technique of Psychoanalysis. New York, International Universities Press, 1955

Goldberg A (ed): The Psychology of the Self: A Casebook. New York, International Universities Press, 1978

Greenson RR: Empathy and its vicissitudes. Int J Psychoanal 41:418–424, 1960

Horowitz MJ: Introduction to Psychodynamics: A New Synthesis. New York, Basic Books, 1988

Jacobs TJ: Posture, gesture, and movement in the analyst: cues to interpretation and countertransference. J Am Psychoanal Assoc 21:77–92, 1973

Kaye K: The Mental and Social Life of Babies. Chicago, IL, University of Chicago Press, 1982

Kernberg OF: Object Relations Theory and Clinical Psychoanalysis. New York, Jason Aronson, 1976

Kihlstrom JF: The cognitive unconscious. Science 237:1445–1452, 1987

Klinnert MD, Campos J, Sorce JF, Emde RN, Svejda MJ: Social referencing: emotional expressions as behavior regulators, in Emotion: Theory, Research and Experience, Vol 2: Emotions in Early Development. Edited by Plutchik R, Kellerman H. Orlando, FL, Academic Press, 1983, pp 57–86

Kohut H: Introspection, empathy, and psychoanalysis: an examination of the relationship between mode of observation and theory. J Am Psychoanal Assoc 7:459–483, 1959

Kohut H: The Analysis of the Self. New York, International Universities Press, 1971

Kohut H: The Restoration of the Self. New York, International Universities Press, 1977

Kris E: Psychoanalytic Explorations in Art. New York, International Universities Press, 1952

Lipton SD: The advantages of Freud's technique as shown in his analysis of the Rat Man. Int J Psychoanal 41:16–33, 1977

Little M: Counter-transference and the patient's response to it. Int J Psychoanal 32:32–40, 1951

Loewald HW: On the therapeutic action of psycho-analysis. Int J Psychoanal 41:16–33, 1960

Loewald HW: On motivation and instinct theory. Psychoanal Study Child 26:91–128, 1971

Loewald HW: Reflections on the psychoanalytic process and its therapeutic potential, in Papers on Psychoanalysis. New Haven, CT, Yale University Press, 1980, pp 372–383

Mahler MS, Pine R, Bergman A: The Psychological Birth of the Human Infant: Symbiosis and Individuation. New York, Basic Books, 1975

Main M, Kaplan N, Cassidy J: Security in infancy, childhood, and adulthood: a move to the level of representation, in Growing Points in Attachment Theory and Research. Edited by Bretherton I, Waters E. Monogr Soc Res Child Dev 50:66–104, 1985

Mandler J: Representation, in Handbook of Child Psychology, Vol 3. Edited by Mussen PH. New York, Wiley, 1983, pp 420–494

Nelson K: Event Knowledge. Hillsdale, NJ, Lawrence Erlbaum, 1986

Ogden TH: On projective identification. Int J Psychoanal 60:357–373, 1979

Papousek H, Papousek M: Early ontogeny of human social interaction: its biological roots and social dimensions, in Human Ethology: Claims and Limits of a New Discipline. Edited by Foppa K, Lepenies W, Ploog D. Cambridge, UK, Cambridge University Press, 1979, pp 456–489

Racker H: Psychoanalytic technique and the analyst's unconscious masochism. Psychoanal Q 27:555–562, 1958

Reik T: Surprise and the Psychoanalyst. London, Kegan Paul, 1936

Ricks MH: The social transition of parental behavior: attachment across generations, in Growing Points in Attachment Theory and Research. Edited by Bretherton I, Waters E. Monogr Soc Res Child Dev 50:211–227, 1985

Robbins M: Toward a new mind model for the primitive personalities. Int J Psychoanal 64:127–148, 1983

Rogoff B: The joint socialization of development by young children and adults, in Social Influences and Behavior. Edited by Lewis M, Feinman S. New York, Plenum, 1987, pp 57–82

Rothenberg A: The Creative Process of Psychotherapy. New York, Norton, 1987

Sameroff AJ: Developmental systems: contexts and evolution, in Handbook of Child Psychology, Vol I. Edited by Mussen PH. New York, Wiley, 1983, pp 237–294

Sameroff AJ, Emde RH (eds): Relationship Disturbances in Early Childhood: A Developmental Approach. New York, Basic Books, 1989

Sander LW: Toward a logic of organization in psychobiological development, in Biologic Response Styles: Clinical Implications. Edited by Klar K, Siever L. Washington, DC, American Psychiatric Press, 1985, pp 20–36

Sandler J: The background of safety. Int J Psychoanal 41:352–365, 1960

Sandler J: Countertransference and role-responsiveness. Int J Psychoanal 3:43–47, 1976

Sandler J: Psychoanalytic technique and "analysis terminable and interminable." Int J Psychoanal 69:335–345, 1988

Sandler J, Sandler A-M: On the development of object relationships and affects. Int J Psychoanal 59:285–296, 1978

Schafer R: Generative empathy in the treatment situation. Psychoanal Q 28:342–373, 1959

Settlage CF: Psychoanalytic developmental thinking in current and historical perspective. Psychoanal Contemp Thought 3:139–170, 1980

Shapiro T: Empathy: a critical reevaluation. Psychoanal Inq 1:423–448, 1981

Sharpe EF: The analysand, in Collected Papers on Psychoanalysis (1930). London, Hogarth Press, 1950, pp 22–37

Sorce JF, Emde RN, Campos J, Klinnert MD: Maternal emotional signaling: its effect on the visual cliff behavior of one-year-olds. Devel Psychol 21:337–341, 1985

Spitz RA: Transference: the analytical setting. Int J Psychoanal 37:380–385, 1956

Stolorow RD, Atwood G, Lachmann F: Transference and countertransference in the analysis of developmental arrests. Bull Menninger Clin 45:20–28, 1981

Stolorow RD, Brandchaft B, Atwood GE: Psychoanalytic Treatment: An Intersubjective Approach. Hillsdale, NJ, Analytic Press, 1987

Thomä H, Kächele H: Psychoanalytic Practice. New York, Springer, 1987

Vygotsky LS: Thought and Language (1934). Cambridge, MA, MIT Press, 1962

Vygotsky LS: Mind in Society: The Development of Higher Psychological Processes. Cambridge, MA, Harvard University Press, 1978

Wertsch JV: Vygotsky and the Social Formation of Mind. Cambridge, MA, Harvard University Press, 1985

Winnicott DW: Transitional objects and transitional phenomena: a study of the first not-me possession. Int J Psychoanal 43:89–97, 1953

Winnicott DW: The capacity to be alone (1958), in The Maturational Processes and the Facilitating Environment. New York, International Universities Press, 1966, pp 29–36

Winnicott DW: The theory of the parent-infant relationship. Int J Psychoanal 41:585–595, 1960

Wolf E: On the developmental line of selfobject relations, in Advances in Self Psychology. Edited by Goldberg A. New York, International Universities Press, 1980, pp 117–130

7

LAWRENCE FRIEDMAN, M.D.

INTRODUCTION

Lawrence Friedman is a graduate of the University of Chicago and received his M.D. from Temple University School of Medicine in Philadelphia, Pennsylvania. He is Clinical Professor of Psychiatry at Weill Cornell Medical College in New York and Adjunct Professor of Clinical Psychiatry at New York University School of Medicine, and he is a faculty member of the Psychoanalytic Institute at New York University Medical Center and of the Chicago Center for Psychoanalytic Psychology. He is an honorary member of the New York Psychoanalytic Society, the Psychoanalytic Association of New York, and the American Psychoanalytic Association. He has given presentations throughout the world and has published widely on the nature of psychoanalytic concepts, theory of technique, and history of philosophy and psychoanalysis. He is the author of *The Anatomy of Psychotherapy*.

In response to my request for a description of his role in American psychoanalysis, he said:

> I don't know how to describe myself, since I have not advocated for or against a style of treatment or made any practical suggestions of my own. On theoretical and philosophical grounds I have tried to elaborate and critique theories of mind and of treatment, and I've been critical of many critics. For the most part, I have been philosophically conservative, and I think commonsensical. My main interest has been to describe the factual, "on-the-ground" outcome of a recommended technique, its trade-offs of advantages and disadvantages. I think (or hope) that peo-

> ple see me as looking beyond the analyst's self-description of his or her procedure to appreciate in common terms the special power that the technique is capitalizing on, and the problems of other techniques that it was designed to avoid. In other words, when it concerns treatment, I like to imagine that people of various outlooks regard me as an appreciator—someone genuinely anxious to see the practical validity of their outlook. But when it comes to metatheory and philosophy, I think I'm seen as cranky and argumentative.

Dr. Friedman has been an important observer and critic of contemporary psychoanalysis. There is no received wisdom that is beyond the scope of his detailed examination, and an examination by Dr. Friedman helps us to recognize hidden values, assumptions, and judgments that enter into our ideas without our acknowledgment. He is a critical enthusiast and an enthusiastic critic who obviously loves psychoanalysis and psychoanalytic ideas and seems to find it almost unbearable to see these ideas handled carelessly by fellow analysts and critics.

WHY I CHOSE THIS PAPER

Lawrence Friedman, M.D.

I don't consider this my best writing. For that, I might have chosen a chapter on sublimation written for *Introducing Psychoanalytic Theory,* edited by Sander L. Gilman. Nor do I consider it my most significant contribution, which, if I've made any, is probably to set the record straight in "Hartmann's 'Ego Psychology and the Problem of Adaptation'" (*Psychoanalytic Quarterly* 58:526–550, 1989). The reason I chose the paper "Ferrum, Ignis, and Medicina" for inclusion in this volume is that it represents my main interest, which is to puzzle out the forces involved specifically, characteristically, and (if taken together) exclusively in a certain kind of procedure. The procedure has been called psychoanalysis (and, derivatively, psychoanalytic psychotherapy). That title, like an athletic trophy, may in the future pass on to a more popular treatment, but my own interest is not in the history of ideas, let alone the history of terms. I believe that the field of forces Freud discovered, and his peculiar way of producing it, will remain the orienting reference point for comment and variation in all thoughtful talking treatments. Time will have its way with other aspects. Mental activity has no one description. Conflict can be detected among many mental aspects. There is no patent even on technical terms. Transference, resistance, and the unconscious are constantly redefined when they are not actually challenged. It does not seem at all likely that we ever had, now have, or will come to have the final story of human growth and development. Mental disorders are understood differently in every age and with every new technology. It would be a rash prophet who would foreclose the invention of more effective and/or more efficient ways to relieve people's misery. Neighboring humanistic and scientific disciplines will advance reasonable claims to our territory. The only domain that historically-defined psychoanalysis has secure title to is Freud's very peculiar treatment setup and the unique light it sheds on the human mind. For that reason, its original nature, which has not yet been exhaustively understood, should be faithfully remembered so that it can be accurately dissected, both by hard reflection and by thoughtful experiment. The psychoanalytic situation is not a comfortable one; people will not be drawn to it by preference. Nor is it a product of nature; people will not come across it time and again by accident. At this critical juncture in psychoanalytic history and education, amid the rich and creative thinking of our day, there is a real risk that we could lose this defining and conceivably unrecoverable practical resource, and for that reason I have chosen this paper.

FERRUM, IGNIS, AND MEDICINA

Return to the Crucible

LAWRENCE FRIEDMAN, M.D.

ANYONE WHO VISITS A meeting of the American Psychoanalytic Association these days will be astonished at the breadth and vigor of its debates. We see intellectual ferment everywhere. But is that all we see? Is it just a variety of arguments—conflict vs. deficit, narrative vs. fact, etc.? Or is there an edifying story here—a story about a journey into our current issues and on to the goal of psychoanalysis in its second century?

Well, yes of course, there's a story... and another story... and, unfortunately, another story, each crafted to celebrate somebody's favorite outcome. In reality, there is no privileged history of anything. So the short answer to my last question is no. There is no road that led here. Psychoanalysis concerned itself with modern issues very early and with original issues again very lately. It has straggled into view over a wide field and it is still straggling. It wasn't a disciplined march. There is no triumphal entry. Sorry.

Now, that's not a very promising beginning; I should start over and be less circumspect. This time I'll weave together highly personal impressions and generalizations and indulge in grand and free confabulation. That's not so reprehensible, really. The art historian E. H. Gombrich

---

Plenary address presented to the American Psychoanalytic Association, Philadelphia, PA, May 20, 1994.

tells us that if we want to achieve a likeness we have to begin by hacking out a rough image and then comparing it to reality. Only by match and mismatch do we reach a faithful representation. So we can't lose, you and I: I will tell you my fable and you will spot my mistakes and we will end up seeing things more clearly.

In order to help you take your position I'll forewarn you of my conclusion. My moral is that today's arguments are efforts to pull the secrets of human nature out of the very fabric of the treatment situation, treatment here regarded not merely as an instrument of discovery but as an isolated wet specimen to be examined.

How can mere arguments reveal facts of nature? Well, consider this: analytic treatment comes about, in the first place, because of the analyst's attitudes. There is nothing else to make treatment happen. If treatment does something unusual to people, then we can learn about people by picking out the attitudes that make treatment happen, and especially by watching how the attitudes sit together and squirm together to get the job done. And where better to observe treatment attitudes sitting and squirming than in our collective controversy over the course of our discipline's history. With psychoanalysis, the history of ideas is not a background study; analytic history literally assembles the tools of treatment, and it is history that paints subtle meaning onto our stock concepts. And history is even more important for our purpose this afternoon: When over the years analysts try, this way and that, to match their attitudes to the task of treatment, they are doing nothing less than palpating the human condition.

Intending no disrespect to other schools, I'll talk only of Anglo-American, Freudian analysis. And I'll pay no attention to the influence of momentary fashions, philosophical and otherwise, because I am discussing not ideas in general, but how attitudes are designed to serve the needs of an established treatment.

Now, it will not escape your notice that when I ask how ideas serve the needs of treatment I am presuming that there is a psychoanalytic treatment out there waiting to be served—I am supposing that psychoanalytic treatment is an enduring structure that can be lit up by turning on various ideas and attitudes, and, further, that we are so familiar with this treatment that we can hold up its physical likeness in one hand and its associated ideas in the other and tell which treatment postures go along with which ideas.

I am suggesting, you see, that Freud did not design a treatment; he discovered one. First he stumbled on the treasure while following his personal aims. Then he modified the personal motives and made them into a behavioral map by which others could find the treatment directly.

The attitudes he recommended, having been reenacted over the years, in essence if not in detail, make Freud's discovery available in every consulting room where it can be repeatedly identified and empirically examined. We can spot psychoanalysis by its gross appearance, especially by the attitudes that produce it. I will try to catch the spirit of those attitudes by imagining their root form at the time of discovery and then noting what sort of tinkering was necessary to turn them into reliable producers of the treatment Freud had stumbled on. I want to trace Freud's attitudes of discovery as they are transformed into attitudes of technique. Then I will speculate on their subsequent fate.

If I am wrong in my assumption—if treatment is just the application to patients of whatever analytic theory happens to be knocking around at the moment—then my method is pointless. So if you doubt that psychoanalytic treatment has an enduring life and shape of its own, please suspend disbelief this afternoon, because I need two heroes for my story of how we got here. One hero is the collectivity of you and your predecessors—no problem there. But the other hero is psychoanalytic treatment itself, and to conjure that one up I must, as I go along, refer to its identifying physiognomy. And let me make it clear that when I say physiognomy I mean just that—the grossly observable features of the treatment situation. Please be prepared for a certain bluntness of language. Remember, it's attitudes that we're trying to get hold of—attitudes that turn treatment on. And to portray attitudes we must paint with a broad brush and use bold colors, because that's how attitudes are identified—certainly not by careful, technical phrases. Indeed, when practitioners insist on putting their attitudes into technical terms they are usually hiding elements of manipulativeness, and that is another, very useful attitude: that of innocent attitudelessness.

Come with me now back to 1895, and look at the experience reported in *Studies on Hysteria* [Freud 1895]. Everyone knows that psychoanalysis grew out of the search for memories, and that Freud's ambition was to make great discoveries. If the historical path to treatment is any clue to its nature, then curiosity must certainly lie at its heart. That needs no argument, so I shall proceed to the next attitude on my list.

So vivid is the image of Freud as Discoverer that we sometimes forget that a proud man here is a proud man there. As a self-proclaimed physician, Freud had pride in his practice and in his person. He hated to have his bluff called. He disliked having patients show him he was wrong when he told them they would go into a trance. He did not want his authority to be dependent on his patient's response (Freud 1917, p. 451). No wonder he welcomed Breuer's cathartic treatment, "a practice," he tells us, "which combined an automatic mode of operation with the satisfaction of scientific curiosity" (Freud 1914, p. 9). Breuer's treatment was automatic in that it was guaranteed by the patient's normal digestion of memories.

In fact, the new treatment followed the patient's own inclination so reliably that hypnosis proved superfluous. And going a step further, Freud discovered that he always got what he was after if he obeyed hints from patients like Frau Emmy v. N. (Freud 1895, p. 63), who wanted him to stop bird-dogging his objectives and listen to hers. Once again following the patient's wishes, Freud made inclinations such as Frau Emmy's into his own fundamental rule.

This new procedure put Freud in an entirely different position: No more praying for a trance. No more begging for simple memories. No more pleading for clues to symptoms. If the therapist has any question at all, it's a mild wondering about the mood of the moment. Now almost anything the patient says will satisfy Freud. Since he no longer hungers for atoms of significance, and since he is expecting only a vague network of thoughts with only a remote reference to his interests, he can't miss: his professional pride and intellectual confidence are no longer at risk. My point is that psychoanalysis, in addition to being a method of discovery, was Freud's way of immunizing his treatment authority. He writes: "It is of course of great importance for the progress of the analysis that one should always turn out to be in the right *vis-à-vis* the patient, otherwise one would always be dependent on what he chose to tell one" (1895, p. 281).

The trick was to endorse the patient's wishes. That's what made the treatment reliable. When he had formerly asked for a particular service, such as falling into a trance or reporting a memory, Freud was at the mercy of his patient, who might or might not grant his wish. The new treatment that Freud discovered required, instead of a particular service, a whole human relationship, and that is something that people have a hard time withholding. Freud could count on it—provided he himself could muster a special interest.

Freud's unguarded description of this special interest reveals its raw nature, which later will be obscured by technical formulas. Freud's fresh, first impression is that the analyst's attitude is quite different from physicianly attention. "I cannot imagine bringing myself to delve into the physical mechanisms of a hysteria in anyone who struck me as low-minded and repellent, and who, on closer acquaintance, would not be capable of arousing human sympathy; whereas I can keep the treatment of a diabetic or rheumatic patient apart from personal approval of this kind" (Freud 1895, p. 265). What sort of attention is this? We can suppose that it involves a human endorsement and a personal (rather than just an ethical) wish to help. Carried forward, the analyst's human commitment and his curative intent remain for us today the most familiar—and certainly the proudest—of his treatment attitudes. And perhaps I would be wise to end my inventory of analytic attitudes right here, having mentioned curiosity, respectful sympathy, and a desire to help.

But I'll be reckless and ask, What did Freud's interest evoke in the *patient*? Although Freud later publicly pleaded that an analyst asks no more than the privilege of a gynecologist, he knew otherwise and said as much upon his first encounter with psychoanalysis. He recognized that he was doing something forbidden to physicians; he was deliberately courting a personal, affective intimacy. The patients "put themselves in the doctor's hands and place their confidence in him—a step which in other situations is only taken voluntarily and never at the doctor's request" (Freud 1895, p. 266).

And Freud was honest enough to recognize that the intimacy he wanted from his patient might be the sort of personal surrender that counts on a love relationship and must honorably be reciprocated with something more than cure: "In not a few cases, especially with women and where it is a question of elucidating erotic trains of thought, the patient's co-operation becomes a personal sacrifice, which must be compensated for by some substitute for love. The trouble taken by the physician and his friendliness have to suffice for such a substitute" (1895, p. 301). In this first glimpse of the situation, Freud remarks that, quite apart from individual transference, a patient will sometimes experience a dread of becoming "too much accustomed to the physician personally, of losing her independence in relation to him, and even of perhaps becoming sexually dependent on him.... The determinants [of this situation] are less individual [than transferences]. *The cause of this obstacle lies in the special solicitude inherent in treatment*" (Freud 1895, p. 302; emphasis added).

Let us be as bold as Freud. His effort to make great discoveries, and also conduct a confident cure, had unexpectedly put in his hands a peculiar power—the power of a psychological seduction. I shouldn't have to—but I've learned that I had better—add quickly that this seduction is unique, careful, modulated, responsible, therapeutically intended, unselfish, and nonabusive. I have no wish to be provocative. I know that many of you find the word *seduction* intolerable—and for very good reason. But since some elements of treatment exist for the very purpose of cushioning that discomfort, we will understand less about treatment if we hide the discomfort in a euphemism.

By seduction I mean an arrangement whereby the patient is led to expect love while the analyst, in Freud's words, plans to provide a substitute for it. Admittedly the love-substitute is something very special, with secrets we have yet to fathom, but it is not the love the patient is imagining. At that early moment in analytic history one of the conspicuous features of treatment was put in place, namely, the analyst's special interest, his constant, exclusive, selfless attentiveness—an attentiveness which I believe (though this is only implied by Freud) will inevitably spark a flickering apparition of the analyst's deep and lasting attachment to the patient. That illusion may be viewed skeptically, or rationalized out of awareness, or fended off, or kept in the background, or wondered about or feared, but it is always a nidus of uncertainty at the center of treatment, placed there deliberately by the psychoanalyst.

That's not the whole story, of course. The patient also rides the analyst's attention back into himself, where he finds a new respect for—and hopefulness in—the rich potential of his own distress. Even if you can't abide my bad language—my talking about illusion and seduction when every well-bred tongue knows how to pronounce "transference" and "regression"—I'm sure you will agree with me that Freud discovered a unique attitude, let us say, of expectant appreciation (an attitude that possesses perfectly extraordinary eliciting power), and you will agree that this attitude is a hallmark of psychoanalytic treatment.

And perhaps you will agree also that part of what makes the analyst's personal interest so unique is that it is allowed to remain ambiguous for years, while any straightforward declaration designed to clear up the ambiguity is deliberately avoided. Though he may question the patient's beliefs, the analyst never *says* what the extent and limits of his caring are. (I need not cite Freud's advice to neither encourage nor discourage transference love.)

Uncertainty about the analyst's attachment is a source of discomfort. But it is not just that; it is also a tactical problem inasmuch as the need for the patient's attachment gives evidence of the analyst's continued obligation to bargain. Freud learned soon enough that, left to themselves, patients would not aim at his target, and he was actually relieved to find, as he tells us, that "free association is not really free. The patient remains under the influence of the analytic situation" (Freud 1923, p. 40).

Thus, patients were still being subjected to suggestion, if not by Freud's words, then by his procedure. And, accordingly, Freud was still in the position of bargaining. For one thing, without hypnosis he would be the one who saw the hidden meanings, and he would have to persuade patients to believe what he saw (Freud 1904). But that was the least of his problems. The bigger problem was that, though he had coopted some of the patient's wishes to his own ends, in fact the only wish he ever really endorsed was the wish to remember; other wishes were always something to be tamed. And taming remained a problem. Patients could refuse to produce evidence. They could stop talking. They could demand an entirely different relationship. The method was not as dependably automatic as it had seemed.

Freud did not flinch from the larger implication. By 1912 he knew he was no longer in the modest business of retrieving memories. He was back in the persuading business. Even just to conduct the treatment he had to persuade patients to live differently, more courageously, more realistically, etc. (Falzeder 1994; Freud 1912). His wanting that from patients made him dependent on them again. Freud saw the trap more clearly than did Jung or Ferenczi, and he resolved to extricate himself. He would use his influence, but in a way that did not entangle him in compromises. Having already learned not to ask, he would now try to not even *want* any particular information. And he resolved to stop entreating patients to get well; he would make them come to him and solicit him. He wrote to Jung: "you still engage yourselves, give away a good deal of yourselves in order to demand a similar response.... [O]ne should rather remain unapproachable, and insist upon receiving" (Falzeder 1994, p. 314). But here's the problem: If the procedure has any point to it, the analyst has to go after *something*. If he is diffident about causes and he's not evangelical about health, what will he pursue?

Freud very early found an attitude that solved this practical dilemma, and successive generations have reproduced the handy attitude. How? By thinking in terms of resistance, which was Freud's behavioral map through this minefield.

The resistance was the something that Freud could be passionate about, struggle with, go after, and still remain a neutral conduit for what the patient ultimately wants and would naturally produce (were it not for the resistance). It was not just a rhetorical trick, *provided* there was something that both he and the patient could fight against. Freud thought there was such a thing: the enemy was a motivated *ignorance* of inner reality that limited the patient's autonomy. By fighting against the ignorance Freud was *freeing* the patient's decision making. In that way Freud could still count on the force of the patient's own wishes to serve the analyst's purpose. The analyst could press his own case without entreating the patient and without manipulating the patient because the patient's ultimate response was *guaranteed*, theoretically, by a third presence—objective truth, truth undistorted by the analyst's and patient's preconceptions and wishful thinking (Freud 1914). Objective truth serves two purposes: In the first place, it is a gratifyingly clear goal for a distressingly undefined partnership. In the second place, truth is a monitor that allows the analyst to exert influence without compromising his liberating purpose. Let me say just a few words about each of these two services.

First, let us consider why it is so important to have a clear goal. Floating above both parties—usually silently—is the unanswerable question of what exactly the analyst's investment is in his patient. Any therapist will be less uneasy if he can point away from that uncertainty to a straightforwardly mutual task of investigation that goes on regardless of the relationship. In other words, a personal ambiguity is balanced by an objective work relationship. And that balance is fostered by the idea that whatever is or isn't real in the relationship, it is all for the purpose of bringing objective truth into sight. Thus, an attitude oriented to objective reality takes some of the vertigo out of the relationship.

Now, about the second way that objective reality serves the analyst—how does it lessen mutual dependency? Freud worked his way out of mutual dependency by balancing his affectionate interest, which led to personal entanglement, against an opposite, disentangling attitude—an attitude that can be fairly characterized as socially adversarial. I say, *socially* adversarial. Obviously Freud was not an adversary of his patient's welfare. That qualifier understood, I will now speak simply of adversarialness. Many have commented on Freud's bellicose treatment images. We are all familiar with his famous martial metaphors. From first to last Freud was in a struggle. If it's a matter of Freud's own writings, I hardly need to argue my case for adversarialness, and in fact, that very word has often been used in personal criticism. But my purpose here is to emphasize the universal service that this adversarial attitude renders to the treatment that Freud discovered.

Let us look back at the original adversarial attitude that led Freud to the treatment. Freud, as I have suggested, was impatient for great discoveries, and, as Schafer has noted, that made him an adversary to patients who barred the way. But let us ask: did Freud become less adversarial when he stopped fishing for memories and started nourishing a whole relationship with his patients? On the contrary, the adversarial attitude became even more essential at that point. For now it was not just the Conquistador who was fighting; it was also the adamant therapist. The researcher's impatience was being trimmed to a different service, a different ruthlessness—one that would sustain the newly discovered treatment. After all, free association was a way of paralyzing the patient's will, and that's a fairly adversarial thing to do. But it is just one example of a general attitude. Through each revision of treatment, Freud was reconfirming and deepening his first lesson, namely that wanting something from a patient defeats the purpose. As I have noted, Freud found that he lost leverage when he engaged patients too wholeheartedly. They would play out their neurosis on the instrument of his therapeutic desire. He had to retain autonomy not just to make discoveries but to keep himself free of the patient's manipulation, and the patient free of his.

By 1912 Freud saw that an allegiance to objective truth would solve the problem: addressing himself to objective truth, he could preserve his independence even while he was involved with the patient's wishes. The patient was wrestling with a transference figure, but Freud was wrestling with resistance to objective truth, and ultimately—I emphasize, ultimately—none of the patient's holds could succeed in making out of the search for truth a repetition of an unhappy old childhood routine. The patient finds that this, the most open intimacy of his life, paradoxically diverts him to objectivity.

And for his part, Freud could make a demand on the patient without offering a piece of himself in exchange (without losing his skin, as he put it). He would offer the truth rather than his own love or approval. The injunction to confront objective truth gave the patient an endless task by which he could endeavor to win the analyst's favor. You know that patients will scan every treatment for a sign of what is wanted of them. What they find in that search is what I will call the demand structure of the treatment. If you don't offer one demand, the patient will perceive another. Freud provided a demand: Let up on your yearnings and aim for objective truth!

And that, in turn, would free the patient. The patient could please Freud only by seeking the truth. And the truth would then make the patient free, because he would be putting himself into a position where he could *choose*, instead of being compelled automatically. The rule of abstinence is simply a corollary of these considerations.

And so from 1912 to 1914 Freud recommended to us the cardinal concepts of transference, resistance, and objective truth so that we might put ourselves into this useful, semiadversarial frame of mind. We welcome what the patient is revealing, but we think he's revealing it in order to conceal something more important. Nothing is more characteristic of psychoanalysts than their inclination to *see through* everything. The adversarial attitude is so ingrained in analysts that it affects their collegial discourse. Just as a patient's cooperation is never innocent of resistance, so a reported treatment can't go well without a zealous observer suspecting an error of collusion. And, justified or not, the profession's response to Loewald and to Kohut was surely influenced by fear that they were diluting a fundamental, adversarial attitude.

I realize that none of you will recognize adversarialness as a feature of your treatment. You are more likely to see what I am pointing to if I ask you to reflect on the balance you keep between analytic credulity and analytic skepticism. Though analysts cannot miss Freud's adversarialness, accompanied as it is by drums and trumpets, their own adversarialness is usually manifested quietly, as analytic flexibility. What I call adversarialness, and what Freud described in similar idiom, refers to the way the analyst sets his face against appeals by the patient, denies bids for validation and reassurance, sternly summons what is most reluctant, rebuffs advances to "buy" any picture of the patient or his fate, waves away comforting roles, and says to everything, in effect, "No; something else." Adversarialness deconstructs the patient's presentation and frees the analyst's imagination. It eyes appearances skeptically and keeps looking for a reality beyond. It shuffles dramas and story lines and deflates lessons and moralizing.

The significance of this last point can hardly be exaggerated. Ordinarily we see people as dramatic figures. Schafer is right: narrative is the way we understand human action. And where our imagination is least constrained, there we make up the simplest and most persuasive stories. We "know" public figures more crisply than we know our spouse. It's more obvious what to do about the national economy than how to deal with the kids. Until we are assaulted by complexity, until we are entangled by love and responsibility, we see a simple, old-fashioned melodrama of good and evil, and when we don't have to act we moralize fiercely.

So we can't help seeing patients that way or they us. Analysts, despite themselves, often view process this way. Once in a while they slip and hear themselves say that their patient is trying to get away with a wicked treatment perversion, or flagrantly abusing the process in some fashion. But then they recapture Freud's adversarial attitude, which says that what's seen is in any case just surface, and they sober up on the objective truth of the mind with its perfectly neutral psychodynamics. A mental mechanism may malfunction, but it can't misbehave. One frequently sees Freud personally alternating this way: his letters express his moralized dramas while his published theory tends to neutralize them.

Moralizing keeps drifting into treatment, as indeed it must, but it is constantly swept out. Of course the analyst must experience his own effort dramatically—no one perseveres in a tough project over years without some agonistic framework. So an official drama of treatment is available—but only one: the crusade against resistance. Yet fighting the resistance is probably the least confining, the least defining, drama that a therapist can act in, because resistance itself is so ill defined. (Compare, for example, the fight against a "false self," which is so much more dramatically specific.) Other than the single image of fighting resistance, no drama is finally accepted by the Freudian analyst. No sense of "what we're doing together" hardens into routine. No patient is finally pigeonholed. The adversarial attitude refuses them all.

The adversarial attitude and the hunt for objective truth—these characterize the whole of treatment. Every time an analyst sees an event as an instance of something larger, he is endorsing Freud's view of the mind as an object. Every time an analyst disengages himself from an ordinary social response, he is utilizing Freud's adversarialness to social offerings and is imitating Freud's reach toward a mental object behind appearances.

So here's my list of attitudes—the founding attitudes of psychoanalytic treatment. Do you recognize this picture? Endless curiosity; endorsement of the patient's thrust; an evocative sort of affection; a faithful intimacy; a nervous dance around an illusion of lasting attachment; a demand that the patient rise above his wishes and face the truth; constant skepticism about all appearances; a lightness about the patient's dramas and the drama of treatment; absence of role and judgment. And I might add, as I mentioned at the start, a studied disingenuousness, that is, an attitude of innocent observation.

Well, what do you say? You say: yes, the portrait does convey a faint likeness and it might look better in a dark corner of the attic. What a dull list of hateful attitudes! What about plain human affection? How about easing pain, defeating demons, mastering fate? Where is the playfulness and creativity, the enlargement of experience? Where is the excitement of surviving risky genuineness? Aren't *these* the daily rewards for which analysts rise in the morning and go to work? And I say, yes, you are right, analysts do go to work for those reasons. They can do that because the *workplace* is there, assured by their taken-for-granted, baseline attitudes. My caricature is an underdrawing of the workplace—or the laboratory, as I shall presently describe it. But even as such, I confess, it lacks one identifying feature that has been the subject of ardent controversy. I must now add a note about what might be called the analyst's attitude of incubation.

We saw that Freud first achieved mastery by hitching his research wagon to the patient's memory machine. But even in 1912 he knew that patients weren't suffering just from retained memories; he knew they also had a general *interest* that is fastened onto their parents. For a while it was tempting to think that adult life is just too difficult for these patients, and that treatment is a halfway house to being a grown-up.

The idea that patients have to grow up in treatment took deeper root when theory expanded in the 1920s. After all, the superego appraises reality not in a factual but in an attitudinal way, and it might well need some growing out of. And that impression was reinforced when, in 1923, Freud allowed that there's a sense in which patients are not split-minded but wholeheartedly oppose their treatment and, indeed, throw their whole selves into every meeting with the world. With that, I think, Freud took his first steps down a dark path at the end of which he would find so few uncorrupted egos that human development came to seem an education in cowardice adapted to a projected world, itself built out of need and fear. (That's my hyperbolic inference from Freud 1937, pp. 234ff.) Don't think for a moment that the theory of signal anxiety did away with the maturational image of treatment. It is true that in later theory infantile stubbornness was no longer the villain. Freud now acknowledged that people have self-protective, good reasons for lagging behind. But the same theory told him that the world we are taught to live in is a fearful world, and if we are to free ourselves from it we have to be brave as well as wise. The need for some sort of growing up in treatment was never absent from Freud's writings, from his first mention of the repetition compulsion to the late picture of a spoiled child who is unduly fearful because he has been overprotected.

This takes us into the realm of world building and world breaking. The constructivist implications of Freud's theory were understood by his coworkers. In the 1930s Hartmann was by no means alone in pointing out that significant reality is largely social reality, and its appreciation often a matter of having a realistic *attitude* or a realistic *perspective* and useful *reflexes,* or a composite *orientation* arranged by a *well-integrated* psychic apparatus. Being realistic involves experiencing "appropriate" *meanings,* some of them quite peremptory.

This was not the kind of mind Freud cared about; it would never be capable of free choice in a field of objective reality. But analysts with more mixed objectives were not so quickly discouraged. It did not displease them to think that psychoanalysis can help patients with their problem solving even if the problem isn't a simple recognition of objective truth. It is largely this problem-solving paradigm that we know as ego psychology, a term that should include Melanie Klein's work.

The reality that these ego psychologists ended up with was an individualized grown-up-ness, though Anna Freud and the North Americans did not discard a factor of neutral perception.

Analysts can't relax there. If treatment aims at an individualized maturity rather than truth, the analyst can no longer act impersonally when he makes his customary demand. The demand structure of psychoanalysis presupposed an objective reality that both parties could turn to and salute. Feeling respect for truth in his bones, the analyst was reassured that his body English would be disciplined, his role responses tentative, his personal influence erasable. If the maturational view took over, treatment might end up as a cloud of encouraging perspectives mixed with bundles of shaping influences. The sympathetic and seductive features of treatment might wash away the spice of challenge.

In this predicament practitioners on both sides of the Atlantic looked to the same principle for salvation: If disciplined analysts will confine themselves to nonmanipulative interpretations, then by definition their personal attitude won't impinge on patients, and the structure of treatment will remain psychoanalytic. In other words, if an interpretation can be objective, then it doesn't matter how confused the notion of reality becomes. The call is to save interpretations and let reality fend for itself. That may seem an odd solution, but it is logical, and in many quarters during the 1950s and 1960s an idealized interpretation was fast becoming the sole repository for the threatened demand structure of analysis.

Therefore it was a matter of analytic life or death that an interpretation should convey nothing but precisely what is hidden, so that it will not transmit the analyst's persuasive attitude.

Now, that is too heavy a burden for any human communication to bear. Thus, in the eyes of those who followed, this brave first effort to preserve the structure of treatment and thereby safeguard the patient's autonomy was seen, instead, as a priestly, rule-bound formalism, smug, authoritarian, and doctrinaire—perfect, in other words, to serve as a foil for rebellion by the next generation (our generation), which, as always in history, turns contemptuously from the Academy back to nature. In this case, nature is the crucible of live treatment.

Thus, after decades of taking the structure of treatment for granted, analysts today are poking at it to see how it's built. They are systematically varying treatment attitudes and watching the results.

Consider, for instance, the objective truth demand. What happens to the rest of treatment if you remove it? Objective reality was the bulwark of analytic skepticism. We were skeptical because reality was hiding behind appearances. Respect for reality buffered the analyst against the patient and the patient against manipulation. Now analysts are trying to think about patients in terms of story lines that are free of objective truth reference. Maybe that will make patients more responsible and creative. Maybe analysts can find a more flexible discipline to replace the old truth demand. For instance, it may suffice for the analyst to simply *decide* to read a psychoanalytic narrative into the patient's history and behavior. Maybe just being firm in that *decision* will anchor the analyst when he is being pulled by the patient's undertow. And maybe the analyst can limit such firm decisions to that one manipulation. We shall see.

That's one experiment. There are others. Analysts are also trying to be *more* objective—for instance, by using interventions that do more neutral pointing and less perspectival describing, pointing for instance to visible and categorical affects, muffled resentments, or shifts in direction.

Some investigators maximize adversarialness: they spare no island of taken-for-granted cooperation—everything is a compromise formation. Others reduce adversarialness: their experiments will tell us whether empathic affirmation reduces the patient's masochistic collusion while yet steering clear of a social relationship. Investigators are tinkering with the old analytic attitude of curiosity. They attend less to pathology and more to the process of preconscious emergence. Even the attitude of passive observation is being experimentally altered, as analysts remind themselves that they are partly making up what they see and partly producing it inadvertently. How will that affect their ability to maintain a level scrutiny?

Despite this widespread innovation, I think all of these controversies are experiments: they do not trash the laboratory. In my opinion, few psychoanalysts would be happy with a treatment that discarded the features I've mentioned, though we may not agree on their names, or the proper balance among them. If you look closely enough, I think you will see that we are all counting on transmitted reflexes and traditions to keep the main features of treatment in place while we experiment with shades and proportions.

And there, I think, lies the answer to that old, embarrassing question: Why did psychoanalysis wall itself up in institutes and reproduce by inbreeding? Freudian theory didn't need to do that. It could have survived nibbling and adulteration—has, in fact, survived that in popular culture and the academy. But the thing that Freud discovered, the thing we know as psychoanalytic *treatment*—that is quite ephemeral. It is solely the product of attitudes. It is that crucible that needed protection.

Treatment structure has no protection outside of tradition. Without special support it might have disappeared forever, exploding into a galaxy of assorted relationships, each one molded according to how it pleased the therapist to see himself. And if treatment is the crucible of psychoanalysis, its preservation was paramount. That is something to be kept in mind today, when the threat is pointedly aimed at the treatment.

Here is my peroration: Besides their other contributions, analysts do basic research. The standard treatment atmosphere is an imaging technique for mind: general features of mind are measured as the analyst notices the attitudes he must invoke to sustain the analytic atmosphere. It is a kind of echo-cardiography of the soul. Of course it does not produce a readout in pixels. Is it then just a speculative enterprise? Not a bit. Attitudes and their impacts are features of the empirical world. As the analyst switches this attitude on and that one off, he records which combinations most brightly light up the unique analytic situation. It is the slight alterations in treatment attitudes that constitute experiments in this peculiar laboratory of the mind, the laboratory that is dedicated to research on the pathway of desire, the nuances of interaction, the limits of freedom, the relationship of cause and reason, the nature of meaning, the meaning of responsibility, and all the special paradoxes of humanness. I really cannot imagine what other form research on these issues could possibly take.

The supreme irony of today's psychoanalysis is that the gravest threat to its existence finds the profession in an unparalleled, efflorescent vigor—I would call it a renaissance. In that respect, at least, you must consider yourselves fortunate.

REFERENCES

Falzeder E: My grand-patient, my chief tormenter: a hitherto unnoticed case of Freud's and the consequences. Psychoanal Q 63:297–331, 1994

Freud S: Studies on hysteria (1895), in The Standard Edition of the Complete Psychological Works of Sigmund Freud [SE], Vol 2. Translated and edited by Strachey J. London, Hogarth Press, 1955, pp 1–319

Freud S: Freud's psycho-analytic procedure (1904). SE, 7:249–254, 1953

Freud S: The dynamics of transference (1912). SE, 12:99–108, 1958

Freud S: On the history of the psycho-analytic movement (1914). SE, 14:7–66, 1957

Freud S: Introductory lectures on psycho-analysis (1917). SE, 16, 1963

Freud S: The ego and the id (1923). SE, 19:13–66, 1961

Freud S: Analysis terminable and interminable (1937). SE, 23:216–253, 1964

8

GLEN O. GABBARD, M.D.

INTRODUCTION

Glen Gabbard is a graduate of Northwestern University and Rush Medical College in Chicago, Illinois, and the Topeka Institute for Psychoanalysis in Kansas. From 1978 to 1994, he held various positions at the Menninger Memorial Hospital of the Menninger Clinic, and he was the Director from 1989 to 1994. Dr. Gabbard has won every significant award in psychiatry and psychoanalysis, including the Adolf Meyer Award and the Distinguished Service Award of the American Psychiatric Association and the Mary S. Sigourney Award for Contributions to the Field of Psychoanalysis; as well, he has received numerous Teacher of the Year awards, held an extraordinary array of visiting professorships, and presented many keynote addresses. He has been an enormous influence in the field. From 1994 to 2001, he was the Bessie Walker Callaway Distinguished Professor of Psychoanalysis and Education in the Karl Menninger School of Psychiatry and Mental Health Sciences, and he is currently Director of the Baylor Psychiatry Clinic in Houston, Texas. He is known as a superb teacher. He is Joint Editor-in-Chief and Editor for North America of *The International Journal of Psychoanalysis.*

Dr. Gabbard is currently the Brown Foundation Chair of Psychoanalysis and Professor of Psychiatry in the Department of Psychiatry and Behavioral Sciences at the Baylor Medical College in Houston, Texas. He has been on the editorial boards of *The American Journal of Psychiatry, The Journal of the American Psychoanalytic Association, Psychoanalytic Dialogues, Psychoanalytic Quarterly,* and *Psychoanalytic Inquiry,* to mention but a few. He is the author of several hundred papers and is preeminent in fields as various as psychoanalytic criticism of the movies, boundary violations, the treatment of borderline and narcissistic patients, and psychoanalytic education. He is the author or editor of 19 books, ranging in content from the study of out-of-body states to his classic *Psychodynamic Psychiatry in Clinical Practice,* now in its fourth edition, with translation into six languages.

Dr. Gabbard is one of the most powerful voices in psychoanalytic education, and one can be sure that every graduating psychoanalyst has studied several of Glen Gabbard's works.

He has described himself as follows:

> I was analyzed by a Kleinian and steeped in Klein, Bion, and British object relations at the Menninger Clinic and the Topeka Institute for Psychoanalysis. I still think of myself as essentially an object-relations analyst by training. I have never felt comfortable with the model of American ego psychology. I find it doesn't help you much with more disturbed patients. In recent years, I have been influenced by relational thinking, constructivism, and also by the interface of psychoanalysis and neuroscience. I would definitely see myself as a pluralist of sorts at this point. Like Joe Sandler, who was something of a mentor to me, I find that we all use private mixed models when we are behind the couch. No one theory can explain all the clinical phenomena that we see.

WHY I CHOSE THIS PAPER

Glen O. Gabbard, M.D.

"Miscarriages of Psychoanalytic Treatment With Suicidal Patients" was first presented as the North American Plenary Address at the 2004 International Psychoanalytical Association Congress in New Orleans. I chose this paper for inclusion in this volume because it represents the convergence of two long-standing interests of mine: the treatment of seriously disturbed patients and professional boundary violations by psychoanalysts and psychotherapists. Those patients who hate us, defeat us, mock us, and torment us also penetrate us in a way that lays bare our vulnerabilities. They make us face the complexity of our motives in choosing our impossible profession. Patients who do not conform to our scripted fantasies of treatment may lead us into unfortunate transgressions that end careers.

Some time after I began seeing analysts and other mental health professionals who had committed serious boundary violations, I started a special program for professionals in crisis at the Menninger Hospital (of which I was Director) in the early 1990s. From colleagues who came to me in despair over their mistakes, I have learned a great deal about optimal technique with disturbed patients. I have also learned that most of those colleagues who violate boundaries are fundamentally like the rest of us. They deserve our understanding and empathy no matter how much we may condemn their behavior. This particular paper examines a miscarriage of treatment by one colleague who was well-intentioned but terribly lost. He reminds us that we are all masters of self-deception. Much of my professional career has been devoted to the idea that by studying the ways in which we may deceive ourselves, perhaps we can prevent harm to patients and destruction of careers.

MISCARRIAGES OF PSYCHOANALYTIC TREATMENT WITH SUICIDAL PATIENTS

GLEN O. GABBARD, M.D.

WHEN THE IPA PROGRAM COMMITTEE bestowed upon me the honor of being selected as the North American Keynote Speaker for the Congress, I spent some time studying the meaning of the theme "Working at the Frontiers." The word "frontiers" inspired visions of danger, of wildness, and of uncivilized regions where the constraints of society no longer apply. One authoritative definition was particularly apposite: "The part of a country held to form the border or furthest limit of the settled or inhabited regions" (Brown 1993, p. 1034). A second definition was even bolder: "A barrier against attack" (p. 1034). One of the questions thus posed for psychoanalysts at this Congress is to identify the nether regions of the psychoanalytic enterprise, where we are vulnerable to attack, beset by wildness and imperiled by the dangers inherent in our work. As I pondered the dangerous frontiers of psychoanalysis, I associated to the psychoanalytic "train wrecks" I have seen when suicidal patients have been seriously mismanaged by well-intentioned psychoanalysts.

My career has been unique in some respects because of my long-standing interest in two discrete regions of the so-called "widening scope" on this sometimes perilous frontier. For many years I carried

---

Keynote address to the 43rd International Psychoanalytical Association (IPA) Congress, New Orleans, LA, July 29–August 2, 2003.

a large caseload of treatment-resistant suicidal patients with severe character pathology who were sent to the Menninger Clinic as a last resort. I also have spent much of my professional life consulting, evaluating, or treating therapists and analysts (at last count over 150) who have committed serious boundary violations with their patients.

I have noted with growing concern how often the most egregious boundary violations are inflicted on some of our most disturbed suicidal patients. While it is easy for us all to cast aspersions on analysts who have lost their way in the dark night of the soul that accompanies the treatment of severely suicidal patients with personality disorders, I suggest that we refrain from a sweeping contempt towards these colleagues and instead attempt to learn something from them. In these extreme "frontier" situations, we often discover the analyst's essential humanness, stripped to the bone like King Lear howling in despair. These colleagues who have soared too close to the sun in their blind omnipotence and emerged scorched and disgraced are far more similar to us than different.

Suicidal patients, by their very nature, touch on a special vulnerability that is an occupational hazard of analysts. Most of us prefer to think of analytic work as something other than a life-or-death matter. We visualize our ideal patient as an intelligent, reflective, attractive person (somewhat like us), haunted by intrapsychic conflict, but strongly motivated to understand. This much-desired patient embraces life and wants to make changes so life can be lived more fully. By contrast, suicidal patients have determined that life has little to offer, and analysis is a dubious proposition. What insight could possibly transform life into a journey worth traveling? These patients quicken the analyst's pulse by rejecting *a priori* the notion that analytic insight has the potential to make life worth living. While we often speak of such "widening scope" patients as residing on the "frontier," my experience as a supervisor of candidates and a consultant to colleagues suggests that these patients are increasingly common and have moved from the frontier to the heart of psychoanalytic civilization.

In this context I will share a cautionary tale of Dr. N, an analyst in his 40s who consulted me many years ago in the aftermath of a horrific boundary violation. Dr. N gave me his permission to publish the details of his case so that others might learn from them.

The Tale of Dr. N

Jenny was a deeply distressed 35-year-old woman when she came to see Dr. N. His first reaction when he saw her in the waiting room was that she was the most beautiful woman he had ever seen. As she began to tell him the saga of her tragic life, Dr. N was moved. At one point in the middle of her tale, Jenny told Dr. N she was attracted to him and asked if they could stop the meeting so they could date. Dr. N clarified that dating was impossible because their professional relationship had already begun, and turning back the clock was not an option. Disappointed but undaunted, Jenny went on to tell Dr. N how her mother had tortured her by locking her in a closet when she was a child. She also described the details of an incestuous sexual relationship with her father from ages 5 to 12. These horrific but poignant accounts moved Dr. N intensely. Despite the adversity of her early life, she was an intelligent woman who had been accepted into medical school only to drop out and become a model.

As the treatment progressed, Jenny's sexualized transference toward Dr. N appeared to dissipate. She became distressed after some of her sessions, however, and passed out on five or six different occasions in the waiting room. Dr. N was puzzled. She seemed depressed and described a lifelong death wish. She also appeared to dissociate frequently. She recurrently voiced fantasies of killing herself after separating from everyone who was close to her. She had a thoroughgoing conviction that she was evil and dirty and was beyond redemption. Nevertheless, she told Dr. N that she felt calm when she was with him and that she had soothing dreams about him. She passed many sessions in silence, during which she would tell Dr. N that he needed to guess what she was thinking.

Jenny arrived in Dr. N's office at a particular time in his life. He had terminated his own analysis one year prior to her beginning treatment with him. He had also had a series of more recent losses in the months preceding Jenny's arrival. His younger sister had died of cancer, one of his closest friends had been killed in a motor vehicle accident, and his fiancée had broken their engagement and moved out of his home 2 months prior to the beginning of treatment. Dr. N was beleaguered and told me that, in retrospect, he probably should not have attempted to treat a patient like Jenny at that particular moment in his life. He clarified that while he was not in love with her, he often felt like an older brother who was protective of her and deeply committed to rescuing her from herself. He felt he had been making headway when she told him that he had helped her to stop living for others.

Things then took a turn for the worse. After about 3 years in treatment, Jenny started to fall silent in the sessions. She eventually told Dr. N that she was terminating treatment and moving away. With a good deal of coaxing from Dr. N, Jenny revealed that she had quit her job and given away prized possessions. With further probing, she finally confessed that she had purchased a gun. She announced to her analyst that death would be a relief. Dr. N became desperate. He began extending her sessions from 1 to 2 hours and saw her at the end of the day so that their sessions went well into the evening. When he met her for double sessions, he only charged her for one.

Dr. N became increasingly worried that her lethality was such that she could no longer be handled as an outpatient. She had been tried on a variety of antidepressant medications with no effect. He suggested that she needed to be hospitalized to save her from suicide. The patient refused hospitalization and refused to see a consultant. Nevertheless, Dr. N sought consultation for himself from a highly respected senior analyst in his city. After hearing the story, Dr. N's consultant agreed that hospitalization was unlikely to be helpful because the patient's suicidal despair was not based on an acute depression that would lift as a result of hospital treatment. Moreover, she was smooth enough to talk her way out of any type of involuntary commitment. She could appear much healthier than she was if she were required to convince a judge to let her go. The consultant encouraged Dr. N to continue working analytically on her underlying wish to die.

The patient continued to insist that she did not suffer from "clinical depression." Rather, she tried to make Dr. N understand that she was an awful person. Reeling from the recent losses in his life, Dr. N grew increasingly frantic. He noted a "desperate passivity" and a sense that his thinking was "muddled." At one point he said he would do anything he could to keep her from killing herself. Jenny replied that the only thing that would help was if he allowed her to spend a night with him in his house. She explained that she had intractable nightmares of physical and sexual abuse and that she longed to have the first good night's sleep of her life. Dr. N refused and explained that sleeping with a patient was unethical. In response to this straightforward explanation, Jenny looked at him coldly and asked, "What is more important? My life or your stupid ethics rules?" Dr. N was taken aback, and after several more weeks of trying to reason with Jenny, he finally conceded to her request to have one night with him. He rationalized that this radical measure might be the only means of keeping her alive. He also noted that from a personal perspective, he simply could not tolerate another loss by death.

On the night of this transgression of professional boundaries, he established ground rules that they would sleep in separate beds and there would be no sexual contact. The patient agreed, but when the time arrived, she came into his bed during the night and asked poignantly if Dr. N could hold her. One thing led to another, and ultimately they had sexual relations. In Dr. N's own words, "She seduced me while I protested that we should keep our pajamas on." He knew that his career could be ruined, but he held on to the fantasy that he might be saving her life.

The next morning Jenny informed Dr. N that she knew all along he would eventually sleep with her. She was confident that men found her irresistible. He told her that what he had done had been wrong and they could no longer see each other. She implored him to go out with her on dates, but he told her it was impossible.

Dr. N consulted with me several weeks after this incident, and he told me that he was tormented by what had happened. Jenny told him that the important thing to her was that he could love her despite what he knew. But he felt tortured and began to realize that there was a malicious, sadistic streak in Jenny that he had overlooked. He told me that he had noted her sadism when she described how she had dumped other men who were madly in love with her. However, he reflected on the fact that he had had a blind spot about her aggression toward *him.*

He described enormous feelings of guilt because he was beginning to recognize that he had actualized her transference fantasy by sleeping with her and therefore repeating the trauma of incest at the hands of her father. Dr. N told me that the moment he became aware that something aggressive was being reenacted was when they were having intercourse. He asked her about birth control. He knew that she had slept with three different men and assumed she was taking oral contraceptives. Jenny told Dr N that she couldn't have children, and she insisted that he should ejaculate inside her. Dr. N had a strong feeling that she was being dishonest because there was no way she could know that she was incapable of having children. He suddenly knew that she was trying to bring him down. He withdrew and felt a wave of nausea come over him. He sensed that he had made a serious error in judgment. In the midst of his anguish, however, he made a revealing comment: "At least I saved her from suicide."

DISCUSSION

This case involving a tragic miscarriage of psychoanalytic treatment will serve as a touchstone to discuss a variety of seriously misguided treatments for which I have served as a consultant. I will also draw on observations I have made serving in a role as analyst or therapist of colleagues who have made egregious boundary violations with suicidal patients. Some points will apply directly to the case of Dr. N, while others will draw on different cases that I cannot discuss in detail for reasons of confidentiality. While the example of Jenny and Dr. N involves sexual boundary violations, I have seen many others that stop short of sexual contact but are nevertheless highly destructive to the patient. In some cases worried analysts have taken suicidal patients into their homes and treated them like family members, invited them on family vacations, gone shopping with them, and shared dinner at local restaurants with them. In other cases analysts have treated the patient for free, engaged in extensive self-disclosure of their own personal problems, and had numerous extra-analytic contacts with the patient in public locations or in the patient's home.

Three caveats are in order before further discussion. First, readers should not dismiss the case of Dr. N as a bizarre aberration that is a rare occurrence. The scenario I have described is disconcertingly common among the boundary violation cases I have seen. Second, sexual boundary violations occur for a variety of reasons, and the mismanagement of suicidality is only one of many scenarios (Celenza and Gabbard, in press; Gabbard and Lester 1995; Gabbard and Peltz 2001). Finally, suicide can be mishandled in ways that do not involve boundary violations, of course, and I do not mean to neglect the importance of those cases by emphasizing the scenario in this particular communication.

DISIDENTIFICATION WITH THE AGGRESSOR

The vicissitudes of rage, hatred, revenge, and murderous fantasies have been well examined in the literature on suicide (Asch 1980; Chavrol and Sztulman 1997; Hendin 1991; Kernberg 1975; Maltsberger and Buie 1974, 1980; Menninger 1933). There can be little question that the act of suicide is enormously destructive to those left in the aftermath. Family members and friends are often enraged at what has been done to them. Suicidal threats in the context of analytic treatment may be experienced as a direct attack on the analyst's competence and person. Indeed, suicide is the ultimate narcissistic injury for an analyst. The patient is, in effect, thumbing his or her nose at the analyst. Analysts and therapists are frequently devastated in the wake of a patient's suicide. When colleagues have consulted with me after one of their patients has committed suicide, some have told me that they are seriously considering leaving the profession. Others have revealed that they think of nothing else for weeks on end as they search their memories for signals that they may have missed from the patient that might have ultimately prevented the suicide from occurring.

The boundary transgressions that occur with suicidal patients are often directly related to the mismanagement of aggression and hatred. This statement holds true to an even greater extent when the suicidal patient is a victim of childhood trauma, as in the case of Jenny. Patients like Jenny, who have engaged in incestuous sexual relations with a father, been locked in a closet by a mother, or been subjected to a multitude of other variations on "soul murder" (Shengold 1979), internalize abusive introjects that haunt them throughout their lives. Dr. N responded to this history and to the clinical presentation in the way that many of us do. He was determined to demonstrate that he was completely unlike the abusive parents by going to extraordinary lengths to save the patient from suicide. This posture on the part of the analyst, which I have elsewhere labeled as "disidentification with the aggressor" (Gabbard 1997), is a desperate attempt to disavow any connection with an internalized representation of a bad object that torments the patient. The analyst may be insidiously invaded by the abusive object and may unconsciously identify with it because of subtle or not so subtle interpersonal pressures from the patient. Many patients who have suffered severe childhood abuse or neglect approach analysis with the expectation that they deserve to be compensated for their tragic past by extraordinarily special treatment from the analyst (Davies and Frawley 1992). The ordinary analytic frame, within which we create an analytic space for the patient, may be experienced as depriving and even sadistic to such patients. They may insist that greater demonstrations of love and concern are necessary to prove that the analyst is not just as monstrous as the parent.

Dr. N, like most of us, was predisposed to avoid being transformed into the bad object that resides in the patient's internal world. As Money-Kyrle (1956) pointed out years ago, many of us enter this field unconsciously attempting to repair our own damaged internal objects from childhood. When we are intent on reparation, and we are then accused of destructiveness instead, our professional reaction formation is challenged in a way that may create extraordinary anxiety. Karl Menninger (1957) once noted that professions dedicated to helping others provide an ideal opportunity to conceal sadism. In some way we are always reassuring ourselves that our motives are beyond question because we have chosen to spend our days in the business of understanding others and helping them to improve their lives. An unconscious agenda of cleansing the dyad of hatred and aggression may cause the analyst to scotomize the sadism in the transference. Retrospectively, Dr. N was aware that he could only see the malicious aspects of Jenny directed toward other men—not toward him.

Because of this blind spot, the patient's sadism was able to "fly beneath the radar" of Dr. N and invade him. The abusive object then resides within the analyst and operates outside his awareness, persecuting him from within. In Dr. N's effort to rescue the patient from suicide, the abusive object took possession of him and engineered a retraumatization of Jenny. To this day, the malevolence transmitted by Jenny and her internal object world continues to torment Dr. N, who worries every day that his career could be ruined if Jenny chooses to file a complaint. In this way, Jenny inserted herself into the analyst and actualized a fantasy that the two of them would never be apart. She thus becomes unforgettable. She resides in him as a kind of foreign body and stains him with the badness that she feels has pervaded her since childhood. Now Dr. N feels similarly "dirty" and damaged.

Hence another way of understanding what transpired between Jenny and Dr. N goes beyond her projection of an abusive object into her analyst. She could be viewed as having projected a self-representation of a dirty and damaged child into Dr. N. In this object relations scenario, she identifies with the internal abusive object and destroys Dr. N in the same way she was destroyed by her parents. Parents who abuse their children may secretly envy their children's innocence (Grotstein 1992) and seek to spoil it through incest. In an analogous manner, the patient, unconsciously identified with the abusive parent, may wish to spoil what is perceived as the analyst's untainted purity by encouraging a boundary violation. To impute these unconscious motives to the patient, of course, does not relieve the analyst of the responsibility to act ethically no matter what wishes are brought to the treatment by the patient.

The analyst's unconscious anxieties are often at the core of the impasses that occur with suicidal patients. These anxieties may relate to an acute sense of one's vulnerability in the face of the patient's intense destructiveness. Many analysts feel that their reputation will be ruined if a patient commits suicide. Others may have primal anxieties regarding abandonment. Rosenfeld (1987) has noted that in impasse situations, analysts may deal with their anxieties by colluding with one aspect of the patient's personality while splitting off or compartmentalizing all other dimensions of the patient. In this manner, psychotic transference–countertransference reactions may become rigidified and the analyst may become paralyzed. The only way out may seem to be a terribly misguided series of unorthodox enactments.

The counterpart of transference hate is, of course, countertransference hate. One of the worst scenarios that results from the analyst's mishandling of aggression is that the countertransference hatred toward the patient goes undetected. This disavowal may lead to enactments that are disastrous (Maltsberger and Buie 1974). Analysts may unconsciously communicate to their patients that they don't wish to see them anymore or actually forget appointments. One analyst even left on vacation for a week without informing her patient of her upcoming absence until the day before her departure. Indeed, some suicides may even be precipitated when patients perceive their analysts as rejecting them (Hendin 1991). Federn (1929) once wryly observed that "only he who is wished dead by someone else kills himself" (quoted in Asch 1980, p. 56). That "someone else" may be the analyst.

Part of the analyst's rage and despair may be in direct response to the patient's failure to get better, thus thwarting the analyst's omnipotent strivings to heal. Celenza (1991) described a therapist who could not tolerate negative countertransference feelings when the treatment was at an impasse and similarly could not abide the patient's negative transference. The therapist embarked on a sexual relationship with the patient as an unconscious attempt to bypass all negative feelings in the patient and himself, hoping to foster an idealizing transference instead. Searles (1979) also noted that sexual involvement with patients may result from the analyst's therapeutic striving. In reaction to frustration at the patient's lack of improvement, the analyst may succumb to the illusion that a magical curative copulation will transform the patient. Dr. N, for example, held on to the magical belief that his submission to sexual relations with Jenny had saved the patient's life.

FAILURE OF MENTALIZATION AND COLLAPSE OF ANALYTIC SPACE

In the kind of collusion enacted by Dr. N and Jenny, the analytic play space collapses. Jenny does not view Dr. N "as if" he is her father. He *becomes* the father, and the incestuous act must be repeated. Dr. N, in turn, loses track of the fundamental aspects of the analytic situation and fails to recognize the "as if" dimension of the countertransference, and simply actualizes the role of the father. In this scenario, Dr. N's object (Jenny) is concretely identified as a projected part of the subject (the analyst). The analyst thus relates to the patient as though the patient is part of the self (Gabbard and Lester 1995). The difference between the symbol and the object is lost, and both members of the dyad succumb to a form of concrete symbolism in which there is a direct equation between the symbol and symbolized (Segal 1957).

In these impasse situations there is a *folie à deux,* a shared psychosis in the transference and countertransference. The psychosis is circumscribed to the dyad and involves a specific, but limited, failure of reality testing that is not generalized to other situations. In fact, Dr. N was able to carry out competent treatment with other patients during the time he was floundering in his treatment of Jenny. This *folie à deux* reflects an attack on the analyst's thinking directly related to the patient's destructive wishes. As Rosenfeld (1987) notes in his discussion of impasses, "Analysts tend at times to get caught up in a certain way of thinking which really implies a not thinking" (p. 43).

In Dr. N's perception of Jenny as a part of the self, he was also demonstrating a failure of mentalization that is common in impasses with suicidal patients. He lost track of the fact that Jenny's view of suicide and suicidality was entirely different from his own. Dr. N was anxious about her suicidal state, viewed it as a crisis, and did whatever he could to talk her out of it. Jenny, meanwhile, thought of suicide as a salvation of sorts. It was a way out of unspeakable despair. She developed it as a child as the only way that she could transcend feeling trapped in an incestuous relationship. Hence, there was an adaptive aspect of her suicidality that actually preserved a sense of mastery and coherence and provided her with the strength to continue living.

In Walker Percy's award-winning 1961 novel *The Moviegoer,* the chronically suicidal Kate offers a lesson to the protagonist Binx Bolling:

> They all think I'm going to commit suicide. What a joke. The truth of course is the exact opposite: suicide is the only thing that keeps me alive. Whenever everything else fails, all I have to do is consider suicide and in two seconds I'm as cheerful as a nitwit. But if I could *not* kill myself—ah then, I would. I can do without Nembutal or murder mysteries but not without suicide. (pp. 194–195)

Suicidality and the act of suicide are not the same thing. The analyst's task is to help the patient distinguish between impulsive actions and fantasy (Gabbard and Wilkinson 1994; Lewin and Schulz 1992). Many patients with severe personality disorders and extensive childhood trauma are truly suicidal, and the risk of suicide must be carefully assessed. I am not minimizing the potential lethality of such patients. The analyst can never be cavalier about suicide threats. What I *am* suggesting is that excessive anxiety about the risk may interfere with the analyst's capacity to think clearly about the functions and meanings of suicidality to the patient. Dr. N's failure of mentalization led to a self-destructive course based on a misreading of Jenny's suicidal intent. Dr. N was unable to assist the patient in constructing a symbolic dimension where fantasy and action are distinct. It is noteworthy in this regard that at a follow-up contact 7 years after the sexual episode, Dr. N learned that Jenny had still refrained from attempting suicide.

OMNIPOTENCE AND LOSS

In an era in which we regard the analyst's psychology as at least as important as the patient's, we must take into account Dr. N's state of mind at the time of the boundary transgression. In the preceding year, he had terminated his analysis, lost his sister to cancer, lost his best friend in a motor vehicle accident, and had been jilted by his fiancée. His grief was fresh and the prospect of another loss, that of his patient, was nothing short of overwhelming to him. Dr. N was struggling with a rawness or a vulnerability that made him particularly susceptible to take responsibility for the patient. He may not have been able to prevent the loss of the loved ones in his personal life, but he had the opportunity to make reparation for his imagined failures with them by saving his patient. In response to his depressive anxieties, manic defenses kicked in and he became determined to save the patient. The omnipotence in this posture escaped his awareness at the time but became increasingly conscious as he reflected back on what had happened. Dr. N wrote to me several years after seeing me: "I remain with the tendency to believe that love can cure, that I can right psychological wrongs through force of will and personal charisma, but I am recurrently reminded of the inevitable limitations/error of that point of view and the need to play with this notion of omnipotent helpfulness and what it means about my own need for help and the patient's need for an omnipotent other." His failure to insist on hospitalization when he was convinced she was about to kill herself is an example of his conviction that only he could save the patient. At the very least, colleagues on a hospital team may have helped him think through alternative strategies and helped him get sufficient distance from the case to reflect more fully on his countertransference collusion.

As with many other cases of serious boundary violations, there appears to have been a unique "fit" between Dr. N and Jenny. He had a largely unconscious need to heal through love and thus enact a specific form of object relatedness—namely, an omnipotent healer and a grateful patient (Gabbard 2000b). Dr. N's parents were divorced early in his childhood, and he spent much of his youth trying to rescue his mother from depression and unhappiness. He always felt that his mother did not date men who were good enough for her. Dr. N noted that Jenny looked a lot like his mother, and, retrospectively, he could see how he was re-enacting his childhood rescue attempt with Jenny. We can speculate that her similarity to his mother might have made her more forbidden and even more enticing. The patient, on the other hand, had an intense need to thwart this enactment and destroy his therapeutic zeal as well as his professional reputation. The more she foiled his efforts to heal, the more he escalated his heroic attempts to change her. The uniqueness of this "fit" was reflected in the fact that Dr. N had never engaged in any other form of serious boundary violation in his career. After the incident with Jenny, he decided to return for more analysis. He reports no subsequent violation in the years since his treatment of Jenny.

Analysts who enter into this type of *folie à deux* with a suicidal patient often forget what analysis is. They become convinced that their analytic knowledge and training is useless; it is their "person" that will save the patient. This paradigm of rescue may take the form of a deficit model, in which the analyst becomes convinced that some type of provision will make up for what is missing in childhood (Gabbard and Lester 1995). In the case of Dr. N, the notion of filling a deficit was concretized in the act of inserting his penis into her vagina. This regression from fantasy to concrete, bodily insertion is emblematic of how analysts in these situations may enter into a psychotic state of mind. This primitive altered state may lead them to take their patients' fantasies and wishes quite literally.

Sexualization in such situations may reflect a frantic defense against deadness. Feelings of non-being are well described in the incest literature (Bigras and Biggs 1990; Gabbard 1992). The incest victim's sense of self is severely damaged in the course of development, and profound feelings of deadness may result. Analysts may experience corresponding feelings, particularly when the patient disengages and becomes absorbed in the task of planning suicide (Gabbard 1992). Sexualization may offer the hope of bringing life and excitement to patient and analyst alike—a futile effort to revivify a treatment that is dormant (Coen 1992; Gabbard 1996).

Sexualization may, however, entail a self-destructive capitulation to the patient. Dr. N was fully aware that he was sacrificing himself to save the patient. Other analysts, too, will masochistically surrender to a suicidal patient as a way of demonstrating the extent of their caring (Gabbard and Lester 1995). Certain of our colleagues become well known for treating "impossible" patients that no other analysts will treat. Although many of these colleagues are gifted analysts, a subgroup appear to be going through their professional lives recreating a situation that often reflects problematic interactions with their own parents. They may be attempting to prove their worthiness to rejecting and emotionally distant parents or to rework early abandonments. By subjugating themselves to the patient, they may harbor a secret grandiosity, even a Christ identification, in which they view themselves as suffering for the sins of others in the service of transforming others. This masochistic posture may reflect a terror of repeating an early object loss in their own lives. Their willingness to risk their own careers may be regarded as the lesser of evils when confronted with yet another loss. In times when personal losses have recently been endured, analysts may be particularly prone to save the patient at all costs rather than to have to face another variation on the object loss that is already terrorizing them.

Dr. N, for example, was willing to violate his ethics code. He extended hours, stopped charging for the additional time, and gratified the patient's wish to sleep with him in a heroic effort to demonstrate that he cared enough to try to save her life. He was fully aware that the result could be the loss of his profession. What was a clear recreation of incest to an outside observer was construed by the analyst as a noble sacrifice.

I have always felt that there is a special irony in the way that boundary violations are rationalized with highly disturbed suicidal patients.

The rationale for the nonanalytic interventions that lead one down the slippery slope of boundary transgressions is that only radical departures from the analytic frame can possibly reach the patient. The irony is that these traumatized and highly disturbed patients are exactly the ones who require a containing but clear "boundedness" in the treatment to avoid the retraumatization and boundarylessness of their childhood situations.

I am not, of course, arguing for rigidity in the approach to disturbed patients with early childhood trauma. I have consistently advocated for flexibility in treating such patients (Gabbard 1997; Gabbard and Lester 1995; Gabbard and Wilkinson 1994). An affirming, empathic holding environment is essential. What I am emphasizing is that in the name of flexibility, egregious transgressions of boundaries are rationalized without regard for the fact that they simply enact the childhood trauma instead of containing it and understanding it through analytic processing.

CONCLUSIONS

What can we learn from these tragic miscarriages of psychoanalytic treatment? We must begin by being clear that we can never blame the patient for the analyst's transgressions. The patient has no professional code of conduct and is entitled to test the limits of the analytic setting. As Betty Joseph once noted, "The patient has every right to try to seduce the analyst. The analyst has no right to allow himself to be seduced" (personal communication, 2001). Nevertheless, the threat of suicide insinuates itself into the analyst's psyche in a way that is unique in our experience. It brings us squarely face to face with the limits of what we can do as analysts. One obvious lesson from these cases is that analysis may not be the appropriate treatment for certain lethal patients, and that other measures must be considered. Another frontier of psychoanalysis is its border with psychiatry. When necessary, we must avail ourselves of the expertise of colleagues who are knowledgeable about psychopharmacology, electroconvulsive therapy, and psychiatric hospital treatment. We all benefit from a more permeable border between psychiatry and psychoanalysis in these cases. At times we may overestimate the power of analytic treatment.

In still other situations, we think too little of analysis. Analysts may be too ready to abandon the power of containment and understanding and propel themselves headlong into ill-advised actions. Dr. N recalled that he had backed off from systematically interpreting Jenny's transference hostility. He sheepishly noted that most of his interpretive work was directed at her relationships with other men. When she became "bored" with the treatment in the second year, he inquired about anger toward him, but Jenny denied any hostility. In the final weeks of the treatment, he told her that he felt tortured. She was superficially sweet in response, telling him that she didn't want to cause him harm or worry. Jenny told Dr. N that he should be proud of keeping her alive as long as he had and that it wasn't his fault that she'd been ruined early in life. He recognized in retrospect that this was "manipulative artifice."

Another lesson to be learned from the careful examination of these cases is that we analysts have a good deal of ambivalence about the practice of psychoanalysis. Our love for analysis is constantly threatened by our unconscious hatred of analysis (Steiner, 2000). We endure a strain in our work that takes its toll. We demand a self-discipline that few other professions can match. The analytic role at times is experienced as a straitjacket from which we long to escape. Dr. N is not alone in his secret fantasy that love might be more effective than treatment. In many cases the hatred is also fueled by deep resentments toward one's training analyst or institute (Gabbard and Lester 1995).

This unconscious hatred of the analytic role and analytic work is often linked, in part, to envy of the patient. The asymmetry of the analytic setting is such that the devotion to the patient's needs and the patient's concerns is an ethical necessity. It is certainly a luxury to have the full attention of another human being four or five times a week for an hour at a time. We analysts may at times long for similar attention. Ferenczi, for example, noted that he was trying to give to his patients what he himself did not receive from his mother (Dupont 1988). The analytic situation, however, creates a worsening of this problem by exasperating the analyst's wound. In other words, as Ferenczi continued to give to his patients, he could only feel his own deprivation more acutely. He ultimately tried experiments in mutual analysis to try to get something back from the patient to meet his own needs. To his credit, he abandoned this experiment when he recognized it was fraught with problems.

Nevertheless, in my years of consulting on boundary violations cases, I have been struck at how often Ferenczi's mutual analysis is invoked as a rationalization for getting on the couch with the patient and self-disclosing the analyst's personal problems. Management of hatred in the dyad also appears to enter into this variety of enactment. Friedman (1995) has pointed out that the relationship between mutual analysis and persecutory hate can be inferred from Ferenczi's writings. Ferenczi recognized that his forced, overly polite manner thwarted the patient's effort to free herself from persecutory hate. Hence he initiated mutual analysis because it allowed him to disclose his hate to the patient and be forgiven for it. Ferenczi felt the analyst needed to accept the projections of the patient's hatred and then confess it to the patient. Unfortunately, he also regarded the hate as essentially unreal and potentially manageable by the analyst's overpowering love. As Friedman (1995) notes, however: "The claim that some form of love can be an adequate and/or curative response to the patient's suffering only escalates the patient's demand for such, placing unbearable pressures on the analyst that induce incredible tension" (p. 973).

Another lesson that follows from Ferenczi and from the case of Dr. N, as well as from other misguided treatments, is that many suicidal patients are searching for a "bad enough object" (Gabbard 2000b; Rosen 1993). These patients desperately need the analyst to contain the abusive introject that eats away at them inside and causes them to suffer. Analysts who won't allow themselves to be transformed into the bad object only invite the patient to escalate their efforts to reach hatred and aggression within the dyad (Fonagy 1998; Gabbard 2001). It is incumbent on the analyst to resist the magnetic pull to disidentify with the aggressor. We must be able to recognize that aspects of the patient are infuriating, annoying, destructive, and abusive, and we must be able to own our reactions. It is the analyst's role to be hated and to understand that hatred, not to projectively disavow unpleasant affect states and see them in parental figures (or others) outside the consulting room.

Dr. N's case also illustrates the fact that consultation, while helpful, is not a panacea. We may choose an analyst who will tell us what we wish to hear. We may corrupt the process by concealing certain aspects of the treatment. We may ignore the consultant's advice. We may secretly believe that no one outside the quasi-incestuous dyad of analyst and analysand can possibly understand the special and unique features of a particular suicidal patient (Gabbard 2000a). Consultation can be of extraordinary value in such cases, but only if the analyst selects a consultant who can see the situation from a new perspective and who is allowed to share that perspective with the consultee.

There is a thin line between altruistic wishes to help our patients and omnipotent strivings to heal them. We must avoid the quasi-delusional conviction that only we are capable of helping a patient and that it is only our unique personhood, rather than our knowledge and technique, that is useful. We must even accept that in our limits as analysts, we will lose some patients. This recognition may help us avoid masochistic surrender scenarios in which we sacrifice ourselves in a blind and grandiose effort to save another.

Many of us neglect self-care in our training as analysts. When lifeguards or water safety instructors are trained, the first thing they are taught is that they themselves must be safe before saving the drowning victim. If this matter is not addressed, two people may drown instead of one. We can benefit from this philosophy in how we train our analysts. We must attend to our personal lives and be sure that our own needs are met before we attempt to rescue others. An obvious message from studying these cases is that suicidal patients may drag us down with them despite our most heroic efforts. It is our duty to assure that we do whatever we can to keep our heads above water.

REFERENCES

Asch SS: Suicide and the hidden executioner. Int Rev Psychoanal 7:51–60, 1980

Bigras J, Biggs KH: Psychoanalysis as incestuous repetition: some technical considerations, in Adult Analysis, in Childhood Sexual Abuse. Edited by Levine HB. Hillsdale, NJ, Analytic Press, 1990, pp 35–41

Brown L (ed): The New Shorter Oxford English Dictionary on Historical Principles, Vol. 1. Oxford, UK, Clarendon Press, 1993

Celenza A: The misuse of countertransference love in sexual intimacies between therapists and patients. Psychoanalytic Psychology 8:501–509, 1991

Celenza A, Gabbard GO: Analysts who commit sexual boundary violations: a lost cause? J Am Psychoanal Assoc (in press)

Chavrol H, Sztulman H: Splitting and the psychodynamics of adolescent and young adult suicide attempts. Int J Psychoanal 78:1199–1208, 1997

Coen SJ: The Misuse of Objects. Hillsdale, NJ, Analytic Press, 1992

Davies JM, Frawley MG: Dissociative processes and transference-countertransference paradigms in the psychoanalytically oriented treatment of adult survivors of childhood sexual abuse. Psychoanalytic Dialogues 2:5–36, 1992

Dupont J (ed): The Clinical Diary of Sándor Ferenczi. Translated by Balint M, Jackson NZ. Cambridge, MA, Harvard University Press, 1988

Fonagy P: An attachment theory approach to treatment of the difficult patient. Bull Menninger Clin 62:147–169, 1998

Freidman J: Ferenczi's clinical diary: on loving and hating. Int J Psychoanal 76:957–975, 1995

Gabbard GO: Commentary on "Dissociative Processes and Transference-Countertransference Paradigms" by Jody Messler Davies and Mary Gail Frawley. Psychoanalytic Dialogues 2:27–47, 1992

Gabbard GO: Love and hate in the Analytic Setting. Northvale, NJ, Jason Aronson, 1996

Gabbard GO: Challenges in the analysis of adult patients with histories of childhood sexual abuse. Can J Psychoanal 5:1–25, 1997

Gabbard GO: Consultation from the consultant's perspective. Psychoanalytic Dialogues 10:209–218, 2000a

Gabbard GO: On gratitude and gratification. J Am Psychoanal Assoc 48:697–716, 2000b

Gabbard GO: Psychodynamic psychotherapy in borderline personality disorder: a contemporary approach. Bull Menninger Clin 65:41–57, 2001

Gabbard GO, Lester EP: Boundaries and Boundary Violations in Psychoanalysis. New York, Basic Books, 1995

Gabbard GO, Peltz M: Speaking the unspeakable: institutional reactions to boundary violations by training analysts. J Am Psychoanal Assoc 49:659–673, 2001

Gabbard GO, Wilkinson SM: Management of Countertransference With Borderline Patients. Washington, DC, American Psychiatric Press, 1994

Grotstein J: Commentary on "Dissociative Processes and Transference-Countertransference Paradigms" by Jody Messler Davies and Mary Gail Frawley. Psychoanalytic Dialogues 2:61–76, 1992

Hendin H: Psychodynamics of suicide, with particular reference to the young. Am J Psychiatry 148:1150–1158, 1991

Kernberg OF: Borderline Conditions and Pathological Narcissism. New York, Jason Aronson, 1975

Lewin RA, Schulz CG: Losing and Fusing: Borderline and Transitional Object and Self Relations. Northvale, NJ, Jason Aronson, 1992

Maltsberger JT, Buie DH: Countertransference hate in the treatment of suicidal patients. Arch Gen Psychiatry 30:625–633, 1974

Maltsberger JT, Buie DH: The devices of suicide: revenge, riddance, and rebirth. Int Rev Psychoanal 7:61–72, 1980

Menninger KA: Psychoanalytic aspects of suicide. Int J Psychoanal 14:376–390, 1933

Menninger KA: Psychological factors in the choice of medicine as a profession. Bull Menninger Clin 21:51–58, 1957

Money-Kyrle RE: Normal counter-transference and some of its deviations. Int J Psychoanal 37:360–366, 1956

Percy W: The Moviegoer (1961). New York, Vintage Books, 1998

Rosen IR: Relational masochism: the search for a bad-enough object. Paper presented to the Topeka Psychoanalytic Society, January 21, 1993

Rosenfeld H: Impasse and Interpretation. London, Tavistock, 1987

Searles HF: Countertransference and Related Subjects: Selected Papers. Madison, CT, International Universities Press, 1979

Segal H: Notes on symbol formation. Int J Psychoanal 38:391–397, 1957

Shengold L: Child abuse and deprivation: soul murder. J Am Psychoanal Assoc 27:533–559, 1979

Steiner J: Book review of *A Mind of One's Own: A Kleinian's View of Self and Object* by R. Caper. J Am Psychoanal Assoc 48:637–643, 2000

9

ARNOLD GOLDBERG, M.D.

INTRODUCTION

Arnold Goldberg received his B.S. and M.D. from the University of Illinois and did his psychoanalytic training at the Institute for Psychoanalysis in Chicago, where he is currently a Training and Supervising Analyst, having served as Director of the Institute. He has been Clinical Professor of Psychiatry at the Pritzker School of Medicine and is Professor of Psychiatry at the Rush-Presbyterian-St. Luke's School of Medicine in Chicago. He has been Visiting Professor of Psychoanalysis at the University of Chicago and is the Cynthia Oudejans Harris, M.D., Professor, Department of Psychiatry, at Rush Medical College in Chicago. His dedication to teaching is underscored by his having been the winner eight times of the Benjamin Rush Award for Best Teacher in Psychiatry of Rush Medical College.

Dr. Goldberg has been Editor of *The Annual of Psychoanalysis;* has served on the editorial boards of the *Journal of the Hillside Hospital, The Psychohistory Review, The Journal of the American Psychoanalytic Association,* and *The International Journal of Psychoanalysis;* and was the Editor of the *Progress in Self Psychology* series. He has lectured widely in this country and internationally, and his named lectureships have included the Edmund Weil Lecture, New York, the Sandor Rado Lecture of the Columbia University Center for Psychoanalytic Training and Research, the Sandor Feldman Lecture of the University of Rochester Medical Center, the Distinguished Psychiatrist Lecture of the American Psychiatric Association, and the plenary addresses of both the American

Psychoanalytic Association and the International Psychoanalytical Association. He has published on a vast range of topics, many of them centered on the evolution and development of new ideas in self psychology. Dr. Goldberg has been a major contributor to the expansion of Kohut's contributions. He has also been interested in the details of analytic process, the psychology of perversions, and the evolution of our ideas of analytic structure. His books include *Models of the Mind: The Psychoanalytic Theory* (with John Gedo), *A Fresh Look at Psychoanalysis: The View from Self Psychology, The Prison House of Psychoanalysis, Being of Two Minds: The Vertical Split in Psychoanalysis,* and *Misunderstanding Freud.* He edited *The Future of Psychoanalysis, Advances in Self Psychology, Errant Selves: A Casebook of Misbehavior,* and 18 volumes of *Progress in Self Psychology.* Dr. Goldberg's contributions are characterized by a deep commitment to philosophical precision, detailed scrutiny of analytic process, and impatience with received wisdom.

He has said of himself:

> I have great difficulty imagining a role for myself in the American psychoanalytic scene, which, for me at least, is more like a patient in need of a physician, while I can only function as a critic without a cure. Psychoanalysis in America is at a moment in history that seems to warrant worry, but it cannot command the attention for proper concern. I was fortunate enough to live through its time of splendor and significance and unfortunate enough to witness its decline. As a devoted Darwinian, I hope it can evolve to another time of strength and survival, but it seems most of us can only watch and hope and try our best to make it interesting.

WHY I CHOSE THIS PAPER

Arnold Goldberg, M.D.

Years of teaching and writing have taught me that the most important point to keep in mind is the understanding of the audience. I chose "Between Empathy and Judgment" for inclusion in this volume because this particular paper was clearly one that was grasped and responded to with some degree of excitement and enthusiasm, both when I presented it orally and when published. Probably in my heart, I felt that other papers had an equal amount of pride in production, but either the anonymous readers of some journal or the obvious sleeper in some audience disabused me of too much parental hubris. I myself have long ago given up on being a good judge of what I write because of my unfailing self-assurance. I just happen to be right on this one.

BETWEEN EMPATHY AND JUDGMENT

ARNOLD GOLDBERG, M.D.

A PATIENT OF MINE, whom I shall call Karl, said that he wanted very much to write a letter to Ann Landers or Dear Abby. He had come to me after seeing several therapists preparatory to his "coming out" as homosexual, and in each case these therapists were on hand to help him implement this decision of his. Because of my own admitted uncertainty about what he "really" was, and for other reasons based on my inquiring and expressing concern about his life apart from his avowed sexuality, he decided to go into analysis with me. In the analysis, he discovered that his homosexual fantasies were serving what were essentially nonsexual purposes, and he soon became for the first time rather actively heterosexual.

A friend of mine who is a gay therapist—that is, someone who is himself gay and primarily treats gays—tells me that my patient is really heterosexual, and this is now what my patient claims, and what he wants to tell Dear Ann and Dear Abby. He wants them to know that one should never urge anyone to declare himself gay or be directed to a gay therapist or to take any such definitive steps until and unless one knows for sure. And so here is the crux of the matter. Karl says that his analysis allowed him to discover what he really was—i.e., he was able to know for sure, and without it, he may well have decided to become gay. That possibility now offends him. He feels that he was very close to a terrible

---

Plenary address presented to the American Psychoanalytic Association, December 1997.

"Between Empathy and Judgment," by Arnold Goldberg, M.D., was first published in *The Journal of the American Psychoanalytic Association,* 47:351–365, 1999.

mistake. Interestingly, he feels there are lots of other aspects of himself that are likewise what he really may be or seems to be or would like to be, and that he wishes he could be made different. He would have liked his analysis to change these for him as well. He wishes that he were more sociable—why hasn't his analysis helped him there? He feels he is somewhat lazy and now insists that analysis should make him more industrious. When I suggest that he seems to be willing to discover and modify some things about himself—like his sexuality, say—and to regard these as a mark of authenticity, while at the same time he comes upon other qualities—say, a certain aloofness in relationships—and considers them somewhat questionably authentic but eminently alterable, he agrees. But he cannot settle for analysis being confined to the mere unlocking of potentials. Is it not meant to do more? Should it not only allow or enable us to be different, but make us so?

Karl says that he thinks analysts feel that a patient is like an unlit Roman candle on the Fourth of July. The analyst lights it and steps to the side to watch, hoping to admire the display. Some Roman candles are splendid, and some are duds. Blame the factory. But surely one needs to take more responsibility for the display, since no one really seems to step to the side. Karl agrees that his own analysis could not be said to have been clearly weighted on the side of heterosexuality, but he has always suspected that I had a bias in its favor. The neutral stance that I claimed was, in truth, more related to a personal confusion of mine than to a principled conviction. He and I shared a goal, and to say otherwise would be to hide behind a cloak of neutrality that seemed more transparent than real. Or so he says.

This variation on the nature-nurture argument has in the past had a rather clear solution in psychoanalysis. Part of the solution is the existence of real physical constraints. We cannot make people taller or shorter, but perhaps when it comes to weight we are a bit less certain. However, as each new evidence of the physical or biological makes its appearance, we tend to retreat. When we learn of the neurological basis for obsessive-compulsive disorder, we come to read the case of the Rat Man with a different eye. When we become convinced of the genetic basis of bipolar disease, we begin to think less of the dynamic formulations once ascribed to it; but when these same genes are called into question, we quickly rethink our psychological position. Thus we become prisoners of the latest and best physical basis for the psyche. And surely sexuality is bedrock—or is it?

The other part of the solution for what can and should be done for patients, and thus what is in their best interest, is our own set of standards and norms. These tell us how people ought to be, and we work to get our patients as close to them as possible. We have all devised some set of developmental steps that we consider normal and therefore desirable. To travel along the correct path of development and achieve a goal that we consider optimal is the blueprint, secret or open, against which we measure our patients. Thus, in our supposed willingness for patients to follow a path of self-fulfillment, we also posit a map that tells us just about where they should end up.

Sexuality and gender seem to be, or should be, easy. For a while there, everyone had to be heterosexual. Of late, psychiatry and (reluctantly) psychoanalysis have moved to a clear espousal of normal homosexuality. For each of these poles there seems to be a pathology as well; i.e., there exists a pathological heterosexuality that serves to cover over or to defend against a variety of painful situations, up to and including homosexuality. The situation is ever more complex. We regularly see heterosexually promiscuous or deviant men or women who struggle against homosexual intimacy, just as we see gay promiscuity defend against heterosexual closeness. At one point in his treatment Karl said that he might have gone either way, and so one surely has to consider bisexuality as yet another aspect of normal sexual performance. Is it really the case that psychoanalysis allows people to determine what they really are, without the analyst also making some determination? Is it not possible that there is no such thing as what a person really is?

In an excellent review based primarily on Ogden's variation of Kleinian thinking, Sweetnam (1996) argues that gender, being dialectical, may feel fixed at certain times and fluid at others. She claims that different psychological positions—the paranoid and the depressive—provide a context for the anxieties, defenses, object relationship, subjectivity, and symbolization that alter the quality of gender experience within a context that goes beyond a linear developmental timetable or the comprehension of singular identifications. Sweetnam's intention is to balance the biological determinism ascribed to Freud with the newly popular cultural determinism of other investigators, by proposing a framework that embraces both fluidity and firmness. The essential point of her effort is to reveal our psychology as constrained, perhaps trapped, between biology and culture, the body and the world.

At any given moment in analysis we seem to be making some judgment of the way things ought to be, and we tend to direct the process according to that judgment. It is a judgment based on what we claim to be correct and real and true. But just as biology seems to help at certain times, so at others cultural factors seem to weigh in. There can be little doubt that people can go more than one way in more than one domain. It seems a bit naïve to say either that we let the patient decide or that we allow normal development to unfold. We are not merely watching. However, once we relinquish our neutral stance as untenable, we are committed to standing somewhere. Lest we too quickly claim an allegiance to a newly popular embrace of "authenticity," we should probably recognize that one can be an authentic scoundrel as well as a saint. Where once we felt that we need only be empathic with our patients, we now find that we cannot help but judge them as well. Sometimes the two stances seem to be at odds, in need of some principle of unity. And so now to the reconciliation of empathy and judgment.

TWO PERSPECTIVES

At the outset I would like to clarify some of the basic positions that I see as fundamental to psychoanalysis. It is first and foremost a psychology devoted to what some philosophers and many scientists have called a first-person perspective—that is, one that centers on a subjective view of the world that says that *I* know, *I* see, *I* experience. The contrasting viewpoint is that of the third person: objective, external, making statements about him, her, or it that sees, knows, and experiences. First-person perspectives are available to introspection, conscious personal scrutiny, and assessment, and are regarded by some as incorrigible, since one is, or should be, the sole determinant of a personal experience. By contrast, a third-person perspective is available to objective, public examination and testing, and is the clear winner in a scientific tug-of-war. To complete the picture, we consider a second-person perspective, the experience that *you* are having, to be graspable by another by way of an inner comparison or vicarious introspection. It has been the sad fate of psychoanalysis to have been ever tempted by a third-person perspective as an ultimate goal to be reached. Most neurophysiologists lay claim to a third-person perspective as allowing a complete description and explanation of any and all brain phenomena and so as the goal of all studies of behavior. But most, if certainly not all, scientists also agree that first- and third-person psychologies are irreducible one to another. There can be no elimination of the "I" experience. Biology and social psychology can never replace depth psychology. These remain complementary but distinct perspectives.

It is worth a moment to explain and justify this thesis of the irreducibility of first- and third-person perspectives, since the tendency to treat depth psychology as a way station to some sought-for biosocial final explanation seems solidly entrenched. Psychoanalysis thus becomes wedged in between biology and social psychology in a scientistic effort to explain from an objective point of view all there is to know about people. But just as no study limited to the makeup of DNA can reveal the final phenotype, so too the study of neuronal pathways demands an experience if we are to identify precisely the fate of this or that brain activity. When we know just how and why the brain produces the color brown, we still need to determine exactly what color is experienced. Nor should we be fooled into thinking that knowing enough about the brain will close the gap. There exists such a gap for both empirical and conceptual reasons. No matter how much we subscribe to the premise that all phenomena are ultimately neural, as surely they are, we need to recognize with equal certainty that psychological phenomena are not thereby eliminated. Indeed, a famed perceptual physiologist has stated recently that "perceptual findings must be considered primary, and if the neurophysiological data do not agree, the neurophysiological data must be wrong" (Uttal 1997, p. 300). The first-person perspective is essential.

On the social side of the ledger is the evidence recently accumulating that calls into question the biological innateness of sexuality, especially as regards women, some of whom seem capable of choosing their sexual identity (Golden 1997). Research seems to suggest that some women who identify themselves as bisexual find they are able to entertain the possibility of choosing to be lesbian or heterosexual. In the presence of powerful social and cultural factors, biology seems to take a back seat. The fluidity of sexuality is, however, perhaps called into question by reports of that ridiculous experiment by Money (*Chicago Tribune,* March 14, 1997), who advised parents to raise as a girl a boy whose penis had been accidentally amputated. After countless surgeries and hormone treatments, the child finally insisted on becoming the boy he knew he was. One may theorize that biology or early imprinting was a factor here, but I suspect that an analytically informed observer could see that simply everyone around the child knew he was a boy masquerading as a girl and that the communication of that fact, however unconscious, was omnipresent. Thus, it seems sometimes that biology rules the day and at other times that social factors predominate. Nonetheless, a first-person psychology remains valid, despite whatever third-person issues are studied and raised, because only such a perspective allows us entry into the personal experiences of the subject. It must be admitted, however, that sole reliance on a first-person perspective has caused problems that continue to plague our field.

The effort to establish psychoanalysis on what was felt to be a firmer, more scientific ground certainly began with Freud's 1895 Project. That effort was taken up later by Heinz Hartmann, who insisted that psychoanalysis was an explaining, rather than an understanding, psychology. Hartmann said that the study of forces in opposition, of energy and its expression, was the scientific ground for psychoanalysis. For him, an understanding of psychology is necessarily unreliable and so fails to be a science. Only an explanation of the causal relations in the mind, he believed, could bring psychoanalysis to its rightful place in science, and these causal connections are made not from reports of subjective experience but rather from (in his words) the actual mental connections. Empathy not only is rife with potential errors, but neglects that part of our personality—the unconscious—that is fundamental to psychoanalysis. Hartmann wanted an objective psychoanalysis that was reliable and capable of validation. His was essentially a plea for a third-person psychology in which our judgments or truths must rule.

The love affair of analysis and objectivity was certainly cooled, if not shattered, by the central role assigned to empathy by Heinz Kohut and his colleagues. Although these two Heinzes were friends socially, ideologically they were quite far apart. Kohut's concentration on empathy as vicarious introspection indeed moved psychoanalysis back into a first-person perspective. This focus has been taken up in countless variations on the theme—from an insistence on seeing things primarily from the patient's point of view to the embracing of a postmodern or relativist position that calls into question the very existence of truth or fact or objectivity. Things are what they are felt to be and not what others say they are. What happened to the patient as a child is not a question of history but of meaning. Rashomon becomes the new cultural symbol of psychoanalysis, as at our conferences "it all depends" becomes an introductory mantra. To see the world from the perspective of the patient is to suspend judgment and to enjoy, perhaps momentarily, a trial identification with the other.

A problem that presents itself in any singular focus on empathy is that it is either a sustained or a momentary inquiry into a conscious experience. When one steps into the shoes of another to vicariously introspect, the material is by definition that which is conscious. A first-person perspective entails experiences that have qualities and are realized. We own our experiences, and they are a conscious part of us. Imagine the difference between a name you cannot remember and one you cannot possibly have known. The first is felt as something that must be brought back into awareness, while the second allows no ownership claims and remains outside the psyche. For those who would limit our data to the empathically accessible, therefore, the role and even the existence of the psychoanalytic unconscious becomes problematic.

To be sure, the complex role of empathy in psychotherapy and psychoanalysis is not diminished by a recognition of its inherent limitations. But we need to add a crucial component to the data obtained by empathy. A component that belongs to the observer, it may be thought of as consisting of preconceptions or perspectives or theories, but it is essentially derived from the eye of the other. It is a judgment. The balance to the purely subjective experience of the patient is offered by the judgments brought by the observer. These are the observer's theories, preconceptions, morality. If the observer believes in the unconscious, it is added to the mix. To gain access to another, we carry ourselves and our beliefs along, and so every first-person perspective, every study of individual meaning, is seen and then changed by the onlooker. (And it needs perhaps to be said that every third-person perspective also carries with it the subjective coloration of the observer.) The psychoanalytic observer, the empathic student of a patient, carries convictions and judgments not only about the patient's reported experiences but also about what is known at first only to the analyst: the content of the patient's unconscious. Initially this is felt by the patient as foreign or separate. The unconscious is experienced not as first-person phenomena but as something alien and apart. To bring it into subjective experience, to realize Freud's "Where id was, there shall ego be" (once considered the work of psychoanalysis) is to move from the third-person perspective on the contents of the unconscious—however conceptualized—to the first-person perspective of subjective ownership and individual meanings. The two Heinzes—Kohut and Hartmann—must be joined in this reconciliation of empathy and judgment.

The autobiography of the analysand is "since Rousseau a construction, not a representation" (Bernstein 1995, p. 70), and into it is introduced what the analyst knows/presumes to be present, primarily if not exclusively, in the patient's unconscious. These additions are the shifts or switches between facts and meanings, objective and subjective, judgment and empathy, that we all live with as we understand our patients while simultaneously judging them. It should perhaps be emphasized that empathy or understanding or first-person psychology is certainly not opposed to judgment or explanation or third-person psychology; rather, the two interpenetrate. A similarly false dichotomy is often drawn between creativity (ascribed, erroneously, exclusively to artistic endeavors) and discovery (falsely attributed exclusively to the scientific). The argument over whether psychoanalysis is an art or a science is played out on the same erroneous basis, as these are ends on a continuum rather than separate domains. To fault the empathic approach by noting its contamination with inferences is as wrong as condemning objectivity by seeing the subjective component in it. These are conceptual errors. Empathy and judgment must penetrate one another, as do discovery and creation. However, since an analysis is an exercise in first-person psychology, we need to see it as what one writer has called "a theory-mediated autobiography" (Bernstein 1995, p. 70). Thus we see that all sorts of theory, from Freudian to Kleinian to Kohutian to Lacanian, can be used for an acceptable redescription of childhood and indeed all personal experience. All these redescriptions may be true, since the autobiography is shaped by those who create it. What emerges from a psychoanalysis is a first-person account of a life, written by two people, an empathic account interpenetrated by the judgments of the other.

CLINICAL IMPLICATIONS

A return to Karl will afford us a better view of psychoanalysis as a first-person psychology. Karl manifested a type of clinical state that some of us have been studying for some time: the narcissistic behavior disorders. Some of my friends, however, both in psychiatry and psychoanalysis, seem genuinely puzzled by this diagnostic category. They either consider it the result of too much empathic immersion or politely ask me just what those words are supposed to mean. My answer to that question is that these are pathological conditions characterized by behavior considered distasteful, abhorrent, or antisocial, and felt by the actor to be performed as if by another person. Thus, a perfectly respectable citizen will periodically find himself stealing something, a perfectly moral woman will find herself picking up strange men in bars, an otherwise honest person will find himself lying. My patient Karl was a voyeur who would fairly regularly find himself looking at men's penises in locker rooms and masturbating with the immediate image or the memory of it. Karl hated himself for this behavior and spoke of its occurrence as if it were done by someone else, as if he could not, and would not, own it. The cases that a group of us have studied show this phenomenon of disavowal rather routinely; a split in the self seems to allow the coexistence of parallel personalities with different sets of goals and ambitions, different values and needs, indeed seemingly different psychic organizations. Typically, one personality is acknowledged and the other despised; i.e., one is understood and the other is harshly judged. That both are conscious gives no clear answer to the problem posed by the split: one is me and the other is him.

In writing of repression, which Kohut called a "horizontal" split,

Freud emphasized the patient's ignorance: "It is a long superseded idea, and one derived from superficial appearances, that the patient suffers from a sort of ignorance, and that if one removes the ignorance by giving him information (about the causal connection of his illness with his life, about his experiences in childhood, and so on) he is bound to recover. The pathological factor is not his ignorance in itself, but the root of his ignorance in his inner resistances; it was they that first called this ignorance into being, and they still maintain it now" (Freud 1910, p. 225). By contrast, the split of disavowal, first noted by Freud in the fetishist (Freud 1927) is vertical rather than horizontal; here the patient both knows and yet does not acknowledge, as would happen if the contents of the unconscious were made known to the patient and were therefore conscious but not really owned or experienced as part of the self. It is thus a matter not of ignorance but of abhorrence regarding what is known. These patients judge themselves, but not like those who suffer guilt from a harsh superego; rather, they treat themselves as others whom they would shun; they see themselves from a third-person perspective and so disown a part of themselves.

We often note that the anxious or depressed patient is *unable* to step aside from a symptom in order to disavow it. By contrast, a patient of mine with an eating disorder spoke of her binges as if in retrospect she very much disliked that person who stuffed herself with Oreos. In treatment, more often than not, the therapist or analyst joins with the patient in this harsh judgment. The college professor who steals books in an unpredictable and uncontrollable manner very much expects the analyst to be as critical of his behavior as he is. Save for those patients whose behavior disorders dominate their psyches, these patients with vertical splits live a life between understanding and judging and ask the same of their analyst. This now becomes a virtual laboratory for a study of the tension between empathy and judgment. The analyst, struggling to understand and not condemn, shares the split of the patient, while almost simultaneously being asked to condemn until understanding is achieved. When one treats a scoundrel, be it a thief, a liar, a voyeur, or an addict, it is foolhardy to claim a neutrality for ourselves. We always take a stand. And some of us even, in turn, judge ourselves harshly or benignly for the stand that we take.

Perhaps one of the more interesting phenomena to have emerged from our study is the wide range of tolerance or intolerance claimed by the analysts in our group. While one of us may be quite content to have a stalker as a patient, another may be totally unable to sustain a therapeutic stance toward such behavior. The analyst who comfortably treats a thief is considered to be himself mildly unusual, but only by some members of the group—until that moment in our discussions when he betrays his own quite corrupt self. And when that moment occurs, he is as astonished as anyone to see himself as a kindred soul to his dishonest patient. The movement from tolerant understanding to critical judgment becomes a rather routine feature of our group discussions, with some members resting more easily in one phase than in another. The dishonesty of one of us is sharply attacked and condemned by the others until, over time, we begin to see the lack of purity, the inherent contradiction, in all of us. What once were sharp lines of demarcation between right and wrong, truth and falsehood, become shaded into vague areas of personal opinion. We seem unable to find our footing as we shift between the parallel selves of our patients, as we discover shades of the same split within ourselves.

The transition from the one perspective to the other is graphically demonstrated by a Lacanian, Slavaj Žižek (1992), who describes the story of a serial killer as told in Fred Walton's movie *When A Stranger Calls.* The film first presents the killer as an unfathomable object, with whom no identification is possible, and then makes a sudden transposition into the perspective of the killer himself. Žižek discusses the two points of view, that of the victim and that of the murderer, and the sudden twist of the movie: "The entire subversive effect hangs upon the rupture, the passage from one perspective to the other, the change which confers upon the hitherto impossible/unattainable object or body, which gives the untouchable thing a voice and makes it speak, in short, which subjectivizes it" (p. 57). Once captured by the identification with a murderer, we find it quite difficult to depart from that position to once again objectify and despise him. We are denied the comfort that we had previously enjoyed of knowing for sure, a comfort best thought of as a warning, since the interpenetration of empathy and judgment makes for the unstable state more proper to the life of a psychoanalyst. We do, however, manage to carve out positions of resolution, and those positions share both the judgmental condemnation suggested to us by Freud in his consideration of the endpoint of analysis, along with the self-empathy needed to restore balance to our ever-present uncertainty and lack of closure. This resolution maintains, however, the interpenetration of judgment and empathy.

EMPATHY, JUDGMENT, AND TREATMENT

Let us consider empathy as discovery, more or less, and judgment as creation. Moving back and forth between empathy, which aims to discover what is there but at times is inaccessible, and judgment, which creates something by bringing in new materials, is both a paradox and a sought-for state. The autobiographies we create are necessarily shaped by the theories we employ—our judgment—to mediate what we hope to discover in our patients by way of empathy. We discover, by using our theories, what is in the unconscious, but we do so by knowing beforehand what is there to be found. Similarly, our patients come to recognize the split-off areas as really belonging to them, as the foreign territory of the repressed and the disavowed, the psyche split off horizontally or vertically is joined with the rest of the psyche. In treating patients with behavior disorders, we become able to be empathic first with one side, then with the other, and ultimately with both. We must, however, realize that seeing things exactly as the patient does makes blind men of us both. We need to remain objective about our subjectivity; we always judge or evaluate our meanings as we step aside and see ourselves as we would see another.

This oscillation between empathy and judgment has a counterpart in our consideration of what we find in a patient versus what we bring to our investigations. With Karl, I knew I wanted to rid him of his voyeurism, but I could also rather easily identify with that activity; I was more puzzled than anything about his both wanting and hating his homosexual longings. Over time, as I became convinced that they represented a sexualization related to the transference, I brought my judgment into his analysis and created a new configuration.

The history of psychoanalytic technique has itself made this journey from discovery to creation. The earliest pioneers in the field were intent on discovering the contents and makeup of the unconscious; the latest contributors, advocates of the various interactive theories, address the jointly created products of analytic and therapeutic work. Most contemporary investigators seem to seek a resolution to the dilemma through some sort of fifty-fifty compromise. No one seems any longer to deny the importance of the analyst's person. Nor is anyone likely to say that the patient's past and unconscious are not to be reckoned with. Unfortunately, the resolution seems often to be reached by means of a popularity poll, and more often than not is generalized to apply to all of our patients. But what I have learned from Karl and so many others is the simple truth that sometimes I matter and sometimes I do not. I may matter when I wish I did not, and when I really wish I did, I often don't. It is different with every patient, just as I am different myself with each of them. One might even say that Karl found what he wanted in me: that peculiar combination of being able both to understand him and to judge him, a combination that differed enough to allow for a change but was close enough to allow a connection. With perfect empathy he would have had no chance; with unrelenting judgment he would have had no space.

Because of the moral issues that are so salient in them, behavior disorders are striking in their appeal to our individual judgments. However, moral concern exists to some extent in every treatment we conduct. It is regularly concealed within our theories and in our particular views of what we consider to be right and proper, normal and expectable. Every form of psychopathology calls forth a variety of beliefs or opinions, which essentially are our prejudices (Warnke 1987). There is no way we can see a patient without our preconceptions and prejudices, but they do not have equal effect on all patients. Sometimes, with some patients, empathy dominates the treatment, while others seem most attuned to our individual inputs: to both our personalities and our theories. Today's psychoanalysts run the risk of attributing either too much or too little to their presence, and, thereby, of losing sight of the individual patient's varying needs. We must always focus on the first-person perspective, which requires that we consider the impact of our input on the patient, but the great need of future psychoanalytic research is to better access which patient has that as a central concern and which as peripheral. We cannot discount the possibility that the idea of our significance may be just another prejudice of ours. Being empathic surely must mean to be able to judge what we mean and what we have brought to our patients. This can neither be disregarded nor made too much of.

Biological and physical constraints, in ourselves and in our patients, become interwoven with subjective experience and the culture in which we find ourselves. The necessary interpenetration of first- and third-person perspectives makes for a continual reassessment of any particular bit of analytic data. There are no pure forms, and probably no fixed percentages of types of input. Sometimes biology matters a lot, sometimes a little. The same can be said for sociocultural factors and for our own contributions as analysts. Co-construction does not mean equal partners. Transference does not mean that we are just doing our jobs with no ulterior motive. Perhaps this is the feature that makes psychoanalysis so interesting, inasmuch as it has a built-in level of uncertainty.

One last antinomy that seems to bedevil our field is one that most analysts find especially obnoxious: the contradiction that supposedly exists between history and fiction. Since Freud we have been urged to liken ourselves to archaeologists, unearthing the hidden and doing so carefully, cautiously, in order to avoid disturbing the past or contaminating the relics. But these relics are but traces of the past, and they demand an imaginative interpretation to allow us to see, in one scholar's terms, "what I would have witnessed, if I had been there" (White 1978). When we form these imaginary mediations (Ricoeur 1988), we interweave fiction and history, fashioning our reconstructions according to one type of preferred story rather than another. This fictionalization of history allows us to construct at times a tragedy, at other times a comic novel. We begin to write our own imaginative interpretations of what is remembered as history but is recast as a present moment.

A very common psychoanalytic event is the retelling of significant episodes from a patient's childhood. Each recall carries with it a new possibility for reinterpretation and perhaps a new and better understanding. For Karl there was the momentous time, after his parents' divorce, when his father came to take his sister and him out for the weekly parental visit. This historical event, characterized by Karl's feigning sleep so as not to join his sister, became the nucleus for a whole set of scenarios. Sometimes Karl hoped his father would return for him alone. Sometimes he fantasied having time alone with mother. Sometimes he would give up his act and race to join his father and sister. As analyst, I would imaginatively revisit the scene and silently write the script that I hoped was history as represented, but realized was being newly written as a sort of fictionalization of history.

Once again we see an interpenetration, here of history and fiction, just as we did with the first- and third-person perspectives, with discovery and creation, and with empathy and judgment. The mix in each instance, however, is to be considered not as contamination but as enrichment.

POSTSCRIPT

The answer to Karl's lament was offered by himself when he came to see me shortly before his marriage and some months after his official termination. It is apparent to any analyst who listens to this tale that my patient's complaint was composed around that remaining bit of transference directed to the parent who had failed to be perfect and to make his son perfect. Karl told me that he still occasionally wanted to look at men, but that that was something he could manage and live with. His gratitude to me was properly tempered with the disappointment that must accompany any treatment. I was pleased and a little hurt, but was comforted by recognizing that analysis as a profession, and as an individual encounter, is a very mixed bag.

REFERENCES

Bernstein JM: Recovering Ethical Life. New York, Routledge, 1995

Freud S: "Wild" psycho-analysis (1910), in The Standard Edition of the Complete Psychological Works of Sigmund Freud [SE], Vol 11. Translated and edited by Strachey J. London, Hogarth Press, 1957, pp 221–227

Freud S: Fetishism (1927). SE, 21:152–157, 1961

Golden C: Do women choose their sexual identity? Harvard Gay and Lesbian Review, Winter 1997, pp 18–20

Ricoeur P: Time and Narrative, Vol 3. Chicago, IL, University of Chicago Press, 1988

Sweetnam A: The changing contexts of gender: between fixed and fluid experience. Psychoanalytic Dialogues 6:437–459, 1996

Uttal WR: Do theoretical bridges exist between experience and neurophysiology? Perspect Biol Med 40:280–302, 1997

Warnke G: Gadamer: Hermeneutics, Tradition and Reason. Stanford, CA, Stanford University Press, 1987

White H: The Tropics of Discourse. Baltimore, MD, Johns Hopkins University Press, 1978

Žižek S: Enjoy Your Symptom: Jacques Lacan in Hollywood and Out. New York, Routledge, 1992

10

JAY R. GREENBERG, PH.D.

INTRODUCTION

Jay Greenberg graduated from the University of Chicago, received his Ph.D. in Clinical Psychology from New York University, and received his certificate in psychoanalysis from the William Alanson White Institute in New York. He is the author of more than 50 papers, and his book *Object Relations in Psychoanalytic Theory,* written with the late Stephen Mitchell in 1983, was a landmark in American psychoanalysis, bringing a clear, cogent, and compelling description of object relations theory to American ego psychology. His voice has been gentle but persuasive, strong but not dogmatic.

Dr. Greenberg is a Training and Supervising Analyst at the William Alanson White Institute in New York and Clinical Associate Professor of Psychology at the postdoctoral program in psychoanalysis at New York University. He has served as editor of *Contemporary Psychoanalysis* and as a member of the North American Editorial Board of *The International Journal of Psychoanalysis*. He has been honored as the invited speaker at almost every significant meeting and organization for psychoanalysts. His numerous awards include the Distinguished Scientific Award of the Division of Psychoanalysis of the American Psychological Association, the Edith Seltzer Alt Distinguished Service Award of the William Alanson White Institute, and many named lectureships. He is an Honorary Member of the American Psychoanalytic Association.

When asked to describe his place in the American psychoanalytic scene, he said the following:

My place in the American psychoanalytic scene today? I'm not sure that's for me to say, but I see myself as someone who's interested in and, to the extent possible, familiar with the work of analysts from a range of different perspectives.

My training, both in graduate school and at the White Institute, was pluralistic, although its overarching orientation was interpersonal. Perhaps because of my training, from the beginning I have been impressed by what analysts from different traditions have in common: our attempt to engage patients in the difficult, often painful work of examining their lives in ways that deepen their appreciation of the meaningfulness of their experience. This shared commitment, peculiar in the broader context of the culture in which we live, makes it both possible and essential to think and theorize about the implications of our different points of view.

My ideas about theoretical convergence and difference underlie the interest in comparative psychoanalysis that has been a part of my thinking from the beginning. In turn, the comparative psychoanalytic approach has shaped the attempts at synthesis that characterize a great deal of my recent work. Because of this, while I respect and value the contributions of many schools of thought, I don't see myself as signing on to the views of any one school. Clinical psychoanalysis is about questioning our analysands' "received wisdom," and our attitudes toward our theories should be the same. Because of this, I am more or less continually rethinking my own ideas and trying to find ways of expressing myself that capture the nuances of what I'm thinking and feeling when I work with patients. I expect myself to keep changing as an analyst, and to embrace the continuous tension between the familiarity of where I've been and the excitement of wherever I'm heading. In my writing I try to communicate both the openness and the tension that I feel are essential to our best work.

It's also worth saying that I rebel against the constraints of psychoanalytic organizations and think that there are too many interesting things for us to say to each other to justify staying behind institutional walls. So I try to talk to as many people as possible, especially to those with whom I disagree, because I think that it is the conversations we can create among analysts who come from different traditions that will keep psychoanalysis vital.

WHY I CHOSE THIS PAPER

Jay R. Greenberg, Ph.D.

I particularly like "Conflict in the Middle Voice" because it touches on a number of problems that are central to the psychoanalytic project but is, quite clearly, still a work in progress. Several themes are addressed but none is fully developed; as I see it, the paper opens many lines of thought but resolves none of them. That keeps me interested and engaged with the ideas in it, because there is a lot more work to be done.

And I think the open questions are generative enough to engage others as well.

I also like the paper because it has the potential for creating a conversation with classicists and other students of the humanities who are interested in ideas very similar to those that we struggle with in our clinical work but who approach those ideas in a very different, often strikingly unpsychological way. Psychoanalysis began with Freud's conviction that creating coherent narratives not only has the potential for explaining neurosis but for curing it. Today, despite our romance with neuroscience and despite our concern over the prodding of managed care companies, I believe that the life histories we develop in our work with patients draw on themes that have been addressed for thousands of years by those committed to exploring human experience in depth. The converging sensibilities and the very different perspectives brought to these themes by scholars and clinical psychoanalysts have great potential for promoting exchanges that enrich all disciplines.

But we must not believe that psychoanalysts can explain the texts; we can only propose readings that stand side by side with other readings. And, perhaps more important, we must be willing to engage with those alternative readings and to learn from them. My discussion of the middle voice—an archaic grammatical form of interest mainly to philologists and, recently, to some postmodern literary critics—is an example of this; it illuminates a crucial psychoanalytic problem in an unexpected way. Similarly, many of the themes that come up in the Greek tragedies, taken on their own terms, can teach analysts a great deal about what goes on in our consulting rooms. We live these themes every day with our analysands and so, more than almost anybody else, we know how alive and how crucial they are in our contemporary world. Because of this experience, psychoanalysts can contribute importantly to the appreciation of ancient texts.

This paper represents a start in these directions; there is much more to say. And that reflects my fondest hopes for anything that I write.

CONFLICT IN THE MIDDLE VOICE

JAY R. GREENBERG, PH.D.

IN THE MIDST OF A crucial scene in Homer's *Odyssey*—the recognition of the returning Odysseus by his childhood nurse, Eurycleia—the narrator inserts what appears on the surface to be a distracting digression. Turning the reader's attention away from the moment when Eurycleia will see a scar on Odysseus' leg, leading her to realize that her master has returned home after 20 years, Homer describes the moment during Odysseus' adolescence when he first got the scar. The wound was inflicted in the course of a boar hunt that took place during Odysseus' visit to the distant home of his maternal grandfather, Autolykos. Heroically, Odysseus located and flushed out the boar, simultaneously being gored by and killing it.

This story, coming at an emotionally tense and narratively climactic moment in the poem, seems so out of keeping with the immediate events that some commentators have thought it to be a corrupt interpolation in the text. Recent scholarship, however, indicates that, to the contrary, it continues and deepens the theme of recognition that Homer is describing. Reinterpretation of a remark in the *Poetics* suggests that no less an authority than Aristotle believed that the story of the boar hunt embodied the central theme of the entire epic (see Dimock 1989).

Homer's digression does not stop with the boar hunt, however. Rather, that episode frames another, earlier one: the naming of Odysseus. This story also involves Autolykos, something of a rogue (his name means "the wolf itself") living on the fringes of society. Described by Homer as a man who "excelled all others in stealing and the art of oaths," Autolykos is probably the right person to name the man who

---

"Conflict in the Middle Voice," by Jay R. Greenberg, Ph.D., was first published in © The Psychoanalytic Quarterly, 2005, *The Psychoanalytic Quarterly*, Volume 74, Number 1, pages 105–120, 2005. Used with permission.

will spend so much of his life away from home, at odds with man and the gods alike. So when he is invited to name his new grandson, he replies:

> Let his name be *Odysseus....*
> the Son of Pain, a name he'll earn in full.
> (Fagles 1996, p. 403, 19.463–464)

This passage requires some explanation. The name *Odysseus,* it turns out, is derived from the Greek verb *odussemai,* which is variously translated as "to inflict pain" or, more strongly, "to hate." But, notably, the name uses the verb in what is called the "middle voice," a form which strikes a balance between active and passive (Bernard Knox in Fagles 1996, p. 514). Greek is one of the few languages that has a unique verb form to express the middle voice, and it is difficult to translate these verbs into languages that do not. It is even more difficult to hold the tension between active and passive that a single word in the middle voice conveys.[1]

Thus, the name given to Odysseus suggests that he will both inflict pain on others and have pain inflicted on him; he will hate and be hated. And, of course, his life bears this out; it is, as Autolykos prophesied, "a name he'll earn in full." The story of Odysseus will be a story of pain inflicted (on Troy, on the Cyclops, on the suitors) and pain endured (the hatred of Poseidon and his 10 years of wandering to get home). The importance of the boar hunt story is clear in this context: it captures a moment—perhaps the first in his life—in which Odysseus simultaneously is wounded by and wounds the other. It is, we might say, the moment at which he grows into his name (see Dimock 1989, p. 258). And for Homeric Greeks, this was a heroic moment.

We can see now why Homer chose to describe these two episodes in the midst of his recounting the recognition of Odysseus; they represent three different perspectives on the question of who the man we have been hearing about really is. Within a relatively few lines, we see him recognized at home, learn the meaning of his name, and are told about

---

[1]Another use of the middle voice implies self-reflexivity, as in "I touch myself." The existence of a unique verb form to convey this experience is of interest to psychoanalysts, but in this paper I restrict myself to the connotation of simultaneous activity and passivity with respect to an external object. For this use, see, in addition to Bernard Knox (in Fagles 1996, notes), Dimock 1989 (pp. 257–260), Mendelsohn 1999 (pp. 33–34), and Peradotto 1990 (pp. 132–134).

a moment that defines his adult character. By this point in the poem, we have heard a great deal about the hero's adventures and exploits. Now, at the moment of homecoming, we need to and are prepared to know more about the character of the man whose story we have been told.

CLINICAL MATERIAL

A patient who had been working hard on problems organized around her inability to value or to enjoy what she has and does—her career, her family, her analysis—said, resignedly, "When I feel excited, something has to happen." In putting things this way, she was primarily referring to a fear that she might act "inappropriately," as she would experience it, on her impulses. She frequently felt that what she said was "blurted out," that she either had or was on the verge of presuming too great an intimacy with others, that she surrendered her professional authority in efforts to promote artificially friendly feelings.

All these were familiar concerns that had been expressed many times over the course of a long analysis. This time, however, what most struck me was that she was speaking in something close to the Greek middle voice. First, consider the phrase "When I feel excited…" This phrase is ambiguous as to the origins of the excitement; she may be excited by someone else, she may be excited about someone else, she may—as a product of fantasy or who knows what else—be describing an experience in her body that is not yet about anybody or anything external to herself.

And notice what happens next: there is a shift in voice to "something has to happen." Here, "I" has—poignantly—disappeared as the subject of the sentence. With this shift, the nature of the event that the patient is anticipating or predicting becomes highly ambiguous. The "something" may be something that the patient *does,* she may express the feeling, or defend against it, or move on to another feeling such as guilt or shame or anxiety. But the shift in voice suggests that she is not sure that what is going to happen next will be an action that she, as subject, will initiate. The "something" that "has to happen" may be an act of hers, but it may also be something that is done to her by somebody else.

In fact, the very idea that "something has to happen" when she is excited may originate with the other who observes her excitement (mother, who tends to squelch it; brother who exploits it; father who claims it; analyst who welcomes it and may even grab onto it as a relief from the patient's overbearing depression). We do not know—and, I suggest, the patient does not know—whether in what happens in the aftermath of her excitement she will be subject or object, an active or a passive participant.

As I understand this analysand, her difficulty in finding a way to live freely and comfortably in the midst of the anxieties that inevitably accompany the experience of—simultaneously—acting and being acted upon is at the core of her intrapsychic conflict. One solution, emptying herself of desire, leaves her feeling victimized by predatory, rapacious others (including, of course, a narcissistically preoccupied analyst whose interest in self-aggrandizement extends to the results of helping her get better, which she accordingly resists). Another solution (less prominent in the presenting picture but certainly latent), in which she sees herself as containing all desire, leaves her feeling like a "wild child," eating up everything that crosses her path, human and otherwise (including, of course, a fragile, vulnerable analyst who might easily succumb to her wiles, and to whom she accordingly gives wide berth). In neither case can she experience herself as both the desiring subject and the desired object. To do so is terrifying.

A few sessions after talking about how something has to happen in the wake of her excitement, this analysand and I lived out her experience in a dramatic way. On the day before the session in question, she and I became more aware than either of us ever had been of how confused she becomes when she wants and needs. This confusion is, almost inevitably, compounded by the response of the person she is involved with. This response never feels right, and so she never feels better. Frustrated and frightened, she becomes angry and spits back at the other person, typically initiating either an argument or a mutual withdrawal that leaves her feeling embittered and untouchable.

Although spelling out the idea of these repeated interactions over the course of the session "makes sense" to her, she cannot get a grip on it, and she tells me that it certainly does not help her feel any better. In fact, she is feeling the confusion that we have been talking about as powerfully as ever. This leaves her feeling desperate, even to the extent of fearing that our long years of work may prove futile.

So she begins the next session by saying that she needs help, that things are miserable. She could complain about all the things that have gone wrong since yesterday's appointment, but she knows that I think this reflects her reaction to the session and that I think she should be talking about what went on between us. Still, she has lost emotional touch with what happened yesterday, even though she knows it is important, so she needs me to help her get back to it. She is stuck.

I agree (silently) with the thought that she needs help talking about what goes on between us, and I am pleased that she is able to ask for help, which is by no means easy for her. But I'm less interested in—and far less clear about—what happened yesterday than I am in how a similar theme is being enacted today. She is stuck in the miseries of her life, which is all she can think about, so she needs my help. But help means bypassing what is consciously on her mind, and pulling her into thinking about what she imagines (correctly) *I* believe she should be thinking about. She remains passive; she cannot imagine even how to begin unsticking herself, which leaves me in the position not only of dislodging her, but of insisting that she address concerns that (in the short run at least) are more mine than hers. I am afraid that this will feel to her like a rape, or at least like a hostile intrusion.

Enthusiastic that we have right in front of us the very thing we have been talking about, I lay out for her what I think is going on, tying it to the feeling of confusion that always comes about when she becomes aware of needing or wanting, and when she has to grapple with the unpredictable reaction of the other. In my own excitement about catching an enactment as it is happening, I certainly use too many words, and perhaps too eager a tone. She, in turn, gets furious; she wanted help understanding what happened yesterday, and here I am blaming her for what is happening today.

So this is where we are left: She comes in aware that she wants my help, but not quite reckoning with the fact that this leaves her at least more or less at the mercy of my reaction to her desire. Furthermore, I am somebody who—despite the well-known cautions of both Freud and Bion—wants *her* in ways that are shaped by our individual histories and by the shared history of our analytic work. Thus, my interpretation, however correct, is a response to her desire to be helped that expresses my own desire to help in a particular way. And in turn her experience of my way of helping is shaped by her ambivalence about wanting to be helped. This ambivalence is in large measure the residue of the history of how her desire has been responded to by those she has desired in the past.

In the present situation, I think it is likely that an aspect of my desire may be that I want to move things along, while she wants to be comforted, to be held in the confusion about her confusion. My desire to move things may be too close to confirming her fear that her desire will be met exploitatively, coopted into the agenda of the other. "When I feel excited, *something* has to happen," and at the moment the something is that her need for help will feed the urgency of my needs—most likely phallic and/or narcissistic needs. We are both living the session in the middle voice. And neither of us, for the moment at least, can get a handle on it.

LIVING IN THE MIDDLE VOICE

There are, of course, any number of compelling explanations for this analysand's experience to be found in her personal history. But this paper is not about personal history; it is about the ambiguities and the anxieties that are inherent in living every moment of our lives as both subject and object, simultaneously. These are the ambiguities that the Greeks captured so well in their use of the middle voice as a grammatical form.

Living in the middle voice is daunting. So, too, is theorizing in the middle voice. The classicist John Peradotto has noted that contemporary readers of Greek texts inevitably have a difficult time holding the implications of middle voice verbs in mind. We tend to think of verbs—and of people—as being either active or passive at any given moment, leading to an artificial dichotomization of experience that impoverishes our understanding (Peradotto 1990, p. 132). This can be a particular danger to psychoanalysts. Because we live constantly in a world of things done by and things done to—consider the dynamics of the hour I described, or of any analytic hour—the tendency to think exclusively in terms of active versus passive, and the accompanying elision of one dimension that Peradotto describes, is particularly palpable. One could construct a compelling history of psychoanalytic theorizing organized around the elisions that various authors have chosen, but that is not the theme of this paper.

I do want to include a brief word about Freud's strategy, which was to speak in the active voice especially in the way in which he framed his theory of conflict. Freud's conflict at its root is intersystemic. Despite later emendations that introduce intrasystemic conflict or the ubiquity of compromise formation, fundamentally the struggle is between desire and restraint, both of which emphasize the intentions and the activity of a conflicted subject. Moreover, on the level of desire, Freudian conflict theory also posits an agent whose libido is directed toward particular objects (mother and father) and whose aims are reasonably stable in contrast to those of the younger child.

It is likely that Freud's preference was personal at its roots. Recall the reason for what was certainly his weightiest conceptual shift: the abandonment of the seduction hypothesis, the enthroning of fantasy, and the consequent substitution of psychic reality for material reality in the etiology of neurosis. Writing to Fliess in 1897, he confides the "great secret that…I no longer believe in my *neurotica*" because he finds it difficult to hold on to the idea that so many bourgeois Viennese men have molested their children. The decisive point, however, is that the seduction theory implies that "in every case the father, *not excluding my own,* had to be blamed as a pervert" (Freud 1897, p. 259; italics added). It was difficult, evidently, for Freud the conquistador to experience himself as the object of others.

Of course Freud's dilemma is my analysand's dilemma as well; it is the dilemma we all live with. In characteristic ways, we rid ourselves of one or another aspect of our experience—sometimes of ourselves as subject, sometimes of ourselves as object—thus limiting what we are able to know. When we keep the idea of the middle voice in mind, we can see that these omissions mark a sense of unease. In this respect, Freud and my analysand are interesting cases in point. Freud retreated from whatever reminded him that he was the object of the intentions of others. This is clear in the way he analyzed his own dreams; consider the striking omission of the acts of his friend Fliess in his account of the so-called specimen dream of psychoanalysis, the dream of Irma's injection (Erikson 1954; Schur 1972). And, of course, Freud generalized this approach, leading him eventually to the wish-fulfillment theory of dreaming itself. This theory gives us a powerful tool for probing our desire, but it leaves no room for appreciating the formative role of unconscious experiences of being acted upon by other people. If we think about the anxieties that are inherent in living in the middle voice, Freud's omission suggests that his theory lends itself to being used as a counterphobic defense.

Compare my analysand's solution. Terrified of what her excitement will lead her or others to do, she empties herself of desire. In contrast to Freud's dreamer—consumed by wishes—she wants nothing at all. As a result, she loses touch with herself as an active subject; she lacks inner direction, because without desire there can be no direction. And, further, because she tends to project desire into others, she is surrounded by people who are filled with want; they want things for themselves and they want things from her. The confusion that plagues her results from this; she does not know where she wants to go, and a great deal of what she feels reflects her reactions to, and her need to cope with, what is done to her.

Both Freud's solution to the problem of living fully in the middle voice and my analysand's solution compromise the fullness of experience; both are reactions to the inescapable anxiety that grows out of the need to live effectively in a world of other people.

CONFLICT AND AGENCY

Homer and the heroes he wrote about in *The Iliad* and *The Odyssey* seemed to have accepted the shared agency captured in the middle voice as a simple fact of life. This comes across most powerfully in epic accounts of the relationship between mortals and gods. There are episodes in both poems in which we find actions that are initiated by the gods alone, others in which the will of humans determines the course of events, and yet others in which agency is shared by god and mortal acting in concert. Neither the author nor the characters involved seem either particularly surprised or particularly troubled by the constantly shifting locus of control.

A few brief examples will illustrate the mix of acting and being acted upon that gives shape to human experience in the epics.[2] In *The Iliad,* Aphrodite snatches Paris away and brings him to the safety of his bedroom as he is about to be strangled by Menelaus; her uncompromised power to do this is acknowledged by all who are involved (Fagles 1991, p. 141, 3.439–441). There are many such incidents, but other events that are instigated by the gods require the collaboration of mortals. In a famous example, when Achilles is about to attack Agamemnon, he is visited by the goddess Athena, who says:

> Down from the skies I come to check your rage
> if only you will yield.
> (Fagles 1991, p. 84, 1.242–243)

Here Athena wishes to restrain Achilles (who has himself been shown to be ambivalent about his urge to attack), but she cannot do so entirely on her own. The hero has it in his power to yield or to resist; what eventually happens will be determined both by the pressure put on him by the goddess and by his own choice. No less than Athena's power to stop the arrow, this shared initiative is a fact of life which is accepted by mortal and god alike.

And, finally, some events in the epics are caused entirely by the will of mortals. In what is perhaps the most dramatic example of this, the entire course of events in *The Iliad* is set in motion by the all too human rage of Achilles, itself a response to Agamemnon's all too human belief in his own entitlement.

Three centuries after the epics were written, in the midst of an enlightenment period during which the Greeks were making tremendous

---

[2]The gods themselves are not immune to being acted upon by humans. They are frequently saddened by human behavior, and they can even be physically harmed by mortals: Diomedes wounds Aphrodite in *The Iliad* (Fagles 1991, p. 175, 5.380ff).

advances in mathematics, medicine, and other sciences (and during which Athens had achieved unprecedented political and military success), the shared agency that had once been simply assumed began to chafe. Human potential—the conviction of the power of mortal intelligence and rationality—seemed unlimited. In this changed intellectual climate, a new literary form, tragedy, emerged quite suddenly. In the tragedies, the belief in shared agency (between mortals and gods, but also among humans themselves) continued. But now the sharing was seen as problematic by the authors of the tragedies and as a source of conflict by the characters in the plays.

The historian of tragedy Jean-Pierre Vernant, noting that tragedy as a dominant literary form arose and declined in Athens over a period of only 100 years, suggests that it reflects the concerns of a society that was moving beyond what he calls "heroic values and ancient religious representations" and toward "the new modes of thought that characterize the advent of law within the city-state" (Vernant 1990, p. 26). In this developing culture there was little room for the kind of unquestioning submission to divine will that we find in the epics; instead, people sought guidance from laws that were invented and enforced by mortals themselves.

Vernant is talking about a historical moment; once the rule of law was firmly established in Athens, great tragedies were no longer written. Drawing on his perspective, scholars in a number of fields have explained the ongoing appeal of the tragedies by noting that they address the difficulties people face when rapid social, scientific, and political changes cause upheavals in traditional ways of experiencing and living in the world. For example, the political theorist Richard Ned Lebow (2003) has suggested that "Tragedy can be understood as a response of modernization.... Changes threaten traditional values and encourage the emergence of new ones" (p. 25).

This formulation resonates with sensibilities that emerge from doing clinical psychoanalysis. There is a striking parallel between the societal changes that, in the views of Vernant and Lebow, form the cultural background for the emergence of a tragic vision and the developmental processes that we analysts live through with our analysands. But there is one notable exception: The historical changes are episodic and may even occur infrequently. The Nobel Prize-winning poet Czeslaw Milosz stressed this infrequency:

> People always live within a certain order and are unable to visualize a time when that order might cease to exist. The sudden crumbling of all current notions and criteria is a rare occurrence and is characteristic of only the most stormy periods of history. (Milosz, quoted in Lebow 2003, p. 25)

This "sudden crumbling" looks quite different from a psychoanalyst's perspective: the breakdown of "current notions" and the demands of "modernization" are, I suggest, analogs of individuation. They parallel what we know as the developmental move from dependency toward increasing autonomy. What Vernant, Lebow, and Milosz are describing on a societal level is a feature of everyday life as we emerge from embeddedness and move toward the creation of our own individual lives. Thus, in contrast to the rare and episodic havoc that is wreaked by cultural modernization, our personal "current notions" are at risk of crumbling on a daily or even minute-to-minute basis as we strive to express ourselves in ways that move us into a world beyond the "certain order" that we have always known.

So, whether we are aware of it or not (and most typically we are not), each of us experiences "the most stormy periods of history" on a regular basis in the course of our own personal development. This points to ways in which the tragic vision poignantly informs and is informed by our own experience.

Consider a motif that is characteristic of the tragedies. Oracles, pronouncements from the gods about the future course of events, are more prominent in the tragedies than in the epics. But despite the frequent occurrence of oracles—and despite the universally acknowledged power of the gods—mortals regularly try to circumvent what has been decreed, often with disastrous consequences. In perhaps the most famous example of this, Oedipus—told *unconditionally* by Apollo's oracle at Delphi that he will kill his father and marry his mother—sets out to take fate into his own hands. He believes that he can, irrespective of the will of the gods, unilaterally determine the course of his life; this is why he leaves home and resolves never to see the people whom he believes to be his parents again. And indeed, for a very long time Oedipus is extraordinarily effective; he saves Thebes by solving the riddle of the Sphinx,[3] and for 20 years he is the godlike ruler of the city. But Oedipus' attempt to assert his will succumbs, ultimately, to the limits of human capacity. Both what he can achieve and (perhaps more important) what he knows are constrained in ways that he could not have imagined at the beginning of the play.

Oedipus' attempt to create a life based on human rationality alone,

---

[3]In his bitter argument with the prophet Tiresias, Oedipus imperiously declares that he has solved the riddle on his own—through the use of human rationality—neither asking for nor receiving any help from the gods.

a life not dictated by and perhaps even lived in defiance of the will of the gods, captures our own struggle to experience personal autonomy. This theme is central in many Greek tragedies; in contemporary psychoanalytic terms, tragic conflict arises from the incompleteness and instability of the experience of agency. And because the extraordinary transitional period during which the tragedies emerged as a literary form resonates with out own personal developmental struggles, tragic themes speak to us across the millennia. Vernant's characterization of the vision of the Greek tragedians captures what we and our analysands live through in every clinical encounter: because agency is not yet fully achieved, all human action is "a kind of wager—on the future, on fate and on oneself.... In this game, where he is *not* in control, man always risks being trapped by his own decisions" (Vernant 1990, p. 44, italics in original).

Listening to the tragedians and translating their lessons into terms familiar to individual psychology require us to rethink what has become the traditional psychoanalytic perspective on the relationship between conflict and the achievement of a sense of personal agency. The impulse/defense theory of conflict requires a subject who already has developed a considerable degree of personal agency—in Freud's own terms, someone who has achieved stable psychic structure. In this view, both agency and conflict are development achievements, and only an active agent can have the sort of structured intentions that define conflict.

In contrast, the sensibility expressed by the use of the middle voice and the tragic vision suggests that the experience of agency itself is ineluctably ephemeral. Agency is a paradox, perhaps the central paradox of human existence, and this breeds conflicts that occupy every moment of our lives. On a daily basis, the tragedians taught, we are faced with the need to act as agents while remaining aware that we live in an interpersonal world in which others (god and mortal alike) are simultaneously asserting their own agency. And we must strive to act autonomously and effectively despite the constraints imposed by our histories (personal, familial, and cultural), and despite the uncertain consequences that our acts will have in the future.

This parallel between individual development and Athenian cultural development suggests an approach to understanding the continuing appeal of the tragedies 2,500 years after they were written, one that is, again, at odds with the received psychoanalytic explanation. Freud's account of this appeal was too intimately involved with his ambition to create the Oedipus complex; he failed to see that a historical reading of the texts could deeply inform psychoanalytic thinking. Today, while nobody doubts the power of his invention, his strategy has made it difficult for analysts to engage readers from other disciplines in conversation. Freud's narrow vision of the nature of conflict—that it always involved inner impulses and defenses against them—shaped his reading of *Oedipus* and was in turn shaped by it.

Thinking about conflict in terms that stay closer to the sensibility of the middle voice and the problems of living within it that are highlighted in the tragic vision suggests that we must consider more than just our own conflicted intentions. We must also take account of the conflicted experiences of being the object of the intentions and reactions of others at the same time that we are experiencing these conflicted intentions.

When we think this way, we discover my analysand as I described her in my vignette. The conflicts of which she is becoming aware in her analysis—and that she and I are living out together—reflect the dilemmas that plague us all: How can we act when we cannot know either the reasons for or the effects of our actions? How can we even desire when we cannot predict the events that our desire will set in motion, because our desire is directed toward a desiring other? My analysand says "When I get excited, something has to happen," and because she cannot know either why she is excited or what that "something" will be, to experience excitement is to place a wager in which everything is on the line.

So, for my analysand to be able to own her desire, she must struggle more effectively with anxieties about the ambiguous origins of her excitement, and with anxieties about the uncertain future that will follow when she acts upon it. And this is not, for her or for any of us, a one-time thing—it is something that must be lived through (sometimes more, sometimes less consciously) in every moment of our lives. Conflict is inevitable, both because we cannot be sure how to act in a way that is most true to ourselves, and because we cannot be sure how others—driven by their own inner imperatives—will act upon us or how they will react to us. The experience of agency, including the awareness of its limitations, emerges from—and recedes back into—this sort of conflict.

Conflicts around the need to experience agency constitute my analysand's deepest dilemma. This is conflict in the middle voice, the conflict of all the tragic heroes who have grappled with the need to act while remaining aware both that they are living out the history of being acted upon and that they are irreducibly uncertain about how they will be acted upon in the future. For my analysand, and for all of us, to own our humanity is to claim our place as an active agent in our interpersonal world and to submit to the agency of others—past, present, and future, in one and the same fateful act.

REFERENCES

Dimock G: The Unity of *The Odyssey.* Amherst, University of Massachusetts Press, 1989

Erikson E: The dream specimen of psychoanalysis. J Am Psychoanal Assoc 2:5–56, 1954

Fagles R (trans): Homer's *The Odyssey.* New York, Penguin, 1996

Fagles R (trans): Homer's *The Iliad.* New York, Penguin, 1991

Freud S: Letter 69 (to Fliess, 1897), in The Standard Edition of the Complete Psychological Works of Sigmund Freud, Vol 1. Translated and edited by Strachey J. London, Hogarth Press, 1966

Lebow R: The Tragic Vision of Politics: Ethics, Interests and Orders. Cambridge, UK, Cambridge University Press, 2003

Mendelsohn D: The Elusive Embrace: Desire and the Riddle of Identity. New York, Alfred A Knopf, 1999

Peradotto J: Man in the Middle Voice: Name and Narration in *The Odyssey.* Princeton, NJ, Princeton University Press, 1990

Schur M: Freud Living and Dying. New York, International Universities Press, 1972

Vernant J-P: The historical moment of tragedy in Greece: some of the social and psychological conditions, in Myth and Tragedy in Ancient Greece. Translated by Lloyd J. Edited by Vernant J-P, Vidal-Niquet P. New York, Zone Books, 1990

11

WILLIAM I. GROSSMAN, M.D.

INTRODUCTION

William Grossman received his A.B. and M.D. from New York University and did his analytic training at the New York Psychoanalytic Institute. He has been Clinical Professor of Psychiatry at Albert Einstein College of Medicine and Training and Supervising Analyst at the New York Psychoanalytic Institute, where he has also taught a variety of courses in psychoanalytic theory. He has served on the Board of Directors and Program Committee at the New York Psychoanalytic Society and as a Trustee and Member of the Curriculum and Education Committees at the New York Psychoanalytic Institute.

Dr. Grossman has been a member of the Editorial Board of *The Psychoanalytic Quarterly, The International Journal of Psychoanalysis, Psychoanalysis and Contemporary Thought, The Journal of Clinical Psychoanalysis,* and the Advisory Board of *Neuropsychoanalysis.* He has been a dedicated teacher to generations of psychoanalysts.

Dr. Grossman's honors include the A.A. Brill Memorial Lecture of the New York Psychoanalytic Society, the Sandor Rado Lecture of Columbia University Center for Psychoanalytic Training and Research, the Freud Anniversary Lecture of the New York Psychoanalytic Institute, and the Heinz Hartmann Award Lecture of the New York Psychoanalytic Institute, to give a partial listing.

Dr. Grossman's contributions are wide ranging, extending from efforts to delineate the core of psychoanalytic clinical work to attempts to place the development of psychoanalysis within the broad arena of a history of ideas and science. His method is to contextualize the beginnings of various issues and then to deal with some of the controversies regarding these issues as thinking about them has evolved. His 1976 paper on penis envy is an example of his capacity to rethink a Freudian concept and place it within contemporary knowledge of child development, gender identity, and cultural influence. Grossman has been a penetrating critic of psychoanalytic concepts and has written significant papers on the concepts of the self, masochism, the role of theory in clinical work, and the relation between theory and technique. He brings an extraordinary depth of philosophical and historical thought to each of his papers.

He says of himself:

> I've addressed the current relevance of some of the issues within the framework and from the point of view I've constructed. As I see it, I've been taking a psychoanalytic view of the development of psychoanalytic ideas.
>
> My other role in psychoanalysis has been as a teacher for many years, both for candidates and the graduates of psychoanalytic institutes. I've been privileged to have been a consultant, reader, advisor, and critic for some of the most important figures in our field as well as providing guidance for younger authors.

WHY I CHOSE THIS PAPER

William I. Grossman, M.D.

I chose "The Self as Fantasy: Fantasy as Theory" for inclusion in this volume because it is a condensed example of my approach to considering psychoanalytic concepts. It provides, first, a nonpsychoanalytic context within which the psychoanalytic ideas on this topic developed and continue to be developed. The paper also says something about the way this concept was being used at the time in psychoanalysis. At the same time, it uses Freud's ideas of mental functioning and theory as fantasy to place the idea of the self in a somewhat different framework as a mental conception and complex construction. This paper pointed the way to a reconsideration of the place of the concept in development and a critique of the contemporary inferences from child observation. This allowed me to introduce the idea of some continuities between animal behavior and the study of human development.

THE SELF AS FANTASY

Fantasy as Theory

WILLIAM I. GROSSMAN, M.D.

THE PROBLEM OF THE self in psychoanalysis stands at the intersection of many traditional philosophical and psychoanalytic issues which might be thought of as lying along two axes. The first axis, by far the older, joins the everyday personal experiences of self—that is, self-awareness, self-consciousness, self-observation, self-esteem, self-determination, and will—with the ancient philosophical dilemmas concerning a variety of themes, such as mind and body, free will, and the relation between the self and the world of things. The other axis is the psychoanalytic axis with the concrete events of the clinical situation and the subjective experience of the patient at one end, and its mosaic of systematic, theoretical concepts at the other end. The concept of self joins these coordinates and the different perspectives they offer. Although for some psychoanalytic purposes we may not need to keep all of these perspectives in view at any one time, we must not forget the everyday personal and philosophical axis. Even in the realm of theoretical examination, ignoring this axis will covertly narrow and redefine the concept

---

Presented at the panel "Psychoanalytic Theories of the Self" at the fall meeting of the American Psychoanalytic Association, New York, December 1980. After this paper was presented, a paper by Spruiell (1981) appeared that both complements and presents alternative ways of looking at the problems presented here.

"The Self as Fantasy: Fantasy as Theory," by William I. Grossman, M.D., was first published in *The Journal of the American Psychoanalytic Association,* 30:919–937, 1982.

of the self. This redefinition will lead to the kind of confusion that has accompanied the use of many terms in psychoanalysis that have been borrowed from the popular language or other sciences and have both subjective and systematic meanings—for example, "instinct" and "ego."

Discussing the interrelation between these two axes enlarges on some thoughts presented in an earlier paper on introspection (Grossman 1967) and in a second paper on anthropomorphism (Grossman and Simon 1969).

The central points of view of this paper are, first, that there is an essential tension in psychoanalytic theory between the subjective and objective points of view regarding patients' experiences. Second, this tension is built into the experience of patients themselves, that is, it is inherent in personal concepts of the self. Third, this tension cannot be avoided in the philosophy of the self or in any theory of the self. Furthermore, any psychology that takes subjective experience as a starting point and as a communication from the patient will be involved in this tension between subjectivity and objectivity. The only points of view which can escape such a tension are those that are strictly behavioristic and treat patients' verbal statements not as communications about themselves, but rather as reports to be correlated with other behaviors irrespective of their subjective meaning to the patient. Fourth, theories derived from direct infant observation may attempt to evade this tension between subjective and objective points of view by assuming that the behavior observed can be treated as equivalent to the mental activities of the infant, and therefore blur the distinction between subjective and objective by placing subjective meaning into behavioral observations.[1]

The poles of the two axes of the self—the everyday-personal-philosophical and the psychoanalytic-clinical-theoretical—might seem at first to represent the poles of abstraction and concreteness. However, this would not do justice to the difference between them. The issue here is rather one of the subjectivity and objectivity of the points of view taken at either pole of each axis. Both the subjectively oriented clinical data on the self and the objectively oriented theory of psychoanalysis include the personal and philosophical ideas of the self. This will become apparent if we now talk about the sources and nature of this subjective-objective duality in psychoanalytic theory.

---

[1]For an excellent philosophical discussion of subjective and objective, see Nagel 1979; for a clinical discussion, see Bach 1980.

There are three sources of this duality. First, we have the views that Freud himself brought to his organization of his earliest psychoanalytic data. Among these is his idea that man has a dual orientation that serves both his species and himself. You will recall that Freud (1914, p. 78; 1915, pp. 124–125) said this explicitly in discussing the sexual instinct, which serves the reproduction of the species and the pleasure of the individual, noting that these two aims were not always to be harmonized (Freud 1916–1917, pp. 413–414). Man's psychology, then, was also to serve his biological destiny (Freud 1914, p. 78). He is both a person and an organism. His psychology serves himself and his society. His hate and love are divided between himself and his objects. His mind contains both himself and others from his past, including what he once was himself. His consciousness faces both outward and inward. In keeping with his views on man's dual orientation, Freud organized the data of the clinical situation according to two kinds of concepts: those derived from a general theoretical orientation to psychology as a branch of biology, and those derived from the categories of experiences of conflict his patients brought to him with their everyday language about their impulses and values.

At an early stage of grappling with such issues, Freud (1905, p. 113) said the theory was biological and that the therapy was psychological. While those to whom he addressed this remark were supposed to be reassured that not all of his thinking was psychological, later critics have been troubled by this very point. However, the use of biological and physical drive and force models for psychoanalysis is not the only problem. More troublesome is Freud's consistent effort to use the same concepts to solve simultaneously the problems of the psychoanalytic situation and what he called "the great problems of biology and philosophy."

The second source of the dual subjective-objective orientation of analysis comes from the position of the analyst as analyst. On the one hand, in his clinical work, he must take the point of view of the patient in order to understand something of the patient's experience and to understand the subjective experiences of childhood which are contained in the present communications and reminiscences of the patient. In other words, he must recognize a unity in the subjectivity of the present and the subjectivity of childhood. At the same time, he must maintain a position of objectivity, being neither caught up in his own subjective reactions to the patient's subjectivity nor, on the other hand, absorbed in his own subjective preoccupations. He takes, then, an objective view of both his own subjective responses and the patient's subjective communications. We call the analyst's objectivity his "psychoanalytic neutrality."

The third source of this dual subjective-objective orientation of analysis comes from the data of analysis itself. That is, the patient's reports, deriving as they do from the personal-philosophical axis of the self, are bound to contain a double orientation. A subjective component expresses imagery, feelings, thoughts, emotions, sensations, urges, desires, tensions, wishes, and memories. A capacity for reflection on subjective experience introduces a more distant viewpoint, an objective mode or perspective (Loewenstein 1963; Sterba 1934).

Thus, Freud constructed a psychoanalytic theory of mind, the analyst constructs the mind of his patient, and the patient constructs his own experience in speaking about himself. That these three activities have a similar form, roughly speaking, that a person speaking about himself is in a situation similar to a theoretician, is built into the psychoanalytic model of mental activity according to which personal accounts and descriptions of self-experience are, in a broad but fundamental sense, theories.

In other words, a patient speaking about himself and reflecting in addition to revealing himself imparts objectifying constructs to his experience. His activity in this way parallels that of the analyst who constructs the mind of the patient with objective neutrality while grasping the patient's subjective experience. It was out of these operations in the clinical situation that Freud constructed psychoanalytic theory. For this reason, all personal accounts and descriptions of self-experience in the psychoanalytic situation are fundamentally theories, but they are theories on the everyday-personal-philosophical axis. On that axis, personal theories have always informed philosophy as philosophy has informed personal theories.

When Freud took the self-reflecting patient and the observing analyst and placed them in the mind as the system Conscious-Preconscious, he viewed all mental products as being, in some sense, theories. For instance, in his paper on "Screen Memories" (Freud 1899, p. 322) he said that memories are selected and formed with a purpose. For this reason, we have memories, not "*from* our childhood," but only "*relating to* our childhood." Freud also referred to secondary revision as the first interpretation of the dream. For Freud, myths are theories and theories are myths (Freud 1913a, 1913b; 1933b, p. 211). In this sense he spoke of the theory of drives as "our mythology" (Freud 1933a, p. 95). Infantile fantasies are theories about sexuality. All mental products, then, are personal constructions. Theory and fantasy serve both subjective, conflict-resolving aims, and objective, reality-orienting aims. According to Freud, both have a similar form. They are composed of elements of the infantile, the actual, and the contribution of regulating interests, goals, and values. Differences between various mental products result from the particular mixture and correspond to the uses for which they are constructed and their relation to reality.

In an open-minded spirit, Freud was willing to acknowledge correspondences between prescientific cosmologies and a variety of psychoanalytic ideas. Most dramatically, he pointed out the similarity of structure between Schreber's delusion and the libido theory. He wrote (Freud 1911), "Schreber's 'rays of God,' which are made up of condensation of the sun's rays, of nerve-fibers, and of spermatozoa, are in reality nothing else than a concrete representation and projection outwards of libidinal cathexes; and they thus lend his delusions a striking conformity with our theory" (p. 78). To this comparison, he adds humorously, "It remains for the future to decide whether there is more delusion in my theory than I should like to admit, or whether there is more truth in Schreber's delusion than other people are as yet prepared to believe" (p. 79). Both Schreber's delusion and Freud's theory are theories of Schreber's self-experience. Delusions are theories, and theories may turn out to be delusions. Freud was later to emphasize that even delusions have a basis in fact, and like constructions in analysis are "attempts at explanation and cure" (Freud 1937, p. 268).

Freud first explains Schreber's delusion in terms of libido theory. He adds to this the suggestion that libidinal disturbance "may result from abnormal changes in the ego" (Freud 1911, p. 75). Whereas it is possible to translate the shifts in libido into statements about "motives," it is not possible to do this with statements about ego states. This corresponds to the issues confronted by the distinctions between motives and causes (Rapaport 1960), personal motivation and impersonal forces (Loewald 1971), actions and happenings (Schafer 1976), reasons and causes (Grossman 1967; Klein 1976), causes and meaning (Rycroft 1966), and implication and causality (Piaget 1971). Many other authors have discussed similar distinctions in theory using different pairs but with the same implication.

Freud (1911) did add a comment that allowed even the ego state to enter the world of personal experience. Many details of Schreber's delusion, he said, "sound almost like endopsychic perceptions of the processes whose existence I have assumed..." (p. 79). This idea, that a disturbance in ego function and structure not only *causes* a particular organization of conscious contents but is actually perceived and represented in consciousness has recurred often among psychoanalytic ideas. Federn's concept of "ego feeling" is an example of this. His ideas were a response to the need for a more elaborate description of self-state experience in his clinical work with psychotics. More recently, Kohut

(1977, pp. 109–110) has used the concept of "self-state dreams," which seems to be a related concept.

If one states that a structural condition or state of the organism, not a motive, intention, or purpose, explains and is represented in the *manifest* mental state, the following possibilities may be considered: First, the organization or structure can be known by direct perception—as Freud suggests, endopsychic perception. Second, the consequences of the functioning of the structure and its disorganization are not actually perceived directly but inferable from their known consequences. The patient complains of pain in his right lower abdomen. The doctor knows it is his appendix. The patient may then say, if he cares to, "My appendix hurts." This would be analogous to Schreber saying, "My libido connections are not working." A third possibility not utilized by Freud, but provided by his theory, is more interesting and makes better sense. Both Freud's theory and Schreber's delusion are in part self-state and object-relations descriptions. The similarity of the forms of the two theories derives from this. If Schreber had described his state in terms of his self in relation to his world, if he had said, as many patients do, that his world had collapsed, his message would have been more intelligible but no less problematic. The self-state description is, according to our theory, constructed in the same way any mental product is constructed, in a manner similar to Schreber's delusion. That is, the self-state description renders feelings, impulses, and ideas in the form of a fantasy construction. In the case of the self-state, the language of this fantasy is everyday language about an everyday fantasy about a fantasized entity, "the self" (Abend 1974; Schafer 1968, 1978). The "self" is the term popularly used to provide an organizational point of reference for inner experiences. It therefore seems to be a concrete entity, and is treated like an experiential "fact" (Spiegel 1959). The "self," then, is a special fantasy with its own language and referents. It is caught up in the popular discourse in the language of self-experience. It is anchored in and derives a sense of immediacy from the bodily experiences, activities, and emotional interactions with other people. The "self" appears to be both supremely subjective yet also an objective organization, an organismic property, discernible by others. This apparent objectivity of "the self" arises from the fact that a person and those around him may equate observable and characteristic behavioral organizations or traits with an internal entity, "the self."

In calling the self-concept a theory or a fantasy, I do not wish in any way to diminish its importance in regulating behavior. It seems to me that our concept of fantasy at times is a rather static one, as though we thought of a fantasy as something like a television picture. Perhaps the model from which the unconscious fantasy was taken, namely, the daydream, gives fantasy this connotation. However, fantasy has, and has always had, a much more important role in our theories: It organizes and directs behavior. Fantasies are complex structures that have an effect on mental organization as well. They are both an aspect of mental organization and have an effect on it. The relation between fantasies, mental contents in general, and structure or organization of mental life was discussed by Rapaport in a paper on the superego. Starting from Hartmann's distinction between the "inner world" and the "internal world," Rapaport (1957) wrote:

> It is the inner world which regulates the orientation in the external world. It is an inner map of the external world. The internal world is the major structures—the identifications, defense structures, ego, id, etc.; they can also be considered internalizations but they are an internal world. Man's inner map of his world is, however, in the force field of the organization of the internal world. The inner map of the outside world has selective omissions and is shaped to the structure of the internal world, that is, of the psychic apparatus.... The relation between the inner world and the internal world is one of the very interesting systematic questions, which may turn out to be the crucial one in the problem of the self. (pp. 696–697)

For Rapaport, the inner world was a substructure of the ego. Yet he was perhaps the only one to consider systematically that the relation between the contents of the inner world, of fantasies, perceptions and so on, and the internal world was one of complex interaction. In fact, he said, changes in the internal world, changes in mental structure *could* certainly be initiated and occur under the influence of the inner world. He made the point too that major structural changes could occur as a result. Structural changes, alterations in defenses and identifications, could in turn change the overall organization of the inner world, as well. I think he was correct in linking this complex relation between the functions of mental content and mental organization with the problem of the role of self-experience in mental life. The point is that although organization and content are useful polarities for purposes of some kinds of classification, it would be a mistake to underestimate the dynamic and structural importance of fantasy structures. It is precisely when we are considering a fantasy structure with such wide-ranging organizational and dynamic importance as the "self-" concept used in psychoanalysis that the structure-content polarity becomes less relevant. I shall only mention, without elaboration, the relation between the self as a concept-fantasy-theory and our ordinary usage of the term self-representation. I regard self-representations as nuclear fantasies of complex structure from which a personal self-concept is synthesized and abstracted (cf. Eisnitz 1980). This conception of self-experiences, and the view of the relation between the concepts of self and self-representation are essentially similar to those of Kernberg (1975, pp. 315–316). He, however, emphasizes the self as a structure and stresses its comprehensive wholeness, while I see these as inherent in fantasies. The difference between the ego as a "structure" and the self as a "structure" is that the "ego" is a technical term, our term, for classifying behavior, fantasy, experience, and so on—what Hartmann and colleagues 1964) called "centers of psychic functioning." The "self," on the other hand, is a term of ordinary personal reference whose theoretical significance lies in the fact that it has significance for patients.

As a fantasy, the details of the "self" may be elaborated, distorted, re-represented, repressed, and otherwise defended against. In short, it may be conscious or unconscious. As the mental representation of the person as his own object, the "self" includes some representation of the person's mind. To be one's own object, after all, involves recognizing one's desires (id), dealing with one's interests in reality—acting on one's own behalf (ego), being what one loves or criticizes (superego). Only in this sense does the self "contain" the mental apparatus.

So far, I have made the point that the concept of the self as a popular and philosophical concept is the source of the self-concept in analysis, which thus derives from the common experience of self-reference. If the self is a fantasy, what is the fantasy about? It is customary to speak of the "self' as referring to certain properties (Schafer 1968), such as agency, that is, the "source" or the "initiator" of action. Self is usually treated as a "place" which would be the locus of experience. It is the "object" of reflection and self-reference, of the self-defining experiences of continuity or recognition of history. It is thought of as the initiator of self-control. The fantasy is essentially embodied in the idea of self-reference, reference to an entity separate from other people—at least to some degree. Along with separateness come the issues of connectedness, similarity, and difference. Other properties and issues could be mentioned, but those will suffice to make my point. Taken together all such elements constitute the framework and dimensions of self-fantasies for all patients, regardless of diagnosis. Spiegel (1959) has emphasized the spatial and perceptual character of self-language. He considers the "self" a reference framework from which one has perspective.

In this discussion, I have been guided to some extent by analyses of the self-concept by Mischel (1977) and Toulmin (1977). Toulmin in particular stresses that the effort to use the noun "self" in a technical, theoretical way, apart from reflexive idioms, never escapes the link to everyday self-reference. "Self" depends on a person's view of himself, which from a psychoanalytic point of view means it is a fantasy. As Stone (1973, p. 54) remarked, the "adult organism" can "preserve the subjective illusion" of reacting as a whole "only with the aid of an elaborate unconscious system, various compromise formations (ranging from dreams to well-marked symptoms or pathological character traits), and, paradoxically, through the operations of the underlying tripartite structural system." In short, "the self" is a "personal myth" (Kris 1956), a myth of which everyone has his own more or less original version.

In presenting the elements and dimensions of the self as a fantasized entity, it should be recognized that these are a kind of framework, the categories of experience of the self. Ordinarily they are not within awareness or a matter of concern. Like the framework of the analytic setting, they are taken for granted unless something happens to focus attention on them. It is precisely those borderline and otherwise narcissistic patients who are in one way or another preoccupied with defining, characterizing, and delineating themselves who are also extremely attentive to and concerned with the setting, the framework, and the details of the analytic situation. In a related context, Anna Freud (1954) wrote of a patient whose interest in psychoanalysis excluded the person of the analyst. What should have been an object relation became an ego interest.

The categories of self-experience are in part the categories used to classify events in the objective, physical world and are a cognitive classification. As cognitive capacities they can be studied systematically, as can their development in the child. Bach (1975, 1980; "Some Notes on Perspective," unpublished, 1976), exploring subjectivity and objectivity, has discussed elaborate clinical material relating to the preoccupation with these issues, especially continuity and perspective, and related the clinical data to psychological studies. Clinical material of this type shows the patient's preoccupation with description and self-delineation and often has a static and lifeless quality. It is as though the narcissistic patients are preoccupied with finding an objective view of their boundaries. The act of describing those boundaries, in fact, immobilizes and excludes the auditor. What gives these preoccupations life again is the exploration of the object relations from which this effort springs. The situation has its parallel in the hypochondriasis which expresses object-related conflicts through somatic preoccupations (Richards 1981). In both cases, a concrete and ostensibly objective anchor has been found for the projected inner conflicts from which consciousness of significant objects is excluded, except secondarily. Similarly, the patient's concern with the framework and details of the analysis displaces the conflict from the person of the analyst. The static quality that boundary preoccupations and hyperobjectivity have contributes to the boredom that may be experienced at times with these patients. According to the view I am offering, the clinical appearance of the preoccupation with the dimensions of self-experience is the manifest content of unconscious conflict. The viewpoint that such phenomena are independent of conflict is based on an overly narrow conception of conflict.

The problem of dealing with material relating to the self in analysis is not resolved by accepting the patient's view that the fantasies about the state of the self, whether conscious or unconscious, describe some actual entity or endopsychically perceived state. Nor, on the other hand, can such descriptions be analyzed by immediately reducing them to caricatures of unconscious drive-related fantasy. The technical handling and interpretation of such self-descriptions are delicate matters. Patients giving such descriptions are narcissistically invested in their accounts and in their particular point of view of themselves. The narration of elaborate "self-observations" often serves as means of relating to others. In other words, self-description may serve many interpersonal functions, such as appeal, reproach, revelation, gift, and so on. By no means the least important is the invitation to appreciate and approve the style, wisdom, and self-knowledge.

Any effort to explore such fantasies, especially in states of tension, may be experienced as an attack. Some interpretations that focus on anxiety, hostility, and conflict, as well as those focusing on issues of closeness and affection, may stir up anxiety in some patients. They may then be experienced as "disintegrating," because for the patient they increase self-doubt by introducing an alien or disapproving point of view into the mind.

Clinically, then, the issue is one of relevance and the way the patient perceives the process of interpretation. If the patient feels the need to control or use the analyst for support, self-esteem regulation, an opposing view of self and the world, need satisfaction, tension regulation, or narcissistic gratifications, he will understand interpretations as serving or failing to serve these functions. Clarification of the "use of the object" (in Winnicott's phrase) will then be of primary relevance.

This will also entail the careful exploration of the patient's point of view. However, his need to protect his way of seeing things may mean that he equates being understood with having his point of view acknowledged before exploration is possible. What is at issue is a fear that his perceptions and fantasies will be condemned and devalued with the valuable parts ignored or submerged by those of the analyst. Elaboration of these problems points to the topic of transference—and character analysis.

These brief remarks on technique are meant only to indicate that the problem of the "self" in analysis is a matter of tactics and technique. Problems of analysis of self-material have been mistakenly regarded as showing the inadequacy of Freudian drive and ego-psychological theory. Rather than a theoretical difficulty, the trouble was a lack of systematic consideration of what goes into the art of the analyst—what Loewenstein called "dosage, timing and tact" and the careful "exploration of the psychic surface." Many of the examples purporting to show the inapplicability of classical theory are really criticisms of "timing, dosage and tact." Mechanical, insensitive or poorly timed interpretations of drive and conflict, sometimes "wild analysis," do not refute theory but expose its misapplications. The fact that such examples of technique are frequent points to a gap in the theory of therapy—the theory of how to apply the psychoanalytic theory of mind to psychoanalytic technique. The interest in problems of ego distortion and narcissistic personality disorders has stimulated the process of making the art of analysis the subject matter of a theory of technique.

Before closing my discussion, I should like to return to the problem of how we develop our psychoanalytic conception of the self and the parallel between psychoanalytic concept formation and the development of personal self-concepts. Our conception of the self in psychoanalysis, in whatever way we choose to formulate it, is built up of some objective observations of childhood and the partly subjective data of psychoanalysis. The value of infant observation lies in the fact that it provides a perspective on behavioral organization. Behavioral organization may contribute to what becomes self-experience by virtue of the fact that adults attribute meaning to it and respond to it as though it represented the activities of a self-aware, self-directed person. Thus the interpretation by the object of this preadapted organization becomes a part of the reflection of the self which helps to constitute it. In some cases these organizations themselves can become the basis of self-reflection, contributing as well to the fantasy of the self. In this way, organization becomes mental content via a fantasy about one's organization. Thus infant behaviors, such as the very early capacity for facial mimicry and for discrimination between persons in the environment, the capacity to respond differentially to different perceptual situations, the repetition of effective actions, are organizations that also guide the responses of people in the environment. What all this behavior shows is the potential nucleus of self-observation (what one may observe of oneself) and the nucleus of the perception of other people's response to oneself. These behaviors may be seen as representing a complex form of primary ego autonomy. Through the process of self-observation and perception of others' response, these primarily autonomous functions may become part of the subjective world. It is clear, however, from *this* description that whatever cognitive capacities may develop in this regard, the actual fantasy of self and of other will be much more complex because of the shaping of such perceptions by the well-known object-related fantasies and the self-fantasy. The fantasy of self-structure may not correspond to an actual structure at all, but rather something more complex in terms of the meaning of these observable organizations for the patient in relation to the objects in his environment.

One of the dangers in using child observation in the construction of our concept of the self in analysis is the too-ready equation of the self-experience of adults, especially disturbed adults, with behaviors having similar form in infancy. Although these two sources of information, objective on the one hand, subjectively oriented on the other—infancy and analysis—form the basis of our self-concept, they can never in fact be combined in such a way as to firmly tie the one to the other. We are in danger then of attributing adult categories of experience such as *experience* of initiative, cohesion, totality, and so on, to an infant who does not yet make sufficient distinction between self and object. We may too readily forget that the capacity for discrimination among objects, differential responses, and even self-recognition in a mirror may occur in animals other than man. Yet we do not readily attribute to such animals anything like a self in the human sense.

The observable behaviors generally considered indicative of the developing self are actually behaviors necessary for adaptation. The essential characteristic converting adaptive behavior into a "self," converting an infant into a person, is a capacity for reflection, for having a self-fantasy. In this connection, Lewis and Brooks-Gunn (1979) distinguish between the "categorical self" and the "existential self."

At the heart of the problem of the self is the question of how the capacity for reflection develops and how the dialogue of the self is engaged. Social dialogue and adaptation appear to begin at birth and also find a striking parallel in the social interactions of family pets. A description of my dog illustrates the extent to which the "self-" concept is built on a combination of socially adaptive behavior and meaning supplied by one participant.

In what follows, it is *not* my intention to parody child observation. I wish merely to underscore the problems of interpreting rich and complex data in a most important area.

My dog behaves differently toward each member of the family. He shows discrimination. He initiates interactions of different kinds—playful, demanding, affectionate. He seeks me out, and if I am attentive and willing to follow, he will lead me to the kitchen, where he will look steadfastly at the biscuit jar. He shows agency and initiative. When he bites my hand in play, he watches my face attentively and lets go if I mimic a painful expression. He distinguishes my discomfort from his, distinguishes "self" from "other." He knows when he is being mocked. If I mimic him when he is whining a complaint, he barks and becomes agitated. Finally, I come up behind him when he is lying on the floor watching me in the full-length mirror as I approach. I raise my foot and bring it down behind his head outside the range of his vision, never touching him. He cringes. Does he recognize himself in the mirror? My reason for telling you about my dog is not to brag about him nor to set an example for you in my joyful and approving mirroring of his achievements. Rather, I am struck by the fact that perhaps some people would be willing to treat these achievements as a manifestation of a self and self-other discrimination, if I were describing an infant rather than a dog. Does my dog have a self? Behavior alone cannot answer this question, and we cannot question the dog. This may be the crucial point in the understanding of the self and in self-understanding. It may not just be a question of being able to speak to answer the question. The process itself of learning to communicate through language may be essential to the capacity to have object representations of self and other. That is, to be objective and therefore truly subjective may depend on this very process as well as on the capacity to symbolize and reflect. So, paraphrasing Wittgenstein, I would say, if my dog could speak I would not understand him, for his experience would be too different from mine. When I speak about the capacity to symbolize, I also have in mind not only the capacity to recall a situation which is not actually going on, but also to imagine situations which have never happened, the capacity to think, "what if."

To put oneself in another's place, to see things from his perspective is to imagine something that has never happened. The building up of self- and object representations, and the development of the capacity for empathy, come from the never-ending repetitions of the effort to change perspective, to be objective with respect to oneself, and to be subjective from the point of view of others. The interpersonal consequences of this effort contribute to the fantasies of the self as well as of objects.

But what of the infant's self? Can the fact that we know he will be a human adult, perhaps a philosopher or a psychoanalyst, help us to empathize with his experience of the wholeness of his self? If an infant could speak, we could not understand him either. As infants get to be older children, we understand better what they are saying. But they can no longer tell us what they wanted to say at the beginning. When the child in us speaks, dreaming or waking, we do not understand. Analysis is the method by which we try to understand the child, but it is no longer the same child. The childhood we reconstruct is virtual, in the sense of a virtual image. It is the part of childhood that is significant now.

We deal with two groups of problems: 1) how to explain to the patient what he is saying, his inability to say it, or why he needs to say it as he does; 2) how to explain the way a child's mind becomes an adult mind. We need to explain both although, at a particular clinical moment, they are not equally relevant. It is a mistake to think we can do without such explanations, even the explanation of how man the animal is related to those other two issues of man the person. If one does not make explicit one's conception of the personal and the organismic (Rubinstein 1976, 1981) the relation will be implicit. In our implicit, unknown, unformulated theories the child's mind once more has free play.

REFERENCES

Abend S: Problems of identity: theoretical and clinical applications. Psychoanal Q 43:606–637, 1974

Bach S: Narcissism, continuity and the uncanny. Int J Psychoanal 56:77–86, 1975

Bach S: Self-love and object-love: some problems of self and object constancy, differentiation and integration, in Rapprochement: The Critical Subphase of Separation-Individuation. Edited by Lax RF, Bach S, Burland JA. New York, Jason Aronson, 1980, pp 171–197

Eisnitz AJ: The organization of the self-representation and its influence on pathology. Psychoanal Q 49:361–392, 1980

Freud A: The widening scope of indications for psychoanalysis: discussion. J Am Psychoanal Assoc 2:607–620, 1954

Freud S: Screen memories (1899), in The Standard Edition of the Complete Psychological Works of Sigmund Freud [SE], Vol 3. Translated and edited by Strachey J. London, Hogarth Press, 1962, pp 301–322

Freud S: Fragment of an analysis of a case of hysteria (1905). SE, 7:7–122, 1953

Freud S: Psycho-analytic notes on an autobiographical account of a case of paranoia (dementia paranoides) (1911). SE, 12:3–82, 1958

Freud S: The claims of psycho-analysis to scientific interest (1913a). SE, 13:165–190, 1953

Freud S: Totem and taboo (1913b). SE, 13:1–161, 1953

Freud S: On narcissism: an introduction (1914). SE, 14:67–102, 1957

Freud S: Instincts and their vicissitudes (1915). SE, 14:109–140, 1957
Freud S: Introductory lectures on psycho-analysis (1916–1917). SE, 16, 1963
Freud S: New introductory lectures on psychoanalysis (1933a). SE, 22:1–182, 1964
Freud S: Why war? (1933b). SE, 22:197–215, 1964
Freud S: Constructions in analysis (1937). SE, 23:255–269, 1964
Grossman WI: Reflections on the relationships of introspection and psychoanalysis. Int J Psychoanal 48:16–31, 1967
Grossman WI, Simon B: Anthropomorphism: motive, meaning and causality in psychoanalytic theory. Psychoanal Study Child 24:78–111, 1969
Hartmann H, Kris E, Loewenstein RM: Papers on Psychoanalytic Psychology. Psychol Issues Monogr 14. New York, International Universities Press, 1964
Kernberg O: Borderline Conditions and Pathological Narcissism. New York, Jason Aronson, 1975
Klein GS: Psychoanalytic Theory: An Exploration of Essentials. New York, International Universities Press, 1976
Kohut H: The Restoration of the Self. New York, International Universities Press, 1977
Kris E: The personal myth: a problem in psychoanalytic technique. J Am Psychoanal Assoc 4:653–681, 1956
Lewis M, Brooks-Gunn J: Social Cognition and the Acquisition of Self. New York, Plenum, 1979
Loewald H: On motivation and instinct theory. Psychoanal Study Child 26:91–128, 1971
Loewenstein RM: Some considerations on free association. J Am Psychoanal Assoc 11:451–473, 1963
Mischel T: Conceptual issues in the psychology of the self: an introduction, in The Self: Psychological and Philosophical Issues. Edited by Mischel T. Oxford, UK, Blackwell, 1977, pp 3–28
Nagel T: Mortal Questions. Cambridge, UK, Cambridge University Press, 1979
Piaget J: Insights and Illusions of Philosophy. New York, New American Library, 1971
Rapaport D: A theoretical analysis of the superego concept (1957), in The Collected Papers of David Rapaport. Edited by Gill MM. New York, Basic Books, 1967, pp 685–709
Rapaport D: On the psychoanalytic theory of motivation (1960), in The Collected Papers of David Rapaport. Edited by Gill MM. New York, Basic Books, 1967, pp 853–915
Richards AD: Self theory, conflict theory and the problem of hypochondriasis. Psychoanal Study Child 36:319–337, 1981
Rubinstein BB: On the possibility of strictly clinical psychoanalytic theory: an essay on the philosophy of psychoanalysis. Psychol Issues 36:229–264, 1976
Rubinstein BB: Person, organism, and self. Paper presented to the New York Psychoanalytic Society, January 27, 1981

Rycroft C: Introduction: causes and meaning, in Psychoanalysis Observed. Edited by Rycroft C. New York, Coward-McCann, 1966, pp 7–22

Schafer R: Aspects of Internalization. New York, International Universities Press, 1968

Schafer R: A New Language for Psychoanalysis. New Haven, CT, Yale University Press, 1976

Schafer R: Language and Insight. New Haven, CT, Yale University Press, 1978

Spiegel LA: The self, the sense of self, and perception. Psychoanal Study Child 14:81–109, 1959

Spruiell V: The self and the ego. Psychoanal Q 50:319–344, 1981

Sterba R: The fate of the ego in analytic therapy. Int J Psychoanal 15:117–126, 1934

Stone L: On resistance to the psychoanalytic process. Psychoanal Contemp Sci 2:42–73, 1973

Toulmin SE: Self-knowledge and knowledge of the "self," in The Self: Psychological and Philosophical Issues. Edited by Mischel T. Oxford, UK, Blackwell, 1977, pp 291–317

12

IRWIN Z. HOFFMAN, PH.D.

INTRODUCTION

Irwin Z. Hoffman received his B.A. from Brandeis University in Waltham, Massachusetts, and his Ph.D. in Clinical Psychology from the University of Chicago. He is a graduate of the Chicago Institute for Psychoanalysis and is Faculty and Supervising Analyst at the Chicago Center for Psychoanalysis and the National Training Program in Contemporary Psychoanalysis. He has served on the faculty of the Division of Psychology in the Department of Psychiatry at the University of Illinois College of Medicine, has been Associate Professor of Clinical Psychiatry at Northwestern University Medical School, Lecturer in Psychiatry at the University of Illinois Medical Center, and Faculty at the New York University Postdoctoral Program in Psychotherapy and Psychoanalysis. He has been the recipient of research grants from the National Institute of Mental Health, the American Psychoanalytic Association Fund for Psychoanalytic Research, the Liddle Fund, and the Mary S. Sigourney Trust for teachers of psychotherapy. He has served on the editorial boards of *Psychoanalytic Dialogues, The International Journal of Psychoanalysis,* and *Contemporary Psychoanalysis.*

Throughout his career, Dr. Hoffman has been an avid teacher, conducting workshops and presenting papers. A few titles will convey some of the range of his interest: "The Incompatibility of the Medical Model and the Therapeutic Community," "Death Anxiety and Adaptation to Mortality in Psychoanalytic Theory," "A Coding Scheme for Studying the Analysis of the Transference" (with Merton M. Gill), "The

Patient as Interpreter of the Analyst's Experience," "The Value of Uncertainty in Psychoanalytic Practice," "Dialectical Thinking and Therapeutic Action," "The Intimate and Ironic Authority of the Psychoanalyst's Presence," "Constructing Good-Enough Endings in Psychoanalysis," "The Myths of Free Association and the Potentials of the Analytic Relationship," and "Forging Differences Out of Similarity: The Multiplicity of Corrective Experience." Recently, many of Dr. Hoffman's papers have been collected and combined with several important new essays in the volume *Ritual and Spontaneity in the Psychoanalytic Process: A Dialectical-Constructivist View* (Hoffman 1998).

Dr. Hoffman has been a leading proponent of the dialectical-constructivist point of view, emphasizing the intrinsic ambiguity of the psychoanalytic situation. In this view, every encounter of analyst and patient is co-constructed, overdetermined, and subject to multiple interpretations. Along with his emphasis on constructed meaning, however, Dr. Hoffman has centered attention on the ritualized asymmetry of the analytic relationship, an asymmetry that gives the analyst a special kind of authority that is integral to therapeutic action. That authority is "ironic" because it is continually challenged through the analysis of the transference and through the exposure of the analyst's human fallibility.

Dr. Hoffman collaborated with Dr. Gill in bringing the primary role of transference and countertransference interactions to the attention of American analysts. In every attempt to explore the patient's experience in the analytic setting, the actual person and characteristics of the analyst have a critical role to play. From this point of view, not only meanings but also possible ways of being are co-created by the analytic couple rather than merely discovered or wholly determined by internal and external pressures. Dr. Hoffman has said, "I am proposing a single psychoanalytic modality in which there is a dialectic between noninterpretive and interpretive interactions" (Hoffman 1998, p. xiii). He emphasizes all the subtle, nonverbal behaviors by which the analyst and the patient reveal themselves to each other. He focuses on the importance of noninterpretive interactions that encourage the realization of latent potentialities of the dyad potentialities for both repetition and new experience that are also continually explored. Dr. Hoffman argues for maintaining "a sense of the dialectic between, on the one hand, the core of analytic discipline, which entails the analyst's consistent self-subordination in the interest of the patient's long-term well-being, and, on the other hand, the analyst's personal subjective participation" (p. xxvii). He has been a strong and innovative force integrating the impact on psychoanalysis of intersubjectivity, constructivism, relational theory, and postmodernism.

WHY I CHOSE THIS PAPER

Irwin Z. Hoffman, Ph.D.

In general, in this paper I integrate the paradigm of dialectical constructivism that I had been working on in the 1980s and early 1990s with the existential issues that were partially the subject of my dissertation (Hoffman 1972) and that were discussed in my paper on death anxiety in 1979 (Hoffman 1998, Chapter 2). Now the social construction of reality is seen within the context of mortality so that it is imbued with a greater sense of urgency as well as a quality of defiance. The quest for meaning and for the affirmation of the worth of self and other is pitted against death, the indifferent universe, and the element of indifference emanating from the "object."

This essay carries the title of my book *Ritual and Spontaneity in the Psychoanalytic Process: A Dialectical-Constructivist View,* in which it is Chapter 9, and includes the most detailed and extended clinical illustration in the volume. A key liminal moment demonstrates the co-creation by analyst and analysand of a quality of relatedness that is new and generative even as the specter of potentially destructive forms of enactment is evoked. The case affords an especially poignant look at the interplay of neurotic and existential anxiety. The patient's primary symptom, a kind of vertigo, could be viewed as rational, whereas the usual sense of balance and confidence that people maintain in their everyday lives could be viewed as illusory, grounded essentially in denial. The case also offers the opportunity to explore the relationship between "drive" and "deficit," with particular attention to the issues highlighted by self psychology and classical theory. The two perspectives in this case play themselves out in a special manner in that the patient had an interest in self psychology that he seemed, at times, to use defensively. The chapter closes with a series of dreams bearing on the termination of the analysis, including one that synthesizes multiple themes, ending finally with an account of the last hour in which analyst and analysand try to co-construct a "good-enough ending" for that hour and for the analysis.

REFERENCES

Hoffman IZ: Parental Adaptation to Fatal Illness in a Child. Doctoral dissertation, University of Chicago, Chicago, IL, 1972

Hoffman IZ: Ritual and Spontaneity in the Psychoanalytic Process: A Dialectical-Constructivist View. Hillsdale, NJ, The Analytic Press, 1998

RITUAL AND SPONTANEITY IN THE PSYCHOANALYTIC PROCESS

IRWIN Z. HOFFMAN, PH.D.

PSYCHOANALYTIC RITUALS

There is a fixed routine in the psychoanalytic process, a routine with the kind of symbolic, evocative, and transforming potential that gives it the aura of a ritual.[1] There are fixed times, a fixed place, and a fixed fee. Each appointment is usually 45 or 50 minutes long. Commonly the seating arrangement is the same every time, whether or not it entails the use of the couch. The couch itself, when it is used, adds to the peculiarity of the situation, to its foreignness, and perhaps to the mystique of the now seemingly disembodied analyst's voice.

In addition to these "extrinsic" factors (Gill 1954, 1984), within the process itself there is a fundamental asymmetry. The patient is invited to "free associate" and thereby, presumably, to expose the structure of his or her emotional life. The analyst remains strangely hidden or anonymous, strangely, that is, relative to the norms of ordinary social conduct. Although analysts vary considerably in the ways that they

---

[1]Catherine Bell (1992) writes that "ritualization is a way of acting that specifically establishes a privileged contrast, differentiating itself as more important or powerful. Such privileged distinctions may be drawn in a variety of culturally specific ways that render the ritualized acts dominant in status" (p. 90).

"Ritual and Spontaneity in the Psychoanalytic Process," by Irwin Z. Hoffman, Ph.D., was first published as Chapter 9 in *Ritual and Spontaneity in the Psychoanalytic Process: A Dialectical-Constructivist View,* by Irwin Z. Hoffman, pp. 219–245.

conceptualize the role of their own subjective, personal reactions in the process, few if any—notwithstanding Ferenczi's experiments late in his life—would advocate the complete breakdown of this asymmetry. If there is room in our culture for that kind of process, it is certainly difficult to imagine what it could mean in the context of a professional service in which one party pays the other for confidential psychological help. Indeed, we are in Ferenczi's debt for exposing the untenability of anything approaching a fully mutual analysis. One of the problems Ferenczi (1932) ran into very quickly was that he couldn't possibly speak freely to RN about what came to his mind and still honor the confidentiality of his experiences with other patients, because those experiences were often precisely what came to his mind (p. 34).

The analytic frame, of course, provides the general boundaries for the relationship, a multifaceted scaffolding of protection for both the patient and the analyst. It sets up the special "potential space" in which the "play" of psychoanalysis can go on (Modell 1990; Winnicott 1971) As Modell says, "Despite the spontaneity and unpredictability of the affective relationship between the analyst and the analysand, there are also certain affective constants that are institutionalized as part of technique and contribute to the frame or the rules of the game" (p. 30). We usually think of these institutionalized constants, combined with the fixed aspects of the setting, as contributing to a safe environment, one that provides the context for the real analytic work (as in the working alliance) or is in itself the vehicle for a good deal of therapeutic action (as in the holding environment). From this point of view, deviations from psychoanalytic rituals might be thought to endanger the atmosphere of safety that they are designed to foster and their nurturant, development-facilitating potential.

DOES THE FRAME CREATE A SANCTUARY?

There are, however, important counterpoints to the view that the analytic frame establishes a standard, safe environment. First of all, the extent to which the setting can be standardized is limited. Psychoanalytic rituals leave a great deal of room for variations in the manner in which they are carried out. Thus, if the rituals *were* adhered to by an analyst in a very rigid way, that in itself would be experienced by the patient as a choice by the analyst, one that would be highly suspect in terms of its motivation. This goes without saying, of course, for the interactions that go on within the context of the frame but are not themselves conspicuously defining of it. What the analyst will say, for example, between 9:00 A.M., when he or she opens the door and says, "Come in," and 9:50, when he or she says, "It's time to stop," is (or should be) clearly less predictable than those starting points and end points themselves. But it is also the case that even the start of the hour and its conclusion leave much latitude for the analyst to convey a range of personal attitudes and moods. Is the analyst smiling, or frowning, or neither? Does he or she say "Hi, Bob. C'mon in," or just "Hello," or nothing—maybe just a slight nod of the head? At the end, does the analyst say, "Our time is up" or "We have to stop now" or "I know this is a difficult moment to stop, but we are out of time for today"?

The conclusion of a session is of special interest. Because it is the last moment, it has special weight. Whatever taste it leaves is apt to linger at least until the next session, which is not to say the taste has to be pleasant. Sometimes it might seem "best" for a session to end on a sour note: depressed or angry or whatever. But it's important to recognize that there is an element of choice, uncertainty, and responsibility associated with the analyst's contribution to the ending. As much as we might like to feel that what we do at the end of a session merely conforms to a standard routine for which we are not personally responsible—a little like merely "following orders"—the conclusion of every session is a joint construction, one that is chosen, in part, by us, however much it is organized around a given, objective boundary.

Suppose a patient says, with about a minute to go, "I feel like I'm going in circles today and not getting anywhere. Frankly, I don't think I've changed much since I started seeing you," and suppose he or she then falls silent. Now there is a half minute or less left. As the analyst, I could wait 20 seconds or so in what might feel like a heavy silence and then simply say, "It's time to stop." We would be ending then on a certain kind of note. I could tell myself that, after all, it's the note the *patient* chose to end on. The patient's action and the clock created that ending, not I. Because it's the ending created by the patient and the standard time limit, it's the "right" one for the patient and me to live with and, perhaps, to explore the next time we meet. Certainly the patient is a major architect of the session's conclusion. To leave it at that, however, would be to deny that in being silent for those last seconds I was *choosing* a course of action and thereby co-creating that ending. First of all, in all likelihood I would not, in fact, know what the time was to the second, but even if I did, I could have said it was time to stop just a few seconds after the patient spoke, or I could have waited about 20 seconds more than I did. These are options that are likely to create three very different endings with very different affective colorations. And then, there is the alternative of actually responding directly to the patient's comment. There are innumerable possibilities, of course.[2] On the side of combatting the mood set by the patient, if it seemed to fit, I could say, "I think it means something that you say that right at the end. In fact, I think that it's your way of expressing your anger about having to leave"; or maybe, "Really? I thought that was a good session and that we accomplished a lot. Aren't you doing that number on yourself and on me that we've talked about many times?" Whatever I said, I would then have the option of saying "It's time to stop" right after I made my comment, or waiting a few seconds to give the patient a chance to respond. The latter might be a risk, because I'd be running over and I'd be concerned about inviting a response and then having to cut the patient off. So maybe I'd say, "Unfortunately, it looks like I'm going to have the last word today, because we do have to stop." The point is that each of these options, the various lengths of silence and the various comments that I might make, constructs a different ending and a different reality. Moreover, in that moment, in that split second which is the moment of choice and of action, there is no way to know what is the "right thing" to do. Indeed, there can be no single "right thing" for the patient or for the relationship. The moment is shot through with uncertainty. First, I don't know just what it means that the patient has said what he or she has said. Second, I don't know the full meaning of whatever inclinations I may have to be silent or to speak. And third, whatever I choose to do, I don't know what opportunities are being lost and what would have happened if I had chosen a different course. The safety afforded by the analytic frame is a qualified one in that it cannot spare the patient or the analyst these uncertainties and the anxieties that attend them.

Ultimately, constructing a "good-enough ending" is the challenge of termination, a separation process that can be decisive in terms of the outcome of the entire analysis. And yet the boundary situations associated with the endings of sessions and with the ending of the analysis as a whole are also like any moment within every session, which is always both structured by analytic ritual and left to the participants to create. Thus in every moment there is a kind of ricocheting going on, a dialectical interplay between ritual and spontaneity, between what is given and what is created, between what is role-determined and what

---

[2]Of course this is a hypothetical example, so the possibilities of what I might say are relatively unconstrained. But even with a real case, there would be infinite possibilities, although they would be encompassed within a narrower range. "Infinite" does not mean "unlimited." As I have written elsewhere (Hoffman 1998, Chapter 3), "there are infinite numerical values between the numbers 5 and 6, but that range excludes all other numerical values" (p. 77).

is personal, between constraint and freedom.

In fact, in a general way, it could be said that in our neuroses we suffer from the dichotomous organization of these polarities, a feeling that the choice is between a suffocating submission to internal and external constraints, on the one hand, and a loss of control in which "all hell breaks loose," on the other. We hope that through analysis it will be possible for us to replace such dichotomous thinking with dialectical thinking, with an integrative sense of the interdependence of apparent opposites. In that light, perhaps, we can reaffirm Freud's aphorism, in somewhat revised form: "where id [and superego were, split off from each other], there ego shall be [mediating their dialectical relationship]" (cf. Freud, 1933, p. 80).

Before moving to a fuller clinical illustration, I'd like to discuss another counterpoint to the view of the frame as a kind of sanctuary. Not only is it not possible for the analyst's behavior to be fully standardized, but also the intrinsic features of the frame are not simply benign. Racker (1968) says that no encounter with the actual person of the analyst is necessary in order for the patient to begin speculating about the complementary countertransference. He says:

> [T]he analyst communicates certain associations of a personal nature even when he does not seem to do so. These communications begin, one might say, with the plate on the front door that says "Psychoanalyst" or "Doctor." What motive (in terms of the unconscious) would the analyst have for wanting to cure if it were not he who made the patient ill? In this way the patient is already, simply by being a patient, the creditor, the accuser, the "superego" of the analyst; and the analyst is his debtor. (pp. 145–146)

But is a reparative motive, which is, after all, relatively benign, the only kind that the patient can plausibly attribute to the analyst for assuming this rather peculiar role? It seems to me there are others that are much more threatening to the patient's sense of safety. Is the analyst not the person who has detected a certain need in the society for understanding, for love, for an idealized object; the one who has scanned the culture (usually with special attention to the white, urban middle class and upper class) and thought, "Why shouldn't I take advantage of this hunger, this craving that a lot of people have for this kind of attachment?" Is the analyst not also the one who has found a way to feed his or her narcissism without being subjected to very much personal risk, or, perhaps, one who fears and craves intimacy and has found a way to have it while still maintaining a good deal of control and distance, or one who enjoys his or her sense of power over the people (if business is good, the *many* people) who want to be his or her special or favorite one? Finally, what could be better than to have all of this hidden under the guise of being the "good-enough parent" who provides, "objectively," a secure holding environment, armed against whatever protests might arise with knowing interpretations of the "neurotic transference"?

These motives, and others like them, comprise the dark, malignant underside of the analytic frame. It is a side that I think we commonly deny. It's rather astonishing, I think, how ready we are to compare ourselves to rather ideal parents, not perfect perhaps, but surely "good enough," and how prepared we are to see the influence of the pathogenic aspects of the patient's past upon the entry into the analytic space of the so-called bad object (cf. Slavin and Kriegman 1992).

The rituals that constitute the frame are undoubtedly essential to the process, and deviations from them are certainly as open, if not more open, to suspicion regarding their self-serving nature as is their religious observance. What I'm questioning is the *neatness of the dichotomy:* adherence to the frame creates safety, deviation from the frame creates danger. Even if the frame is mostly beneficial, it does not create a perfect sanctuary because, as I have said, it cannot eliminate the analyst's personal participation as a co-constructor of reality in the process and because its defining features are, in themselves, suspect.

Psychoanalytic rituals provide usefully ambiguous grounds, not only for new experience and development, but also for neurotic repetition.[3] Acknowledging this reality has at least two important clinical implications. First, the patient's conscious and unconscious objections to analytic routines, even his or her rage about them, must be taken seriously. By that I mean *more* than that we have to get into the patient's world and see it from his or her point of view. That attitude can be subtly patronizing, to the extent that we consider the patient's perspective to stem from deficits or even from unresolved conflicts originating in childhood, and to the extent that we hope that the patient will eventually come to see things from a more developmentally advanced perspective. Instead, I mean that we recognize what may be objectionable about the frame, even from the point of view of a mature, "healthy" adult, so much so that we may wonder what kind of pathology would result in a person being willing to go along with it at all! The one in need is the one who may be driven to accept an invitation to be exploited, and the analytic arrangement can be construed, quite plausibly, as extending such an invitation. A second clinical implication of acknowledging the malignant aspects of the frame, in

[3]See Hoffman 1998, pp. 2–3, on Macalpine 1950.

addition to recognizing a place for an unobjectionable *negative* transference (cf. Guidi 1993) and for reasonable resistance, is that such acknowledgment provides theoretical grounds for considering the benign potentials of momentary deviations from the standard routine. A readiness to deviate in certain limited ways may offset the exploitative meanings that can get attached to maintaining the frame in an inflexible manner. There is no way for the analyst to know, with certainty, what course to pursue with respect to the balance between spontaneous, personal responsiveness and adherence to psychoanalytic rituals at any given moment, nor can the balance that is struck be one that the analyst can completely control. The basis for the patient's trust is often best established through evidence of the analyst's struggle with the issue and through his or her openness to reflect critically on whatever paths he or she has taken, prompted more or less by the patient's reactions and direct and indirect communications.

With these ideas as background, let's take a closer look at a piece of clinical experience.

CONFRONTING A PHOBIA WITHIN THE ANALYTIC SETTING: A SERENDIPITOUS OPPORTUNITY

A patient, Ken, is in my private, downtown office on the 21st floor for the first time. For about three years we had met four times per week at my office at the university, which was on the seventh floor. In that office there was one small window at the foot of the couch. Here, there are two enormous windows on the wall across from the couch to the patient's right, about 6 or 7 feet away. The patient is terrified of heights. The theme of high places is at the center of a complex knot of symptoms, an amalgam of depression, anxiety, obsessional tendencies, and phobia. Ken has had full-blown panic attacks just contemplating certain situations that involve heights, not to mention being in them. On one occasion, he traveled to another city for a meeting where he was to make a presentation on a subject of great interest to him. At the last moment, to his dismay and embarrassment, he had to back out, because to get to the room where the meeting took place he would have had to walk across a corridor with a railing overlooking an atrium. But his reactions are variable, and sometimes he has managed very well in situations that could have been disabling. In general, he is a very competent, resourceful person, a mental-health professional himself and a psychotherapist.[4] Ken is also a devoted husband and father of three young children.

At the university office, Ken had generally felt comfortable. He had rarely felt anxious during a session. Sometimes he would get anxious after a session while waiting for the elevator, which was next to a window. Often he would take the stairs rather than wait. He had told me of a fantasy of coming back to the office to ask for some ill-defined help. He had thought of my comforting him or perhaps waiting with him at the elevator, but he never acted on that impulse. In general, he had always been respectful of the conventional limits of the analytic situation and had made good use of it as a context for expressing and exploring the things that troubled him. In many ways he was an ideal analysand, reporting many dreams and experiencing and reflecting upon transference issues in the here and now and in terms of genetics.

Changes in my schedule and Ken's made it more convenient to have first one, then two of our four sessions in my downtown office. The idea of meeting there was broached for the first time by me, anticipating a day when the university would be closed because of a holiday but when I would be working in my practice. Ken actually declined that invitation, but he subsequently brought up the possibility himself because he wanted to take advantage of the opportunity to tackle his fear of heights within the context of the analysis. We did, however, discuss the fact that once the option was made available, Ken felt some internal pressure to try it, along with a sense that I might want him to. And it is true that I thought this might be a serendipitous development. The combination of the two locations could provide the opportunity to confront the phobia directly, as Freud (1919) suggested was necessary with such symptoms, but with the advantage of having that confrontation woven into the analytic routine itself. The latter would include alternation between the "safer" and the more "dangerous" settings.

So, here we are at the end of this first session on the 21st floor. Ken has managed to get through this hour without a major attack of anxiety or vertigo. He was quite anxious at the beginning, although it was not as bad as he had anticipated, especially with the window shades pulled down, something I had done in advance at Ken's request. He said, "I was afraid I would be drawn to the windows and I would become like a robot or an automaton, unable to control myself. And then what would you do? Would you stop me? Of course, I feel that you would." I say that he may have a wish for an experience in which I stop him physically from doing some-

---

[4]In an earlier draft of this essay, this information was disguised. After reading it, the patient said he felt that the disguise took too much away from the atmosphere of the process and that it was not necessary

thing self-destructive. He says he feels that would be a demonstration of will and strength for his benefit. He reports a dream. "There is a truck with long boards of wood. Somehow I go underneath all the wood boards. They started to slide out of the truck on top of me and I realized I could be crushed. But I got out and I didn't panic. I don't remember whether there was anyone else helping. I think I just got out myself." He spontaneously thinks of the unloading of a truck as a metaphor for the analysis. Then he associates to his father. He thought of him as husky and strong physically, but he always felt threatened by him rather than comforted. He says his father "always wanted to win," whereas he, as a father himself, enjoys roughhousing in a playful way with his own children. I say, "Meeting with me here has a lot of meaning for you I think. It's probably not just the height as such that is affecting you." The patient says, "I could get into resenting it, having to put myself through this. But I do have a sense that we are in this room *together* and that in general we are in the process together, and that helps." Now this much-anticipated and dreaded first time is over. I say, "It's time to stop." Ken sits up. He seems a bit shaky. Then he looks at me and, rather to my surprise, he says, "I don't feel *too* bad, but I wonder if you'd mind walking to the elevator with me?"

MOMENT OF TRUTH: THOUGHT IN ACTION

I think it's good to stop at points like this to consider the analyst's position, because, as an exercise, it's useful to consider the kinds of attitudes the analyst may have toward the patient's request without the benefit of hindsight.

The instant the patient's question is posed I am called upon to act. There is no way that I can "call time" to think it over. If I hesitate or if I say, "Well, wait, let's think about this for a moment," or "Maybe you could say a little more about what you're feeling," I am of course *acting* in a particular way. There is no way to just think about it without acting, and however I act will have some sort of complex meaning to myself and to the patient. The commonsense idea, one that is highly valued psychoanalytically, that I should think *before* I act is of little or no help in this respect. It certainly will not do to say, "Let's think about it and talk about it more tomorrow and then we'll see." The moment of truth is now. What I do will express *something* about me, about our relationship, and about the patient. While it cannot be action following thought in a linear way, it might, nevertheless, be action that is saturated with thought or thought-full.

Does it make any sense to ask what is the right thing or the best thing for the analyst to do? Many would say, "It depends." More needs to be known about the patient, his history, his dynamics, the status of the transference, and the nature of the process in this very session. I have told you so little, after all, of what I know or knew, so little, one might say, of what was "going through my mind." But even if I could explicate all of the issues pertaining to that list of considerations about the patient, to what extent would that put us in a better position to decide what I should have done and with what attitude? Is an accurate assessment of the patient's state of mind possible? And if it were possible, would it be enough?

The alternative to the view that the analyst should act simply in accord with an assessment of the patient takes it for granted that the analyst acts in relation to a complex, only partially conscious, organization of his or her own thoughts and feelings. In the moment of action there is no sharp split between what is personally expressive and what is in keeping with one's technical principles or diagnostic assessment. Expressive participation and psychoanalytic discipline are intertwined (Hoffman 1998, Chapter 7). If there is a "right" or best thing for the analyst to do, it might be something that is *integrative* of as many considerations about the *relationship* as possible. From the point of view of a supervisor or consultant, for example, the information that is relevant would have to include the nature of the analyst's experience. And the suggestions that a supervisor would make would take account of the analyst's involvement in the process. The supervisor might say, "Given that the patient was apparently experiencing such and such and that you [the analyst-supervisee] were experiencing such and such, might it have been useful to do or say this or that?" Let me emphasize that I'm not saying that this "given" in the analyst's experience should be immune from criticism. After all, there are certain attitudes and perspectives that we try to cultivate so that the probability will be higher that our experience will at least include certain properties: empathic listening, for example, theoretically informed understanding, critical reflection on our own participation, and so on. In fact, part of my purpose in this paper is to convey my own sense of the optimal analytic attitude, one that allows for a range of countertransference experiences that can be used constructively to promote the process.

SOME BACKGROUND: A CHILDHOOD OF SCARCE LOVE AND DREADED IMPULSE

Certainly, as I said, I have conveyed only a small fraction of the information about the patient that was relevant to my action at that moment.

In fact, what I could formulate to myself at that time, not to mention what I can recapture from memory, is probably only a fraction of the information I was processing. Considerations of confidentiality limit even further what I can convey to you accurately. Finally, whatever information is selected and however it is organized constructs a story line of some kind, a particular narrative account among the many that might be pertinent and even compelling (Schafer 1992). With those qualifications, here are a few more highlights from the patient's history.

Ken was an only child. His mother was alcoholic, estranged from her unsympathetic, self-centered husband, painfully lonely, and often depressed. When the patient was 15 years old she killed herself, using a combination of drugs, a plastic bag over her head, and gas sucked in from a Bunsen burner from the patient's chemistry set. The patient came home from school one day and found the house locked. A note on the door suggested he go to a neighbor's house until his father came home. Later, the father and the patient descended the winding stairs to the basement where they found the mother's body. There was a note addressed to the patient that read: "I had to do this. I couldn't take it anymore. You go on and have a happy life. You're great." In this act, the mother constructed, not a "good enough" ending, surely, but a catastrophic one for her son to carry with him for the rest of his life.

The patient's father was a salesman. He was very narcissistic, full of a kind of bravado, a macho style that was decidedly unempathic in terms of its responsiveness to the patient's needs and sense of vulnerability. The father's "competitiveness" was so extreme it often deteriorated into virtual abuse. Here's one telling story. In playing one-on-one basketball when the patient was in his early teens, the father, who was much taller, was happy to block all the patient's shots and win the game ten to nothing. Indeed, Ken, who was a quiet, sensitive type and something of a bookworm, often felt his father didn't particularly like him. In fact, Ken thought his father preferred two of his nephews, both of whom liked hunting and fishing, activities that were quite abhorrent to the patient.

Ken had only scant and fragmentary memories of his mother. What was particularly striking was that he had vivid memories of parts of her body, distinct images of them in the bathtub, for example, especially her breasts, which he admired. He had more difficulty remembering her face, not to mention difficulty recapturing a sense of her as a whole person. Toward the end of the first year of the analysis the patient recalled a moment in his early teenage years when, looking at his mother passed out drunk in her bed, while his father was out of town on one of his many business trips, he thought to himself, "Why don't I just have sex with her and get her pregnant? Maybe that will enliven her and make her happy." Ken also had conscious wishes that his mother would die, which were countered, in part, by his realizing that her death would leave him alone with his father. Many times he fantasized wishfully and anxiously about his father being killed in a plane crash and not returning from one of his trips. At times, he was also very afraid of his father. On one occasion he refused to go on an amusement park ride with him for fear that his father would push him out of the elevated car to his death.

Thus, perhaps an important aspect of the atmosphere of the patient's childhood could be characterized as one that was full of the dangers of eruption of incestuous, patricidal, matricidal, and infanticidal impulses. We developed a picture of his environment as one in which he felt that he was left alone with dangerous temptations. He had a sense that it was all too easy for him and others to act on impulses that were destructive to him, to them, or to both. It felt as if he had only his own will to prevent an action that could be disastrous, and his own will often did not seem up to the challenge. He had his parents as models, after all. In the end, through an act signifying the ultimate abdication of responsibility, his mother left him with a terrible choice. He could try to demonstrate that one could be moved by forces beyond one's control to do oneself in. If he threw himself out the window, or more precisely, if he succumbed to what he experienced as a force drawing him out the window, he could say, "This must be how it was for her; she loved me but could not stop herself." But if he stopped himself with thoughts like, "What will become of those I care about, including my children?" he was left with the agonizing question as to why she couldn't or wouldn't have done the same for him.

A WALK TO THE ELEVATOR: AN EXPERIENCE IN "LIMINAL" SPACE

Let us return now to Ken's request. Notice that it occurs after the "official time" is up. Now we are in that interval that occurs in every analytic hour between the ending of the formally allotted time and the moment the patient leaves the office. I think it's a particularly interesting time because it is both inside and outside the frame. It occupies a place akin to what the anthropologist Victor Turner (1969) identifies as "liminal." Turner (1969) writes, "Liminal entities are neither here nor there; they are betwixt and between the positions assigned and arrayed by law, custom, convention, and ceremonial" (p. 95). Although Turner is interested in liminality as it is reflected specifically in the rites of passage of certain tribal cultures, what he has to say about it can be generalized to other aspects of social life (cf. Fourcher 1975). Indeed, the basic dialectic that *underlies* social life is *exposed* under the conditions of liminality. This is the dialectic of spontaneous, egalitarian relatedness, what Turner calls "communitas," and structured, hierarchical role-relatedness:

> It is as though there are two major "models" for human interrelatedness, juxtaposed and alternating. The first is of society as a structured, differentiated, and often hierarchical system of politico-legal-economic positions with many types of evaluation, separating men in terms of "more" or "less." The second, which emerges recognizably in the liminal period, is of society as an unstructured or rudimentarily structured and relatively undifferentiated comitatus, community, or even communion of equal individuals who submit together to the general authority of the ritual elders.... [F]or individuals and groups, social life is a type of dialectical process that involves successive experience of high and low, communitas and structure, homogeneity and differentiation, equality and inequality (pp. 96–97).

And further, very much in keeping with my view of the analytic process, Turner writes that "wisdom is always to find the appropriate relationship between structure and communitas under the *given* circumstances of time and place, to accept each modality when it is paramount without rejecting the other, and not to cling to one when its present impetus is spent" (p. 139).

So when the time is up we enter that peculiar, liminal zone that is "neither here nor there." I think it's useful to consider it not only for its own sake, but also because it exposes more clearly the dialectic between ritual and spontaneity within the process as a whole. The strategy is analogous to learning about so-called normal mental processes by studying psychopathology. In this instance we have not only the period in the office after the time is up, which, after all, is ironically a part of normal analytic routine, but also the prospect of time spent with the patient outside the office. In these two liminal zones, the one more outside the ritual than the other, the personal-egalitarian aspect of my relationship with Ken is highlighted and partially extricated from the role-defined hierarchical aspect, so that the tension between the two is felt more acutely than usual.

I responded to Ken's request immediately, simply by saying "Sure," and we walked to the elevators. My immediate feeling was that it would have been extremely stingy of me to decline or even to hesitate, since it had been such an ordeal for Ken to tolerate the session in this office. I knew, after all, that the idea of meeting at this location was initiated originally by me. Also, the patient's request, an aggressive initiative on his part, was out of character. It was a risk for him to make it, and I thought he might well feel not only disappointed, but also humiliated if I said no. I certainly didn't want to be like his father blocking his shots in basketball. That danger seemed greater to me than the dangers of complying. Also, because the request was so unusual, I felt inclined to give the patient the benefit of the doubt and respect whatever creative wisdom might have prompted it. Another consideration might have been that I felt that, over time, I had conveyed enough of an impression of personal availability to contribute to the patient's readiness to make the request. In any case, as Ken and I waited in the hallway we made a little small talk about the elevators, the express type versus the local type, which stopped at which floors, which he came up on, and so on. After a couple of minutes, one opened up and Ken stepped in. We shook hands just as the doors began to shut. It was not our customary way of parting. I'm not sure which of us reached out first.

Before getting to the patient's retrospective view of the experience the next day I want to stop to talk a bit more about the episode at the elevator, an example of an "extra-analytic" interaction. How do we conceptualize the nature of the interaction in the hallway? On the surface it could hardly be more mundane. Just a little, rather uninteresting small talk. But as we are waiting there is a little tension in the air, a touch of awkwardness, and a feeling that what's happening has a little extra "charge." Would we say that the analyst, ideally, would feel entirely comfortable in that situation? Would we say that the patient, too, would be comfortable the closer he was to completing his analysis? My own view is that regardless of the specific personalities of the participants, and regardless of the amount and quality of analytic work each has under his or her belt, there is a residue of tension that is *likely* because here, in the hallway, outside the psychoanalytic routines of time, place, and role-defined interactions, the analyst emerges out of the shadows of his or her analytic role and is exposed, more fully than usual, as a person like the patient, as a vulnerable social and physical being.[5] At this moment, in Turner's terms, "communitas," a sense of equality and of mutuality, moves into the foreground while role-determined, hierarchical structure shifts to the background. This reversal of figure and ground is likely to feel conflictual because both parties have much invested in the

---

[5]This heightened sense of visibility can occur within the customary hour too, at times, as might happen if the analyst moves to open a window or changes the furniture arrangement or the place where he or she sits.

analyst's relative invisibility. The analyst's capacity for an encompassing perspective and for constructive use of his or her special expertise is enhanced by the protections against narcissistic injury that a position of relative anonymity affords. This aspect of the ritual provides some rational ground for the analyst's authority in relation to the analysand. Beyond those rational grounds, however, there is an irrational component to that authority, a certain element of mystique[6] that gives the analyst a special kind of power. Only with that magical increment of power does the analyst stand a chance of doing battle with pathogenic object relations that were absorbed before the patient was old enough to think, or most importantly, to think critically. And only the analyst's relative anonymity can allow the patient to invest him or her with that magical power, one that represents, in more or less attenuated form, the power of the longed for omniscient, omnipotent, and loving parent.

So, it's not surprising that there is a little tension and a little awkwardness accompanying the small talk as we wait for the elevator. But it would be misleading to say that the special authority of the analyst, both its rational and its irrational components, are dissolved in these circumstances. Let's not forget that a reversal of figure and ground does not mean that one side of a dialectic is sacrificed in favor of the other. Rather, the two poles, that of spontaneous, egalitarian, informal participation and that of authority-enhancing, role-related, formal participation, continue to work in tandem, synergistically, the one potentiating the impact of the other. On a personal level, many relational themes are being played out, more than I can mention here, and more, indeed, than either participant could be aware of back then, or even now in retrospect. For one thing, this is a kind of transgression that I am joining the patient in, a bit of mischief in relation to the psychoanalytic "authorities," the tribal "elders," but also in relation to those authorities as they are internalized as part of my own (and maybe the patient's) psychoanalytic conscience. There is also a sense, however, that the transgression is a minor one, a forgivable one, even, perhaps, a constructive one. We both know that we will be back inside the analytic frame the next day and we both fully expect that this very interlude of escape from it, this relatively" "frameless" experience, as Grotstein (1993) calls it, will probably be subjected to routine analytic scrutiny. We will then be able to ex-

[6]The authority and the mystique are *ironic* because the grounds for them have been largely eroded in our culture and because within the process itself they are subjected to critical scrutiny in the analysis of the transference (see Hoffman 1998, Chapters 1 and 3).

plore the latent meanings of our interaction in the hallway as though it were part of the manifest content of a dream (cf. Kern 1987).

Aided partly by this expectation, at the very moment that I transgress I am aware, implicitly, that the patient and I are also trying to construct a *noncatastrophic* transgression, a *nonincestuous, nonsuicidal, nonhomicidal* violation of the rules. We are trying to differentiate this illicit act, stepping out the door together, from stepping out of the 21st-floor window, from being drawn into an incestuous abyss with the mother, from killing the mother, from killing the father, from being killed by the father, from the mother killing herself. In these scenarios, the patient may be either in the parent's or in the child's role, casting the analyst into the complementary position. All these potential differentiations—in which, hopefully, something new will emerge out of the shadows of something old—all these possibilities have special power, not only because they have been or will be understood analytically, but also because in the background it is the analyst who is participating in them and authorizing them. By making more vivid the patient's sense, as Ken puts it, "that we are in this together," by being, for the moment, a person conspicuously like the patient himself, by trusting the patient's conscious judgment, by extending myself beyond what is most comfortable for me (which reciprocates the patient's extension of himself in coming to my private office), by spending some time with the patient that is not paid for, by all of these simultaneous actions and others, I have at least a fighting chance, as the analyst, operating with the mantle of authority that is uniquely mine by virtue of my ritually based position, of overcoming the soul-murdering impact of the parents' conduct. I have a chance of reaching the patient with messages such as, "You are a person of worth; you have a right to be fully alive; you don't have to be buried alive under those wood boards; your feelings matter; you deserve respect as a unique individual; you can have concrete impact on me without destroying me or yourself; your desire, even when it runs counter to what is conventionally sanctioned, is not necessarily deadly; indeed, that desire has the potential to do more good than harm."[7] In sum, I am in a position to offer the patient a profound kind of recognition and affirmation. What is transformative, however, is not this action alone, but a continual struggle with the tension between

---

[7]The point bears a rough similarity to that of Strachey (1934) on the therapeutic action of mutative interpretations via the analyst's acceptance of the patient's "id-impulses."

spontaneous responsiveness and adherence to psychoanalytic ritual and a continual effort, in Turner's (1969) words, "to accept each modality when it is paramount without rejecting the other" (p. 139).

Now let's return to the particulars of the process and consider the patient's experience of the episode as he reported it the next day, now in the relative comfort of the university office.

THE PATIENT'S REFLECTIONS: CO-CONSTRUCTING NEEDS AND WISHES

"When I asked you to walk me to the elevator I wondered if you were irritated. But I felt you were being friendly and supportive in the hallway. I had very mixed emotions about asking you to do that, because I was actually feeling good enough. It wasn't a necessity. I didn't feel like I had become liquid and needed you to pour me into the elevator. Yet I was afraid if I didn't ask I might just be overwhelmed at the last minute. Then I was also conscious that maybe I was testing you a little to see how flexible you would be. That doesn't feel real terrific. A little dishonest maybe." I asked, "Did you plan on it beforehand?" Ken replied, "Yes, as a kind of contingency plan. But then it got to be sort of a superstition." I said, "So it was important in itself, just the wish that I go with you." Ken replied, "Yes, and *without* the excuse of my being terrified."

The patient then expressed interest in how my career was going. He wondered whether my colleagues, if they knew about it, would approve of my walking with him to the elevator. He also expressed concern about the sincerity of my action. Maybe its self-aggrandizing purpose was to impress others with, and congratulate myself for, my independence of mind. He thought maybe his doubts were carried over from his mistrust of his parents. He grew up feeling there was something uncertain about the extent and quality of their interest in his well-being. His mother seemed very pleased by his excellent grades, but did not want him to tell others about them lest they become envious. So the grades became a kind of guilty secret between them and a special gift just for her. His next associations were the following: "You know, something was going on with me then sexually too. I was looking up little girls' dresses and there was the sex play with the little girl next door. We were taking turns in the closet, dropping our pants and exhibiting ourselves. It was such a small house. How could my mother not know what was going on in the back bedroom?"

There are many issues raised by this vignette. What I want to emphasize is the fact that the patient spontaneously brings up the possibility that his own behavior was manipulative *after* I complied with his request. In effect he says that he might have been disguising a forbidden, oedipal wish, one that had the potential to jeopardize my "marriage" to the analytic community, as a developmental need. He also comments, however, that if he didn't ask, "he might have been overwhelmed at the last minute." It is easy to imagine that he might have panicked if he had asked and I had said no. I think it's probable that the sense that there was something dubious about the request might not have developed or jelled enough for the patient to verbalize it to himself, much less to me. So the act of acceding to the patient's request facilitates the emergence of his sense that the request might not have been necessary, whereas a refusal to accede to it, or even signs of reluctance, might have fostered a feeling in him that I was withholding help when he desperately needed it. One might say that the way the analyst responds influences the kind of experience that is created or "constructed" within the patient at that moment. One of the central implications of "constructivism" in psychoanalysis is just this: namely, that the patient's experience does not emerge in a vacuum but is, rather, partly a result of what the analyst is doing or conveying (Hoffman 1998, Chapters 5 and 6; Mitchell 1991). The interaction of the experiences of the participants is constructed in that sense, not just in the sense of interpretation that attaches meaning to those experiences "after the fact," so to speak. Before that, there is the active construction of the "fact" itself.[8]

That the patient reflects on the illicitly wishful aspects of his request and then associates to "forbidden" sexual acts in his childhood is of special interest, because the entire episode is occurring against a backdrop of struggle between myself and the patient in which I was usually the one to suggest that his symptoms had *partly* to do with unresolved conflicts about sexuality and aggression, whereas he took the position that his problems stemmed more simply from not feeling sufficiently appreciated and loved. Once he summed up two years of analytic work by saying that he thought the heart of what he was learning in analysis was that he wanted people to like him, a formulation that I thought fell a bit short of the complexity and profundity of my own interpretive contributions. Sometimes Ken would report extraordinarily evocative dreams, full of images of sex and violence in a somewhat disinterested manner, almost as though he was bored by them. Meanwhile, I'd be bursting with ideas

---

[8]No "backward causation" is implied here. The issue is the construction of experience as it is developing through the interaction, what I have called the "prospective" aspect of constructivism (see Hoffman 1998, Chapter 6).

about what they might mean. We came to understand this scene as an enactment in which the patient was like his sexually enticing but inert, semiconscious, inebriated mother while I was in a position like the one he was in as a child: left alone with my psychoanalytic "drives." So, to put it a bit schematically, I was caught in a dilemma: I could interpret actively and be experienced as a kind of rapist, or I could be more passive and compliant and be experienced as one who, through a kind of benign neglect, allowed the patient to drift along, identified with his mother, in his own semiconscious, anesthetized state.

I might add that Ken had a great deal of interest in psychoanalysis and had read a lot of Freud and of Kohut. He never could quite locate me because, although it was clear to him that I was not Kohutian, I did not seem to fit his preconceptions of what a Freudian would be like either. It pleases me that in the course of the analysis he seemed to come to an understanding of himself that involved some kind of integration of the two perspectives, an integration reflecting, not surprisingly, something more like my own viewpoint. He still thought, however, somewhat to my disappointment, that self psychology could encompass the integration we had developed. So in the end we had negotiated a compromise, although, thankfully no doubt, we still had our share of healthy differences.

EXISTENTIAL AND SYMPTOMATIC PANIC

It is not hard to understand the patient's panic as a symptom, one that can be interpreted in a variety of ways. One that I referred to earlier is that it reflects Ken's sense, fostered by a variety of traumatic events and themes in his life, that he and others might not be able to inhibit acting upon enormously destructive impulses. One might say that the patient felt that he was always in danger of losing his sense of his own humanity, that he could at any moment become a robot, a monster, or a very destructive, instinctually driven animal. Interestingly, one of the first things he said to me was that he was pleased to see that I had a book by Kohut in my bookcase because he didn't want to be perceived as "a bundle of drives." The patient was obsessed with certain horrifying images, one of which was of a woman whose normal outward appearance concealed a completely mechanical apparatus under the skin. Another image that preoccupied him was that of a certain type of reptile, or a type of toad, the slimiest and ugliest he had ever encountered. He was disgusted by these images but sometimes couldn't get them out of his mind. The force of gravity came to represent the force of his own instinctual life pulling him down, pulling him into an incestuous snare with his mother who, figuratively, was continually calling to him from her grave.

In the transference, the patient's panic got organized around a conflict between a longing to be taken over by me and fiercely competitive ambitions. A central task was to differentiate the possibility of my benign influence (through consideration of interpretations, through absorption of my regard for him, and through selective identifications) from what the patient seemed to experience unconsciously as an emasculating homosexual submission.[9] The complementary task was to differentiate expressions of his own healthy ambition and competitiveness in our relationship from murderous inclinations. Full-scale panic attacks, accompanied by a kind of vertigo, would often occur in the office when I was saying something that the patient felt was important for him to consider. Sometimes the governing unconscious paradigm seemed to be "kill or be killed" or "rape or be raped," reflected symbolically as a conflict within the patient between speaking in a controlling way and passively listening. At times, the patient's urgent need to block my speaking, to block my "shots," as it were, took the form of a full-blown panic attack. As I spoke, he'd raise his hand and say, "Stop, please." Then, shuddering, he'd turn on his side and face the back of the couch.

These were just a few of the dynamics underlying the symptom that we explored. But to think of Ken's panic only as a symptom obscures its existential, universal implications. Symptoms are often thought of as involving partial misappraisals of what is possible in the present associated with experiences that were not optimal and not necessary in the course of development. Many would say that these difficulties can be alleviated in analysis by a combination of new understanding and a corrective interpersonal experience, an experience that facilitates development and that obviates the need for the symptom as a way of dealing with psychological predicaments. Even if we no longer think of the therapeutic action of analysis as a matter of simply making the unconscious conscious, but rather of "negotiating," opening up, and promoting new ways of being in the world, we are also not likely to consider the route to health to be one that entails, ironically, a certain increment in self-deception. If it's not simply a matter of making what is unconscious conscious, we'd nevertheless be averse to thinking that it's a mat-

---

[9] The issues appear to be related to what Freud (1937) referred to as "biological bedrock," the repudiation of femininity, which in men takes the form, according to Freud, of an inability to allow themselves to be influenced by their analysts (presumably male) because such influence is equated with castration.

ter of making what is conscious unconscious! Yet I think there is a kernel of truth in that seemingly paradoxical idea.

Human consciousness brings with it the awareness that to invest in and care about ourselves and others entails, not only the risk of devastating loss, but absolute knowledge of its inevitability. Our challenge is to be fully engaged in living, even though we know we are heading right toward the edge of the cliff and that there is no way to avoid going over it.[10] Ken is right; we *are* going out that window. There is a sense in which catastrophic anxiety, utter debilitating terror, is always rational and the absence of it is always irrational.[11] That is, to invest in and enjoy life means, in some measure, avoiding thinking about death; it means drawing the blinds, it means huddling up against a protective wall, against the back of an analyst's couch. Of course, there is an irony here because the irrational becomes rational when we recognize that that avoidance is our most sensible course. We might as well build our "sandcastles" (Mitchell 1986) because the alternative leaves us alone with the vertigo of meaninglessness. With full acknowledgement of their looming presence, we nevertheless have to turn our *attention* away from our mortality and from a haunting sense of our ultimate insignificance in order to make living possible at all. The universal bad object is out there for all of us as nothing but the human condition. To combat it we band together in groups, in families, in communities, in cultures, to make and sustain our sense of worth. As part of that spectacular effort that is as natural to human beings as building nests is to birds, we imbue the mind-bodies of our children with love before they are able to think critically. We lock in their sense of worth in such a way that they can withstand the assault of reflective consciousness and yet join us in the business of socially constructing some kind of sustaining reality (Berger and Luckmann 1967; also see Nagel 1986).

This locking-in of self-worth is precisely what my patient, Ken, did not get enough of from the critical authorities, namely, his parents, in the critical period when he needed it most and was most open to it. Not only did he not get enough love and affirmation in that phase to buffer his awareness of the void that surrounds us all, but in the end, his mother,

---

[10] Jessie Taft (1933), the Rankian, writes, "To put it very simply, perhaps the human problem is no more than this: If one cannot live forever is it worth while to live at all?" (p. 13).

[11] Freud, unfortunately, never took death anxiety seriously in his theory building, an omission that has all the signs of defensive denial (Hoffman 1998, Chapter 2; Becker 1973).

as a consequence surely of her own unspeakable suffering, removed whatever porous shield her presence may have offered against the harsh reality of an indifferent universe. She, in her anguish, presented him instead with a devastating message, one that is not manifestly in her suicide note and that, if anything, makes a mockery of it. That unspoken message calls attention to the tenuousness of the prototypical bond of mother and child and therefore, simultaneously, to the tenuousness of the child's sense of selfhood. Whatever the sincerity of her intentions, the mother's overt pronouncement, "You are great," carries with it the covert message "You are nothing," a message that exposes the fact that the crucial background supports for our sense of meaning and worth are not divinely authorized. Rather, they are nothing more nor less than human constructions, grounds for living that people have the power to build and to destroy. To know that, of course, is to know immediately that our sense of meaningful selfhood is partly illusory. If, as Mitchell (1986) has written, "narcissism entails the attribution of illusory value" (p. 108), one may ask just what attribution of value is *not* illusory?[12]

In the face of the crushing reality of death, what remains is a need to turn away from it enough to affirm life, and the route to such affirmation (beyond what can be accomplished by parents with children) often entails the magic of ritual. Funeral and memorial services and other ritualized aspects of mourning are among those social practices that function most clearly as attempts to combine support for grieving with buttressing the conviction of the bereaved that it makes sense for them to go on with their lives. Freud himself, despite his rationalism, came to recognize the irrational component in the therapeutic action of psychoanalysis. In the *New Introductory Lectures* (Freud 1933), in the same passage in which he said, "where id was, there ego shall be," Freud discussed the psychological impact of "mystical practices" and commented, undoubtedly grudgingly, that "it may be admitted that the therapeutic efforts of psychoanalysis have chosen a *similar line of approach*" (p. 80; italics added).

FRAGMENTS OF TERMINATION

I shall close by reporting a few of Ken's very rich dreams in the termination phase of his analysis. About five months before the end he re-

[12]See Mitchell (1986) following Winnicott on "going out to meet and match the moment of hope" in analysis (p. 115).

ported a dream in which he was on a field where "they had let loose a whole bunch of animals from the zoo: armadillos and one animal I made up, this big scaly thing like an anteater. It had big folds of skin all over it. The skin was so scaly that I couldn't see the face. And I just found it disgusting." In the same session Ken reported a dream in which he was walking around in a downtown street, feeling aroused and wanting to masturbate. He felt he was close to an orgasm but that he first had to find a woman with whom he could make eye contact, someone who would look at him with a warm and lively expression. In these dreams we can see the tension between the patient's horror of a mindless life of the flesh and his groping for a way to integrate his own sexuality with interpersonal engagement and personal wholeness.

With regard to the patient's difficulty allowing *me* to be the one who could help him to achieve that integration, not long before, the patient dreamt that he was eating some kind of fish with maggots in it that turned into something like fruit-fly larvae. He took some into his mouth but then spit them out, feeling disgusted and like he wanted to throw up. We talked about the patient's aversion to incorporating something from me, perhaps very specifically a particular line of interpretation having to do with sexual conflict, but more broadly, whatever I, as a man, had to offer him. Then about a month before the end, the patient reported the following dream:

> I was down in the basement. Someone was trying to get in with a drill. The basement in the dream is like a fortress. There is a big door with a deadbolt and a key lock. Somebody is drilling a hole in it. And I am standing there by the door thinking I can almost see the point of the drill coming through. And I think it was you out there. And I have the idea that if I can put my finger on the point of the drill you'll know I'm in there and that I'm alive. And I'm thinking that it's dangerous. [Laughs] This gets so phallic as I speak. I don't know how big the drill is. If you stand too close to it, it could run right into your body. So the fears are there, and yet somehow it also feels like it's going to be OK.

So here is the patient identified with his mother and yet struggling to differentiate himself from her. He's in the basement where she killed herself, and there I am outside, perhaps like he was outside when he came home from school that awful day when he found the door locked. But now there is some kind of rescue operation going on. In order to be saved, to make contact, he has to touch that phallic object, he has to let himself be reached and touched by my own attempts to break through to him. To do this he has either to overcome the sense that the contact is necessarily sexual, or better, to be less threatened by whatever sexual and aggressive dimensions there may be in our encounter. Finally, he has to let me reach him, despite his having felt impotent to reach his mother. Here he has to overcome a need he feels to absolve himself by proving that such "awakenings" are simply impossible.

And apropos of my theme in this essay, the moment of contact in the dream occurs in a moment of trespass. Someone is breaking into the basement of Ken's home. An intruder is entering where, presumably, he has no place, where he does not belong. The law is being broken, the patient's private space is being violated. Surely this cannot be a precedent, a prescription for a way of living. Locks on doors are there for safety, there to create environments in which we can live with some semblance of security, even environments in which we can create illusions of security, in which we can hide from the terror of annihilation. But there are times when our "security systems" reach a point of diminishing returns and they need to be deactivated, if only temporarily. So it is with the analytic frame. It's there to protect us, to create an environment that is especially conducive to both exploration of meaning and affirmation of worth. But it has its dark, suffocating side, especially when it is taken too seriously and adhered to too zealously. Thus, the ideal holding environment becomes one in which the frame itself is fully understood to be a construction, a set of ritual activities that are enriched by their integration with the analyst's personal, spontaneous participation. Such participation sometimes takes the form of limited departures from the frame, excursions into liminal space, although more commonly it involves qualities of naturalness and spontaneity that are mingled with the ritualized, role-determined aspects of the process. Analysis then becomes a model for living, a rich dialectic between plunging into experience and reflecting on its meaning (Becker 1973, p. 199). It entails for the analyst an integration of being with the patient as a fellow human being, sharing the same kind of personal vulnerability, and being, *ironically,* the very one who is idealized and authorized by the culture and by the patient himself or herself to bestow upon the patient a sense of personal significance and worth, the kind that stands a chance of overcoming the most profound kinds of childhood injuries, even as they are joined by the inexorable insults of the human condition.

ADDENDUM

In the last hour, Ken brought me a gift, a fossil sculpture reminiscent of a time when he and his father went hunting for fossils, a memory that was recovered now for the first time and that was one of the very few fond memories he had of his father. The gift, also interpreted by the patient as symbolic of the excavations of the analysis, was accompanied by a note, one that was a far cry, needless to say, from the one the mother left upon her "termination." Ken's note read, in part, "I can't describe all that you've meant to me. You know anyway. I'm going to continue to try to let you into my life." After I said it was time to stop, we stood tentatively in that liminal space, a moment in time that was both "inside" and "outside" the analysis. As I reached out to shake Ken's hand, he said, "If you don't mind, I'd rather have a hug." We embraced and said goodbye, thereby co-constructing, hopefully, a good-enough ending for that last hour and for the analysis.

REFERENCES

Becker E: The Denial of Death. New York, Free Press, 1973

Bell C: Ritual Theory, Ritual Practice. New York, Oxford University Press, 1992

Berger P, Luckmann T: The Social Construction of Reality. Garden City, NY, Anchor Books, 1967

Ferenczi S: The Clinical Diary of Sandor Ferenczi (1932). Translated by Balint M, Jackson NZ. Edited by Dupont J. Cambridge, MA, Harvard University Press, 1988

Fourcher LA: Psychological pathology and social reciprocity. Hum Dev 18:405–429, 1975

Freud S: Lines of advance in psycho-analytic therapy (1919), in The Standard Edition of the Complete Psychological Works of Sigmund Freud [SE], Vol 17. Translated and edited by Strachey J. London, Hogarth Press, 1955, pp 159–168

Freud S: New introductory lectures on psycho-analysis (1933). SE, 22:7–182, 1964

Freud S: Analysis terminable and interminable (1937). SE, 23:216–253, 1964

Gill MM: Psychoanalysis and exploratory psychotherapy. J Am Psychoanal Assoc 2:771–797, 1954

Gill MM: Psychoanalysis and psychotherapy: a revision. Int Rev Psychoanal 11:161–179, 1984

Grotstein JS: Boundary difficulties in borderline patients, in Master Clinicians Treating the Regressed Patient, Vol 2. Edited by Boyer LB, Giovacchini PL. Northvale, NJ, Jason Aronson, 1993, pp 107–141

Guidi N: Unobjectionable negative transference. The Annual of Psychoanalysis 21:107–121. New York, International Universities Press, 1993

Hoffman IZ: Ritual and Spontaneity in the Psychoanalytic Process: A Dialectical-Constructivist View. Hillsdale, NJ, The Analytic Press, 1998

Kern JW: Transference neurosis as a waking dream: notes on a clinical enigma. J Am Psychoanal Assoc 35:337–366, 1987

Macalpine I: The development of the transference. Psychoanal Q 19:501–539, 1950

Mitchell SA: The wings of Icarus: illusion and the problem of narcissism. Contemp Psychoanal 22:107–132, 1986

Mitchell SA: Wishes, needs, and interpersonal negotiations. Psychoanalytic Inquiry 11:147–170, 1991

Modell AH: Other Times, Other Realities: Toward a Theory of Psychoanalytic Treatment. Cambridge, MA, Harvard University Press, 1990

Nagel T: The View from Nowhere. New York, Oxford University Press, 1986

Racker H: Transference and Countertransference. New York, International Universities Press, 1968

Schafer R: Retelling a Life: Narration and Dialogue in Psychoanalysis. New York, Basic Books, 1992

Slavin MO, Kriegman D: The Adaptive Design of the Human Psyche. New York, Guilford, 1992

Strachey J: The nature of the therapeutic action of psychoanalysis. Int J Psychoanal 15:127–159, 1934; republished 50:275–292, 1969

Taft J: The Dynamics of Therapy in a Controlled Relationship (1933). New York, Dover, 1962

Turner V: The Ritual Process: Structure and Anti-Structure. Chicago, IL, Aldine, 1969

Winnicott DW: Playing and Reality. New York, Tavistock, 1971

13

THEODORE J. JACOBS, M.D.

INTRODUCTION

Theodore Jacobs is a graduate of Yale University in New Haven, Connecticut, and the University of Chicago School of Medicine. He did his psychiatric residency at the Albert Einstein Medical College in New York, where he now is Clinical Professor of Psychiatry. He is a Training and Supervising Analyst at the New York Psychoanalytic Institute and the New York University Psychoanalytic Institute. He is a Child and Adolescent Supervising Analyst at the latter. He has been on numerous editorial boards, including *The Psychoanalytic Quarterly; Psychoanalytic Inquiry; The Journal of Infant, Child, and Adolescent Psychotherapy;* and *The Journal of Clinical Psychoanalysis.* He is currently on the Board of Directors of *The Psychoanalytic Quarterly.* He is a Past President of the Association for Child Analysis. Dr. Jacobs has been a visiting teacher and lecturer at many psychoanalytic institutes here and abroad and has presented a number of named lectureships, including the Sigmund Freud and A.A. Brill lectures at the New York University and New York Psychoanalytic Institutes.

Dr. Jacobs is the author of more than 50 papers and chapters on a variety of psychoanalytic and psychiatric topics and is the author of *The Use of the Self: Countertransference and Communication in the Analytic Situation* and coeditor of the volume *On Beginning an Analysis.* His work on a detailed examination of countertransference and the analysts' continuing their experience during the analytic session helped to open a new chapter in American psychoanalysis.

Jacobs has said of himself:

I've always regarded myself as someone who respects and honors the classical tradition. In fact, I deplore the fact that so much that is valuable in the in-depth exploration of the individual psyche is being lost in today's relentless focus on interaction, enactments, and the two-person psychology that is so much in vogue.

At the same time, I felt in my training that certain fixed positions of my teachers who ignored or disparaged the interactive dimension of analysis and the contribution of the analyst's subjectivity to the analytic process represented a closed-mindedness, often out of bias or for political reasons, that detracted from rather than enhanced our field. Accordingly, I began to think and write about my own countertransference experiences—in part because there were so many of them—in an effort to get on the table what was not being discussed in our training.

I found that many of my colleagues shared my feelings that a centrally important aspect of analysis was being ignored.

It so happened I began to write about these things just at a time when there was an opening up of analytic thinking with regard to matters of countertransference, interaction, intersubjectivity, and the like. It was as though a torrent of pent-up feelings about these issues was suddenly released in the mid-1970s and 1980s.

So although I was one of the first Americans to write openly about countertransference and the analyst's inner experiences, I simply was in the forefront of a wave that swept our field. I do not consider myself a pioneer in any sense of the word, but a classical analyst who began to write about an aspect of analysis that all of us knew operated in every treatment.

WHY I CHOSE THIS PAPER

Theodore J. Jacobs, M.D.

I chose "On Misreading and Misleading Patients" for inclusion in this volume because it brings together a number of issues that have interested me and also contains some of my current thinking about these questions.

For many years, I have been interested in the ways that subtle, and covert, aspects of countertransference affect the emerging material and the analytic work. I have also been interested in the way we analysts deal in sessions with such countertransference influences on the analytic process. In particular, I have been concerned about the way that in the face of mistakes we often have a need to deny our errors, consciously or unconsciously, leading the patient away from this material and thereby entering into a collusion with patients that has a damaging effect on the analytic process.

I am also interested in the impact on treatment of revealing, rather than concealing, our errors and the way that this kind of revelation affects the therapeutic alliance and the ongoing work. And, in a broader sense, I am interested in the way that unconscious communications are experienced by analyst and patient and how, technically, these can be identified and explored fruitfully as a centrally important, if sometimes overlooked, aspect of analytic work.

ON MISREADING AND MISLEADING PATIENTS

Some Reflections on Communications, Miscommunications, and Countertransference Enactments

THEODORE J. JACOBS, M.D.

IN CONTRAST TO THE earlier conceptualization of countertransference as an obstacle to analytic work (Reich 1951), contemporary views of countertransference (Ehrenberg 1997; Levine 1997; McLaughlin 1981, 1987; Renik 1993; Schwaber 1992; Smith 1999), emphasize its central role as a pathway to the unconscious of both patient and analyst.

While this perspective has been invaluable both in correcting the one-sided and limited view of countertransference that prevailed for many years and in underscoring the importance of the analyst's subjectivity as a means of understanding the patient, the current focus on this aspect of countertransference has led to some diminution in contributions that explore aspects of its other face—its problematic side.

Some contemporary authors, extending Brenner's view of countertransference as a compromise formation, maintain not only that countertransference represents the product of multiple, conflicting forces

"On Misreading and Misleading Patients: Some Reflections on Communications, Miscommunications, and Countertransference Enactments," by Theodore J. Jacobs, M.D., was first published in *The International Journal of Psychoanalysis*, 82:653–669, 2001.

operating in the mind of the analyst, but that every instance of countertransference simultaneously facilitates and interferes with the analytic work (Smith 1999).

While this is a theoretically plausible and an understandable extension of the contemporary view of countertransference as a multiply determined entity that can exert a number of effects on the analytic process, the idea that every countertransference response functions in this dual way has yet to be convincingly demonstrated.

Moreover, although this view may be theoretically correct, unless one can demonstrate how a piece of countertransference behavior both facilitates and retards the analytic work and the extent to which each effect operates in a session, such a perspective is, clinically, of limited value. In fact, by not making clear that the obstructing and facilitating effects of countertransference are rarely of equal importance and that in a given session, one of these forces may have a far greater impact on the process than the other, such a view of the clinical manifestations of countertransference can be misleading.

Clearly there are instances in which the analyst's countertransference behavior is so disruptive—even destructive—and so derails the process that whatever facilitating effect it may also have, is, to all intent and purposes, a negligible factor in what is taking place in the clinical moment. The same is true on the positive side. At times the analyst's subjectivity, including particular countertransference responses, may have the effect of advancing the treatment. In such situations the positive effect of the countertransference is the central clinical fact that requires exploration and interpretation. At that moment any other effects that the countertransference may have induced, including the possibility that it covertly increases resistance in some manner, while not unimportant, are, from a clinical vantage point, secondary to the change that has taken place in the analytic process.

To determine the actual effect of countertransference on analytic work, as opposed to theoretical considerations, it is important not to confuse theory with the realities of the clinical encounter. Pragmatically, it is also important to assess the extent to which a countertransference response has actually enhanced or has retarded the analytic process. Failure to make these distinctions and assessments has the effect of clouding, rather than clarifying, the clinical picture.

In this paper, my focus will be on the clinical situation and on one facet of countertransference, its troublesome side; on an aspect of countertransference, in fact, that is easily overlooked. I am referring to situations in which particular needs, conflicts and biases of the analyst, not infrequently rooted in narcissistic conflicts, lie embedded within, and are concealed by, his quite proper and correct interventions; interventions that are derived from well-accepted theory and long-established techniques.

To illustrate these matters, I will offer several clinical examples in which issues of this kind led me to carry out troublesome countertransference enactments. In two instances these enactments were quite unconscious, and were it not for the patients' responses to them—in one case by confronting me with my behavior, in another by developing a symptom closely related to it—in all likelihood I would not have become aware of the impact of my actions.

In the third example, my behavior was also carried out spontaneously and, initially, outside of conscious awareness. Soon thereafter, however, I realized that the intervention that I had just offered was itself an enactment which misled the patient by deflecting her attention from behavior of mine that I did not wish to confront. Despite this understanding and the opportunity it gave me to make an immediate correction of my error, for reasons that I will discuss, I did not do so.

My purpose in describing these clinical vignettes is not solely to illustrate the way in which countertransference elements may be woven into the fabric of the analyst's interventions. I will also discuss several controversial issues raised by the clinical material.

One such issue concerns the analyst's countertransference reactions and whether or not they are inevitably enacted in sessions. That is, whether, as Renik (1993) maintains, such responses can neither be identified nor contained by the analyst prior to their being expressed in action.

On the basis of my clinical material, I will discuss this question from the standpoint of two pathways that countertransference reactions can take. While these means of communicating countertransference responses are not mutually exclusive and, in practice, regularly exist in some combination, at any given time, for reasons that have largely to do with forces operating in the mind of the analyst, one pathway may become the predominant one.

One form of countertransference, enacted outside of conscious awareness, is expressed primarily through nonverbal means. The other, which can be enacted through a variety of channels, initially registers in consciousness as an affect, thought, fantasy, or memory. As I will discuss presently, it is the latter form of countertransference expression that the analyst may, through self-monitoring, be better able to contain rather than enact, while the former type, nonverbal reactions, expressed unconsciously in quite automatic fashion, conforms more closely to Renik's description of countertransference responses that can neither be identified nor controlled prior to being enacted in sessions. I will also comment on the relationship that not infrequently exists between the two types of countertransference reactions and the way in which the handling of one may affect the extent to which the other is enacted in sessions.

In connection with one of the cases that I will report, I will also touch on the thorny question of the handling of certain types of countertransference reactions; those in which, to avoid issues that cause him pain or embarrassment, including, and most especially, errors that he has made, the analyst intervenes in a way that misleads the patient by deflecting her attention away from the issue at hand. While for the most part such countertransference enactments are carried out spontaneously, only to be discovered later—if, in fact, the analyst recognizes them at all—they may also be consciously, and quite deliberately, performed. When troublesome countertransference behavior of this kind occurs, the question arises as to whether frank acknowledgment by the analyst of his actions and open discussion of the impact that his error has had on the patient advances the analytic work or, as some colleagues hold, unnecessarily burdens the patient and the treatment with the analyst's own issues. In connection with a case example, I will offer some thoughts about this difficult problem in technique.

Current thinking in psychoanalysis, supported by child observational research studies (Emde 1988; Fonagy and Target 1996; Stern 1985), has clarified the central role played by perception of the other, both in the development of self and object representations and in ongoing psychological functioning of the adult. In the analytic situation, through the work of such colleagues as Aron (1996), Ehrenberg (1997), Gill (1982), Hoffman (1983), Levine (1997), McLaughlin (1981), Natterson (1991), Poland (1992), Renik (1993), Schwaber (1992), Stolorow and Atwood (1992), and others in the United States, and Casement (1985), Feldman (1993), Joseph (1985), Sandler (1990), and Steiner (1993) in England, we have come to recognize that the patient's experience of the analyst, often registered outside of awareness, regularly influences the emerging material and the developing analytic process.

It goes without saying that as perception is strongly colored by transferences and projective identifications, the patient's view of the analyst requires thorough exploration. Our entirely correct—and indispensable—efforts to utilize this analyst-centered material (Steiner 1993) as a pathway to the unconscious of the patient, however, may, at times, cause us to overlook something else of importance: the way in which the patient's conscious responses to, and thoughts about, the analyst are defensively utilized to screen out and suppress certain accurate, but anxiety-provoking, perceptions of him and the covert countertransference elements contained in the analyst's communications.

While active questioning of the patient about her perceptions of the analyst or other active means of searching out this information—a technique favored by a number of colleagues (Aron 1996; Ehrenberg 1997, Renik 1993)—can be effective in eliciting those perceptions that are conscious, or can readily be made so, others that have registered subliminally or have undergone repression are ordinarily not accessible in this way. Often it is only through dreams, daydreams, or hints embedded in the patient's associations that such perceptions can be uncovered. To accomplish this it is necessary for the analyst to employ the kind of receptive, open-ended technique involving much quiet listening that fosters regressive movements in the minds of both participants and favors the emergence of such material.

In addition to certain correctly perceived countertransference reactions, not infrequently defended against by patients are their perceptions of particular traits, attitudes, and values of the analyst, which are inevitably transmitted in the course of analytic work. When, as often happens, such perceptions evoke anxiety or other troubling conflicts in patients, they are repressed or otherwise excluded from consciousness.

It is not the patient alone, however, who defends against the emergence of these perceptions. For reasons of his own, the analyst, too, often wishes to avoid the patient's conscious recognition of and comments about certain of his personal qualities as well as those countertransference reactions that he regards as constituting lapses of control or other embarrassing errors.

Often overlooked, too, in the process of exploring the transferences and projective identifications contained within the patient's experience of the analyst is material that may be exerting an important effect on the treatment; material transmitted by both parties that refers to unconsciously established rules and agreements about their relationship and about what may, and may not, happen in the analysis. Like the unconscious collusions that often lie concealed behind the patient's suppression of his accurate perceptions of the analyst, the failure to identify and confront these tacit agreements often represents the living out of mutually shared needs of patient and analyst; needs that, not infrequently, center for each on the avoidance of anxiety and the maintenance of emotionally important self-representations.

In what follows I will try to illustrate how such unconscious communications may, at times, operate in the clinical situation.

Some years ago I began the analysis of an intelligent and articulate but quite inhibited young woman. My work with her illustrated some of the difficulties inherent in our ideas about what constitutes confirmation of an interpretation.

Raised in a joyless atmosphere by anxious and depressed parents, Ms. C was herself a bundle of fears. Extremely cautious in everything she did, she was convinced that any venture that she undertook would end in disaster. In analysis she risked little and months would go by without her daring to express a thought about me. Her life, too, was bound and constricted by her anxious expectations. Without enthusiasm, she carried out a daily round of routine activities unleavened by the slightest pleasure.

Ms. C's resistance to change was such that the smallest movement in treatment met with powerful opposition. This fact, together with an absence of much in the way of dream or fantasy material, gave the analysis a weighty, plodding quality. After a time I found that I did not look forward to sessions with Ms. C. In fact, in the middle of an hour, I would sometimes become aware that my musculature was tense and that I was sitting with my body rotated away from her. Aware of these reactions, I would try to attend more closely to what my patient was saying, hoping to catch a whisper of the unconscious in the reports from the field that characterized her sessions.

In our sessions Ms. C would appear not only depressed, but defeated. She gave the impression that for her life was an unending burden. In presenting herself in this way, Ms. C was not only giving expression to her state of mind but was also transmitting a complex communication about our relationship and about the role in her life that she hoped I would play.

Ms. C's childhood experiences had convinced her that the only way to obtain help from her parents was to be in trouble; that is, to be sick, miserable, or otherwise incapacitated. It was the only approach that elicited even a hint of a caring response. Thus, in Ms. C's tone, manner, affect and posture, she was communicating to me a mute appeal for help and nurturance.

By presenting herself as she did, however, Ms. C was also warding me off; protecting herself against the emergence of threatening erotic feelings and ensuring that I would not find her a sexually appealing woman. Although it became clear that Ms. C very much wanted me to be attracted to her and, at times, unconsciously carried out seductive movements on the couch as an expression of that wish, the sexual stirrings that she experienced in sessions terrified her. Thus by feeling and appearing continually miserable and unhappy, Ms. C was not only making certain that she would not act on her sexual feelings, but unconsciously, was bringing on punishment both for her sexual wishes and for the envy, competitive feelings, and resentment that she also harbored toward me. A number of these elements, and my response to them, were contained in the hours that I will describe.

One day as Ms. C was speaking of her limited life and despairing of ever breaking out of her shell—a feeling that more frequently than I cared to acknowledge I found myself sharing—an unexpected image appeared in my mind. I envisioned a small oval object, grayish-brown in color and rather delicate looking, with something alive inside. At first I could not identify this object, but after a moment or two I recognized that it was a cocoon. Then it occurred to me that this image must have arisen in response to the material of the hour. Taken with this idea—and using it, as I later realized, to screen out certain anxiety-provoking feelings of my own—I recognized no other source of this fantasy.

In fact, without actually using the word *cocoon,* Ms. C had been representing herself as living within such a protective shell. With sadness and little hope that she could actually do so, she had also expressed a yearning to emerge from this self-created prison.

Utilizing the material of the hour and the fantasy I had in association to it, I offered the interpretation that Ms. C seemed to be expressing the idea that she lived in a cocoon that she was struggling to break out of. This notion of herself, I added, seemed not only to be a long-standing one that had helped shape many of her experiences in life, but was her way of expressing feelings that she was having right now with me in this session. It was also a view of herself, I said, that she seemed to want me to share.

In response, Ms. C was silent for several minutes. Then she curled into herself, pulled up her legs, and lowered her head. The thought occurred to me then that with these movements she was pantomiming being wrapped into a cocoon. While this may, in fact, have been true, I failed at that time to recognize the aversive nature of Ms. C's movements. Feeling hurt by what I had said, she was retreating into a protective shell.

Ms. C then spoke about how trapped she felt in sessions. She needed me, she said, but she felt all bound up by fear of me and of my disapproval. She wished to express herself, to tell me how she really felt in sessions, to let herself go and to break the bonds that encased her, but she was too afraid of me and her feelings about me to do so. This is the way it was in her family. Terrified of making waves and especially of incurring the wrath of her father, for years she sat on her feelings and felt totally squelched. Then Ms. C told me of her childhood interest in butterflies and how she had wished that she could be such a free and beautiful creature. In reality, however, she said, she knew that she was nothing but a dingy moth trapped in the cocoon of this treatment and the cocoon of her family. But while the cocoons of nature eventually fall away, hers had become rigidified and hardened; in essence, it was a tomb from which there was no escape.

I recall being pleased with this piece of work and with an intervention that had not only elicited a confirming response, but had put the patient in touch both with an immediate experience with me and with a long-standing, ongoing fantasy. What I did not recognize at that time was that in addition to the meaning that I had suggested, Ms. C's actions, as well as her words, expressed a defensive wish to retreat from feelings of hurt and anger that she experienced at my remark, one that she took to be a put-down of her as a woman. In retrospect, I thought that in her movements, she was also conveying a wish for me to comfort her and, by positioning her legs in the way that she did, unconsciously attempting to interest me sexually.

The scene now shifts to a session that took place a week later. Because of a family obligation that conflicted with one of her analytic hours, Ms. C had announced earlier in the week that she would have to miss that session. Later in the hour in which she made this announcement, I pointed out what I thought to be a significant omission based on aspects of Ms. C's character—her fear of asking for anything for herself and of my disapproval and rejection if she did so. I mentioned that she had not brought up the possibility of a change of appointment. She acknowledged that this was so, and after exploring her underlying feelings of guilt and unworthiness, as well as the shameful fantasies of entitlement that give rise to her fears, she summoned up her courage and asked me if I had another time available. In fact, I did, and Ms. C gratefully accepted the new appointment. Both she and I, I believe, recognized that in addition to confronting her avoidance, my intervention constituted the offer of a gift. It was, in short, an enactment on my part that had to do both with my wish to reach out to Ms. C and, unconsciously I suspect, make amends for the opposite wish; the desire to flee the situation and not have to contend with someone who, all too often, could make me—and unconsciously was seeking to make me—feel as inadequate and despairing as she herself felt.

Emboldened by my offer of a substitute appointment, which meant to her that I found her to be a person of some value, Ms. C became braver in the next session. That hour, in fact, was unlike any that had occurred before. In it Ms. C spoke with surprising openness.

"I appreciate what you did today," she began, "you did not have to change the appointment. You didn't even have to bring up the subject. I wouldn't have. You could have used the free hour for yourself, to read the paper or to sleep late. I appreciate the consideration you showed. It makes me think that maybe you like me after all. Maybe I'm not just a pill and a bore." Ms. C paused, then went on.

"There is something I've been meaning to say to you but I haven't been able to until now. It's about something that has upset me. I don't know if you realize it, but sometimes you get irritated with me. Not that I blame you. If I were you, I'd be bored out of my mind. But when you feel that way you can be critical. Then you are liable to put me down, not in a big way, but in a subtle, analytic way. Like when you said I exist in a cocoon. I was upset by that. I felt like saying, "Don't we all live in cocoons? Don't you live in a cocoon with your practice and your nice house and your professional associations? I don't notice you going out to state hospitals to deal with really troubled patients. You have your own little life—we all do. I guess you are right in one way, though. Your cocoon is of your choosing. Mine is part of my illness. It is true that as a kid I used to imagine being as lovely as a butterfly, but I know now that I never will. One day, though, I am going to break out of my cocoon, and maybe one day you'll break out of yours."

What had happened was clear. On one level, Ms. C understood and confirmed the interpretation I made; and her associations demonstrated, as I had imagined, that we had indeed shared an unconscious fantasy. But on another level, she was wounded by the interpretation, which she experienced as a subtle attack on her. For some time I was puzzled by her response. Then I thought about her words. I had been impatient with her, she said, impatient and annoyed. In my mind I reviewed the session and tried to recapture my mood of that day and what it was that I was feeling. The session, I remembered, had begun on a heavy note. Ms. C had looked morose and she was silent for quite a while. I recalled sitting quietly and patiently but also experiencing a familiar kind of weighty feeling. Ms. C had begun several recent sessions in this way and they had not been very productive. Use of my own feelings of heaviness, boredom, and growing helplessness as a guide to understanding and interpreting certain inner states that Ms. C was experiencing and, through projection, was invoking in me, while useful in helping her gain insights that she did not have before, did not result in any discernible movement in my patient. Ms. C recognized the truth of these observations, but this understanding was not accompanied by much alteration either in her mood or in the sustained silences that emanated from it.

The hour I spoke of was heading in the same direction, and although I was not consciously aware of experiencing annoyance or irritation at the time, I have no doubt that such feelings—which were never far from the surface and had been growing in recent weeks—came through in my interpretation.

On reflection, I recalled that some weeks earlier Ms. C had spoken with self-contempt of feeling like an insect or, worse, a larva waiting to hatch. Thus, on one level my use of the cocoon imagery unconsciously echoed my patient's negative view of herself. In using this imagery I was, I believe, not only unconsciously retaliating for the feelings of inadequacy that Ms. C was able to evoke in me, but playing into her defensive need to keep me at a distance and to cause me to experience her as an unattractive woman.

This is not to say that this intervention was not reasonably accurate and useful. I think that it was and Ms. C's response indicated that this was so. But equally important, I believe, is that my intervention also concealed an inner response of mine that was related to covert communications taking place in the hour. This interplay between patient and analyst involved Ms. C's silences and her largely uncommunicative behavior on the one hand and my frustration at her tenacious resistances and inability to make greater progress on the other. Ms. C heard that aspect of my message that spoke to my feelings of frustration and anger as well as the one that addressed her long-standing fantasy. Because she was afraid of her aggression, afraid of any confrontation with me, she suppressed her reaction to the critical message and gave voice only to the one that, although useful in its own right, was also less threatening. What is of interest also is that it was only after I had agreed to change her hour, an act that to Ms. C served as evidence that I cared about her, that she was able to discuss that part of her reaction to my interpretation that had gone underground. Had she not done so, I would have had no reason to question my belief that on the basis of an unconscious communication I had done nothing other than offer an interpretation that had provided a piece of insight and had advanced the analytic process.

On reviewing the transactions that had taken place between Ms. C and myself, I realized that my focus had been almost exclusively on our verbal exchanges. I had paid comparatively little attention to the array of messages that were being transmitted nonverbally as accompaniments to, commentaries on, and sometimes contradictions of the verbal material.

Now in order to better understand what had transpired, and was continuing to transpire, between Ms. C and myself, I began to pay close attention, not only to the covert meanings contained within our words, but to these nonverbal messages. Conveyed through posture, gesture, and movement, in facial expressions, in the tone, syntax, and rhythm of speech, and in the pauses and silences that punctuated the hours, these unconscious communications anticipated both subsequent conscious recognition in patient and analyst of the affects and fantasies to which they referred and the later verbalization of this material.

As I observed Ms. C and myself in interaction, I became aware of certain patterns in our movements. Often reciprocal and cueing off one another, these movements were enacted in a repetitive manner, almost like a familiar dance.

It became clear, for instance, that in connection with the mobilization of certain emotions Ms. C and I engaged in predictable behavior. Thus, in sessions if we began to feel negatively toward one another—not a rare occurrence in light of Ms. C's tenacious resistances and the feelings of frustration that they evoked in me—each of us would unconsciously and automatically carry out particular movements.

Typically, for instance, during periods of silence Ms. C would rotate her body slightly to the left, fold her arms across her chest, and turn her head toward the wall.

On my side, I became aware at such times that I would turn my body slightly to the right, away from Ms. C and in a direction opposite to her movement. I would also lean back in my chair and, for brief intervals, would close my eyes when listening.

After a period of time ranging from several minutes to a half-hour or more, not infrequently Ms. C would again reposition herself. She would draw up her legs, flex her knees, and let her arms fall to the side. At the same time, she would roll onto her back so that she was no longer facing the wall. Then she would begin to speak in a quiet, modulated voice and in a tone that seemed placating or appeasing. At these times, there was about her a muted, but definite, seductive quality.

In response, I would find myself turning back toward Ms. C. I would lean forward in my chair and when offering an intervention would speak in a tone that came close to matching hers.

In addition to my effort to communicate understanding and empathy in this way, there was in my action, I believe, a resonant response to Ms. C's seductive behavior.

Although at the time I did not appreciate the significance of these nonverbal enactments, which conveyed negative emotions, efforts at repair, and a covert sexuality between Ms. C and myself, later, upon reflection, I realized that they anticipated the conscious registration of emerging feelings in both patient and analyst. They operated, in other words, as an early signal system for affects that were approaching but had not yet reached consciousness. Many years ago, Felix Deutsch (1952) demonstrated that certain nonverbal behaviors regularly predicted and anticipated the appearance of particular themes in the patient's subsequent material.

If, as happened later in the analysis, I was able to observe these nonverbal communications in Ms. C and myself and decipher their meaning, it often became possible to gain access to the underlying affects and fantasies. Gaining conscious awareness of these responses, in turn, helped me both to better contain them and to utilize them interpretatively.

When, on the other hand, I overlooked the nonverbal interactions taking place in sessions, the related affects often grew in intensity with the result that the increased feeling of pressure from within not infrequently led to the kind of troublesome countertransference enactments that I have described.

Awareness of the kinds of covert messages that may be concealed within our so-called correct interpretations may throw some light on another familiar clinical entity—the negative therapeutic reaction. While it is well known that both unconscious guilt and the need to maintain an object tie with a masochistic parent may contribute to the development of this reaction, other factors that play a role in its formation are often overlooked. I will illustrate what I mean with this brief example.

Ms. A was an angry woman who, when she began analytic psychotherapy with me, announced that she was simultaneously taking on her third husband and third analyst. Her two previous marriages and two previous tries at analysis had all ended in failure. Weary and battle-scarred, her husbands and analysts had all thrown in the towel.

Ms. A's anger began in childhood and for understandable reasons. Her mother died suddenly when she was 4 and, unable to care for her, her father had sent her to live with an aunt. This woman had little interest in, or tolerance for, children and she openly resented the burden that had been placed on her. Feeling deeply rejected by this aunt and unwanted in her home, the child thought repeatedly of running away. This she never did, however, because, among other reasons, there was no other place for her to go.

In our work together, Ms. A was difficult and provocative. Endlessly critical of me, she also repeatedly threatened to break off treatment. For the most part I was able to maintain my composure in the face of these attacks, but there were times when her behavior got under my skin.

One day when my patient was particularly angry, had accused me of being antagonistic to her, and once again threatened to leave treatment, I offered a transference interpretation that attempted to link past and present. Because I did not provide what she felt she needed, I said, Ms. A was experiencing me as the mean-spirited aunt of her youth whom she deeply resented; it seemed to me, I added, that to pay me back she was trying to induce in me the very same feelings of frustration and anger that she had experienced at her aunt's hands. Then I went on. Just as she threatened to leave her aunt but never did because she was the only mother Ms. A had, she repeatedly threatened to leave me but had not done so because of her conviction that there was no one else she could rely on; that I was the only therapist in the city who could work with her.

Ms. A's reaction lingers in memory. She broke down, cried bitterly, and remained depressed for several days thereafter. It took neither of us long to understand what had happened. Ms. A had responded, not to my transference interpretation, which on one level was correct enough, but to the true meaning of my message. Tired of the battle, and with my patience[1] worn thin, I had unconsciously sent Ms. A a familiar message; the same message, in fact, sent by her husbands, her previous analysts, and her aunt and father before them. I had invited her to leave.

As in the case of Ms. C, nonverbal communication played out in posture, gesture, and movement in this treatment offered early clues to nascent affects in both patient and therapist, affects that, on my side, were eventually enacted in this unhelpful way. Whenever, for instance, Ms. A launched one of her typically veiled attacks on me, her words would be accompanied by particular actions. As she spoke, Ms. A would move toward the edge of her chair, her upper body would be thrust out and angled forward, and her head, with chin leading, would follow suit. The posture was one of belligerence, but curiously mixed with a kind of provocativeness that at times I experienced as covertly sexual.

I, on the other hand, would sit leaning back in my chair; leaning as far back, in fact, as I possibly could in what clearly was an involuntary retreat from Ms. A's poorly concealed aggression and provocative behavior.

After she had given vent to her feelings, in this way Ms. A would straighten up, slide backwards in her seat, and appearing drained, would remain quiet for several minutes.

In response, I would move forward, my body no longer angled backwards, and I would resume my usual listening posture. These seesaw movements, backwards and forward, advance and retreat, commu-

---

[1]At this point in an earlier version of this paper I committed the parapraxis of writing the word *patient* instead of *patience,* a clear illustration of how enduring countertransference feelings, stimulated by memories, can infiltrate and affect the operations of the ego even years after treatment was ended.

nicating anger, a breach between Ms. A and myself, and efforts to heal that breach, punctuated the sessions and were reliable markers for what at any given time was transpiring between my patient and myself.

Had I been able at the time to understand the importance of such movements, it would have been possible, I believe, for me, early on, to identify and explore the underlying feelings of irritation and rising anger experienced by both patient and therapist before they spilled over into the kind of verbal enactment that was the cause of much trouble in this treatment.

If, in fact, such nonverbal elements can be identified and explored as they appear, it is often possible for the analyst, through introspection and attunement to what is rising from within, to monitor, better contain, and early on make interpretive use of some of his countertransference responses rather than unconsciously enacting them and attempting, after the fact, to grasp the meaning and significance of such enactments. Increasing the scope of his awareness, then, to include the movement patterns of patient and analyst as they engage in the analytic hour is, I believe, a valuable tool in the analyst's ongoing efforts to turn his subjective reactions into useful insights rather than automatic actions.

This example and others like it raise a question about our patients' negative reactions to interpretations that seem correct. How often, one wonders, do such reactions represent accurate readings of the analyst's unconscious meaning?

I would like now to describe another clinical example, one in which my need to protect my self-esteem at a particular moment in an analysis led to a skewing of the analytic dialogue, to the development of a tacit agreement not to broach a potentially painful and embarrassing issue, and to make use of an analytic intervention as a decoy aimed at shifting the focus of the patient's attention. As I have mentioned, this kind of enactment, which involves a collusion with the patient, serves protective functions for both participants in analysis and may exert a profound, and even decisive, influence on the course of outcome of the analytic work.

Some years ago, in the early days of the women's movement, when most male analysts wore their chauvinism like a comfortable old cardigan, a militant young feminist came to see me. She did so quite warily and reluctantly, accepting the recommendation of a teacher who had been in treatment with me only when a valued friendship ended because of her poorly controlled aggressive behavior. That she did so for target practice, however, soon became evident, for from the moment Ms. N stepped foot in my office she unleashed a blistering attack on Freud and his testosterone-heavy theories, on analysis as male propaganda, and on me as one of its sexist practitioners. Finally, leaning forward in her chair and looking for all the world like a bull about to charge, she hurled a challenge at me.

"I'm into consciousness-raising," she announced. "What are you into?" Taken aback, I did not know what to say. For several seconds I stared at her blankly. Then a response popped into mind.

"Unconsciousness-raising," I replied.

That exchange pretty much summed up the situation between Ms. N and myself. From the outset a major disagreement divided us. For Ms. N, the pain and suffering that she experienced and the unhappiness in her life for which she sought relief stemmed from a single source—society's discriminating attitude toward women. I, on the other hand, was interested in promoting the idea that in addition to this harsh reality the inner world of fantasies and beliefs that Ms. N developed as a consequence of her unique psychological experiences played a role in her troubles.

It was a standoff, and as the result of this non–meeting of the minds for some months progress in the analysis could be measured by the thimble-full. In time, however, things began to change. Largely, I think, because we came to understand one another, Ms. N and I finally reached an accommodation. I learned to listen to and appreciate her realities, external as well as psychological, and to convey that appreciation to her, and she, grudgingly, allowed that the particular way in which she put things together in her mind might have influenced her thinking about herself and others.

We still had our troubles, though, and one problem centered around the feeling of boredom that I sometimes experienced during Ms. N's sessions. Although her capacity for self-reflection gradually improved, Ms. N was given to much externalization. It was not rare for her to focus on the shortcomings of others and to complain at length about the way that she was treated by friends and family. Leaving no detail to the imagination, she would cite every fault, foible, and blemish of the miscreants who had used her badly. A particular target of hers was her father, who sounded to be a vain, bigoted, and devious man who fancied himself a scholar and a gentleman and who sought, through lies and rationalizations, to induce others to believe in this deluded self-image.

While the material relating to Ms. N's father and other family members was assuredly important, after a while it became so familiar, the same complaints and stories so often repeated, that I found myself experiencing fatigue in sessions. Recognizing that strong emotions must be lurking behind this reaction of mine, I undertook what self-reflection I could and came into touch with the feelings of anger and annoyance that Ms. N's clearly defensive behavior was evoking in me. While useful in providing some insight into what was transpiring beneath the analytic surface, this approach had little effect on my responses to Ms. N.

I felt a clear sense of relief, then, when, in the second year of treatment some new and rather dramatic material made its appearance in Ms. N's sessions. This material had to do with the strong possibility that my patient, as a young child, had been sexually fondled by a male teenage cousin who occasionally babysat for her. Although, generally speaking, I am wary of the idea that such experiences are the key to neuroses, I was interested in exploring the sequelae of this episode. I thought that the fantasies it had evoked and the transformations in memory it had undergone over the years might help account for Ms. N's persistent and irrational anxiety over physical contact with men, a symptom for which I did not, at that point, have an entirely satisfactory explanation.

Keenly interested in this newly emerging material and eager to hear more about it, I was frustrated and disappointed when, soon after making a transient appearance in Ms. N's associations, it disappeared from view. It was as if the repressive forces that had originally overtaken it had, once again, driven it underground; and although I worked as actively as I could with the defenses that I thought were keeping the relevant affects and memories out of conscious awareness, they remained under cover.

Instead of speaking of the material that was new and possibly of great significance in her development, Ms. N returned to the old complaints, wrapping herself in them as though they were a suit of used clothing.

Once again I found it difficult to keep attuned to her; once again I experienced tedium. During one early morning hour following a night in which I had had little sleep, I was particularly restless. As often happens when I am tired, I moved about more than usual in my chair. I twisted, I fidgeted, I shifted positions, all no doubt in an effort to stay alert. Finally, as Ms. N was droning on about one of her tight-fisted relatives, I found myself reaching for the notebook that I keep at my side to record an occasional dream, an intriguing sequence of associations, or other material that I may wish to review. There was nothing in what Ms. N was saying, however, that I really wished to record. Nonetheless, I had reached for the book and fingered its binding. Then I opened it to the section reserved for Ms. N and glanced at an old note that I had written. All this I did as a distraction. I was bored and tired and I wanted some stimulation, some relief from the feelings of dullness and vague uneasiness that I was experiencing. In the process of thumbing through the notebook and glancing at the previous note, I had tuned my patient out and had missed a few sentences of what she was saying. I had managed to blank them out.

Although my movements were carried out quietly, they were not so quiet that Ms. N did not hear them. At first she said nothing and simply carried on with her dissection of the penny-pinching relative. There was something different in her voice, however. She was speaking in a routinized way, like an actor reciting his lines while thinking of an unpaid rent bill.

Then, suddenly, Ms. N was silent. For several minutes she did not speak.

"Something's happened," I said. "Something seems to be blocking you."

"I didn't think that you were interested in what I was saying," Ms. N replied. "I thought that you were distracted. I heard noises."

"And what did you make of what you heard?"

"I don't know. There were odd sounds, like you were stroking something or fingering something. Then it sounded as though you were opening a book and turning pages."

As Ms. N spoke, I recalled something that she had told me some time before; that as he read her a goodnight story her cousin's fingers would begin to play over the pages of the book. Then, slowly, he would reach out, touch her thigh, and move his hand toward her genital area.

"I thought that you had no interest in what I was saying," Ms. N went on, "that I was totally boring and that you had picked up a book and were leafing through it. Either that or you were just playing with it to amuse yourself."

"'Stroking it,' you said before."

"Yes, that, too. I heard rubbing noises. Maybe that's the way shrinks get off in sessions when they are bored. They rub their books instead of their dicks. That's their perversion." After a moment of silence, I spoke.

"Such sounds are familiar to you," I said.

Then Ms. N fell silent again. When she resumed speaking her voice contained a note of resignation.

"Okay. I get it. You think I thought that you were like my cousin, George; ready to make a move, ready to reach for my crotch. I wasn't aware of that, but maybe I did. Actually I wouldn't put it past any shrink. Most of them end up screwing their patients one way or another. You guys are a pious lot, but sneaky. Patients get abused in therapy all the time."

Ms. N went on to speak at some length of her distrust of analysts, especially males, and of her suspicion that I might turn out to be as devious as most men who, one way or another, use women. Then toward the end of the session she spoke once more of the night-time scene with her cousin, repeating what she had told me and recalling for the first time that she had a crush on him and felt very excited in his presence. Then she added that there was probably something to the fact that she had come to believe that all men, basically, were like George; charming, exciting, but not to be trusted. Rising from the couch she added a final note.

"It's true," she said, "that lying down scares me. I don't see you and I don't know what you are about. When you start moving around I get jittery. I don't know what might happen next. In that sense I've probably gotten you and George all mixed up in my mind. But what bugs me, what really makes me crazy, is when I begin to think that you are like my father. Not only that I imagine that you are like him, but that you really are like him."

After that session, Ms. N's distrust of me increased. Her resistances hardened and silences dominated the sessions. When she did speak, what she said was mostly reportage; dispatches consisting largely of descriptions of other people and accounts of events at work. She had gone into hiding and the reason for this was clear. In some part of her Ms. N knew that I had deceived her with a piece of psychoanalytic sleight of hand. Out of boredom, anger, and a wish to escape from those feelings, I had turned away from Ms. N and tuned her out. I had not been doing my job, the job she was paying me to do and for which I had signed on. Seeking distraction from inner tensions, I had been caught out. Ms. N sensed what was happening. Rather than acknowledging the truth of her perceptions, however, and thereby experiencing the feelings of shame and guilt that would accompany such an acknowledgment, I had led Ms. N down another path. For reasons of her own that had much to do with her fear of a threatening confrontation, she went along with me.

It so happens that the path on which I set her needed to be explored and both of us knew it, and that exploration had its own value, for significant memories concerning a traumatic and influential childhood experience were, in fact, triggered by my behavior in making covert noises. Moreover, although I had not recognized it at the time, my behavior was part of a pattern of interaction taking place between Ms. N and myself.

Through the quality of her verbalizations, repetitious, reality-oriented, focused on details, Ms. N was not only employing powerful resistances against the emergence of threatening affects, particularly sexual feelings towards her analyst, but with concealed aggression, was causing me to experience the kind of frustration and disappointment that characterized her experiences with her father, with George, her cousin, and with other important men in her life. With some concealed anger of my own, I had responded to her behavior by turning away from her and shutting her out. Only later did I realize that my anger had much to do with Ms. N's teasing behavior and that a sexually tinged and sadomasochistic interaction had been taking place between us.

In addition, outside of conscious awareness, both of us, I believe, were enacting a scenario that had to do with the George episode. Ms. N had set the stage by bringing up sexual material, holding it out, as it were, in front of me, and then withdrawing it. Then, in an unconscious effort to evoke the now submerged material, I, in essence, became George; that is, a male sitting behind Ms. N, holding a book and, like a reader, slowly turning pages. In this way—perhaps both in response to a fantasy of Ms. N's that was communicated to me and out of some anger and frustration of my own—I was recreating a threatening scene from my patient's childhood. All of this—and more—needed to be, and eventually was, interpreted and usefully explored. But as important as these factors were, it is also true that both patient and analyst made use of them to avoid confronting what, for each, was a more anxiety-provoking issue.

By moving rapidly to the past we entered into a collusion in which the apparent analytic investigation of an important childhood experience was used in the service of mutual avoidance. Utilizing a particular kind of body English, I had turned Ms. N away from the truth. In doing so I had, in fact, become what she feared most that I would be, an untrustworthy person. Ms. N's remark at the end of the hour summed up the situation succinctly. As a consequence of the deception that I had initiated I had become not only the father in the transference but a man who, in actuality, had behaved like Ms. N's father. Until I could return to this incident, replay it with my patient, and help her understand what had truly happened, she would not be able to trust me.

It was necessary to look again at what had occurred, and through an appropriate intervention, let Ms. N know that her perceptions had been correct.

When in a subsequent session, I detected a reference to the incident in question in Ms. N's associations, I drew her attention to her ongoing concern with it and sought to continue exploration of her thoughts about what had happened. This approach yielded little, however, nor did interpretations of anxiety about speaking frankly about the episode.

Recognizing the untenable position in which Ms. N had been put—she had, in reality, been gaslighted (Calef and Weinshel 1981)—and realizing that meaningful work in analysis could not take place under these circumstances, I felt it important to address the issue more directly. I therefore asked Ms. N if she had any awareness of the fact that her perceptions had been accurate and that she had correctly identified the sounds she heard as my thumbing through a notebook. I also said that I had become distracted, that my attention had wandered, and that, embarrassed by my behavior, I focused Ms. N's attention on the childhood experience with George rather than deal with the effects of my own actions. Ms. N replied that she had sensed what had happened but had quickly dismissed that thought from her mind when I moved away from the present situation and alluded to the George episode. The whole experience, she said, was too frightening. She felt I was evading something but could not confront me with my evasion. She was too afraid of the consequences—too afraid that I would become furious and send her away.

By offering this intervention, I not only raised the question of how Ms. N had dealt with her original perception, but I confirmed that it had been accurate. I am well aware that not all analysts would have dealt with the matter in this way. Many colleagues would have been content to work exclusively with the patient's defenses, fantasies, and projections and to leave the reality of what occurred ambiguous.

In fact, not a few analysts contend that to acknowledge a mistake to a patient rather than simply exploring the patient's perception of what occurred in an hour is a serious error. Maintaining that such self-disclosures are often motivated by feelings of guilt, by a need to confess, by the hope of obtaining forgiveness from the patient, or by a wish to undo the error made, these colleagues hold that disclosures of this kind essentially serve the analyst's needs and unnecessarily burden the patient with the analyst's issues.

There is much truth to this argument and to the corollary idea that it is the analyst's responsibility, to the extent possible, to monitor his countertransference responses and to utilize them in the service of understanding. It is true, too, that the danger of using the patient to serve the analyst's needs, always present, is increased in situations in which the analyst experiences distress over an error that he has made and, unconsciously, may seek relief by revealing his mistake to the patient. There is also the possibility that the analyst's actions in disclosing his mistake may have the effect of limiting or foreclosing the patient's exploration of her perceptions of what occurred in the hour.

While these considerations are clearly important and must be taken into account whenever the analyst is faced with the question of disclosing a mistake that he has made, there are times, I believe, when not to disclose an error that has been perceived by the patient and that has had an adverse effect on the treatment is itself a mistake and creates a serious—and sometimes insuperable—problem in the treatment; one that, in fact, places a heavy burden on the patient.

Such behavior on the part of the analyst compounds the error already made and puts the patient in an impossible, and often destructive, bind. Realizing that the analyst does not want her to know the truth, she has to suppress or deny what, in fact, some part of her knows to be true. She is being asked, in other words, to enter into a collusion with the analyst and, along with him, to be the bearer of a secret that can have a deforming effect on the analytic process. Moreover, the patient may, and often does, experience the analyst as being unwilling, or unable, to face up to his own errors, seeking instead, to conceal that fact behind the protective cover of proper and quite correct analytic technique. Such a situation, I believe, cannot foster growth. It can only lead to deception, collusions, and increased distrust, both of the analyst and of the patient's own perceptions.

Once the air was cleared and Ms. N and I had dealt with what had actually happened between us, we could do what we should have been doing all along—exploring more fully the transactions and covert communications taking place between us that had led, on the one hand, to my experiencing boredom and fatigue during Ms. N's hours and, on the other, to her need to present herself in a way that contributed to the evocation of such reactions.

Later on we had a chance to explore other relevant issues; Ms. N's reaction to my evasion, her own need to evade the truth and not confront me with her perceptions, and the response she had to my finally acknowledging what had happened. Each of these reactions was important as they contained views of me, initially as weak and vulnerable, then as more hardy and able to face harsh realities, that were meaningfully connected with long-standing self and object representations. Of particular importance in this regard was Ms. N's shifting perception of her father, a talented and effective, but thoroughly devious, businessman with whom she was unconsciously identified.

On Ms. N's part, then, this enactment constituted a reemployment of an important mode of defense; the unconscious denial of an accurate perception whose conscious recognition would have led to the mobilization of rage and to consequent inner turmoil based on the fear that to reveal her feelings would result in the loss of a person that she both loved and needed. It was this conflict, involving me at the moment, but related in the past both to her father and to her beloved cousin, George, that Ms. N handled through a familiar enactment, one whose interpretation proved to be a very significant experience in her analysis. Its effectiveness came, I believe, from the immediacy of the experience with me and from Ms. N's recognition of how, out of fear, she had denied what she knew to be true.

What I have wished to illustrate in this example, then, is the way that, as analysts, we often manage to sidestep issues that cause us pain, embarrassment, or anxiety. Not infrequently concealed within our well-accepted analytic techniques and timely interventions are subtle expressions of envy, rivalry, and aggression toward our patients. Hidden, too, in our interpretations, and often well rationalized, may be our needs to maintain our position of authority and superiority. Even more troublesome at times are the unrecognized sexual feelings that may be stimulated in sessions as well as feelings of love and dependency that we commonly experience in the course of our work. We are somewhat better, in fact, at recognizing and confronting negative feelings than positive ones. The vast majority of papers on countertransference deal with conflicts over aggression. Very few touch on the vicissitudes of loving and sexuality in an analytic treatment.

Other potential sources of tension and anxiety in the analyst, too, may be avoided. Often overlooked and not confronted as important influences on our work are our attitudes toward money and its importance to us; the effect on us of growing older; the impact of our personal losses and disappointments on our approach to patients; and the role that our status in our institutes and in the profession plays in affecting our sense of ourselves and the way we function in the clinical situation.

It is our petty faults, too, that we have trouble acknowledging and integrating into our clinical work; our moments of meanness, of spiteful retaliation, of boastfulness, of greed, of inattention, of self-justification, and of small-minded competitiveness with colleagues. Often we shut out recognition of these traits in ourselves and effectively manage not to be aware of them. When we are unable to do that, we may find ways of ignoring them, setting them aside, and avoiding the hard task of confronting the impact that they have on our patients. Instead we may find ourselves focusing on the patient's material. As that pathway is so readily available, so integral a part of analytic work, we may not be aware of how we can pick up themes and trends in what patients say that are relevant to their conflicts, interpret them accurately and with insight, and to all appearances do a useful piece of analysis. What we are doing in those situations, however, is not only useful (which on its own terms, it clearly is); we are also utilizing what might be called an analytic screen; that is, using our skills and insights, in part, to avoid an uncomfortable truth—that our personal shortcomings, whether they take the form of a lapse of attention, an unnecessarily critical comment, a failure to recognize the truth of a patient's perception, or a momentary need to upstage him, exert a powerful influence on all that occurs at any given time in the treatment situation.

In short, it is our natural and normal self-esteem needs operating as ever-present forces in analysis as they do in life that may, at times, constitute a significant source of difficulty for the analyst. While contending with such personal responses is an inevitable, even necessary, part of doing analytic work, our ongoing efforts to understand and explore not only our conflicts but also issues of self-esteem as they may be subtly conveyed both in our interventions and in our omissions can be a valuable source of fresh insights. Unrecognized or not confronted, however, such problems may lead to the kinds of unconscious collusions and avoidances that I have attempted to describe in this paper.

On my side, my enactment clearly served defensive purposes. It spared my self-esteem, for I was deeply ashamed of my behavior, and helped stave off the intense self-criticism that was on the verge of being released. Thus, it served as a rationalized effort to avoid a narcissistic injury, a maneuver not unknown to analysts as well as their patients.

But there was also a less conscious determinant of my behavior, a factor that I became aware of only later, when, at home, I reflected on what had happened. As an adolescent, I had experienced seductive behavior on the part of a female relative who, in her own way, had acted in a manner not unlike Ms. N's. After some time in this situation, I found myself responding in kind. When this girl would try to engage me, I would ignore her—pretending to listen, but, in fact, tuning her out.

It was this old response, among others, that was activated, I believe, in my work with Ms. N and that I enacted in the session I have mentioned. Clearly, I was more frustrated with, and annoyed by, her behavior than I knew, a reaction that, in part, was linked to a piece of my own history. As I have mentioned, Ms. N had unconsciously been teasing me by dangling intriguing sexual material in front of me and then withdrawing it. It turned out that she had often acted in this way with boyfriends and with her father, a pattern of behavior that represented an identification both with his teasing behavior and that of her cousin, George. Interpretation of this aspect of her behavior opened up channels of memory and Ms. N recalled a number of incidents in which she attempted to turn the tables on others, teasing and mocking playmates and siblings as she had been teased and mocked by men whom she loved.

In summary, what I have tried to present in this paper are some thoughts about the way in which the two people in the analytic situation, often acting in concert, may selectively screen out certain realities having to do with aspects of the analyst's person, his attitudes and his behavior. Unrecognized and unacknowledged, these subtly and often unconsciously expressed qualities are not infrequently embedded within our quite proper and correct theories and techniques. It is there that we must look for and uncover them, for left to do their work they can undermine our best efforts. Fostering the kinds of errors and collusions that I have described in this communication, they can have a profound effect on the course and outcome of the analytic work.

REFERENCES

Aron L: A Meeting of Minds: Mutuality in Psychoanalysis. Hillsdale, NJ/London, Analytic Press, 1996

Calef V, Weinshel E: Some clinical consequences of introjection: gaslighting. Psychoanal Q 50:44–65, 1981

Casement P: Learning From the Patient. New York/London, Guilford, 1985

Deutsch F: Analytic posturology. Psychoanal Q 20:196–214, 1952

Ehrenberg D: The Intimate Edge: Extending the Reach of Psychoanalytic Interaction. New York/London, Norton, 1997

Emde R: Development terminable and interminable, II: recent psychoanalytic theory and therapeutic consideration. Int J Psychoanal 69:283–296, 1988

Feldman M: The dynamics of reassurance. Int J Psychoanal 74:275–285, 1993

Fonagy P, Target M: Playing with reality I: theory of mind and the normal development of psychic reality. Int J Psychoanal 77:217–233, 1996

Gill MM: Analysis of Transference. Psychological Issues. Monograph 53. New York, International Universities Press, 1982

Hoffman I: The patient as interpreter of the analyst's experience. Contemp Psychoanal 19:388–422, 1983

Joseph B: Transference: the total situation. Int J Psychoanal 66:447–454, 1985

Levine H: The capacity for countertransference. Psychoanalytic Inquiry 17:44–68, 1997

McLaughlin J: Transference, psychic reality and countertransference. Psychoanal Q 50:639–664, 1981

McLaughlin J: The play of transference: some reflections. J Am Psychoanal Assoc 39:595–611, 1987

Natterson J: Beyond Countertransference. Northvale, NJ, Jason Aronson, 1991

Ogden TH: The concept of interpretive action. Psychoanal Q 63:219–245, 1994

Poland W: Transference: an original creation. Psychoanal Q 61:185–205, 1992

Reich A: On countertransference. Int J Psychoanal 32:25–31, 1951

Renik O: Analytic interaction: conceptualizing technique in light of the analyst's irreducible subjectivity. Psychoanal Q 62:553–571, 1993

Sandler J: On internal object relations. J Am Psychoanal Assoc 38:859–880, 1985

Schwaber E: Countertransference: the analyst's retreat from the patient's vantage point. Int J Psychoanal 73:349–361, 1992

Smith H: Countertransference, conflictual listening and the analytic object relationship. J Am Psychoanal Assoc 48:95–126, 1999

Steiner J: Problems of psychoanalytic technique: patient-centred and analyst-centred interpretations, in Psychic Retreats: Pathological Organizations in Psychotic, Neurotic and Borderline Patients. London, Routledge, 1993

Stern DN: The Interpersonal World of the Infant. New York, Basic Books, 1985

Stolorow R, Atwood G: Contexts of Being: The Intersubjective Foundation of Psychological Life. Hillsdale, NJ, Analytic Press, 1992

14

JUDY L. KANTROWITZ, PH.D.

INTRODUCTION

Judy Kantrowitz is a graduate of Sarah Lawrence College and received her Ph.D. from Boston University in Clinical Psychology. She then did analytic training, first as a research candidate and then as a full clinical candidate, at the Boston Psychoanalytic Society and Institute. She was Associate Clinical Professor of Psychiatry at Tufts Medical School and is currently Associate Clinical Professor of Psychology in the Department of Psychiatry at Harvard Medical School and at the Beth Israel Hospital. She is a Training and Supervising Analyst of the Boston Psychoanalytic Institute.

Throughout her career, Dr. Kantrowitz has had a major research commitment, working with the Sander 25-Year Follow-Up Study of Children, the Research Advisory Board of the International Psychoanalytical Association (IPA), and the Task Force on Outcome and Efficacy of the American Psychoanalytic Association. She has seamlessly combined clinical work, teaching, and research in a prospective longitudinal study of the outcome of psychoanalysis and later on the outcome of psychoanalytic training, and she is currently involved in a study of the problems of confidentiality in psychoanalytic scientific communication and the ramifications on the analytic process when patients read about themselves. She is a member of the Research Advisory Board of the IPA and has been a member of the Editorial Board of *The Journal of the American Psychoanalytic Association* and a reader for *The International Journal of Psychoanalysis* and *The Analytic Quarterly*. Her work on the patient-analyst match has had a major influence on psychoanalytic thought.

Dr. Kantrowitz is a dedicated teacher of medical students, psychoanalytic candidates, and psychology students. She is the author of more than 60 papers and reviews and many honorary lectures, including the Charles Fisher Memorial Lecture of the New York Psychoanalytic Institute, the Franz Alexander Lectureship of the Southern California Psychoanalytic Institute and Cedars-Sinai Residency Program, and the Felix and Helene Deutsch Scientific Paper Award of the Boston Psychoanalytic Society and Institute.

Dr. Kantrowitz has written two books: *The Patient's Impact on the Analyst* and *Writing About Patients: Responsibilities, Risks, and Ramifications.*

She has said of herself:

> When I was an analytic candidate in the late 1960s and early 1970s, most of my teachers presented a view of psychoanalysis where the analyst was a "blank screen" and countertransference was something to be understood and worked out in training analyses and would then no longer be active in work with patients. I could not accept either of these ideas; they defied common sense. So when I needed to do a research project in order to see analytic patients (back in those days psychologists could only analyze patients if they could justify it as necessary to inform an academic area), I proposed a project to study the relationship between patient suitability and analytic outcome. I took the characteristics that we had been taught would make "good" analytic patients and assessed them through both interviews and projective tests prior to analysis and then reinterviewed and retested these patients one year after termination of analysis to evaluate how these patients had changed. I also interviewed their analysts after the termination to learn their view about the treatments. In the subtext of these interviews, many personal characteristics, attitudes, and conflicts were revealed.
>
> My finding that no patient characteristics alone or in combination accounted for the outcome now has been replicated in many studies. What I then went on to explore was the effect of overlapping or clashing characteristics and conflicts between patient and analyst. When analysts remained "blind" to similarities or failed to understand patients because they were too different (e.g., when similar conflicts were dealt with by different defenses or similar defenses protected them from different conflicts) analytic work often stalled. In addition, I found that analysts' characteristics that could be facilitating at one point in analysis might be impeding at another. In other words, not only were analysts not blank screens or interchangeable, who they were crucially contributed to what was analyzed and with what depth it was pursued. My work, therefore, contributed to changes in views about the importance of the personal characteristics of the analyst, the value of self-analysis, and the use of countertransference understanding to benefit both patient and analyst. My work was published beginning in the mid-1980s at a time when other classically trained psychoanalysts were becoming open to similar conceptualizations. My ideas about the match between

patient and analyst affecting the course and outcome of analysis are similar to those of relational theorists, but my emphasis is to return what is discovered interpersonally to its intrapsychic origins so that what becomes known can be owned and boundaries between what is self and other can be more clearly appreciated. What the analyst learns about him- or herself will certainly benefit the patient but does not become a focus for the dyad.

WHY I CHOSE THIS PAPER

Judy L. Kantrowitz, Ph.D.

I chose "The External Observer and the Lens of the Patient-Analyst Match" for inclusion in this volume because I believe it integrates ideas that I have been developing over 25 years. Following a completion of the longitudinal outcome project, I studied psychoanalytic treatments, in both formal research studies and my own clinical work, and found data that confirmed what I had seen as common sense; that is, of course, that the characteristics of the analyst affected analytic work. By the mid-1980s, many analysts were expressing similar views; two people, not one, determined the course and outcome of psychoanalysis. Of course, that was one reason why we had been unable to predict the outcome of analysis by assessing only the patient. The match between the conflicts and characteristics of the patient and the analyst influenced the course and outcome of psychoanalysis. Countertransference did not dissolve with personal analysis and was a phenomenon to learn from, not to be avoided. Today all this is commonplace.

Over the next decade and a half, the concept of the match continued to be of great clinical use to me. It is a perspective I use when I supervise, and it is the first place I look to elucidate my own countertransference when I confront impasses in doing analytic work. Often, I find a familiar aspect of myself that I have overlooked that has an unfortunate overlap with an issue of my analysand. But if the stalemate is not overcome, I talk with a colleague to help me find what I cannot see. Almost always what I learn relates to an area of interdigitation between my patient and myself. Once analysts are experienced enough, it is this kind of countertransference that I find most often interferes with their work. In the paper that follows, I have tried to illustrate how the concept of the patient-analyst match can be used both to overcome impasses and to deepen analytic work.

THE EXTERNAL OBSERVER AND THE LENS OF THE PATIENT-ANALYST MATCH

JUDY L. KANTROWITZ, PH.D.

IN THE COURSE OF analyzing patients, certain phenomena catch analysts' attention and make them wonder what they are not seeing and why this is occurring. The most notable of these occasions are when analysts become aware of intense countertransference reactions, when they find themselves repeatedly caught in enactments, and when analyses become stalemated. Sometimes analysts have not understood an aspect of the patient's difficulties, but for experienced, skilled analysts most often the problem resides in the transference-countertransference (Chused 1991; Davies 1994; Ehrenberg 1992; Hoffman 1983, 1994; Jacobs 1991; Kantrowitz 1992, 1993, 1995, 1996; McLaughlin 1981, 1991; Pizer 1992; Poland 1988; Renik 1993; Sandler 1976; Schwaber 1983, 1992; Spillius 1994). At these times, analysts often, formally or informally, seek the view of a colleague to illuminate the situation.

Overlapping conflicts between patients and analysts that emerge in the transference-countertransference are interferences that analysts most often recognize. The effects of characterological overlaps are apt to be subtler and their disruption to the work less easily detectable. Therefore, they may stay unrecognized unless something external forces them into conscious attention. When analyses are seemingly going smoothly, analysts are not as likely to discuss them or seek the view of colleagues. After formal training ends, there is no built-in expectation that analyses will be discussed. Analyses then may remain totally private communications between patient and analyst, subject to the

---

"The External Observer and the Lens of the Patient-Analyst Match," by Judy L. Kantrowitz, Ph.D., was first published in *The International Journal of Psychoanalysis,* 83:339–350, 2002.

strengths and limitations of the particular pair. Unless analysts find a format to discuss their cases, such as a peer supervision group, a mutual supervision with a colleague on a regular basis, or an ongoing consultative relationship, there are likely to be areas of blind spots in some aspect of their analytic work. These blind spots may or may not impose a significant impediment to analytic progress, but in some more nuanced way they are likely to influence the process.

This paper focuses on the important effect of reporting clinical experience to a colleague or a group of colleagues. The reporting of this material, which in all other respects remains totally confidential, is undertaken to obtain an outsider's perspective. The outside view is sought so that the analyst can acquire awareness and insight into what otherwise would likely remain removed from consciousness. The concept of the match between patient and analyst may provide a particularly useful lens in this process. I will define my understanding of match as a perspective for insight about the effect of the patient-analyst dyad on the analytic process. I will offer three illustrations of its beneficial value in the context of a third party's perspective on the analytic pair.

Considering the effect of match between patient and analyst provides one way of conceptualizing the impact of their interaction on the analytic process. I am not trying to define a "good" or "bad" match but rather to clarify how considerations of the nature of the match can illuminate aspects of analytic work. Focus on the match call attention to specific aspects of character, defense, or conflict elaborated in the transference-countertransference interaction. Match highlights the similarities and differences between the participants. Similarities may lead to understanding but also to blind spots and defensive collusion. Differences may lead to curiosity and exploration but also failures in empathy and engagement; either may facilitate or impede the process. The effect of the match may change during the course of treatment. Factors that initially benefit engagement in analytic work may later impede it.

While my definition of match includes all the multifaceted ways that patient and analyst overlap in conflict, character, and experiences, it is in the area broadly called character that the concept of match may prove most useful. Attitudes, values, beliefs, cognitive style, and strategies of adaptation and defense are components of character that are likely to influence the course and depth of the work. A focus on similarities and dissimilarities alerts the colleague, supervisor or consultant to manifestly non-conflictual, or at least non-anxiety charged, areas of overlap or disjunction between patient and analyst that may affect analytic work.

When the countertransference reaction has its roots in the analyst's character and conflicts, then whether or not the match is impeding will depend on how much the analyst's character is modifiable. However, unless they are aware of the obstacle, analysts cannot begin to modify habitual characteristics or dynamic conflicts that interfere with analytic work. Sometimes patients point out these interfering factors to their analysts. And sometimes analysts listen, pay attention, and change (Hoffman 1983). But analysts cannot rely on their patients' providing this feedback. Even when invited, not all patients will do so. In addition, the areas I am considering are ones that analysts are less likely to inquire about since they remain outside of their view. Therefore, an invitation for feedback from a party external to the analytic dyad affords an opportunity for a fresh analytic perspective. Making analysts aware of "blind spots" can make them a focus of analytic scrutiny that may then decrease countertransference intensity or enactments and reopen the process if a treatment is stalemated. It may also lead the analyst to more extended self-scrutiny, greater self-awareness, and potentially to psychological growth.

Thinking about the patient-analyst transference-countertransference, and especially characterological issues, in terms of the match between analyst and patient provides the colleague, supervisor or consultant with a particular lens for focus on the interactions. The external observer can view how their conflicts, their characteristics, their styles and the meaning of them, mesh or clash. Match offers an overarching perspective that can be used to evaluate the effect of the distance between patient and analyst in terms of their similarities and differences. Since depending on the phase of the analysis, matches of similarity and dissimilarity are sometimes beneficial and at other times obstacles within the same dyad, considering the effect of the match permits an assessment of whether it is useful or detrimental for the analytic process at any given time. Awareness of the consequences of overlap or divergence affords the analyst the opportunity to make a correction in attitude or stance.

An analyst's awareness that a "blind spot" results from the effect of overlapping characteristics creates a Janus-faced problem. Too vigilant a focus on the uniqueness of the patient's experience may result in the analyst's distancing from an affective resonance. The same analyst might spontaneously provide such emotional attunement for a patient whose history was less similar. For example, an analyst whose parent was overstimulating may resist an empathic identification with a patient who experiences him as an overstimulating parent in the transference. Resistance both to being identified as the hurtfully over stimulating parent, and to reexperiencing the pain of being overstimulated in identification with the patient, create a countertransference reaction. The analyst may then affectively distance himself in a way that the patient experiences as a rejection. This pain goes beyond the inevitable pain of frustrated yearnings since it is based on a perception, albeit preconscious, of what Racker (1968) has called the analyst's countertransference predisposition. In other words, the analyst was predisposed to react in this manner to this situation with any patient.

The other danger is too great an immersion in an affective resonance; it may prevent an awareness, and then exploration, of important dissimilarities. Taking the same example, an analyst, rather than resisting identification with a patient who has been overstimulated as he was, may empathically join with this state. Then, for example, he may erroneously assume the intensity of experience was similar. This assumption may result in his failing to understand or explore a traumatic state. The patient's more blatant or subtler experience may be obscured. In these instances, the transference-countertransference blind spots that develop may limit or even prevent important areas of analytic work.

The effect of overlapping characterological factors can best be illustrated when an analyst's work with several patients is considered. For example, a now graduate analyst was described by three of her four supervisors as talented. They specifically emphasized her working like a more experienced analyst in her awareness and monitoring of her countertransference. The fourth supervisor, who had supervised the third case, also praised her work. However, this supervisor noted one area of countertransference interference which considerably impeded the analyst's work with this patient.

While overall the analyst had a well-conceptualized understanding of the patient's difficulties and in many ways a tactful and sensitive approach in her interpretations, she tended to side with and reinforce the patient's self-critical approach, which was severe. The patient had been helped therapeutically in many areas and grown in self-understanding. The analysis, however, seemed slower and more labored than with her other patients. The analyst was open and welcomed most supervisory observations and suggestions, which were usually smoothly incorporated and increased her analytic skill. However, this was not the case in regard to comments about her approach to her patient's self-criticism. The analyst did not become defensive; she listened; she seemed ready to "accept" criticism and become self-observing, but for a long time she also seemed unable to significantly modify her approach with this patient.

The supervisor and this analyst had an open, respectful relationship. They talked about the difficulty the analyst was encountering. The supervisee acknowledged that self-criticism had been an area of considerable work in her own analysis. While she was much less self-critical than previously, she could easily believe that she was joining her patient's self-critical stance; she knew she still tended to be this way in relation to herself. The analyst seemed always to be on the side of the critic whether against herself or the patient. She treated the patient as she treated herself because she identified with her. The problem was that it was so seamless that she most often didn't see that it was occurring until after the fact, when it was pointed out. The supervisee continued the supervision on this case after graduating. She was consciously aware she needed help in lessening her own harshness with herself as well as monitoring its impact on her work.

In the discussion of the committee prior to her graduation, the other supervisors were very surprised about the analyst having this difficulty. They each then reflected that the cases they supervised were patients who did not suffer from excessive self-criticism. Under these circumstances, the analyst's residual conflict and characterological defense were not stimulated in the analytic work. While it seems a significant area to remain so clearly activated in her work, all who knew and worked with her believed her to be a very competent analyst and capable of further growth in this area. However, the implications are that unless or until she works out this issue, there are certain patients with whom she will be mismatched.

The second example comes from a series of supervisory consultations, during which an analyst became aware of the different impact of her assertive style on two patients who had patently dissimilar characterological adaptations to their conflicts around aggression. In the course of this work, the analyst increased her understanding of her own characterological conflicts and modified her style in a manner that facilitated the work.

The first patient came from a relatively stable family where all the members were successful in their ambitions. She was alone and felt adrift. She sought treatment for her long-standing depression.

The analyst began this case with high hopes. Her patient was bright, in pain, and seemingly motivated to understand herself. A history of small but painful early disappointments emerged. For example, she had not been chosen for a part in a school play; a friend preferred another's company to hers. Later boys who liked her were never the ones she liked. Her current life seemed similar. What she wanted she did not get. What she had seemed unsatisfactory. The analyst empathized with her disappointments and they gradually traced her hurts back to her sister's birth when she was four and how hard she had taken losing her role as the youngest and only girl. They found and elaborated their understanding of slights the patient felt from the analyst. But nothing seemed to move or change in the patient's life or her mood.

The second patient came from a family where there had been little emotional support. The father drank heavily, was erratic in his employment, and was occasionally abusive to the patient's siblings. The mother was seen as depressed and ineffectual. Having worked from an early age to contribute to the family income, the patient had dropped out of college several times due to financial pressures. She had boyfriends but did not speak of any special relationship. She too sought treatment for her long-standing depression.

The analyst began this second case with great trepidations because of the patient's chronic deprivation and unstable family history. This patient also recounted many stories of hurt and disappointment, but her focus quickly shifted to her attempts at mastering situations. The analyst interpreted her move away from dysphoric affects. The patient could acknowledge moving away from painful feelings. The work continued with deepening exploration of her feelings of anger, hurt, fear, and longings to be taken care of. Her backing away from these painful feelings by throwing herself into outside activity was continually addressed. The underlying conflict was explored. Her dysphoric experiences became more fully and intensely expressed in the analysis. Over time, the patient began to describe more enjoyment in her life. She got a better job, thought about returning to school, and began seeing a man who interested her.

It seemed to me from her presentations that this was a competent, well-trained analyst. She was attuned to her patients. What she said conveyed a clear understanding of her patients' states, affects, and defenses. She understood the first patient's retreat from narcissistic vulnerabilities and the second patient's retreat from painful affect. With each patient she was also able to shift and focus on issues as they surfaced. The first patient did seem more difficult to treat. But was it only the patient's entrenched stance that created the problem?

As I listened to the analyst describe her patients, I was struck by her style. She was forthright, direct, pulled no punches in how she conveyed her thoughts, but was still tactful. She could be described as feisty. Clearly, she enjoyed being assertive and feeling the power of mastering with her mind. Her style had a similarity to her second patient's who also met troubles head on. If her problem was that she hadn't been staying with her painful feelings, this patient was now going to try to do this. In contrast, her first patient tended to retreat from assertion. Her aggression was turned on herself; she maintained a muted kind of victim stance. With this kind of patient the challenge was to analyze rather than accept the invitation for sadomasochistic interactions. The analyst did not seem to get caught in enactments, but the work did not deepen as it had in the second case. She did not seem as fully affectively engaged in the process with the first patient. In a subtle way, she maintained a greater distance. Her work lacked the zest she conveyed with the second patient.

The assertive style of the analyst seemed to fit too well the first patient's underlying fantasies that she was someone who could and would be pushed around, which she unconsciously extrapolated to not being treated well or respectfully. The analyst's manner allowed her to be seen as one more person who would bruise the patient. Perhaps the patient identified the analyst with her competent and disappointing mother whom she in turn wanted to disappoint. By failing to use the interpretations actively, she could disappoint her analyst. The fact that they analyzed these occurrences meant less to the patient than the "feel" that they were continually happening in tone. Once I shared this observation with the analyst, she became aware of it herself.

After several consultations focusing on this aspect of her style of intervention and its impact on the patient, she felt something ease between them. When she returned for a consultation several months later, she described an hour in which the patient saw herself as less helpless. The analyst then began to more actively question her contribution to incidents in which the patient felt injured. She began to see more clearly the countertransference that she enacted.

The analyst stated that work with this patient made her aware of how little tolerance she would have for being in a passive, victimized position that her patient described and put the analyst into. It had led her to wonder whether unconsciously she been impatient with her analysand for being willing to remain in this role and thus frustrating the analyst. She wondered if she had become even a little more assertive than usual, as if to say, "Don't ever think I will join you in that passive position." Now, more conscious of her style through the consultations, she thought her approach may have softened somewhat.

The analyst's comfort and even pleasure in her assertive style may be in part a defensive use of her aggression, a possible reaction formation to her own masochistic tendencies. If this speculation is correct, there still was no evidence that this difficulty interfered with her effective professional work or enjoyment of life. The conflictual aspect of her aggression seemed bound in her character in a way that became manifest in my contact with her only when stimulated by this particular kind of interaction. The countertransference aspects, once recognized, were worked with by the analyst. Her self-reflection enabled her to respond to the patient in a manner that was sufficiently different that the patient also was able to make some shift in her stance. The patient-analyst match with the first case illustrates an initially problematic overlap which was eased by the analyst's becoming aware of the difficulty and being able to alter her stance somewhat.

The analyst's comfortable assertive style seemed to facilitate the second patient's work. She used her technical skill to direct the focus of the treatment, but her particular manner also resonated with and supported the patient's own assertive push for mastery. Listening to her report the hours, I could hear them enjoy the "toughness" in getting to work. Yet this was not a toughness that took them away from facing dysphoric affects; rather it was employed to help confront and withstand it. Perhaps at a later point in the treatment, the patient's and analyst's similarity in style will prove an impediment to reaching softer affects, but at this stage of the treatment it seemed an aid in deepening the treatment and freeing the patient in her life.

An example of a match that was beneficial for the major part of an analysis but became problematic in the latter phase of treatment was brought for consultation to a group of which I was a member. This was a small conference in a city distant from the place where this analysis was occurring.

The patient was herself a gifted clinician. She was sensitive and articulate. Both her personal and professional life seemed rich and engaged. She never had any treatment until well into her thirties. When she sought analysis it was manifestly to enhance her skill as a therapist. However, the patient was aware that she did not feel the confidence in herself that her functioning would seem to deserve. Shortly after beginning analysis, she recovered a memory of a traumatic occurrence. The trauma was not of the magnitude of a sexual abuse, but it involved feeling unprotected and betrayed in a way too painful to allow into her consciousness until the analysis. Both her fear and her fury had been repressed and she had developed a reasonableness in her approach to life. In analysis, she freely moved among the past, her present life, and the transference. She experienced and expressed affection and desire and annoyance and anger both toward people in her life and toward her analyst. She made good use of dreams and actively explored the real world. She loved her husband, enjoyed and struggled with her children, had good friends and seemed gifted in her work. She seemed not only an ideal analytic patient but remarkably adapted in her life.

However, like Stein's (1981) patients who hide the fullness of their passions behind an unobjectionable positive transference, this patient was "too reasonable." The analyst addressed this issue steadily after the early years of analysis. From this focus emerged a realization of how thoroughly the patient's precocity hid her anxieties. She had described panic reactions as an adolescent, but there had been no hint of this in her adult years. While she could be angry with her analyst, this did not precipitate great anxiety. The only hint of real distress was shown in how quickly her competitive, rivalrous feelings that stimulated aggressive impulses toward the analyst were dispelled as they were balanced by homosexual desires and attendant anxieties. It was hard to know which conflict was central as each was employed as a defense against the other. The alternating focus kept her from going too deeply into either conflict. The analyst interpreted all these shifts and explored and helped her to expand her affective experiences.

After the analyst presented this material, one of the conference members believed that the patient was suffering from "annihilation anxiety." He thought the patient was very fortunate to have an analyst who had stayed so closely attuned to her state. While he agreed the patient was psychologically well organized he perceived there was an underlying terror.

Two years later, the analyst again presented this case to this conference group. In the year following the first presentation, the patient began to have terrifying dreams; memories of childhood nightmares were revived. Panics around separations were then remembered with the accompanying affect. However, separations from the analyst, while always some source of distress, actually seemed less, rather than more, troubling. Throughout this period, the analyst retained the same stance of reflecting, interpreting, and generally staying closely in resonance with the patient's state as the patient's conflicts became more fully apparent and affective experience intensified.

On this occasion, her colleagues were much less sanguine about the analyst's stance. While there was an understanding that the analyst was being sensitive to the patient's vulnerabilities, most of the group now believed that she was too closely joining the patient's state. There was not enough "asymmetry" in her stance. This position deprived the patient of the transference experience of aloneness which was essential to analyze her anxiety and panic in relation to separation.

The analyst's first reaction was to be surprised, having thought the work was slowly but progressively deepening. However, she quickly grasped the point her colleagues were making. She recognized her characterological tendency to assume a stance of "joining" rather than standing at a greater distance from the patient's state. While she had been aware that she was employing this stance with the patient, the fact that this joining might be preventing rather than facilitating analytic work, had not occurred to her. She saw this as a striking "blind spot" on her part.

Later the analyst reported what had then occurred. On returning from the conference, she was able to subtly shift her stance. Rather than beginning her interpretations of the transference with statements such as " It sounds as if you feel" or "think that I feel" she stated, "You *imagine* that I feel that...." The analyst described the patient immediately registering the difference and experiencing a painful and frightening sense of aloneness. With the analyst present but less emotionally holding her hand, the patient relived her sense of having been abandoned to overwhelming intense anxiety; she recovered memories and feelings of childhood terror. In her fury with the analyst for affectively leaving her alone to face this state, she revived her childhood fury as well as fear. Fantasies that she would be the only person left on earth as well as panic that she would disappear were then linked with her fury and destructive impulses. Her fury then was understood to be at the heart of her terror. Her destructive fantasies became the basis for her unconscious construction of why she had been abandoned. As she worked her way through these painful and frightening feelings and fantasies, she also understood that "joining" and being in resonance with others, something which made her very good at her work with patients, had served a protective, defensive function. It had kept her from the experience of being alone and facing the anxiety embedded in this lifelong conflict. Her joining had been a way to reassure herself that she was a person others would want to be with, a caring, empathic person, not a competitive, destructive one. Following this analytic work, her freedom of feeling was greatly increased and the analytic work moved into the termination phase.

From the description, it is apparent that the analyst and patient had similar therapeutic and personal styles. They both tended to join the affective experiences of others, especially their patients. One could speculate that the analyst identified with the patient. Their similarity in style as well as their choice of profession may have increased this affinity. For the patient, a central conflict lay hidden behind this characterological adaptation. The deeper layers of meaning of this style for the analyst were not presented. However, in reporting back the changes that occurred in the work following her shift in her stance, she indicated that her increased awareness of their similarity led to insights that had personal reverberations.

In this example, a similarity of style and its defensive function facilitated the analytic process during the earlier part of the treatment by creating a feeling of affective resonance and an atmosphere of safety; later this similarity impeded analytic work. Recognition of the blind spot enabled the analyst to see the masking effect their overlap created and to shift her stance. The analyst's conscious focus on understanding this area of similarity expanded not only the patient's analytic work but also the analyst's self-understanding and experience of conflict and affect. Attention to the blind spot then resulted in the psychological change for both participants.

Taking an aerial view, as if in a consultation, analysts may use the lens of the match with their patient to explore how similarities and differences between them may be affectively charged in ways that the analyst was not aware of. Analysts may use the idea of patient-analyst match as a device for furthering their self-analytic work. But there are limits in this focused pursuit, as there are in all self-analytic enquiries. The analyst's view of this dyad with the patient will necessarily be restricted by the analyst's own blind spots and other countertransference phenomena.

As analysts we no longer believe in the perfectly analyzed analyst (Abend 1986). No analysis is ever complete, though some are more far-reaching than others. There is always more to learn about both personal strength and limitations. Patients help analysts expand their self-knowledge (Kantrowitz 1996). But patients are part of the dyad and subject to the same potential blind spots in the interactions. The introduction of an outside point of view can more reliably broaden understanding and bring insight. If it becomes a focus of attention, a match between patient and analyst that an analyst has been unaware of as an impediment to the work may thus become an opportunity for growth in both participants.

In the past, experienced and skilled analysts were thought to seek consultations only when they believed there was an interference in their analytic work. Contrary to this public perception, many analysts have always maintained some form of ongoing dialogues about their work with other analysts (Kantrowitz 1998). These discussions take place in many different formats. Some analysts have peer groups that have met for many years. Other analysts engage in a mutual supervision which, over time, may have many similarities to mutual analysis in the focus on each other's blind spots. Many other analysts prefer to maintain a more formal consultation relationship; this may be a planned, ongoing arrangement or a more infrequently initiated contact.

The introduction of an external observer provides an objectivity not possible from within the dyad. For this feedback to be meaningful it must, like an effective interpretation in analysis, resonate affectively as well as cognitively with the analyst. No matter how many colleagues concur on a view, unless the analyst is receptive to the perspective offered, it will not be assimilated. Ideally, the analyst will not be too defended to take in this information. Under these conditions, the new view will serve to increase the analyst's self-awareness which, in turn, will lead to deeper analytic work.

The views of external observers, of course, are also influenced by their own subjectivities. Their characteristics and conflicts will interface with the analyst's, just as the analyst's does with the patient's. Therefore, the mesh or clash of character and conflict for the analyst-consultant dyad is potentially liable to the same conditions of blind spots as the patient-analyst pair. In addition, who the analyst selects as a peer supervisor, peer group, or consultant will be influenced by the analyst's own proclivity for comfort or challenge in relation to her way of working (Kantrowitz 2002). Experienced analysts know the views and approaches of their colleagues. To a large extent, they are choosing how much similarity or difference in theory, technique, and personal style they wish to encounter when they make their selection. In other words, even with conscious motivation to be vigilant about self-deception, the possibilities for its continued occurrence remain great.

It is easy to be lulled into thinking that continued discussion of analytic cases with one person or group will protect against blind spots. While reporting one's work in this manner certainly increases the likelihood of expanded self-awareness, it is not a guarantee. Analysts who present in such forums need to feel both safe enough and motivated enough to expose their work, their countertransference feelings, thoughts, and fantasies. They also need to stay alert to the effect of the feedback on the analytic pair and on themselves personally. Too little or too strong a reaction that does not lead to self-reflection, insight and some shift in ideas, attitudes, or stance might suggest the need for a different external observer. New eyes and ears may discover something still hidden.

Neither patients' nor analysts' comfort or discomfort with their engagement is a reliable indicator of analytic benefit. A longitudinal study of analytic outcome showed the match of patient and analyst to be the single factor which illuminated the areas of analytic impasse (Kantrowitz et al.1989, 1990). Sometimes neither party was aware of the blind spot. Both believed the analyses to be very successful, but comparisons of pre- and post-psychological tests showed a major area to be unchanged. For example, their mutual valuation of creativity led to an analyst's interpreting a patient's fantasy of "pouring molten lead" on people as "free expression of fantasy"—and failing to recognize or analyze the aggression.

The efficacy of the match can change during the course of analysis. Therefore, feedback offered at one point of analysis may be very different from that offered at another phase. The same study illustrated how an analyst's calm, accepting attitude helped a very anxious, skittish patient gradually feel safe enough to begin to explore her feelings and fantasies but later permitted her to avoid actively grappling with her sexual conflicts. These findings make clear that analysts need to keep discussing their case with others over time in order to remain aware of the effect of the dyad.

In addition to helping the practicing analyst become aware of blind spots, a focus on the patient-analyst match is a useful tool in teaching. Listening to candidates present their cases, it is often possible to discern how similarities and differences in the dyad may be enhancing or limiting of the analytic process. Currently, young analysts are open to recognizing the inevitability of their personal influence on analytic work. They do not seem so burdened by ideas of personal perfection nor do they seem to expect that their own analyses will remove all traces of personal conflict. As a result, they appear to be less narcissistically vulnerable in discussing their countertransference reactions and are more comfortable with observing newly seen aspects of themselves than candidates have in earlier eras (Kantrowitz 2003). These newly discovered aspects are usually manifested in their attitude, style or stance toward the patient, as it is reflected in their presentations in seminars and supervision.

Often candidates' professional and personal curiosity about the dyad and themselves increases as the overlap in the analytic pair becomes clear. Once an awareness of an underlying conflict emerges, the transference-countertransference is revealed and can be understood by them. The perspective aids them in appreciation of the effect of unconscious factors and of how conflict can be embedded and hidden in character, For example, one candidate was aware he was uncharacteristically reluctant to change the time of a patient's hour and took a seemingly "tough" stance in relation to all the issues of the analytic frame. In contrast, during the actual analytic hours, he often seemed to work with an affective resonance in relation to the patient that bordered on a merger. In the course of presenting this material, he came to recognize that while his conflicts and their intensity were far less than his patient's, he and the patient shared a yearning for intense closeness that they both defended against with a "tough guy" stance. This awareness seemed to allow him to be both less "tough" in relation to the frame and to maintain more distance during the actual analytic hours.

Still another use of the perspective of the match is in the evaluation of candidates' learning needs. As the first example in the paper illustrates, reviewing a candidate's work with more than one patient may make it apparent that a personal difficulty interferes with some cases but not others. This discovery can be brought to the candidate's attention by supervisors. Then, together, candidate and supervisors can be alert for the manifestation of this problem in clinical work. With greater awareness, the candidate may then be able to integrate this insight in a manner that allows some shift in the analytic process.

In summary, different people bring out different aspects in each other in life, in analysis, in consultation/supervision, and in teaching. Analysts need to keep in mind that ego-syntonic ways of organizing experience may conceal aspects of their interactions with their patients that impede analytic progress. Some peers and consultants may provide a new perspective while others whose outlooks are too similar may not. The same is true of supervisors and teachers. On the other hand, third-party views that are too different may not be able to be integrated and, therefore, are not of use. To little or too much similarity or difference affect both the course of analysis and of learning. However, when an external observer can use the lens of the match to stimulate an analyst's curiosity about overlapping areas between patient and analyst that have led to enmeshment or clashes, then previously overlooked aspects of the analyst may become available for self-analytic scrutiny. The concept of the match points out meaningful overlaps and disjunctions that can be used to increase awareness of similarities and differences and how they may affect analytic work in different ways at different phases of treatment. This awareness can help us better assist ourselves, our patients, our students, and our colleagues when we serve as their consultants in relation to analytic work.

REFERENCES

Abend SM: Countertransference, empathy, and the analytic ideal: the impact of life stress on the analytic capability. Psychoanal Q 60:563–575, 1986

Chused JF: The evocative power of enactments. J Am Psychoanal Assoc 39:615–640, 1991

Davies JM: Love in the afternoon: a relational reconsideration of desire and dread in the countertransference. Psychoanalytic Dialogues 4:153–170, 1994

Ehrenberg D: The Intimate Edge. New York, WW Norton, 1992

Hoffman IZ: The patient as interpreter of the analyst's experience. Contemp Psychoanal 19:389–422, 1983

Hoffman IZ: Dialectical thinking and therapeutic action in the psychoanalytic process. Psychoanal Q 63:187–218, 1994

Jacobs T: The Use of the Self: Countertransference and Communication in the Analytic Situation. Madison, CT, International Universities Press, 1991

Kantrowitz JL: The analyst's style and its impact on the psychoanalytic process: overcoming a patient-analyst stalemate. J Am Psychoanal Assoc 40:169–194, 1992

Kantrowitz JL: The uniqueness of the patient–analyst pair: elucidating the role of the analyst. Int J Psychoanal 74:893–904, 1993

Kantrowitz JL: The beneficial aspects of the patient-analyst match: factors in addition to clinical acumen and therapeutic skill that contribute to psychological change. Int J Psychoanal 76:229–313, 1995

Kantrowitz JL: The Patient's Impact on the Analyst. Hillsdale, NJ, Analytic Press, 1996

Kantrowitz JL: A different view of the therapeutic process: the impact of the patient on the analyst. J Am Psychoanal Assoc 45:127–153, 1997

Kantrowitz JL: Pathways to self-knowledge: self-analysis, mutual supervision, and other shared communications. Int J Psychoanal 80:111–132, 1998

Kantrowitz JL: The triadic match: candidate, patient, and supervisor. J Am Psychoanal Assoc 50:919–968, 2002

Kantrowitz JL: Tell me your theory. Where is it bred? A lesson from clinical approaches to dreams. J Clin Psychoanal 12:151–178, 2003

Kantrowitz JL, Katz AL, Greenman D, Morris H, Paolitto F, Sashin J, Solomon L: The patient-analyst match and the outcome of psychoanalysis: the study of 13 cases. Research in progress. J Am Psychoanal Assoc 37:893–920, 1989

Kantrowitz JL, Katz AL, Paolitto F: Follow-up of psychoanalysis five-to-ten years after termination, III: the relationship of the transference neurosis to the patient-analyst match. J Am Psychoanal Assoc 38:655–678, 1990

McLaughlin JT: Transference, psychic reality and countertransference. Psychoanal Q 50:637–664, 1981

McLaughlin JT: Clinical and theoretical aspects of enactments. J Am Psychoanal Assoc 39:595–661, 1991

Pizer S: The negotiation of paradox in the analytic process. Psychoanalytic Dialogues 2:215–240, 1992

Poland WS: Insight and the analytic dyad. Psychoanal Q 57:341–369, 1988

Racker H: Transference and Countertransference. New York, International Universities Press, 1968

Renik O: Analytic interaction: conceptualizing technique in light of the analyst's irreducible subjectivity. Psychoanal Q 62:523–553, 1993

Sandler J: Countertransference and role-responsiveness. Int Rev Psychoanal 3:43–48, 1976

Schwaber E: Perspective on analytic listening and psychic reality. Int Rev Psychoanal 10:379–392, 1983

Schwaber E: Countertransference: the analyst's retreat from the patient's vantage point. Int J Psychoanal 73:349–362, 1992

Spillius E: On formulating clinical fact to the patient. Int J Psychoanal 75:1121–1132, 1994

Stein M: The unobjectionable part of the transference. J Am Psychoanal Assoc 29:869–920, 1981

15

OTTO F. KERNBERG, M.D.

INTRODUCTION

Otto Kernberg was born in Vienna, Austria, received his B.S. and M.D. from the University of Chile, and graduated from the Chilean Psychoanalytic Institute. In the course of an extraordinary career, he has at various times been Professor of Psychopathology in the School of Social Work in Santiago, Chile; Rockefeller Foundation Fellow at Johns Hopkins University; Director of the Menninger Memorial Hospital in Topeka, Kansas; Professor of Clinical Psychiatry at the Columbia University College of Physicians and Surgeons; Professor of Psychiatry at Weill Cornell Medical College; Director of the Personality Disorders Institute; and Training and Supervising Psychoanalyst at the Columbia Center for Psychoanalytic Training and Research. He is a Past President of the International Psychoanalytical Association.

A few of his many honors include The Heinz Hartmann Scholar designation of the New York Psychoanalytic Institute, the Freud Anniversary Lecture of the Psychoanalytic Association of New York, the Austrian Cross of Honor for Science and Art, an Honorary Doctorship at the University of Buenos Aires, the Distinguished Service Award of the American Psychiatric Association, the Mary S. Sigourney Award for Distinguished Contributions to Psychoanalysis, Sigmund Freud Lecturer at the University of Vienna, and numerous visiting professorships throughout the world. He is the author of 20 books, some with coauthors, and over 200 single-authored papers and another 200 coauthored papers. He has been in the forefront of the advance of objection relations theory and the scholarly exposition of Klein, Bion, and Rosenfeld for American analysts. His broad view of psychoanalytic theory and technique has led to his clinical, theoretical, and experimental advances in understanding narcissistic and borderline pathology and small and large group processes.

He has said of himself:

> I am convinced that the mainstream psychoanalytic approach, powerfully represented in American psychoanalysis, is a fundamental contribution to the contemporary understanding of psychopathology, the nature of psychic structures, and, potentially, the ways in which psychological dynamics and neurobiological dynamics eventually will have to approach each other. From the viewpoint of treatment, a strong emphasis in American psychoanalysis on its application to a broad spectrum of psychoanalytic psychotherapy techniques will assure, I believe, the practical relevance of psychoanalytic science and profession. I also very much identify with the position of academic psychoanalysis in the United States that aspires to collaboration and integration with psychology and psychiatry, and to assure the place of psychoanalysis as a fundamental behavioral science.
>
> My personal commitment to these ideals and objectives is reflected in my combining the work in psychoanalytic and psychotherapeutic techniques with my dedication to empirical research in the psychopathology and psychoanalytic psychotherapy of personality disorders. I demonstrate these commitments in teaching activities for a broad range of mental health professionals, as Training and Supervising Analyst at the Columbia Psychoanalytic Center for Training and Research, Professor of Psychiatry at Cornell, and involvement with international clinical, educational, and research institutions.
>
> I am firmly convinced that the major efforts of both the American Psychoanalytic Association and the International Psychoanalytical Association have to be directed toward expanding psychoanalytic research along a broad spectrum of approaches centered in empirical research, and a radical innovation of psychoanalytic education. Psychoanalytic Institutes must open up the training of psychoanalytic candidates in the direction of research interests and methodology, establish interdisciplinary and interinstitutional research networks, and bring into psychoanalytic institutes the excitement of exploration of the boundaries of psychoanalysis with the neurobiological and social sciences. At the same time, I am planning to continue to explore the organizational problems of psychoanalytic institutions, particularly the excessively traditionalist aspects of psychoanalytic education that have left major educational problems unresolved over many years. I see my personal role regarding all of these tasks and objectives more in conceptual contributions and publications rather than in an active political role: I believe, in that regard, that I have carried out my duties over the past 30 years.

WHY I CHOSE THIS PAPER

Otto F. Kernberg, M.D.

I selected my paper "Recent Developments in the Technical Approaches of English-Language Psychoanalytic Schools" because it presents an updated summary of the three major currents of psychoanalytic technique, namely, the "mainstream" school represented by the gradual integration of the ego psychology, Kleinian, and Independent British approaches; the relationists school, represented by the combination of the interpersonal, intersubjective, and self psychological approaches; and the French school, represented by the non-Lacanian French approaches. The French approach, although only thinly represented in English-language contributions, has been a major influence and of growing importance in Latin America as well as in the Latin-language psychoanalytic societies of Europe and the French Psychoanalytic Society in Canada.

Studying the internal developments within each of these schools, it becomes apparent that significant rapprochements are occurring between technical currents that have common basic principles, while divergences emerge clearly in the different basic principles of these three major psychoanalytic approaches. My paper attempts to spell out these basic technical principles that have evolved in these respective schools, and their contrasting nature.

By presenting the historical development of these convergences and divergences, I also illustrate the gradually evolving nature of psychoanalytic technique in the light of accumulated clinical experience. Although empirical research within these various approaches and comparing them is still badly missing, the clinical experience of consecutive psychoanalytic generations constitutes an empirical field that tends to modify these approaches over time, often in the face of a rather dogmatic resistance that attempts to hold on to one specific viewpoint. In short, this paper attempts to show where we are today, and to outline the actual controversies and development that are signaling in what direction we are going.

RECENT DEVELOPMENTS IN THE TECHNICAL APPROACHES OF ENGLISH-LANGUAGE PSYCHOANALYTIC SCHOOLS

OTTO F. KERNBERG, M.D.

THE CONTROVERSIAL DISCUSSIONS IN the British Psychoanalytic Society between 1941 and 1945 (King and Steiner 1991), ending with a "gentlemen's agreement" among Melanie Klein, Anna Freud, and Sylvia Payne, constitute, in my view, the starting point of contemporary developments in technique within the English-speaking psychoanalytic communities—particularly the North American and British ones. Those controversial discussions led to a clearer definition of the respective approaches of the ego psychology group, led by Anna Freud, now called "contemporary Freudians"; the Kleinian approach, led by Melanie Klein; and the "middle group" approach, inspired by the theoretical approaches of Balint (1968), Fairbairn (1954), and Winnicott (1958, 1965), now called the "British independents." At first, these controversial discussions initiated a sharp differentiation of analytic approaches, perhaps most clearly reflected in the traditional Kleinian approach in Great Britain, on the one hand, and the ego psychology approach, under the influence of Hartmann and his group in the United States, on the other.

"Recent Developments in the Technical Approaches of English-Language Psychoanalytic Schools," by Otto F. Kernberg, M.D., was first published in *The Psychoanalytic Quarterly,* 70(3)519–547, 2001.

OVERVIEW OF PSYCHOANALYTIC TECHNIQUE ACCORDING TO VARIOUS SCHOOLS OF THOUGHT

The traditional Kleinian approach—intimately linked to the revolutionary exploration of primitive object relations and primitive defensive operations described by Klein (1945, 1946a, 1946b, 1952, 1957), her stress on the earliest preoedipal levels of development, and the clinical application of Freud's theory of the death drive—was characterized by the following features: an approach to clinical material from the viewpoint of a focus on the maximum level of anxiety expressed by the patient at any particular point, the effort to interpret the patient's unconscious fantasies at the deepest level, and an ongoing exploration of primitive object relations within the frame of the paranoid-schizoid and depressive positions (Segal 1973, 1979, 1981).

Kleinians insisted on the following techniques: early, consistent, and comprehensive analysis of transference developments; exploration of the development of an unconscious world of internalized object relations in the transference; and linkages of such transferences with primitive fantasies involving bodily aspects and the interior of the mother's body. Kleinian authors proposed that unconscious fantasy, involving instinctually dominated, primitive object relations, represented at the same time primitive impulses and the defenses against them, so that unconscious fantasies were considered to be the mental correlates of drives. Kleinians have made fundamental contributions to countertransference analysis (Racker 1968).

In contrast, *the ego psychology approach* focused on latter levels of development, centered on interstructural conflicts and the centrality of the oedipal situation, and the analysis of unconscious conflict as represented by impulse-defense configuration, with a particular focus on the defensive structures of the ego—including character defenses and the analysis of such defenses as they become resistances in the analytic treatment situation. The dominance of the consideration of the structural theory (the so-called second topic within French psychoanalysis) as the basis for interpretation also implied the importance of superego defenses and the role of unconscious guilt. Fenichel's (1941) text entitled *Problems of Psychoanalytic Technique* was the fundamental statement of the technical approach of ego psychology, later expanded in Greenson's (1967) classical text and in Rangell's (1963a, 1963b) and Brenner's (1976) contributions. Fenichel spelled out the economic, dynamic, and structural criteria for interpretation; stressed the importance of interpreting always from the side of the ego, from surface to depth; and emphasized the interstructural relations of the conflict between defense and impulse. Fenichel's work remained the definitive summary of ego psychology technique well into the era of the contemporary Freudian approach in the United States.

The British independents, the original "middle group," acknowledged their roots in both ego psychology as represented by Anna Freud, and in the Kleinian approach, particularly the latter's emphasis on internalized object relations as a guiding principle for psychic development, structure formation, and analytic technique (Kohon 1986; Little 1951; Stewart 1992). The British independents stressed the exploration of affective developments in the analytic situation, the importance of preoedipal stages, the centrality of countertransference analysis, and the consideration of early traumatic situations as bringing about a "basic fault" (Balint 1968) that might require modification in technique with regard to tolerance and interpretive management of severe regression.

The analysis of transitional phenomena and of the true and false self, comprising Winnicott's (1958, 1965) contributions, as well as the systematic analysis of the relationships with "bad internal objects" stressed by Fairbairn (1954), converged in an emphasis on analysis of the transference, although transference analysis was not the exclusive focus. The British independents made use of Kleinian contributions to the understanding of primitive object relations and primitive defenses, particularly projective identification, but they also recognized the implications for psychopathology of more advanced levels of development, as well as the impact of later developmental stages on intrapsychic structure and the analytic situation. Because the independents occupied an intermediate position between the approach of ego psychology and that of the Kleinians, their boundaries have been more difficult to define; by the same token, they contributed fundamentally to the gradual rapprochement of ego psychology and Kleinian approaches in the last 20 years.

In fact, the most impressive development of analytic technique within the English-language analytic community, in my view, is the gradual rapprochement of these three viewpoints, as the separate groups have learned about each other's ideas in their confrontations at international meetings, and as practicing clinicians have gradually recognized the therapeutic limitations of whichever theory they attempt to apply. Thus, new generations of analysts have reshaped the respective technical formulations.

CONTEMPORARY KLEINIAN PSYCHOANALYTIC TECHNIQUE

Within the Kleinian school, Rosenfeld's (1964, 1987) analysis of the narcissistic personality, applying Klein's (1957) contributions in *Envy and*

Gratitude to a particular character pathology that had proven to be remarkably resistant to classical analytic technique, implicitly introduced the concept of character analysis—so central to ego psychology—into Kleinian technique. The development of this approach in Steiner's (1993) book on psychic retreat expanded Kleinian analysis to pathological personality organization, and introduced an explicit focus on the here-and-now analysis of characterological resistances. While Bion's (1967a) work focused mostly on primitive transferences of severely regressed patients, his questioning of the authoritarian stance of the analyst, distilled in his famous recommendation to analyze without memory or desire, also raised implicit questions about the categorical style of interpretation of traditional Kleinian analysis (Bion 1967b, 1970).

The Kleinian mainstream, represented particularly by the group led by Segal (1973, 1979, 1981, 1986), Joseph (1989), and Spillius and Feldman (1989), and reflected in the fundamental *Melanie Klein Today* (Spillius 1988) volumes, proposed fundamental changes in Kleinian technique: the focus on unconscious fantasy was maintained, but shifted from its concern with anatomical organs to stress on the functions of primitive fantasy. The interpretive style became less categorical; less focused on aggression, destructiveness, and envy; and more attuned to the dominant level of anxiety in the here and now, rather than the assumed deepest level of anxiety. Increasing attention was paid to projective identification as it affects transference and countertransference, and to the patient's implicit expectations reflected in the analyst's being tempted to move into certain interventions, with an increased focus on nonverbal behavior and on interactions in the here and now.

All of these developments moved Kleinian analysis in the direction of ego psychology, without explicit acknowledgement of this shift. Nevertheless, Kleinian interpretations were no longer dealing as much with bodily fantasy as with the present level of mental functioning of the patient and his or her level of symbolization (Segal 1981, 1986; Spillius and Feldman 1989). In the United States, Ogden (1982, 1986, 1989) introduced a Kleinian approach, with some Winnicottian aspects added to the analytic approach to psychotic patients.

THE CONTEMPORARY FREUDIAN APPROACH

Simultaneously, within the *contemporary Freudian approach,* a number of analysts in Great Britain (J. Sandler 1976, 1987; J. Sandler et al. 1992;

J. Sandler and A.-M. Sandler 1984), as well as a variety of American ones within the ego psychology tradition, began to include an object relations perspective in their theoretical formulations and technical interventions. Modell (1976, 1990), influenced by Winnicott, introduced an object relations approach. Authors dealing with borderline psychopathology and severely regressed patients in general, such as Jacobson (1971), Kernberg (1976, 1984, 1992), Searles (1979), and Volkan (1976), introduced an object relations approach focused on the consequences of earliest internalizations for primitive defenses and object relations, and particularly on the clinical implications of splitting mechanisms and projective identification, including concepts and technical approaches from the Kleinian and British independent schools.

J. Sandler and A.-M. Sandler (1998), in an implicit critique of the ego psychology tradition of interpreting "pure" drive derivatives in the context of analysis of the defenses against them, stressed that unconscious fantasy includes not simply derivatives of libidinal and aggressive drives, but specific wishes for gratifying relationships between the self and significant objects. They proposed that unconscious fantasy thus takes the form of wishes for specific relationships of the self with objects represented by fantasized, desirable relations between self-representations and object representations. According to this view, the expression of impulses and their derivatives is transformed into a desired interaction with an object, and a wishful fantasy includes the reaction of the object to the wishful action of the individual. In the transference, the patient expresses behavior dedicated to the induction of complementary actions on the part of significant objects, at the same time being unconsciously attuned to the "role responsiveness" of the analyst. The analyst's countertransference, codetermined by the patient's transference developments and by the unconscious role responsiveness of the analyst, facilitates the actualization of unconsciously fantasized object relations in the transference. This provides the analyst with a powerful tool for the interpretation of unconscious fantasy in the here and now.

J. Sandler and A.-M. Sandler (1998) described the continuities and discontinuities between the most primitive realizations of unconscious fantasy in hallucinatory wish fulfillment and delusion formation, the complex layers of unconscious and conscious daydreaming, and the unconscious and conscious illusory transformation of the perception of present reality. They clarified, in a contemporary ego psychology theoretical frame, the differences between the ego as an "impersonal" set of structures vis-à-vis the "representational world" (constituted by representations of self and object and of ideal self and ideal object). Affectively invested internalized object relations are actualized in the transference not only in specific, fantasized desires and fears emerging in free association, but also—and significantly so—in the character traits that emerge as transference resistances, very often in the early stages of analysis. J. Sandler and A.-M. Sandler stressed the central importance of affects as the link between self and object representations in any particular fantasized interaction between them, thus expanding the theoretical formulations originally laid down by Jacobson (1964).

The clinical rapprochement of ego psychology with the Kleinian approach is signaled most impressively by Schafer (1997) in *The Contemporary Kleinians of London,* an extremely careful, critical, and yet obviously sympathetic exploration of key contributions from the contemporary British Kleinians addressed to a North American audience. A new mainstream of analytic technique within the English-language analytic community seems to be evolving.

THE INTERPERSONAL OR RELATIONAL APPROACH IN PSYCHOANALYSIS

At this point, I must introduce an additional perspective that complicates everything said so far. *The Analysis of the Self* (Kohut 1971), together with Volumes I and II of *Analysis of Transference* (Gill 1982; Gill and Hoffman 1982), starting from completely different theoretical perspectives and reaching very different conclusions, represented, nevertheless, a significant new current in North American analytic thinking. This current gradually established a relationship with the culturalist analytic approach in the United States, which, beginning with Sullivan (1953), had persisted as a tradition parallel to the analytic community of the International Psychoanalytic Association, and which now surfaced as the *contemporary interpersonal* or *relational* approach in analysis. Self psychology, the intersubjective approach, and the relational and interpersonal orientations together constitute a major alternative to the analytic mainstream within the English-language analytic community (Greenberg 1991; Greenberg and Mitchell 1983; Mitchell 1988, 1997; Stolorow et al. 1983, 1987).

Kohut's (1971, 1977, 1984) self psychology had significant implications for analytic technique. In contrast to Rosenfeld's (1964) and my own recommendations (Kernberg 1984) regarding technical approaches with narcissistic personalities, Kohut proposed that narcissistic pathology constituted a specific pathology, intermediate between psychosis and borderline conditions, on the one hand, and neurosis, on the other, differentiated by the specific idealizing and mirroring transferences of these patients. These transferences reflected the activation of an archaic, rudimentary self whose narcissistic equilibrium could be safeguarded only by the interest and approval of current replicas of traumatically missing selfobjects of the past. The analyst's task is to facilitate the consolidation of the grandiose self. Later, more mature forms of the self, reflected in self-esteem and self-confidence, can develop upon that initial groundwork. The analyst, instead of operating from a position of technical neutrality, must operate within a self/selfobject relationship, within which the tolerance of the patient's idealization and the facilitation of adequate mirroring permit the healing process to occur. Idealization of the analyst replicates the normal process of the transmuting internalization of the idealized selfobject into the ego ideal, thus facilitating the consolidation of the tripartite structure.

Narcissistic psychopathology, in the self psychology view, develops due to the traumatic failure of empathic mothering functions and the corresponding failure of the idealization of the selfobject to flourish. It constitutes a developmental arrest, with a fixation at the level of the archaic infantile grandiose self and an endless search for idealized selfobjects needed to complete structure formations. As a consequence, these patients experience repeated, severe traumatizations as their needs and expectations are not met, traumatizations that are reactivated in the transference and thus are subject to interpretive resolution. The corresponding analytic technique implies that narcissistic idealization of the analyst must be permitted to occur in the unfolding of the idealizing and mirror transferences. The patient's reliving of early traumas by experiencing him- or herself as misunderstood by the analyst must be explored by means of the analyst's empathic recognition of this disappointment and the analysis of the patient's experience of the analyst's failure to meet the patient's needs.

The analyst's inevitable failure to avoid narcissistic traumatizations of the patient brings about temporary traumatic fragmentation of the grandiose self, narcissistic rage, severe anxiety, and hypochondriasis. Traumatization that is severe and unrepaired may lead to the evolution of delusion formation of the grandiose self, with a paranoid form of grandiosity. It is essential, therefore, that the analyst explore how he or she failed the patient due to a lack of appropriate empathy. For Kohut, self/selfobject relations can never be fully resolved, because they constitute a normal need throughout the lifetime.

The technical approach derived from Kohut's theory focused sharply on the here-and-now relationship in the context of an exploration of the potentially traumatic effects of a breakdown in the analyst's empathy. With its de-emphasis of such classical analytic concepts as the importance of unconscious aggression, the centrality of the oedipal conflict and of infantile sexuality, and its rejection of technical neutrality, self psychology constituted a major challenge to the dominant ego psychology approach within American psychoanalysis.

The fact that is was possible to "contain" self psychology within the overall scientific, professional, and administrative structure of the American Psychoanalytic Association (in contrast to the earlier rejection of the culturalist school) had fundamental consequences in bringing to an end the dominance of ego psychology within the educational structure of North American analysis. Paradoxically, this development opened the field to the modifications of ego psychology, inspired by the object relations theory that had evolved as a consequence of the exploration of severe psychopathologies and the related focus on preoedipal pathology, primitive object relations, and defensive operations.

As part of this opening during the last 30 years, and in parallel to the incorporation of self psychology and neo-Kohutian contributions within the American Psychoanalytic Association, the fundamental contributions of Mahler (Mahler and Furer 1968; Mahler et al. 1975) to the developmental analysis of normal and pathological separation-individuation, as well as their implication for the treatment of borderline conditions, became generally accepted, and my own efforts to integrate ego psychology and object relations theory became less controversial. Independently, Loewald (1960, 1980) introduced an object relations perspective into his exploration of the psychoanalytic process.

At the same time, insofar as self psychology stressed the importance of early deficits—in contrast to the universal etiologic importance of unconscious conflicts—a broad spectrum of authors explored the implications of early deficits in severe psychopathologies for analytic technique and its modifications. Simultaneously, Ogden (1982, 1986, 1989) applied British independent and Kleinian approaches to the treatment of patients with severe psychopathology, and the focus on "projective identification" was no longer a sign of "anti-American" activity.

MODIFICATIONS IN THE PSYCHOANALYTIC "MAINSTREAM" VIEWPOINT

Gill and Hoffman (Gill 1982, 1994; Gill and Hoffman 1982), starting from a basis in traditional ego psychology, made modifications in the light of their empirical research on the analytic situation, creating further theoretical and technical shifts in the thinking of North American analysts. Gill demonstrated convincingly that transference phenomena are ubiquitous from the beginning of the treatment, and stressed the importance of transference analysis from the very start, in contrast to the cautious approach to transference analysis in traditional ego psychology. Furthermore, in radically questioning the traditional ego psychology concept of transference as primarily what might be called "a distortion of the present by the patient's past," he postulated that "transference is always an amalgam of past and present, and is based on as plausible a response to the immediate analytic situation as the patient can muster" (Gill 1982, p. 177).

> This view implies a shift to the position that the analyst is per force a participant-observer (Sullivan's term) rather than merely an observer. It also implies a shift from the view of the reality of the analytic situation as objectively definable by the analyst to a view of the reality of the analytic situation as defined by the progressive elucidation of the manner in which that situation is experienced by the patient. (Gill 1982, p. 177)

The transference, in short, is a result of the interaction between the patient and the analyst, and Gill therefore stressed the importance of honest self-scrutiny on the analyst's part. This represented an important, implicit critique of the authoritarian imposition of the analyst's view as part of his or her interpretive function. Gill's proposal also implied that the analyst cannot study the analytic situation objectively, and that the analyst's view of reality must be defined, as mentioned above, by "the progressive elucidation of the manner in which that situation is experienced by the patient."

This "constructivist" view of the transference stands in contrast to the "objectivist" view of it on the part of most American ego psychology and all British approaches; it sharply focuses the analyst's attention on the here-and-now interaction with the patient in terms of the reality aspects of this interaction, without limiting that attention to the reproduction of the patient's unconscious fantasies. It represents a definite shift from a "one-person psychology" to a "two-person psychology," and to a focus on the actual conscious and unconscious interactions between patient and analyst as the major focus of the analytic endeavor, with an emphasis on transference and countertransference analysis that implicitly privileges the patient's subjective experience.

This constructivist orientation was developed further in the intersubjective approach of Atwood and Stolorow (Atwood and Stolorow 1984; Stolorow 1984, 1992; Stolorow and Atwood 1979; Stolorow and

Lachmann 1980; Stolorow et al. 1983, 1987), and established theoretical as well as technical relations with the interpersonal or relational approach of Greenberg and Mitchell (1983). A broad spectrum of analytic approaches within what might be called an overall *self psychology–intersubjective–interpersonal framework* evolved in the United States (Bacal 1990; Levenson 1972, 1983, 1991; Mitchell 1988, 1993; Mitchell and Aron 1999; Mitchell and Black 1995). At a clinical level, the focus of self psychology on self/selfobject transferences as a major matrix of analytic treatment has implied a movement away from the technical neutrality that characterizes the traditional ego psychology, Kleinian, independent, and contemporary mainstream analytic approaches to which I referred earlier.

Post-Kohutian self psychology, analyzing within a frame of providing selfobject functions, has evolved into an emphasis on emotional attunement as a basic attitude, in order to help the patient clarify his or her own subjectivity in the light of the analyst's empathic, subjective immersion in the patient's experience, and with acknowledgment of the intersubjective reality established in the interplay between the patient's and the analyst's subjectivities (Schwaber 1983). The selfobject function of the analyst is translated into his or her interpretive function in clarifying the patient's affective experience. Both deficit models and conflict models of psychopathology may be combined in this emphasis on a sustained empathic immersion of the analyst in the patient's evolving subjective experience. This approach accentuates an "antiauthoritarian" attitude of the analyst, questions the privileged nature of the analyst's subjectivity, and questions the function of the analyst's technical neutrality and anonymity.

The focus on the analyst's role in compensating for past deficits, for overstimulation or understimulation of the patient's archaic self, and for the absence or lack of soothing by parental figures—with a consequent frailty of the development of the self—may derive from a self psychology perspective, but stems also from the application of a model of the infant-mother relationship that focuses on deficits and conflicts derived from separation-individuation.

The interpersonal perspective derived from culturalist analysis, originating in Sullivan's (1953) contributions, focuses on the development of the self as intimately linked with interpersonal experiences. Personality development, in this view, is intrinsically linked with the interpersonal field, as psychic life is continuously remodeled by past as well as new relationships, rather than being determined by fixed structures deriving from past unconscious conflicts. This concept of the personality as developing in a relational matrix (rather than expressing conflicts between drives and defenses against them) requires a focus on the intersubjective field in the relationship between patient and analyst. This new relational matrix, fully explored and interpretively modified, can bring about emotional growth via the patient's integration of these new affective interpersonal experiences.

A major consequence of this overall shift in analytic perspective is the questioning of the traditional, objectivist view of the analyst's subjectivity in facing the patient with his or her transference distortions and their origins. In the constructivist model, exploration of new affective relational developments in the analytic situation is the basic source of mutual understanding of patient and analyst, and the patient's incorporation of this affective experience is seen as a major therapeutic factor. A further consequence of the emphasis on the privileged subjectivity of the patient is the movement away from the interpretation of the aggressive aspects of the transference. If aggression is due to the breakdown of a positive relationship in the patient–analyst interaction and the loss of empathic attunement, it may be traced to that loss, rather than to intrapsychic conflicts in the patient.

Some authors consider self psychology a partial object relations theory focused on the positive, growth-promoting aspects of the relational matrix, not necessarily in conflict with the consideration of the introjection of negative object relations as well. One final and quite characteristic aspect of all these object relational and intersubjective approaches is the relative de-emphasis on sexuality and the oedipal complex, with major importance accorded to the early mother–infant relationship and the traumata of separation-individuation.

The general consolidation of what I have described as the psychoanalytic mainstream has gradually brought the three traditional currents of the British Psychoanalytic Society closer, to the extent that, in my experience, when hearing clinical presentations by British analysts, it is no longer easy to differentiate those with a contemporary Kleinian background, an independent background, or a contemporary Freudian background. In the United States, the traditional ego psychology approach has maintained its relative distinctiveness in the work of important contributors to the contemporary Freudian approach, such as Blum (1979, 1980, 1985), Jacobs (1991), Levy and Inderbitzin (1990), Pine (1990), and particularly Busch (1995) and Gray (1994). In fact, Busch and Gray may be considered the outstanding exponents of the development of the contemporary Freudian approach in the United States, maintaining a relatively classical ego psychology technical approach, but with a significant shift in their analysis of resistance.

The traditional ego psychology approach—that is, analysis of the patient's material from the viewpoint of the ego and from surface to depth, uncovering, at each step, the layers of defenses protecting against unconscious drive derivatives (which in turn might eventually be integrated into defensive operations against still deeper aspects of unconscious drive derivatives)—gradually led to an increased focus on the conscious and preconscious aspects of the patient's functioning in the analytic situation, and/or the external reality in which this mode of functioning was also manifest. The focus on manifestations of defensive structures as clinical resistances often led to an analysis of resistances as unconsciously motivated opposition to the analyst's effort to uncover unconscious fantasy and motivation. "Resistance analysis" implied, under these circumstances, a quasi-authoritarian stance on the part of the analyst, who pointed out to the patient that he or she was "resisting" interpretive efforts. In all fairness, this viewpoint did not do justice to the subtle implications of Fenichel's (1941) and Greenson's (1967) contributions, in the sense of analyzing the unconscious motivation of resistances. In practice, however, "overcoming of resistances" often led ego psychology technique to a potentially adversarial stance in the treatment situation.

Against this tradition, Gray (1994)—and Busch (1995), in following Gray's footsteps—stressed the importance of analyzing the motivation of the patient's resistances, focusing on his or her preconscious reasons for the mode of functioning that the analyst considered to have an unconsciously defensive purpose. Implicitly, exploration of the reasons for the patient's defensive operations led to the underlying object relations activated in the transference, and permitted the resolution of defensive operations without an "overcoming" of the resistances. Busch proposed that his approach might also be utilized in analytic work with severe personality disorders, where severe ego distortions interfere with standard analytic technique, and the patient's expression in action rather than in free association might then be explored in terms of the purposes and defensive functions of such actions, gradually helping the patient's ego to reflect on underlying fears and fantasies.

Perhaps the most radical expression of a "purified" ego psychology approach in the United States—as contrasted with the gradually integrating movement of the analytic mainstream—is represented by Brenner's (1998) proposal to do the following: to drop all considerations of interstructural aspects of the patient's intrapsychic life; to disregard the tripartite structure (or "second topic," as it is termed in French analysis); and to focus exclusively on drives, unconscious conflicts, and compromise formations between drive derivatives and defensive functions.

One might illustrate the wide divergence of recent developments in technical analytic approaches in the United States by contrasting this minimalist development within ego psychology to what might be considered the most radical expression of the intersubjective approach, as seen in the work of Renik (1993, 1995, 1996, 1998a, 1998b, 1999). Renik proposed a selective communication to the patient of aspects of the analyst's countertransference, in order to make the patient aware of how he or she is perceived by the analyst, and of the impact of the patient's personality upon their interaction, thus facilitating analysis of the intersubjective aspects of transference and countertransference. Renik's proposed technique also accentuated the desirability of an antiauthoritarian approach to interpretation.

Before I proceed to summarize the two major currents of English-language psychoanalytic approaches to technique, as reflected in what I have called the mainstream approach and the intersubjective one, it should be stressed that, naturally, each individual analytic contributor would be justified in pointing out that his or her particular approach cannot be completely subsumed in one or the other of these currents; major differences remain among authors who, from a very broad perspective, might be ordered along the lines I am suggesting. However, while such a summary necessarily has to do injustice to specific differentiations, it provides an overview of how psychoanalysis is evolving at this point within the English-language communities.

CHARACTERISTICS OF THE TWO MAJOR CURRENTS OF THE ENGLISH-LANGUAGE PSYCHOANALYTIC MAINSTREAM

Following are the characteristics of the *contemporary psychoanalytic mainstream.*

- Early and systematic interpretation of the transference. This includes the "total transference" of the Kleinians (Joseph 1989; Spillius 1988), the "present unconscious" of J. Sandler and A.-M. Sandler (1998), and Gill's (1982) analysis of resistances against the development, recognition, and elaboration of the transference within an ego psychology perspective.
- A central focus on countertransference analysis and its utilization in the interpretation of transference as a consistent aspect of analytic work, embracing the contemporary "totalistic" concept of countertransference as consisting of all the analyst's emotional reactions to the patient.

- Systematic character analysis, without necessarily mentioning this by name. The analysis of transference resistances as characterologically based defensive operations that reflect an implicit unconscious object relationship emerges in the ego psychology approach (such as is reflected in Busch's [1995] and Gray's [1994] work), in the Kleinian approach (as the analysis of "pathological organizations" [Steiner 1993]), and in the pathological patterns of relationships in the independent school. Kris's (1996) ego psychology contributions to the analysis of free association also imply such a focus on characterologically determined distortions of free association.
- A sharp focus on unconscious enactments in transference and countertransference developments, with emphasis on unconscious meanings in the here and now, as part of the analysis of the transference from surface to depth in ego psychology. Resistances are conceived as object relationships, not simply as impersonal mechanisms. This corresponds to the Kleinian focus on functions in contrast to anatomy in the patient's fantasies, and the analysis of "total transference" (Joseph 1989; Spillius 1988).
- An emphasis on affective dominance. This was first stressed by the independents, but is now considered essential in both contemporary Freudian and contemporary Kleinian approaches.
- A predominance of models of internalized object relations. Even Brenner (1998), a bastion of ego psychology, abandoned the focus on the tripartite structural model in a recent publication on technique.
- Technical neutrality. In contrast to self psychology's explicit abandonment of the emphasis on the analyst's concerned objectivity, and in opposition to the two-person model of the intersubjective school, the contemporary psychoanalytic mainstream focuses precisely on that objectivity, through implicitly stressing a "three-person" model. This three-person model emphasizes the double function of the analyst as immersed, on the one hand, in a transference-countertransference relationship, and on the other, as maintaining an objective distance, from which observations and interpretations of the patient's enactments of internal object relationships can be carried out. A related concept, stressed by ego psychology but implicitly present in other approaches as well , is that of the therapeutic alliance, or conflict-free aspects of the relationship between patient and analyst. As Deserno (1990) pointed out, this therapeutic alliance or relationship is a relative concept—limited, at one extreme, by the danger of conventionalized agreements between patient and analyst that imply a joint blind spot regarding cultural bias, as opposed to another extreme in which the transference is considered to be an infinite regress, and the very

possibility of an objective approach to it from a position of technical neutrality is denied.

- Emphasis on the multiplicity of "royal roads" to the unconscious, in the sense of an assumption of multiple surfaces of defensive formations that lead into the dynamic unconscious, and the fact that affective dominance may point to very different aspects of the material (memories, dreams, acting out, fantasies, and so on)—all of which, under concrete circumstances, constitute a royal road to unconscious fantasy.
- A concerned avoidance of indoctrination by categorical styles of interpretation, and stress on the patient's active work in exploring unconscious meanings with the help of tentative interpretations by the analyst.
- An increased questioning of linear models of development, since the condensation of experiences from multiple developmental levels present themselves as compressed matrixes of experience or behavior that can only gradually be disentangled and separated into different historical events. It may well be that this technical development reflects an indirect influence from French psychoanalysis.

Following are the characteristics of the technical approaches of the *intersubjectivist–interpersonal–self psychology* schools.

- A constructivist approach to the transference, as opposed to the traditional objectivist one. The transference is a compromise formation, and the unavoidable subjectivity of the analyst justifies questioning the possibility of an objective view of it. In this regard, transference develops in parallel to countertransference, which is also a composite of analyst-determined and patient-determined influences. The analysis of the transference is the construction of a joint understanding of the intersubjective structure of the patient-analyst relationship, and both patient and analyst have to accept the influence of unconscious factors in their understanding and interpretation of this relationship.
- Technical neutrality is rejected as an illusion and an expression of the authoritarian position of the analyst. During treatment, the analyst is perceived by the patient as having all the answers, and may easily be seduced into such a position. Within a self/selfobject position of the analyst, technical neutrality is clearly precluded as a potentially traumatizing and destructive effect on the consolidation of a normal self. An empathic orientation is central in the analyst's attitude. The analyst's "anonymity" represents a disguised position of authority, and maintains an idealization that cannot be analyzed.

- A deficit model of early development is recognized explicitly or implicitly, in the sense of failure in early attachment or of a loving dedication on the part of the parenting object, or of other failure of caretakers to meet the patient's dependency needs in early infancy or childhood, leading to insecure attachment and traumatophylic transferential dispositions. Resistances are really mini-traumatic experiences, and the analyst has to consider the possibility of either an excess or a lack of sufficient stimulation in the treatment situation as a traumatic experience for the patient. The self develops within a relationship matrix that is constantly revised and newly traumatized, and the transference repeats such experiences, leading to a focus on the patient's subjectivity and its privileged position.
- Aggression is not seen as a drive or de-emphasized as such. Many authors within this approach perceive aggression as a consequence of a failure in the early infant–mother relationship. Self psychologists usually interpret the emergence of aggression in the transference as consequence of a failure in the analyst's empathy. Neither is primitive sexuality emphasized as a drive; sadomasochism is at times considered a consequence of insecure attachment. Here, object relations theories are perceived as standing in opposition to drive theories.
- The treatment is conceived as a new object relationship, within which the real personality of the analyst is as important as his or her interpretive work. Communication of the countertransference, under certain conditions, may facilitate a new experience of important or fundamental therapeutic value for the patient.

THE FRENCH PSYCHOANALYTIC APPROACH

I referred earlier to the *French psychoanalytic approach* as the third major current of contemporary psychoanalytic formulations, with its corresponding differentiated technical approach. At this point, it may be helpful to briefly summarize this approach, which definitely represents an alternative approach to other analytic techniques and, in my view, provides an external perspective that may enrich the English-language psychoanalytic community. Here I am reserving the term *French approach* for those attributes that, from an outsider's perspective, appear as common characteristics of the French language analytic societies and institutes that are included in the International Psychoanalytical Association, in contrast to the Lacanian approach, which has nevertheless left deep traces in what I consider to be the French mainstream (De Mijolla and De Mijolla-Mellor 1996; Green 1986, 1993; Laplanche 1987;

Laplanche et al. 1992; LeGuen 1974, 1982, 1989; Oliner 1988).

With these caveats, I would summarize the main technical characteristics of the French mainstream, in contrast to both the English-language mainstream and the intersubjective approaches, as follows:

- A general opposition to the concept of *technique* as contrasted with analytic *method,* in order to stress the highly individualized, subjective, and even artistic aspects of analytic practice.
- A strong focus on the linguistic aspects of analytic communication, including the search for nodal points where unconscious meanings may be expressed as metaphor or metonymy—in other words, symbolic condensations or displacement. The assumption is that unconscious influences determine the symbolic significance of linguistic distortions, and constitute a privileged road into the assessment of unconscious conflicts. More recently, affective implications of symbolic meanings expressed in language have been stressed.
- Consistent, subtle observation of the transference, but without a systematic interpretation of it. Rather, there is a punctuated, sparing interpretation of it, in the interest of avoiding an authoritarian distortion of the transference by too-frequent interpretive interventions.
- Leaving aside, rather than paying special attention to, the resistances of the ego, which represent seductive ego functions attempting to shield unconscious fantasy. In this context, intellectual explanations are carefully avoided.
- Direct interpretation of deep, symbolized, unconscious conflicts, while addressing the patient's preconscious through evocative, non-saturated interpretations. Such evocative interpretations are seen as indirectly addressing the patient's unconscious: effective interpretations of preconscious material induce unconscious resonances.
- Simultaneous consideration of somatizations and nonverbal behavior (enactments) in one integrative statement, on the basis of the analyst's combined consideration of the patient's preconscious fantasy and the countertransference. If the patient's behavior cannot be linked with his or her discourse, it is not interpreted.
- Efforts to avoid being seduced by the patient's conscious constructions regarding the realities of daily life. Excessive consideration of external reality risks transforming analysis into therapy.
- Direct interpretation of presymbolic psychosomatic expression of unconscious conflicts. This is a specific approach of the school of Pierre Marty (1980).
- Analysis of the patient's expectation that the analyst is the subject of presumed knowledge. In other words, the symbolic function of the

idealized oedipal father, supposed to protect the patient from the deepest aspects of castration anxiety, is analyzed.

- Focus on archaic sexuality, particularly the archaic aspects of the oedipal complex that develop in the preoedipal symbiotic mother–infant relation. Insofar as the father is always present in the mind of the mother, preoedipal relations are always perceived as resistances against oedipal conflicts. This approach also implies a pervasive consideration of the role of castration anxiety.
- Opposition to linear conceptions of the origin of development. This is accompanied by a strong emphasis on the *après coup,* that is, the retrospective modification of earlier experiences, including a two-stage model of psychic trauma, implying that later experiences may modify earlier ones in a traumatic direction, and/or that only after secondary incorporation of an experience which could not be metabolized does such an experience acquire the meaning of a psychic trauma. There is a focus on analysis of the condensation of psychic experiences from different times into synchronic expressions, and diachronic, narrative developments—repeating the oscillation between synchronic and diachronic expressions in the transference—are emphasized.
- A "progressive" vector of the interpretation, implying a future-directed elaboration of the oedipal complex as one aspect of interpretive interventions. Interpretations are made to open the way, rather than to establish the truth.
- Acceptance of the irreducible basis of earliest transferences, derived from the mother's enigmatic messages. These messages reflect the unconscious erotic investment by the mother of the infant, which will only retrospectively be interpreted as such in the infant's development of primary unconscious fantasies representing the archaic oedipal complex. These transferences may be interpreted, but the final, unconscious repetition of the experience of enigmatic messages from the analyst, the transmission of "unconscious" to "unconscious," has to be respected. (This is a major emphasis in Laplanche's [1987] work.)
- Finally, and very fundamentally, emphasis on the analysis of preconscious fantasy, and on analyzability as based in the development of the capacity for such preconscious fantasy—in contrast to the incapacity to tolerate psychic experience in this psychic realm, and its expression in somatization or acting out. Therefore, the retransformation of acting out and psychosomatic expression into preconscious fantasy constitutes a major technical goal in cases where the patient's tolerance of intrapsychic experience (of a traumatic kind) is limited. This is a major point raised by Marty (1980) and Green (1986).

Implicitly, the French psychoanalytic approach described above is critical of both the English-language analytic mainstream and of the intersubjective viewpoints. The French approach sees a risk of superficiality deriving from the focus on conscious material and clarification of reality life circumstances within ego psychology. French authors would also be concerned about cognitive indoctrination of patients by means of systematic transference analysis, and the acting out of countertransference as a consequence of such systematic transference analysis. The French approach is critical of what is considered to be a neglect of early sexuality and the archaic oedipal complex in the English-language schools, and the French are particularly critical of intersubjectivity as a seduction into a superficial interpersonal relationship, the denial of Freud's theory of drives, and the implicit supportive psychotherapeutic intervention that occurs when the analyst presents him- or herself as an ideal model, with unconscious acting out of countertransference as a major consequence.

CONCLUSION

I have attempted to describe the development of the three major approaches to psychoanalytic technique among English-speaking analysts, and to show how their cross-fertilization during the past 30 years has affected them. In contrasting these three viewpoints with the French mainstream, I have suggested ways in which each of them may be flawed or incomplete. If the trend toward mutual modification of previously hotly defended differences continues, one might expect a degree of convergence in the French and English schools in the years to come.

REFERENCES

Atwood G, Stolorow R: Structures of Subjectivity: Explorations in Psychoanalytic Phenomenology. Hillsdale, NJ, Analytic Press, 1984

Bacal H: Does an object relations theory exist in self-psychology? Psychoanalytic Inquiry 10:197–220, 1990

Balint M: The Basic Fault: Therapeutic Aspects of Regression. London, Tavistock, 1968

Bion WR: Second thoughts, in Selected Papers on Psychoanalysis. New York, Basic Books, 1967a

Bion WR: Notes on memory and desire. Psychoanalytic Forum 2:272–273; 279–280, 1967b
Bion WR: Attention and Interpretation. London, Heinemann, 1970
Blum HP (ed): Psychoanalytic technique and theory of therapy. J Am Psychoanal Assoc 27(suppl):41–70, 1979
Blum HP (ed): Psychoanalytic Explorations of Technique. New York, International Universities Press, 1980
Blum HP (ed): Defense and Resistance: Historical Perspective and Current Concepts. New York, International Universities Press, 1985
Brenner C: Psychoanalytic Technique and Psychic Conflict. New York, International Universities Press, 1976
Brenner C: "Beyond the Ego and the Id" revisited. J Clin Psychoanal 71:165–180, 1998
Busch F: The Ego at the Center of Clinical Technique. Northvale, NJ, Jason Aronson, 1995
De Mijolla A, De Mijolla-Mellor S: Psychanalyse. Paris, Presses Universitaires de France, 1996
Deserno H:. Die Analyse und das Arbeitsbundnis. Eine Kritik des Arbeitsbündniskonzepts. Munich and Vienna, Verlag Internationale Psychoanalyse, 1990
Fairbairn WRD: An Object-Relations Theory of the Personality. New York, Basic Books, 1954
Fenichel O: Problems of Psychoanalytic Technique. New York, Psychoanalytic Quarterly, 1941
Gill M: Analysis of Transference: Theory and Technique, Vol I. Madison, CT/New York, International Universities Press, 1982
Gill M: Psychoanalysis in Transition. A Personal View. Hillsdale, NJ, Analytic Press, 1994
Gill M, Hoffman IZ: Analysis of Transference, Vol II. New York, International Universities Press, 1982
Gray P: The Ego and Analysis of Defense. Northvale, NJ, Jason Aronson, 1994
Green A: On Private Madness. London, Hogarth Press, 1986
Green A: Le travail du négatif. Paris, Les Editions de Minuit, 1993
Greenberg J: Oedipus and Beyond. Cambridge, MA, Harvard University Press, 1991
Greenberg JR, Mitchell SA: Object Relations in Psychoanalytic Theory. Cambridge, MA, Harvard University Press, 1983
Greenson R: The Technique and Practice of Psychoanalysis, Vol I. New York, International Universities Press, 1967
Jacobs T: The Use of the Self: Countertransference and Communication in the Analytic Situation. Madison, CT, International Universities Press, 1991
Jacobson E: The Self and the Object World. New York, International Universities Press, 1964
Jacobson E: Depression. New York, International Universities Press, 1971

Joseph B: Psychic Equilibrium and Psychic Change. London/New York, Tavistock/Routledge, 1989
Kernberg O: Object Relations Theory and Clinical Psychoanalysis. New York, Jason Aronson, 1976
Kernberg O: Severe Personality Disorders: Psychotherapeutic Strategies. New Haven, CT, Yale University Press, 1984
Kernberg O: Aggression in Personality Disorders and Perversion. New Haven, CT, Yale University Press, 1992
King P, Steiner R: The Freud-Klein Controversies, 1941–45. London/New York, Tavistock/Routledge, 1991
Klein M: The Oedipus complex in the light of early anxieties (1945), in Contributions to Psychoanalysis, 1921–1945. London, Hogarth Press, 1948, pp 339–390
Klein M: Notes on some schizoid mechanisms (1946a), in Developments in Psycho-Analysis. Edited by Riviere J. London, Hogarth, 1952, pp 292–320
Klein M: Notes on some schizoid mechanisms. Int J Psychoanal 27:99–110, 1946b
Klein M: The origins of transference. Int J Psychoanal 33:433–438, 1952
Klein M: Envy and Gratitude. New York, Basic Books, 1957
Kohon G: The British School of Psychoanalysis—The Independent Tradition. London, Free Association Books, 1986
Kohut H: The Analysis of the Self. New York, International Universities Press, 1971
Kohut H: The Restoration of the Self. New York, International Universities Press, 1977
Kohut H: How Does Analysis Cure? Edited by Goldberg A, Stepansky P. Chicago, IL, University of Chicago Press, 1984
Kris A: Free Association. Hillsdale, NJ, Analytic Press, 1996
Laplanche J: Nouveaux fondements pour la psychanalyse. Paris, Presses Universitaires de France, 1987
Laplanche J, Fletcher J, Stanton M (eds): Seduction, Translation, Drives. London, Psychoanalytic Forum, Institute of Contemporary Arts, 1992
LeGuen C: L'Oedipe originaire. Paris, Payot, 1974
LeGuen C: Practique de la méthode psychoanalytique. Paris, Presses Universitaires de France, 1982
LeGuen C: Théorie de la méthode psychoanalytique. Paris, Presses Universitaires de France, 1989
Levenson E: The Fallacy of Understanding. New York, Basic Books, 1972
Levenson E: The Ambiguity of Change: An Inquiry into the Nature of Psychoanalytic Reality. New York, Basic Books, 1983
Levenson E: The Purloined Self. New York, William Alanson White Institute, 1991
Levy ST, Inderbitzin LB: The analytic surface and theory of technique. J Am Psychoanal Assoc 38:371–392, 1990

Little M: Countertransference and the patient's response to it. Int J Psychoanal 32:32–40, 1951

Loewald H: On the therapeutic action of psychoanalysis. Int J Psychoanal 58:463–472, 1960

Loewald H: Papers on Psychoanalysis. New Haven, Yale University Press, 1980

Mahler M, Furer M: On Human Symbiosis and the Vicissitudes of Individuation. New York, International Universities Press, 1968

Mahler M, Pine F, Bergman A: The Psychological Birth of the Human Infant, Symbiosis and Individuation. New York, Basic Books, 1975

Marty P: L'Ordre psychosomatique. Paris, Payot, 1980

Mitchell S: Relational Concepts in Psychoanalysis: An Integration. Cambridge, MA, Harvard University Press, 1988

Mitchell S: Hope and Dread in Psychoanalysis. New York, Basic Books, 1993

Mitchell S: Influence and Autonomy in Psychoanalysis. Hillsdale, NJ, Analytic Press, 1997

Mitchell S, Aron L: Relational Psychoanalysis: The Emergence of a Tradition. Relational Perspectives Book Series, Vol 14. Hillsdale, NJ, Analytic Press, 1999

Mitchell S, Black M: Freud and Beyond. New York, Basic Books, 1995

Modell AH: The "holding environment" and the therapeutic action of psychoanalysis. J Am Psychoanal Assoc 24:285–307, 1976

Modell AH: Other Times, Other Realities: Toward a Theory of Psychoanalytic Treatment. Cambridge, MA, Harvard University Press, 1990

Ogden T: Projective Identification and Psychotherapeutic Technique. New York, Jason Aronson, 1982

Ogden T: The Matrix of the Mind: Object Relations and the Psychoanalytic Dialogue. Northvale, NJ, Jason Aronson, 1986

Ogden T: The Primitive Edge of Experience. Northvale, NJ, Jason Aronson, 1989

Oliner MM: Cultivating Freud's Garden in France. Northvale, NJ, Jason Aronson, 1988

Pine F: Drive, Ego, Object, Self. New York, Basic Books, 1990

Racker H: Transference and Countertransference. New York, International Universities Press, 1968

Rangell L: The scope of intrapsychic conflict. Psychoanal Study Child 18:75–102, 1963a

Rangell L: Structural problems in intrapsychic conflict. Psychoanal Study Child 18:103–138, 1963b

Rayner E: The Independent Mind in British Psychoanalysis. Northvale, NJ, Jason Aronson, 1991

Renik O: Analytic interaction: conceptualizing technique in light of the analyst's irreducible subjectivity. Psychoanal Q 62:553–571, 1993

Renik O: The ideal of the anonymous analyst and the problem of self-disclosure. Psychoanal Q 64:466–496, 1995

Renik O: The perils of neutrality. Psychoanal Q 65:495–517, 1996

Renik O: Getting real in analysis Psychoanal Q 67:566–593, 1998a

Renik O: The analyst's subjectivity and the analyst's objectivity. Int J Psychoanal 79:487–497, 1998b

Renik O: Playing one's cards face up in analysis: an approach to the problem of self-disclosure. Psychoanal Q 68:521–539, 1999

Rosenfeld H: On the psychopathology of narcissism: a clinical approach. Int J Psychoanal 45:332–337, 1964

Rosenfeld H: Impasse and Interpretation: Therapeutic and Anti-Therapeutic Factors in the Psychoanalytic Treatment of Psychotic, Borderline and Neurotic Patients. London, Tavistock, 1987

Sandler J: Countertransference and role responsiveness. Int Rev Psychoanal 3:43–47, 1976

Sandler J: From Safety to Superego: Selected Papers of Joseph Sandler. New York, Guilford, 1987

Sandler J, Sandler AM: The past unconscious, the present unconscious, and interpretation of the transference. Psychoanalytic Inquiry 4:367–399, 1984

Sandler J, Sandler AM: Internal Objects Revisited. London, Karnac, 1998

Sandler J, Dare C, Holder A, Dreher AU: The Patient and the Analyst: The Basis of the Psychoanalytic Process. Madison, CT, International Universities Press, 1992

Schafer R (ed): The Contemporary Kleinians of London. New York, International Universities Press, 1997

Schwaber E: Psychoanalytic listening and psychic reality. Int Rev Psychoanal 10:379–392, 1983

Searles HF: Countertransference and Related Subjects: Selected Papers. New York, International Universities Press, 1979

Segal H: Introduction to the Work of Melanie Klein. London, Hogarth Press, 1973

Segal H: Klein. Glasgow, Fontana/Collins, 1979

Segal H: The Work of Hanna Segal. New York, Jason Aronson, 1981

Segal H: The Work of Hanna Segal: A Kleinian Approach to Clinical Practice. London, Free Association Books, 1986

Spillius EB: Melanie Klein Today: Developments in Theory and Practice, Vols I and II. London/New York, Routledge, 1988

Spillius EB, Feldman M: Psychic Equilibrium and Psychic Change. London/New York, Tavistock/Routledge, 1989

Steiner J: Psychic Retreats: Pathological Organizations in Psychotic, Neurotic and Borderline Patients. London/New York, Routledge, 1993

Stewart H: Psychic Experience and Problems of Technique. London/New York, Routledge, 1992

Stolorow R: Aggression in the psychoanalytic situation: an intersubjective viewpoint. Contemp Psychoanal 20:643–651, 1984

Stolorow R: Contexts of Being: The Intersubjective Foundations of Psychological Life. Hillsdale, NJ, Analytic Press, 1992

Stolorow R, Atwood G: Faces in a Cloud: Subjectivity in Personality Theory. New York, Jason Aronson, 1979

Stolorow R, Lachmann F: Psychoanalysis of Developmental Arrests. New York, International Universities Press, 1980

Stolorow R, Brandchaft B, Atwood G: Intersubjectivity in psychoanalytic treatment: with special reference to archaic states. Bull Menninger Clin 47:117–128, 1983

Stolorow R, Brandchaft B, Atwood G: Psychoanalytic Treatment: An Intersubjective Approach. Hillsdale, NJ, Analytic Press, 1987

Sullivan HS: The Interpersonal Theory of Psychiatry. New York, WW Norton, 1953

Volkan VD: Primitive Internalized Object Relations. New York, International Universities Press, 1976

Winnicott D: Collected Papers: Through Paediatrics to Psycho-Analysis. New York, Basic Books, 1958

Winnicott D: The Maturational Processes and the Facilitating Environment. New York, International Universities Press, 1965

16

EDGAR A. LEVENSON, M.D.

INTRODUCTION

Edgar Levenson graduated from the New York University College of Arts and the College of Medicine. He did his psychiatric residency at Bellevue Hospital in New York and his analytic training at the William Alanson White Institute in New York, where he is a Supervising and Training Psychoanalyst. He was Director of the Young Adult Treatment Service at the William Alanson White Institute and Chief Investigator on a National Institute of Mental Health grant for a demonstration clinic for college dropouts. He served as Director of Clinical Services and Chairman of the Council of Fellows of the William Alanson White Institute. Dr. Levenson is a Clinical Professor of Psychology at New York University and was an Associate Clinical Professor at the Albert Einstein College of Medicine. To name but a few of his many awards, he was the first recipient of the William Alanson White Award for Merit, an Honorary Member of the American Psychoanalytic Association, recipient of the Edith Alt Award for Distinguished Service at the William Alanson White Institute, and a Distinguished Life Fellow of the American Psychiatric Association. He has served on the editorial boards of *Contemporary Psychoanalysis, Family Process,* and *The International Journal of Psychoanalytic Psychotherapy.* In addition to his many papers, Dr. Levenson is the author of *The Fallacy of Understanding: an Inquiry Into the Changing Structure of Psychoanalysis, The Purloined Self: Interpersonal Perspectives in Psychoanalysis,* and *The Ambiguity of Change: An Inquiry into the Nature of Psychoanalytic Reality.*

Dr. Levenson has been one of the pioneers of interpersonal psychoanalysis, and his work has been significant in the shift from a one-person to a two-person psychology. He has throughout his career maintained a stance of skepticism toward the clinical relevance of theoretical abstraction and has insisted that therapeutic praxis must be experience driven. Although his views have changed with his experience, he has consistently pointed to the significance of the social context, past and present, in understanding the clinical situation.

WHY I CHOSE THIS PAPER

Edgar A. Levenson, M.D.

I am grateful to the editors for including me in this compendium. "The Pursuit of the Particular: On the Psychoanalytic Inquiry" was first published in 1988, and I have continued to write on aspects of interpersonal psychoanalysis, especially in the realm of that most elusive of holy grails, the praxis. However, this paper seemed to me most representative of my particular version of interpersonalism, and it does contain the seeds of most of my later writings. I also hoped it might be accessible to readers who are less well informed about the interpersonal literature because, alas, psychoanalysts mostly read and reference within their own bailiwick.

I also consulted with several colleagues, most notably Drs. Victor Iannuzzi and Erwin Hirsch, both of whom are often clearer about what I've said than I am. All seemed to concur on what was necessarily a compromise choice.

THE PURSUIT OF THE PARTICULAR

On the Psychoanalytic Inquiry

EDGAR A. LEVENSON, M.D.

IT STARTS SIMPLY ENOUGH. The patient, a divorced man in his forties, is conflicted about taking his preteen daughter on a whitewater rafting trip. The conflict, as he sees it, is not of his making, but caused by the oppositional pulls of his daughter and his live-in womanfriend. He has been with her for almost 2 years, and she is—understandably—increasingly upset with his apparent inability to make up his mind, to marry her or to end the relationship.

Daughter and housemate both are very jealous of his attentions and very competitive; barely tolerating each other on those occasions when he has tried to take them together on vacation. He feels that his daughter's childishness is, at least, age-appropriate; and he resents his womanfriend's importuning and sulking. Although he has already researched possible trips (fairly difficult ones, by the way), he is quite reluctant to raise the issue with Penelope (as I shall call her). Why? Because he wants her to understand and "not mind." How about *not* persuading her, allowing her to be angry, and doing it anyhow? That seemed like a novel idea, his having grown up in a milieu of dreadful reasonableness. His mother was always able to "appeal to his commonsense and good judgment." He was that exemplar of parental coercion, "a reasonable child." And he has become a reasonable adult. It seemed to him, then, uncontestable that a decision should be discussed in an atmosphere of

---

"The Pursuit of the Particular: On the Psychoanalytic Inquiry," by Edgar A. Levenson, M.D., was first published in *Contemporary Psychoanalysis*, 24(1):1–16, 1988.

good will and arrived at by consensus. That there could be a genuine, unreconcilable difference of viewpoint and that life might proceed in the face of the other person's disagreement, and even ill will, seemed to him a novel enterprise. One might reasonably deduce that under his facade of amiability, there would be considerable anger and obstructionism.

On first blush, Penelope *did* seem unreasonable. But there was some faint, ephemeral suggestion that he was enjoying the contretemps. This was not said to him, since it seemed too arbitrary and unsubstantiated a position for me to take, based solely on my impression of an occasional errant glint in his eye, a flash of what I read to be glee. He would have, not unreasonably, heard it as a covert instruction; my championing Penelope's position; namely that there was something hostile and provocative in his behavior.

After this session, he did confront Penelope, firmly informing her that this is what he wished to do; he needed to spend some time alone with his daughter, and if Penelope did really want to go on a whitewater trip, he would go with her alone some other time. To his surprise, she did not protest, or even seem very upset.

That night, he had a dream: He was sitting by the bank of a rapidly flowing river, full of rocks. To his horror, he saw women's bodies, looking quite decomposed, floating down the river. Then he realized the women were alive and that he must do something to pull them out. He awakened in great anxiety.

Since the rushing river was an obvious reference to the forthcoming trip, it was evident to him that some battering of women—real and/or fantasied—was taking place; whether inadvertently or deliberately remained unclear. But, it *was* his dream, ergo *his* perception. It seemed likely, to the analyst, that the dream revealed an unconscious intent; that he was setting up a battle between the two women, causing both of them to lose their composure (to de-compose). This interpretation was made largely to explore the possibility that this is what we might both be thinking, rather than to confront him with an incontestable truth. As Winnicott put it, if one says nothing, the patient gets the impression one understands everything (Winnicott 1965).

I had already learned that Penelope was timid, not very adventurous. He was sure that she would hate a rafting trip. On his first impulse, to invite them both, his fantasy (probably correct) is that she would cower terrified in the bottom of the raft while he and his daughter whooped with joy. Furthermore, he elaborated, she hated any kind of water sport, and would not go swimming at all. She had been a expert swimmer until she'd suffered a head blow in a dive, was knocked semiconscious and nearly drowned. She has a posttraumatic phobia. The idea of being in water over her head terrifies her still, and her current claim to adventurousness seems to be a matter of rivalry besting fear.

Why hadn't he mentioned all this to me before? Didn't he think it might have some bearing on the overdetermination of the present incident? He conceded that this must be so. Again, there was the same glint in his eye, an *augenblick*—something fishy flashing under his agreeable surface. At that point, I remembered—uneasily—that he had, in fact, at one time mentioned it to me; it was not really news that she was terrified of water. Why hadn't *I* remembered that immediately when he mentioned the proposed rafting trip? I had some sense of an unconscious collusion on my part. It did occur to me that I had not myself much love for water or water sports and that whitewater rafting was very low on my list of priorities. I had, indeed, declined to accompany *my* wife on just such a river rafting trip.

Still, something about his choosing this way of spending time with his daughter made me uneasy. There was something preening about it and small-spirited. Couldn't he have found an activity which did not play off against Penelope's fears? On the other hand, why was she so eager to go? Was he supposed to make her fears disappear? Is she competing as a sibling with his daughter? Why was my first response that his motive is disruptive; perhaps that has to do with my competition with him, or my feelings about his doing something that would frighten me. (It is worth noting that while we were discussing his motivations, three white-collar executives were drowned on just such an expedition.) Was he playing off against my feelings? Were we competing? Am I correct about him or is it a countertransferential misreading? Could it not be both?

Since dreams are metaphors, not portents, it is also entirely possible that this dream was more simply reflecting his deeply held conviction that to go against or to deprive a mother substitute was, *a priori,* a murderous act—a fantasy certainly potentiated by Penelope's masochistic stance. Perhaps he would like to kill them both for unnecessarily complicating his life. Or is it that he believes that women would not survive in the mainstream of his potency? Most significantly, why does he have the dream *after* she has agreed, rather amiably, to his going off with his daughter?

It becomes apparent that this simple, commonplace argument with his womanfriend has become far more complicated than first viewing would have suggested. In a word, the surface presentation, the primary text, had been fragmented. Rather than having constructed a plausible or true version of this event, it has been *de*-constructed. Like a pebble dropped in a pond, explicating this singular event has set off a series of recursive horizontal (i.e., into his contemporary space) and vertical (into his history) ripples which now include, not just the patient and his players, but also the analyst. An inquiry which, at first blush, held forth the promise of exposing the "truth" of this man's motives, deteriorates into a series of narrative possibilities, all of which must be true, cannot be untrue, and yet leave us without that satisfying sense of closure—of, "Ah-hah! that's it!"

One might say that the event is "overdetermined" in the classical sense; inasmuch as the singular event is motivated by converging unconscious impulses. This may well be so; but then what is one uncovering, and to what end? Is it a critical underlying dynamic, or the extending reticulating network of relationships inherent in this most commonplace of occurrences?

As the level of complexity rises, as the amount of data increases; the urge to make sense of it, to make coherent information out of raw data becomes overwhelming. Every analyst knows the feeling, the sense of increasing urgency that builds as one listens to the incident. What does it mean? How can it be comprehended? Freud, Sullivan, Kohut, Winnicott dance like visions of sugarplums in the analyst's head.

As any clinical conference will attest, a well explicated case presentation will elicit almost as many clinical perspectives as there are people in the room (assuming a reasonably eclectic audience). It is striking that no one ever seems to have difficulty conceptualizing—from some metapsychological stance—an understanding of the case material, once the extended data is available. Well, as the Sufis like to say, "No problem is too difficult for a theoretician."

Since analysts differ so blatantly in their theoretical formulations, we must assume that our commonality—if it exists at all—must lie in some other area. When we talk theory, we often sound as if we were in entirely different worlds of discourse: when we listen to clinical material, a certain collegiality does emerge.

When observing experienced analysts of different persuasions approach a single clinical presentation, one is struck with their dissatisfaction with the data available. They do *not* immediately lay their metapsychology as a template on the clinical material. Each wants an elaboration of the data, more data, new data, which would reveal a different patient, one created in his/her imagery. Moreover, a Kleinian colleague, whose metapsychology may sound to a pragmatic interpersonalist like sheer phantasmagoria (or is it fantasmagoria?), when presented with clinical material may be nevertheless extremely astute and helpful. Much the same point has been made in Grosskurth's biography of Melanie Klein, wherein a number of prominent analysts (Meltzer,

Segal, Wedeles) describe her as a sensitive and pragmatic observer. To Hyatt Williams, for example, she said, "Simply trust your capacity to listen"—certainly advice Sullivan would have found exemplary (Grosskurth 1986).

What then do they all do in common? *They ask some good questions.* It is my contention that the impulse of the analytic process emerges from just this forcing of data; i.e., the deconstruction of the patient's prepared text, the clinical material, rather than the analyst's explanation of the plethora of data which emerges. I suspect that this is the analytic *vis a tergo,* the driving force, regardless of the metapsychological imagery used. In short, one is not simply collating a lot of information which can then, leisurely, be composed by analyst and patient into a "good story"—one which fulfills their requirement for an aesthetic, plausible and inclusive version of events (Spence 1982). The very act of fragmenting the patient's fictionalized version of his/her life causes anxiety and promotes the transferential carryover. Why this should be so is not so clear to me. The traditional view is that by speaking of that which is supposed to be left unspoken (inattended, repressed), one is pushing *against* the defenses, forcing an enrichment of the defensive surface story, and provoking the transfer of both the content and the defenses into the analyst-patient relationship. But I suspect that what is "repressed" is not so straightforward or linear, and that defenses are not so clear about what they are defending against. It may not be all that reasonable. The very breakdown of narrative order, the temporary chaos which is provoked, may, in itself, be vital to a creative process, a reorganization of experience into far more complex and flexible patterns.

I am claiming that the real task in therapy is *not* so much making sense of the data as it is, but resisting the temptation to make sense of the data! Data, as I am defining it, being either free-associations, fantasy, dreams or carefully formulated interpersonal experience in the Sullivanian mode, the famous "detailed inquiry" (Sullivan 1954)—in all, anything that is subject to interpretation. As Peirce put it, "A sign is something by knowing which we know something more" (Eco 1984, p. 167).

Analysts tend to lean toward either fantasy or relational experience as a primary source of data. It seems likely to me that they both represent vital, but apposite, cognitive functions in the patient, two different ways of experiencing the world. Most analysts work pragmatically within an amalgam of both, at some disregard of their doctrinaire positions. However one conceptualizes data, there remains the crucial debate, in psychoanalytic circles, as to how and why that data works; i.e., whether it is scientifically valid (provable, true, veridical) or whether it is hermeneutically valid (narratively plausibly true, an exercise in interpretation). I find it hard to imagine how psychoanalysis can *not* be hermeneutical. Hermeneutics being, by definition, the study of interpretation. And, since psychoanalysis' primary instrument *is* interpretation, we are all, like it or not, involved in an hermeneutical undertaking.

Can this be true? Don't we distinguish between "insight therapies" and "relational therapies"; i.e., therapies that cure by insight or by relationship (Pulver 1987) ? Hasn't interpretation lost its hegemony in psychoanalysis? Even those therapies which conform to a relational model (using Greenberg and Mitchell's category) must believe that it is the interpretation of what transpires in therapy which specifies psychoanalysis (Greenberg and Mitchell 1983). It is a serious error to confuse the relational model—a structure—with relation*ship*—a psychotherapeutic instrument. To do so is to confuse psychoanalysis with a corrective emotional experience in the context of a benign relational psychotherapy. In that variety of psychotherapy, the patient improves because he/she is having a *de novo* restitutive experience with the therapist. Not a bad thing, in itself, but not psychoanalysis. As Winnicott wrote, "If our aim continues to be to verbalize the nascent conscious in terms of the transference then we are practicing analysis: if not, then we are analysts practicing something else that we deem appropriate to the occasion. And why not?" (Winnicott 1965, pp. 166–167).

The interpretation of what is conceptualized as resistance and transference is the core of the psychoanalytic process, as Freud defined it, and I believe that still remains valid. It is the resistance of the patient, and the partial failure of either insight or restitutive experience, which permits the development and analysis of transference. Psychoanalysis works in the way that psychotherapies fail. By failing to convince, by promulgating disorder, psychoanalysis allows for the development of transference. Putting emphasis on empathic or holding efforts, as do some versions of object relations theory, does not obviate that these efforts are directed toward obtaining regressive material in the therapy, by some version of a forcing inquiry; and is *not,* primarily, a general therapeutic attitude directed toward the patient. To quote Winnicott:

> The advantage of a regression is that it carries with it the opportunity for correction of inadequate adaptation-to-need in the past history of the patient, that is to say, in the patient's infancy management.... Whenever we understand a patient in a deep way and show that we do so *by a correct and well-timed interpretation* (my italics), we are in fact holding the patient and taking part in a relationship in which the patient is in some degree regressed and dependent. (Winnicott 1987, p. 167)[1]

Or, as Goldberg, a self psychologist, put it:

> Only the patient who feels understood will be able to profit from an interpretation about the understanding person i.e., the analyst who is a transference object. Interpretation involves both understanding and explanation. Understanding alone leads to addiction. Explanation alone can lead to compliance. (Goldberg 1987, p. 184)

I chose these two quotes (I don't believe either Sullivan or the Freudians require documentation of this position) to emphasize my point that psychoanalysis is, for all of us, an interpretive discipline, and therefore falls under the rubric of hermeneutics. The question is, what do we mean by interpretation? The answer is not so self-evident.

A brief review of "hermeneutics" supplies some interesting answers, since in contemporary psychoanalytic usage, hermeneutics is perceived in a rather limited way. Hermeneutics, one notes, is named after Hermes, the messenger of the Greek gods. Hermes brought the word of the Gods, usually Apollo, to the oracle at Delphi, who managed to make it more or less intelligible to humankind, but always with an ambiguity which left choice of decision to the supplicant, sometimes—not so unlike psychoanalysis—with disastrous results. King Phillip of Macedon lost his crown and his life when he opted for too optimistic a version of the Delphic utterance. So, interpretation did not make anything clearer, it offered yet another level of meaning.

In its medieval usage, hermeneutics was the instrument of the Church and its function was to reveal the multiple meanings of the canonical writings to its contemporaries; i.e., the focus was on the discovery of textual meaning. To quote Umberto Eco, "*Non nova sed nove*—no new things but the same things—increasingly retold in a new way" (Eco 1984). The authority legitimizes the interpretation. But how can the authority legitimize the interpretation when the authority is legitimized by the interpretation. This paradox is known, in hermeneutic circles, as the hermeneutic circle. Eco states that "The rules for good interpretation were provided by the gatekeepers of the orthodoxy, and the gatekeepers of the orthodoxy were the winners (in terms of political and cultural power) of the struggle to impose their own interpretation" (p. 151). There is in this, at least for psychoanalysts of a certain age, a ring of mournful familiarity.

---

[1]A reading of Margaret Little's account of her analysis with Winnicott suggests that he did not stick very firmly to that position. A great deal went on which seems more relationship than relational (Little 1985).

To quote Brenner, as an example of this first level of hermeneutics, on case material, "Dr S' interventions were guided [quite correctly—EAL] by his understanding of his patient's lifelong problems, problems which were currently active as determinants of her behaviour and associations at the time reported" (Brenner 1987). Period! There is no doubt entertained about what the problems are, or the analyst's accuracy: the task is to make the canonical interpretation mutative, to get it to work.

In this century, first Dilthey, and then Heidegger shifted the hermeneutical emphasis from the discovery of canonical (from the Greek; the rule, the law) truth to the creation of an emergent truth, a mutual truth. "Language is the place where things come authentically to begin (Eco 1984, p. 154)." This second level of hermeneutics is what psychoanalysts ordinarily refer to as "hermeneutical." The therapist and patient create mutually a "good" story; one of many possible combinations and permutations of the data. The story works, not because it is the only truth, but because it is plausible and because it is *their* story, their emergent truth. Spence, as I've said, is the most outspoken proponent of this narrative truth over canonical truth, and so, to a lesser degree, are Schafer and Ricoeur (Ricoeur 1977; Schafer 1976; Spence 1982). Parenthetically, the word, hermeneutics, is not in Spence's index.

Now, to get to my main thesis, there is a third, and more radically secularized hermeneutics called *deconstruction,* to which I have been alluding in the earlier clinical material. "Critical texts must be read in a radically different way, not so much for their interpretive 'insights', as for the symptoms of 'blindness' which mark their conceptual limits" (Norris 1982, p. 23). Or, to quote Eco, "The text does not speak any longer of its own 'outside'; it does not speak even of itself; it speaks of our own experience in reading [deconstructively] it.... The text as symbol is no longer read in order to find in it a truth that lies *outside;* the only truth is the very play of deconstruction" (Eco 1984, pp. 154–155).

Deconstruction is ordinarily associated with Jacques Derrida and his contemporary school of very esoteric criticism (Norris 1982). However, there have existed versions of deconstruction long before his. The most famous being the Jewish mystical movement, the Kabbalah. Let me compare two amusing and brief excerpts, one from the *Zohar,* the thirteenth century kabbalistic scripture, and the other from a contemporary clinical case presentation.

The *Zohar* takes the famous Genesis story of Abraham and Isaac: "and it came to pass the Elohim tested Abraham." The story of Abraham's ordeal is well known. God tested Abraham's faith by requiring the sacrifice of his son, Isaac. The standard exegeses of this story are well known, including Kierkegaard's four different versions of Abraham's leap of faith, his acceptance of the judgment of God and the judgment *as* God's (Kierkegaard 1985). Rabbi Shim'on, in the *Zohar,* takes another tack. He deconstructs the story line by line. Each deconstruction shifts the meaning of the story. The "detailed inquiry," a painstaking historical accounting which would have done Sullivan proud, reveals that—astonishingly—Isaac was no boy, he was already 37 years old! So then Elohim tested Isaac, not Abraham. After all, Isaac did not have to comply. If Isaac had said, "I refuse, " his father could not have been held responsible. Isaac, by his acquiescence, becomes the equal of Abraham. Still, Genesis does say that Elohim tested Abraham, not Isaac. Another level of interpretation takes place. Note that there is no end to the recursive layering of meanings. God has no single meaning. As the *Zohar* says, "There are levels within levels" (Matt 1983, p. 82) and, "In any word shine a thousand lights." Or, as Winnicott so beautifully put it, "Every interpretation is the glittering object which excites the patient's greed" (Clancier et al. 1987).

Now, consider this brief example from a clinical report. The patient, a single young woman, is with considerable embarrassment telling the analyst a sexual fantasy.

> There's a doctor a Mad Scientist and his nurse and he ties me down to—do things to me. The fantasy has to do with—something—it has to do with getting bigger breasts.... The Mad Scientist would do something to give me bigger breasts. I wanted bigger breasts very much.... I had to submit to the Mad Scientist like I was his slave and he was (sic) my master. I try not to think about the fantasy.... I don't want to dig into it....

She then goes on to talk about her master/slave feelings, talking about the fantasy but not really telling it. The analyst says, "You want me to be the Mad Scientist Doctor forcing and hurting you and making changes in you." She denies it. No, she says (with what sounds like injured dignity), "I want you to use your knowledge and your understandings to change me. I have to reject that. I can't agree with you on that" (Silverman 1987).

Note that the patient tells (very guardedly) a fantasy. The therapist interprets in terms of his understanding of transference and dynamics: to wit, this is a transference fantasy—he is the Mad Scientist. His interpretation is consistent with canonical Freudian doctrine. Transference is perceived as a variety of resistance to an insight interpretation. Indeed, Gill says, unequivocally, "All resistance manifests itself by way of transference" (Gill 1982). The interpretation is made to show the patient that she is avoiding insight by projecting the fantasy onto the therapist; ergo, "you see me as the Mad Scientist." This projection protects her from hearing the mutative insight interpretation which would deal with the meaning of the fantasy, presumably her incestuous and sadomasochistic dynamics. Thus insight is the goal, transference is a resistance to insight and must be interpreted away from the therapist and back into the material. The mutative interpretation is not the interpretation of transference, but the interpretation of meaning, which she rejects as a further resistance to insight.

What would Rabbi Shim'on say? How mean is the Mad Scientist if he is giving her what she wants, big breasts? What's so marvelous about big breasts, anyhow? Why breasts, not legs or behind? How will that change her world? Does she believe that men will then be interested in her? Does she want interest, especially on those terms? Does her mother have big breasts? What will the Mad Scientist actually do? Will it hurt? Just what *is* the fantasy? How come if she is so submissive, such a slave, that nothing the analyst says seems to impress her? How is it that, in the transcript, she talks for a while and then says something like, "It makes no sense" or, "I feel sheepish" and then pauses—and virtually each time, the therapist comes forward with an interpretation—which she then proceeds to ignore. Who is controlling whom? The questions proliferate and the clarity decreases; but, for all that, a new sense of vitality enters the exchange.

Now, it appears that the analyst *is* the Mad Scientist. Why? Not because he says so, or theory demands it; but because he *acts* like the Mad Scientist. He is trying to force her to take on something she wants, but will not ask for, get for herself (she could go to a plastic surgeon) or accept gracefully from another person. The analyst has become her invention as much as the obliging Mad Scientist. Note that now transference may be conceived of as their behavior together, not as a distortion projected onto a neutral analyst. His countertransference becomes, not the irritation he admits feeling with her, but his inability to see the extent to which they replay her fantasy. He does not see that every time he ventures an interpretation which is supposed to "work"; he *is* the Mad Scientist, giving her, against her will, what she really wants.

From this perspective, the interaction of patient and therapist is a replay, an isomorphic recreation of the content of her fantasy, occurring as she tells it. It is this remarkable recursive, mirror-image quality of their interaction, which, in my view, gives transference its power, its ability to create a "show and tell" playground. The transference becomes a highly intensified replay of the material under discussion (Levenson 1983). Please note that the transferential replay is in no way simpler or clearer than the fantasy she is presenting. Interpretation still retains an infinity of possibilities.

In both the Kabbalistic story and the second version of the case presentation, the method is essentially deconstructive. The goal is not to arrive at the Truth, nor to create a collaborative narrative, but to open up the text. In Kvarnes and Parloff's (1976) book *A Harry Stack Sullivan Case Seminar,* it is interesting to listen to the participants struggle, at the time, and 25 years later, with, "What did Sullivan do?" It seems to elude them. If one examines what he said, or rather asked, one is struck with how Kabbalistic the method was, the relentless and unfocused questioning. As Ryckoff put it in the *Case Seminar:*

> You can hear Sullivan pinning you down—"Do you know this? What happened then?" He keeps pinning you down all the time. It would make me leery of sticking my neck out to make a broader generalization based on an intuitive sense of what was going on. Because then he would say, "Where the hell is your data?" (Kvarnes and Parloff 1976, p. 38)

All psychoanalysts would agree, for different reasons perhaps, that the patient's surface presentation is riddled with blind spots, inattentions, scotomata, is indeed a veritable swiss cheese of avoidances—all out of anxiety. Any inquiry which threatens to focus that which is left out will certainly mobilize defenses, which traditionally, as I've said, are understood to take the form of transference (Gill 1982). What is avoided is, by no means, necessarily a single underlying dynamic: defenses can operate just as well against a mosaic of dynamic implications. Note that in the example of the Mad Scientist fantasy, one does not arrive at "The Meaning" of the fantasy, but rather at its relevance, its subtle harmonic resonance throughout her life, which not unlike psychoanalysis, is not so straightforward. I trust that this formulation of defense is loose enough to allow for different versions of defenses and what is defended against; and, that we might agree that any therapeutic effort which did not mobilize this tension would be foredoomed. This is not what seems implied in the version of a "good story" arrived at mutually as Spence would have it, by suggesting that "unpacking," or "glossing" the patient's text is in the service of constructing a mutually satisfying narrative truth (Spence 1982). To repeat, I am stating exactly the opposite; namely, that the forcing of data is to deconstruct the story, to create a chaotic flux of meanings, from which new meanings may emerge, forged in a transferential crucible of considerable tension.

From my position, those meanings would be endlessly recursive, a hall of mirrors. However, it is inconceivable that, in any psychoanalysis, data could emerge that any one of the present crop of metapsychologies could not satisfactorily encompass. Can one imagine a Kohutian, a Sullivanian, a Winnicottian listening to a clinical report, scratching his/her head and saying, "I don't know what to make of that?" Metapsychologies of any subtlety supply both an explanatory context for present behavior and a developmental framework. Clearly, we cannot establish the superiority of any theory *qua* theory over another, or we would not be in our present state of disarray. They all fail to pass Popper's test of falsifiability (Popper 1959). They cannot be shown to be wrong, so they cannot be shown to be right. All one can say of a theory is that it is elegant, parsimonious, and internally consistent. What we can—and frequently do—claim for our theories are superior clinical relevance, better results, "cures" of superior substance. These, alas, must largely be taken on faith.

If metapsychologies cannot be challenged as theory, and clinical results are very difficult to quantify or prove, what are we left with? There are a wide diversity of clinical positions held by analysts of high repute. For every Kohutian claim of success, there is a Freudian who attributes the alleged cure to "unanalyzed positive transference." Even in one's own clinical experience, it is very difficult to assess results. Perhaps the patient improved for some reason other than one's theoretical posture.

Moreover, I suspect one really only learns well one way of doing therapy. Is it possible really to accumulate sufficient analysis, supervision, and didactic course training to master more than one way of working? Grasping the concepts is one thing, acquiring the clinical skills inherent in two different and incompatible perspectives of treatment may be near impossible. To paraphrase Heraclitus, one never lies down on the same couch twice!

Ultimately, one's choice of metapsychological posture may well be idiosyncratic—one does what suits one best. And, for the very same reason, what often at first works as a powerful therapeutic device rapidly deteriorates into an obstreperous countertransference as the therapist, enthralled with his/her own metapsychology, falls victim to that most insidious and seductive of temptations, "manipulating the transference." Clinical data remains the only viable antidote to an overdose of metapsychology.

People come to analysts for all sorts of reasons; to get better, to prove they are unlovable, to destroy the power of the analyst, or their mates or parents (the malevolent transformation)—even to perfect their neuroses. Paying fees and coming on time does not a patient make. It takes a great deal of mobilization to change the novitiate into a patient, and that mobilization comes from the inquiry. Metapsychology applied to a non-patient flakes off like oil paint applied to an unprimed canvas.

It is in supervision, that thorny metapraxis, that these issues become most clear. Supervisors are often selected by candidates at analytic institutes because of their theoretical positions: e.g., one goes to "Doctor A" to work on the uses of counter-transference. Yet, "A" often finds that not enough is going on in the observed therapy to demonstrate his/her particular interests.

I think it a reasonable axiom of supervision that a puzzled or immobilized analyst is an analyst with insufficient data in hand. This is not necessarily, as it is often presented, a matter of countertransference, but may be a consequence of characterological resistances to change which antedate the development of transference. To repeat, I am suggesting (or, reminding) that transference is a consequence of a pressured inquiry. It is not a general manifestation of a character defense (every difficulty the patient puts in the way of change), but a specific reaction to the therapist provoked by the inquiry. Once a transference has been developed, *then* it might reasonably be claimed that countertransference is what one does not think to ask: what is "inattended."

Novice analysts usually have no difficulty whatever making very sophisticated assessments of data fed to them. Most people on a post-doctoral level can conceptualize well enough theoretically. Any senior analyst who doubts this has never presented his/her own case material to a class of junior colleagues. What distinguishes the virtuoso performer from the beginner, in this field, is not metapsychological sophistication—which is often no more than locker-room expertise—but the ability to make a patient move, *work!*

In summary, I am positing that, however construed, for all of us the enrichment and deconstruction of the patient's story is our most powerful instrumentality. Even those analysts who pursue that Will o' the Wisp, the mutative interpretation, must begin with a free-associative deconstruction. It is not, *per se,* psychoanalysis, but it is the absolute precondition for psychoanalysis. To use an analogy, it is like the water that turns the millstone, to grind the grain. Albeit metapsychology grinds exceedingly fine, it is still the containment of the analytic milieu and the pressure of the inquiry which provides the force to turn the wheels. One can easily observe the dissipation of that force when acting-out occurs, when the frame is violated. The therapy grinds to a stop, like the mill with a broken dam. Psychoanalysis proper is the analysis of resistance and transference; but transference, however strictly or loosely defined, is not an automatic benediction of sitting in the same room with a patient, of having the patient's character structure impinge on you. It is a consequence of the pressure of the inquiry. The transference is not a slice of life; it is a highly intensified, isomorphic version of what the patient is exploring.

The Kabbalists say that the mystery of God lies in the particular. I am suggesting that the "mystery" (the secret core) of psychoanalysis also lies in the pursuit of the particular, and the peculiar deconstructed mosaic of data (not a coherent narrative) which emerges, whether presented in the form of fantasy, free-association, or Sullivan's "detailed inquiry." The common denominator among experienced psychoanalysts of widely divergent doctrinary beliefs, may well be the ability to elicit sufficient data, under sufficient pressure, to allow psychoanalysis to take place at all. As Masud Khan said, "We are all the servants of the patient's process" (Khan 1969). Our diversity in metapsychology may be less important than our common ability to mobilize—indeed *capture*—that healing process in the patient. What that healing process is is far from clear. Change comes in mysterious ways, perhaps better chronicled by William James and James Joyce, than by analysts. I do believe that psychoanalytic change does not arrive by the construction of a coherent narrative, nor a corrective emotional experience, nor by way of the "Rumplestiltskin" fallacy—i.e., cure that comes by naming the name, nailing down the "right" dynamic.

All we can do, and it's a great deal, is set the stage for change. To repeat, my therapeutic algorithm consists of a fixed and contained frame, a deconstructive inquiry which potentiates defenses and leads to a much augmented version of the patient's operations in the relationship with the therapist. It is there that the working-through takes place; for me not a simple clarification of dynamics, but a very complex, analogic experience which we can comment on, but never fully grasp conceptually. It is not that I believe that metapsychology is irrelevant, or that it is not important for the analyst to have an ontological belief system. Certainly no one operates in a metapsychological vacuum. Nor would I deny that I must have (as Greenberg has pointed out) my own pervasive premises about what really matters developmentally and in adult life (Greenberg 1987). I am *not* removing metapsychology from psychoanalysis. I *am* saying that I don't believe it is the motivating power of psychoanalysis, but rather a spectrum of metaphors for capturing and containing the imploding force of the deconstructive inquiry. It is an effort to make sense of what is happening; and, it is just this "making sense" that I am against. To tolerate the fragmentation of meaning is to create new meaning. I am convinced, to pursue my analogy, that getting the wheels turning is ultimately far more important than what one grinds.

REFERENCES

Brenner C: A structural theory perspective. Psychoanalytic Inquiry 7:167–171, 1987

Clancier A, Kalmanovitch J: Winnicott and Paradox. London, Tavistock, 1987, p 66

Eco U: Semiotics and the Philosophy of Language. Bloomington, Indiana University Press, 1984, p 150

Gill M: Analysis of Transference, Vol I. New York, International Universities Press, 1982, p 29

Goldberg A: A Self Psychology Perspective. Psychoanalytic Inquiry 7:181–187, 1987

Greenberg J: Of mystery and motive. Contemp Psychoanal 23:689–704, 1987

Greenberg J, Mitchell M: Object Relations in Psychoanalytic Theory. Cambridge, MA, Harvard University Press, 1983

Grosskurth P: Melanie Klein. New York, Alfred A Knopf, 1986, pp 449–450

Khan M: Introduction, in The Hands of the Living God: An Account of a Psychoanalytic Treatment. Edited by Milner M. New York, International Universities Press, 1969, p xxxi

Kierkegaard S: Fear and Trembling. Harmondsworth, UK, Penguin, 1985

Kvarnes R, Parloff G: A Harry Stack Sullivan Case Seminar. New York, WW Norton, 1976, p 38

Little M: Winnicott working in areas where psychotic anxieties predominate: a personal record. Free Associations 3:9–42. London, Free Association Books, 1985

Levenson E: The Ambiguity of Change. New York, Basic Books, 1983

Matt DC: Zohar, The Book of Enlightenment. New York, Paulist Press, 1983, p 72

Norris C: Deconstruction, Theory and Practice. New York, Methuen, 1982

Popper K: The Logic of Scientific Discovery. London, Hutchinson, 1959

Pulver S: Epilogue. Psychoanalytic Inquiry 7:289–299, 1987

Ricoeur P: Freud and Philosophy. New Haven, CT, Yale University Press, 1970

Schafer R: A New Language for Psychoanalysis. New Haven, CT, Yale University Press, 1976

Silverman M: Clinical Material. Psychoanalytic Inquiry 7:147–165, 1987

Spence D: Narrative Truth and Historical Truth. New York, WW Norton, 1982

Sullivan HS: The Psychiatric Interview. New York, WW Norton, 1954

Winnicott DW: The aims of psychoanalytic treatment, in The Maturational Process and the Facilitating Environment. New York, International Universities Press, 1965, p 167

Winnicott DW: Holding and Interpretation. New York, Grove Press, 1987, p 192

17

LESTER LUBORSKY, PH.D.

INTRODUCTION

Lester Luborsky is a graduate of Pennsylvania State University and received his Ph.D. in Psychology from Duke University. He received his psychoanalytic training and did research at the Menninger Foundation in Topeka, Kansas. He has spent most of his professional career at the School of Medicine of the University of Pennsylvania, where he has been Professor of Psychology in Psychiatry since 1968. He is the author of over 400 publications and the winner of numerous awards, including the American Psychological Foundation Gold Medal Award for Lifetime Achievement in the Applications of Psychology, the Mary S. Sigourney Award for Contributions to the Field of Psychoanalysis, the Distinguished Research Career Award from the Society for Psychotherapy Research, the Distinguished Scientific Contribution Award from Division 12 of the American Psychological Association, and the American Psychoanalytic Association Award for Distinguished Psychoanalytic Theory and Research. He has been an important member of the governing bodies of many national organizations as well as visiting professor at numerous medical schools.

Dr. Luborsky has engaged in a range of research that demonstrates the validity of conducting empirical research on psychoanalytic propositions and the feasibility of doing research in analytic settings. He is a pioneer in developing ways to measure psychoanalytic concepts. He has authored a manual to operationalize supportive-expressive treatment methods, which derive from psychoanalytic principles. His innovative measures include the Core Conflictual Relationship Theme (CCRT) method, the Symptom-Context method, measurements of the adequacy of the therapist's response to the patient's communication, measurement of the patient-therapist match, and rating scales for patient improvement.

Dr. Luborsky led an extraordinary range of investigations and development of techniques in perception, personality, addiction, psychosomatics, psychotherapy, and psychoanalytic research. A few examples include the development of a reliable psychological health-sickness scale, now known as the Global Assessment Scale; measures of accuracy of interpretation in psychotherapy; demonstration of the contribution of psychotherapy to usual drug counseling and methadone maintenance for opiate addicts; the first validation of the central concept of transference (i.e., the patient's relationship to the therapist parallels the patient's general relationship pattern); and numerous studies of the validity of the CCRT.

In response to my request for a statement about himself, Luborsky responded with the following:

> My work has been extremely influential, with a career spanning over 60 years and with more than 400 publications. My long-term involvement has been with the construction of new measures and manuals, now 36 of them. Among my discoveries are 27 "firsts," such as the first objective measure of the transference, the CCRT methods, the first controlled symptom-context study (from which I developed the Symptom-Context method), the first observer-rated health-sickness scale measure, and the first helping-alliance observer-judged measure. Because of my contributions, I've received various awards related to the field—major awards include the Research Scientist Award of NIMH and NIDA for 31 years, Distinguished Professional Contribution Award of the American Psychological Association, and the Sigourney Award for Contribution to Psychoanalysis.

WHY I CHOSE THIS PAPER

Lester Luborsky, Ph.D.

This paper, "A Relationship Pattern Measure: The Core Conflictual Relationship Theme," is one of the first introductions of the CCRT method to the field. It was published in *Psychiatry,* a journal with mass appeal not only in the psychological field but in the scientific field in general, and it has been cited by other major contributors to the field. This article is of particular importance because the study of the CCRT helps to assess transference patterns, Freud's grandest concept. By using this method, we not only learn about the patient's interpersonal conflicts but also about his or her intrapersonal conflict as well and how the patient translates this interrelationship schema to his or her interactions with the therapist. The relationship conflicts of the patients can be quantified and extrapolated from therapy sessions. This method not only is significant for research but also has many implications for the clinical environment. Also, by isolating the particular conflicts, we can examine their relations to other factors. An example of a commonly studied factor in relation to the CCRT is symptom formation, which has led to more discoveries and has aided in psychosomatic research. Overall, it is crucial to understand the patient's underlying schemas for relationship conflicts in order to correct them.

A RELATIONSHIP PATTERN MEASURE

The Core Conflictual Relationship Theme

LESTER LUBORSKY, PH.D.

PAUL CRITS-CHRISTOPH, PH.D.

RELATIONSHIP PATTERN MEASURES ARE recently developed systems for measuring the main relationship patterns expressed in psychotherapy sessions or in other interviews. They are precise measures of the kind of pattern that dynamic psychotherapists have estimated clinically ever since the start of such therapies. This paper will a) describe a relationship pattern measure b) illustrate it, and then c) compare it with one or more other relationship pattern measures. Beyond these purposes our aim is to indicate the values of these new methods for personality and psychotherapy research.

A dozen of these measures have appeared at an exponential rate since 1976, and this outpouring reflects both clinical and research needs

---

Paul Crits-Christoph is Professor of Psychology in Psychiatry and Director, Center for Psychotherapy Research, University of Pennsylvania, Philadelphia, PA.

This research was supported in part by National Institute of Mental Health grant R01 MH39673, Research Scientist Award MH40710 (L.L.), the Fund for Psychoanalytic Research of the American Psychoanalytic Association, and the Program on Conscious and Unconscious Mental Processes at the University of California, San Francisco, sponsored by the John D. and Catherine T. MacArthur Foundation.

for them. They are listed here in order of year of appearance: Luborsky (1976), CCRT; M. Horowitz (1979), Configurational Analysis; Teller and Dahl (1981), Frame Method; Carlson (1981), Script Method; Gill and Hoffman (1982), Patient's Experience of Relationship with Therapist; L. Horowitz et al. (1983), Consensual Response Formulation; Schacht et al. (1984), Dynamic Focus; Grawe and Caspar (1984), Plan Analysis; Weiss and Sampson (1986), Plan Diagnosis; Bond and Shevrin (1986, unpublished), Clinical Evaluation Team; Perry (1986), Idiographic Conflict Summary; Maxim (1989), Seattle Psychotherapy Language Analysis Schema.

One of the best known versions of a central relationship pattern is the transference pattern, which when identified serves to guide the therapist's techniques in psychodynamic psychotherapies (Luborsky 1984). At least for the Core Conflictual Relationship Theme (CCRT) measure, there are cogent parallels between Freud's (1912) observations about the "transference template" and the observations from the CCRT (Luborsky et al. 1986, 1988).

Because so many of these measures are rapidly becoming available, it is important to begin the process of comparison among them. In fact, as yet there are still no published comparisons among the measures. Within the set of papers presented here, these five measures are compared: the CCRT, the Role Relationship Models, the Dynamic Focus or Cyclical Maladaptive Patterns (CMP), the Idiographic Conflict Formulation (ICF) and the Plan Diagnosis (PD). For each comparison the CCRT is included. Each of the five methods has some aspects in common with the others; the most common shared element is the presence of a wish type of component. There was no special selection factor that led to comparisons among the five discussed in this set rather than among some of the others, beyond the availability of a proponent of the method to do the work of the comparative study. One other method has been included in a comparison study—the Patient's Experience of the Relationship with the Therapist (PERT) (Gill and Hoffman 1982), which has been compared with the CCRT by Kächele et al. (1988). The paired comparisons showed the formulations from the two methods to be moderately similar.

The listing of these new methods includes only those methods with a guided clinical judgment and quantitative content analysis system for making inferences about the pattern based on psychotherapy sessions or on other forms of interviews. See also the broader review by Singer and Salovey (1991). Not covered in the list is the large area of research on estimating the main relationship pattern by questionnaire methods, which mainly had its heyday from 1955 to 1976. This material has been reviewed elsewhere (Luborsky et al. 1986), and its clinical applicability has been more limited than the methods we are about to review.

PERSPECTIVES ON THE CCRT

This paper will give an account of the Core Conflictual Relationship Theme method (CCRT) (Luborsky 1976, 1977) and will provide a case example of its application. The CCRT is the oldest of the genre of relationship pattern measures applied to sessions. It has benefited from a concerted effort at psychometric development, although much more remains to be done (Luborsky and Crits-Christoph [1990]). The purpose of this account is to facilitate a comparison with a closely related method, called Role-Relationship Models (RRM), which is a sector of the Configurational Analysis Method (Horowitz 1979, 1987). That method overlaps in one aspect with the CCRT but is much broader—for example, as its name implies, it assesses role-relationship models. A companion paper on RRM follows this one, including a description of that relationship pattern method and a comparison with the CCRT as applied to the same patient's psychotherapy sessions. The comparison paper will point out the assets and liabilities of each method so that prospective users of the methods can make an informed choice in attempting to meet the requirements of different types of applications.

CCRT METHOD AND SOME OF ITS THEORETICAL BASES

The procedures of the method follow the CCRT Guide (Luborsky, Edition of 3/27/85; Luborsky and Crits-Christoph, in preparation). The method is an assessment system for reliably drawing inferences about relationship patterns from relationship narratives. These narratives are parts of sessions in which the patient spontaneously presents episodes about relationships, hence they will be referred to as "relationship episodes" or "REs." A minimum of 10 REs is a desirable number to provide a basis for deriving the CCRT. The steps in the CCRT method were chosen because they represent a kind of formalization of the inference process used by clinicians in adducing transference patterns. Within each RE, the CCRT judge makes inferences about types of: a) wishes, needs and intentions, b) responses from other, and c) responses from the self. Then, to be sure the inferences are being made at the most appropriate level, the same judge goes through the process a second time and redraws the inferences. The final CCRT is an assemblage of the most frequent types of wishes and responses across all the REs.

These are the basic assumptions of the theory as they are reflected in the method:

1. *The data base:* A basic assumption is that a rich data base from which to infer the CCRT relationship patterns arises from narratives about episodes in relationships as well as from enactments during the session of relationships with the therapist.
2. *The categories:* It is an integral assumption that the CCRT consistently covers two broad classes of components: a) wishes, needs, and intentions in relation to another person, and b) consequences of two kinds, responses from the other person and responses from the self. This division into two components may roughly correspond with Freud's duality of id impulses versus ego functions or, in more modern language, the dimensions of motives and drives versus control and executive functions. The output of the method contains aspects that are related to self schemas as well as to self-other schemas.
3. *The reliance on frequency* (i.e., redundancy across narratives): The CCRT relies heavily on the frequency of the specific types of each of its three kinds of components: the wish directed toward the other person and the two varieties of responses, from the other person and from the self. The CCRT's core is based on the types of components with the greatest frequency. Greater frequency is assumed to indicate greater centrality within the relationship schema. Frequency probably corresponds fairly well to intensity, as discussed in Murray (1938) for the scoring system for the TAT.
4. *The level of inference:* The level of the inferences from the narrative data about the types of each component varies from superficial (in a nonpejorative sense)—that is, close to the patient's statements—to moderately inferential. It is an important assumption that the "moderately inferential" inferences are essential because they more readily generalize across narratives and therefore form a large part of the final CCRT.
5. *The stability of the theme:* The CCRT method guides the delineation of a relationship pattern that has considerable evidence for its stability over time as demonstrated empirically (Luborsky et al. 1985).
6. *The inclusion of conflicts within the theme:* It is a basic assumption that a good relationship pattern measure should include the central relationship conflicts. The CCRT is expressed in a format that reflects two main classes of conflicts: those between wishes and those between wishes and the responses of other and the self.
7. *The inclusion of the symptoms among the Responses from Self:* An assumption that is built into the format for the CCRT is that the symptoms are classed as Responses from Self. Therefore the symptoms are often helpfully understood within the context of the CCRT and in part as a product generated by this context. As the case example

will illustrate, a wish might be experienced as running up against a frightening response from another person that makes one feel helpless, and the conflict might contribute to the development of a symptom, as hypothesized in Freud's (1926) theory.

CASE ILLUSTRATION

The data for the illustration of the method are transcripts of a time-limited (24 weekly sessions) psychoanalytic psychotherapy of Mr. A, a patient with a social phobia.

At the time of the therapy Mr. A was in his early 30s. He was the middle child of a professional father and a homemaker mother and had been married for several years. His wife was a partner in their small design firm. He entered psychotherapy with the hope of overcoming moderately severe agoraphobic symptoms that were interfering with his work and marriage. At the start of psychotherapy he was anxious and phobically restricted about air travel, highway travel, unfamiliar restaurants, and related situations. (For a more detailed description, see Horowitz 1989.)

In order to compare the CCRT and the RRM, our Pennsylvania group and Horowitz's San Francisco group independently applied their measures to the same transcripts of videotaped psychotherapy sessions, Sessions 4 and 17.

RESULTS

The CCRT Method With Tailor-made Categories

There are two main methods of categorizing inferences from sessions: the tailor-made and the ready-made (or standard) categories to be described later). The usual CCRT scoring system is called tailor-made because the judge tries to derive categories of inferences that have the best fit with the data from each patient's sessions. The categories do not have to fit other patients but need fit only the particular patient under investigation.

For the CCRT analysis of Mr. A three independent judges did the analysis on the relationship episodes of two sessions. A sample of 5 REs of the 10 REs is given in Table 1. The results of the analysis are given in Table 2. Since the CCRT is based on the highest frequency of each, the frequencies in Table 2 are listed in order of average frequency from most to least. For examples, for Judge L the wish, need, or intention is "to

TABLE 17–1. Precis of first five relationship episodes (RE) (Session 17)

RE 1 *Wife*	I didn't go on the trip with wife and partner. Feel I've failed. I couldn't push self to go, so I blame self. Also I'm using my fear as a weapon.
RE 2 *Therapist*	I was uncomfortable since we spoke last session. We spoke of developing my own pace. But then the session ended at 60 minutes! I felt a quick temper and suspiciousness of you for ending it then.
RE 3 *Father*	I relied on father's interpretation of what to do, but sometimes he didn't know what he was talking about. He said, to succeed, wear suits and ties. I was angry and confronted him. I didn't feel bad about what I said to him.
RE 4 *Fiancée*	The girl I almost married in college had a distinct concept of the role I was supposed to play in her life. It was the reason our relationship fell apart and I got out of it. It was the time in my life when I started feeling ill in restaurants so I stopped going. My work was a constant battle about what I was supposed to do.
RE 5 *Father*	I was living out what father taught us about success and careers. It is hard to rebel against father. The idea of "rebellion and trying to prove to him I can succeed" is a hard idea to hold on to. I'm scared of saying "I don't believe what you said"—it would be hurting him. He'd feel he'd failed because I'm in treatment.

carry on in my own way; to oppose pressures to do things from those who I am close to; to stand up against them," and this wish appears in 7 out of the 10 REs found in the two sessions (5 REs were found in each session); for Judge M, the wish is "to do what I want without giving in to the wishes of the other person"; for Judge P the wish is "to stand up for what I want with others; to not go along with wishes of other." It is impressive by inspection alone that each of the three judges has made similar inferences about the types of each component.

The Tailor-Made CCRT: Agreement of Judges by Paired Comparisons

But what is "impressive by inspection" may not be so to the relentless researcher whose wish is to know exactly how much is really similar. To satisfy this wish we relied on a paired comparisons method in which each formulation by each judge is compared with the formulation of the other judges on the same case as well with formulations from other cases. This method is similar to the "agreement judge" system in Levine

TABLE 17–2. Patient A: CCRT for three judges using tailor-made categories from relationship episodes (REs) in Sessions 4 and 17

Judge L	RE[a]	Judge M	RE[a]	Judge P	RE[a]
Wish 1					
To carry on in my own way; to oppose pressures from those I am close to.	7	To do what I want without giving in to others' wishes.	8	To stand up for what I want; to not go along with others' wishes.	9
Wish 2					
To please and not hurt the other.	4	To not hurt the others, so I try to live up to their expectations for me.	4	To be close to others: to communicate and share.	6
Negative response from other					
Control me, pressure me, expect me to conform to their ideas.	6	Constrains me, cuts me off.	4	Unreceptive	3
		Expects me to do things his way.	3	Doesn't understand me.	3
				Leaves me	3
Negative response from self					
Feels helpless.	5	Angry, frustrated, resentful.	7	Not able to assert self, go along with others.	6
Phobic symptoms (anxiety, etc.)	4	Nervous, upset, anxious.	5	Anxious.	5
Self-blame.	4				
Positive response from other					
Supportive and reassuring.	5	Accepting, nonjudgmental.	2	Understands me.	1
				Likes me.	1
				Receptive.	1
Positive response from self					
Assertive, fight other's ideas.	4	In control, not anxious.	3	Do something about what I want (assert self).	4

[a]The number of REs that show the CCRT category.

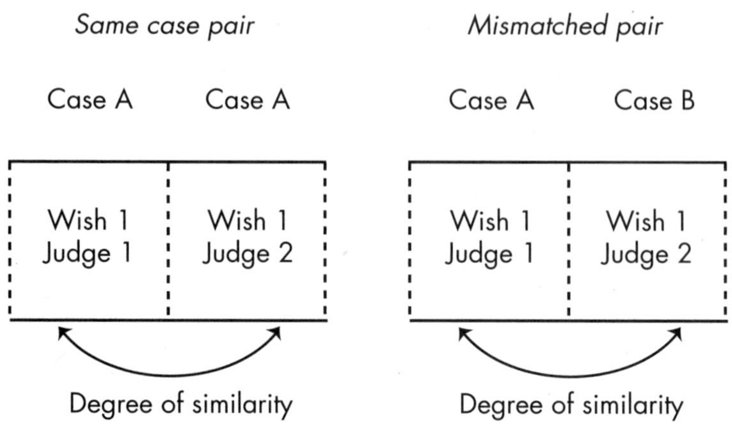

FIGURE 17–1. Diagram of paired comparisons method for determining degree of similarity.

and Luborsky (1981) and in Luborsky et al. (1985). The paired comparisons method provides information on the difference in the levels of similarity of the tailor-made categories for the same-case pairs versus those for the mismatched pairs. This method (see Figure 1) is especially suitable for dealing with tailor-made categories; we cannot use the more conventional reliability methods for such categories.

To describe the method in more detail as it was applied to Mr. A's sessions: In addition to the CCRT formulations obtained on this case by each of the three judges, four other CCRTs randomly selected from other cases were used for comparison purposes. Each of the seven CCRT's was paired with all the others, making a total of 21 pairs. The agreement judges rated the similarity for each pair using a 1 to 7 rating scale (1=completely different, 7=completely identical). The agreement judges, of course, were blind about which cases each CCRT came from.

The intraclass correlation coefficient (pooled judges) was used for assessing the agreement of judges on their similarity ratings. It was calculated to be .73. The agreement judges' ratings were then combined, and the average of the three "same-case" CCRT pairings was compared to the average similarity of the three CCRT formulations for the phobia case paired with the CCRTs from "mismatched" cases. The mean similarity for the same-case pairings was 5.5; for the mismatched-case pairing it was 2.8 (the means are significantly different at $P<0.01$ level by paired t-test). Therefore, we have shown by this method that judges agree with each other significantly more when the formulation by each judge is compared with the formulation of the other judges on the same case than when the pair includes formulations from different cases.

The Standard Categories CCRT

The provision of the set of uniform standard categories within which all inferences can fit should increase the reliability of the CCRT scoring, both for the agreement of different judges wish each other and the agreement of one judge with himself from occasion to occasion. We recommend a combination of both tailor-made and standard categories systems: The judge should consult the standard category list after the usual CCRT tailor-made scoring and select categories that are most similar to each one derived from the tailor-made system.

The standard category list, derived empirically, is based on 16 cases (Luborsky, Edition #1, 6/10/85). The CCRTs for all patients in the normative group are derived from psychotherapy sessions. All of the patients were in long-term psychotherapy: 10 in psychoanalytic psychotherapy and 6 in psychoanalysis. The set is an assemblage of those categories that best describe the core theme components expressed in the REs of the sample of 16 patients. The categories are organized logically, psychologically, and conveniently for ease of application by the judge.

Some of the standard categories are similar to those in the Thematic Apperception Test (TAT), according to the scoring categories of Murray (1938) and Aron (1949). We did not deliberately try to make categories that were the same as those in the TAT, but some of the similarity results from the use of narratives about relationships in both the CCRT and the TAT.

The basic characteristics of the CCRT standard categories are as follows:

1. These categories are the ones that most frequently fit the REs of the cases in the normative set of 16 nonpsychotic patients in psychodynamically oriented psychotherapy.
2. The categories are readily discriminable from each other, i.e., an attempt was made to keep them from overlapping each other.
3. The adjectives used within each category description are synonymous, or nearly so.
4. The order of the list of categories for each of the three CCRT components in somewhat similar; where possible, the category with the highest mean frequency is presented first. This organizational principle is intended to ease the judge's task in finding a particular category.
5. The same words are used for the same type of category for each of

the three components. For example, Wish: To reject the other's *domination;* Response of Other: *Dominates;* Response of Self: Feels *dominated.*

Instructions for applying the standard categories: 1) For each RE, the judge first applies his or her own tailor-made inferences and then chooses the standard categories that fit these inferences best. The selections are made from the list of categories for each of the three components. 2) It is desirable for the judge to give two choices if two are reasonably fitting. However, only one is to be given if the second would be far-fetched. Sometimes no category is reasonably applicable since the standard list is not comprehensive. 3) It is valuable to rate the degree of applicability of each category scored.

Results with the standard categories for Mr. A: The judges tended to agree in their selection of categories (Table 3). For the wish component of the CCRT, all three judges selected two categories about equally and with higher frequency than other categories (mean of the three judges). These two wishes were closely related in meaning: 1) To assert one's independence and autonomy. 2) To overcome other's domination; to be free of obligations imposed by others. Other categories, conceptually less related to the main ones, were selected by the three judges with slightly lower frequencies: 1) To achieve, be competent, be successful. 2) To please the other person. 3) To get help, care, protection and guidance from others. Two judges selected the same most frequent negative response from other: dominating, controlling, interfering, intimidating, intruding. For positive response from other, all three judges selected "accepting, approving" most frequently: For the negative response from self, "anxious, tense, upset" was selected most frequently by all three judges. For the positive response from self, the category "assertive, express self assertively, gain control" was selected with highest frequency by all three judges.

Comparison of Mr. A's Tailor-made CCRT with Standard Categories CCRT

When we compare the same judges' selections of standard categories with their own tailor-made categories for Mr. A, we find first that the two main types of standard category wishes are clearly represented in the two main types of tailor-made wishes. The wish that is most obviously the same in both methods is the tailor-made "to oppose" (Judge L), "to do what I want without giving in" (Judge M), "to stand up for what I want with others" (Judge P). All three of these appear to be similar to the most prevalent wish in the standard categories, "To overcome other's domination; to be free of obligations imposed by others; to not be put down by others."

TABLE 17–3. Patient A: CCRT for three judges using standard categories from 10 relationship episodes (REs) in Sessions 4 and 17

		Judges		
		L	M	P
		RE[a]	RE[a]	RE[a]
Assertive, independent wishes				
1	To assert my independence and autonomy	7	7	10
1a	To overcome other's domination; to be free of obligations imposed by others; to not be put down by others	7	7	9
1b	To achieve, be competent, be successful	5	4	4
Submissive, dependent wishes				
2	To please the other person; to avoid hurting the other person	4	4	2
3	To get help, care, protection and guidance from the other person	4	3	5
Negative responses				
Other:	Dominating, controlling, interfering, intimidating, intruding	6	5	3
Self:	Anxious, tense, upset	5	7	10
	Helpless, less confident, ineffectual ("I do not know how to do things")	5	5	8
	Frustrated	2	6	4
	Angry, resentful, hating	2	5	5
Positive responses				
Other:	Accepting, approving	3	2	2
Self:	Assertive, express self assertively, gain control	4	5	6
	Gain self-esteem, feel affirmed, self-confident	3	4	4

[a]The number of REs that show the CCRT category.

The standard and tailor-made methods' results are also similar to each other for the responses from other and responses from self, with only a few exceptions.

DISCUSSION

In the course of applying the CCRT method to Mr. A's psychotherapy sessions, we found that when three independent judges used the CCRT in its usual tailor-made form, they agreed with each other considerably. Their good level of agreement is consistent with our reliability studies

(Crits-Christoph et al. 1988; Luborsky et al. 1986). Furthermore, the interjudge agreement was even more obvious after the judges translated their CCRTs into standard categories (Luborsky et al. 1985).

The formulations from the CCRT can help in the understanding of relationship conflicts that are important in symptom formation, especially for patients like Mr. A, who have obvious recurrent symptoms.

Our CCRT methods suggest that the patient's social phobic symptoms can be understood as a resultant of the conflict between opposed wishes. The more expressed type of wish (part of the assertive wishes in Table 3) is in conflict with another, simultaneous but less often expressed type of wish (part of the submissive wishes in Table 3). This clash of simultaneously experienced, opposed wishes may set the stage for the appearance of the phobic symptoms. The social phobia could also be a resultant of another direction of conflict: that between the potential expression of these opposed wishes and the responses from other and self, especially responses from other.

Although it is commonplace for clinicians to suspect that psychological conflicts spawn symptoms, rarely are systematic methods used to examine this interaction. The CCRT methods can assist in any such examination. Other researchers are also attempting to delineate the relationship conflicts and their possible connection to the symptoms. Some of the systematic methods are even simpler than our own, such as the one being developed by L. Horowitz (1983), based on a relationship problem questionnaire whose results are correlated with the patient's symptoms. We look forward to comparing his questionnaire method with our own methods.

In trying to surmise what new realms of application might be profitable to inspect, we recognize that thus far we have relied on only one kind of contemporary psychodynamic psychology. It emphasizes the centrality of a) "understanding intentionality [i.e., wishes] from the point of view of the person" (Klein 1970), and b) understanding the consequences (i.e., responses) to these intentions in relation to others and to the self. We might progress in our search if we expanded our perspective by engaging in comparisons with versions of contemporary nondynamic psychology—for example, Kelly's (1955) analysis of relationship grids, and the new cognitive psychologies (M. Horowitz [1991]).

REFERENCES

Aron BA: Manual for Analyses of the Thematic Apperception Test. Berkeley, CA, Willis E Berg, 1949

Bond J, Shevrin H: Similarities and differences between methods of formulating a patient's psychodynamically relevant relationship schemas. Unpublished manuscript, University of Michigan, 1986

Carlson R: Studies of script theory: adult analogs of a childhood nuclear scene. J Pers Soc Psychol 40:501–510, 1981

Crits-Christoph P, Luborsky L, Dahi L, et al: Clinicians can agree in assessing relationship patterns in psychotherapy: the Core Conflictual Relationship Theme method. Arch Gen Psychiatry 45:1001–1004, 1988

Freud S: The dynamics of transference (1912), in The Standard Edition of the Complete Psychological Works of Sigmund Freud [SE], Vol 12. Translated and edited by Strachey J. London, Hogarth Press, 1958, pp 97–108

Freud S: Inhibitions, symptoms, and anxiety (1926). SE, 20:77–175, 1959

Gill MM, Hoffman IZ: A method for studying the analysis of aspects of the patient's experience of the relationship in psychoanalysis and psychotherapy. J Am Psychoanal Assoc 30:137–167, 1982

Grawe K, Caspar F: Die plan Analyse als Konzept und Instrument für die Psychotherapieforschung, in Psychotherapie: Makro-und Mikro Perspechriven. Edited by Baumann U. Cologne, Germany, Hogrefe, 1984

Horowitz L, Weckler D, Doren R: Interpersonal problems and symptoms: a cognitive approach, in Advances in Cognitive-Behavioral Research and Therapy, Vol 2. Edited by Kendall PC. New York, Academic Press, 1983

Horowitz MJ: States of Mind: Analysis of Change in Psychotherapy. New York, Plenum, 1979

Horowitz MJ: States of Mind: Configurational Analysis of Individual Psychology, 2nd Edition. New York, Plenum, 1987

Horowitz MJ: Relationship schema formulation: role-relationship models and intrapsychic conflict. Psychiatry: Journal for the Study of Interpersonal Processes 52:260–274, 1989

Horowitz MJ (ed): Person Schemas and Maladaptive Interpersonal Patterns. Chicago, IL, University of Chicago Press, 1991

Kächele H, Luborsky L, Thoma H: Ubertragung als Struktur and Verlaufsmusterawei Methoden zur Erfassung dieser Aspekte, in Der zentrale Beziehungskonflikt. Edited by Luborsky L, Kächele H. Ulm, Germany, PSZ-Verlag, 1988

Kelly GA: The Psychology of Personal Constructs, Vol 1. New York, WW Norton, 1955

Klein G: Perception, Motives and Personality. New York, Alfred A Knopf, 1970

Levine FJ, Luborsky L: The Core Conflictual Relationship Theme method: a demonstration of reliable clinical inferences by the method of mismatched cases, in Object and Self: A Developmental Approach. Edited by Tuttman S, Kaye C, Zimmerman M. New York, International Universities Press, 1981

Luborsky L: Helping alliances in psychotherapy: the groundwork for a study of their relationship to its outcome, in Successful Psychotherapy. Edited by Claghorn JL. New York, Brunner/Mazel, 1976

Luborsky L: Measuring a pervasive psychic structure in psychotherapy: the Core Conflictual Relationship Theme, in Communicative Structures and Psychic Structures. Edited by Freedman N, Grand SS. New York, Plenum, 1977

Luborsky L: Principles of Psychoanalytic Psychotherapy: A Manual for Supportive-Expressive (SE) Treatment. New York, Basic Books, 1984

Luborsky L: A guide for scoring the Core Conflictual Relationship Theme (CCRT). Edition 3/27/85

Luborsky L: A standard list of scoring categories based on the CCRTs of a normative group. Edition #1, 6/10/85

Luborsky L, with collaboration of Mellon J, Crits-Christoph P: An aid to reliability studies of the CCRT: Standard Scoring Categories. Edition 7/12/85

Luborsky L, Crits-Christoph P: Understanding Transference: The Core Conflictual Relationship Theme Method. New York, Basic Books [1990]

Luborsky L, Mellon J, Alexander K, et al: A verification of Freud's grandest clinical hypothesis: the transference. Clin Psychol Rev 5:231–246, 1985

Luborsky L, Crits-Christoph P, Mellon J: The advent of objective measures of the transference concept. J Consult Clin Psychol 54:39–47, 1986

Luborsky L, Crits-Christoph P, Mintz J, Auerbach A: Who Will Benefit from Psychotherapy? Predicting Therapeutic Outcomes. New York, Basic Books, 1988

Maxim P, Sprague M: Metacommunication of Interactive Sequences in Therapy. Seattle, University of Washington Press, 1989

Murray H: Explorations in Personality. Oxford, UK, Oxford University Press, 1938

Perry JC: A comparison of three methods of assessing psychodynamic conflicts. Proceedings, annual meeting, Society for Psychotherapy Research, June 1986

Schacht T, Binder J, Strupp H: The dynamic focus, in Psychotherapy in a New Key: A Guide to Time-limited Dynamic Psychotherapy. Edited by Strupp H, Binder J. New York, Basic Books, 1984

Singer J, Salovey P: Organized knowledge structures in personality: schemas, self schemas, and scripts. A review and research agenda, in Person Schemas and Maladaptive Interpersonal Patterns. Edited by Horowitz M. Chicago, IL, University of Chicago Press [1991]

Teller V, Dahl H: The framework for a model of psychoanalytic inference. Proceedings of the Seventh International Joint Conference on Artificial Intelligence 1:394–400, 1981

Weiss J, Sampson H: The Psychoanalytic Process. New York, Guilford, 1986

18

ROBERT MICHELS, M.D.

INTRODUCTION

Robert Michels graduated from the University of Chicago and Northwestern University Medical School and did his analytic training at the Columbia University Center for Psychoanalytic Training and Research in New York, where he is on the faculty as a Training and Supervising Analyst. He has throughout his career combined full-time academic positions with an extraordinarily active role in psychoanalysis. He is one of the more eminent figures in American psychiatry as well as psychoanalysis. He is the Walsh McDermott University Professor of Medicine and University Professor of Psychiatry at Cornell University in New York and has been Barklie McKee Henry Professor and Chairman of the Department of Psychiatry at Cornell University Medical College, Psychiatrist in Chief of the Payne Whitney Clinic and the Westchester Division of the New York-Presbyterian Hospital, and Stephen and Suzanne Weiss Dean of the Cornell University Medical College and Provost for Medical Affairs, Cornell University. To name but a few of the positions he has held, he has been President of the American Board of Psychiatry and Neurology, President of the American Association of Chairmen of Departments of Psychiatry, President of the American College of Psychiatrists, and has served on numerous committees of the American Psychoanalytic Association. He was a member of the Board on Biobehavioral Sciences and Mental Disorders of the National Academy of Sciences, Institute of Medicine, and has been on the editorial boards of *The American Journal of Psychiatry, The International Journal of Psycho-*

analysis, The Journal of the American Psychoanalytic Association, The New England Journal of Medicine, and *The Psychoanalytic Quarterly,* to name but a few. He has been recognized with many awards, including the American Psychiatric Association Distinguished Service Award, the American College of Psychiatrists Distinguished Service Award, the American Psychiatric Association Seymour D. Vestermark Award, and the George E. Daniels Award of the Association for Psychoanalytic Medicine, as well as numerous named lectureships and visiting professorships. He is the author of more than 200 papers.

He is preeminent throughout the psychiatric and psychoanalytic communities for the incisiveness and scholarly depth that he brings to clinical, theoretical, administrative, and political issues of central importance to psychoanalysis and psychiatry. Dr. Michels has been a major influence on a generation of young analysts who have benefited from his unique combination of dedication to psychoanalysis, devotion to psychiatry, and an amazing critical capacity to enlighten our areas of fuzzy thinking, complacency, and philosophical and ethical sloppiness.

Dr. Michels submitted the following note about himself:

> I was trained in North American ego psychology with an adaptational spin, and with anti-metapsychological and Sullivanian supplements. I became interested in self psychological, hermeneutic, constructionist, and clinical aspects of Bion-Klein, with Lacanian and Winnicottian additions. Finally, I moved to an explicitly pluralistic approach (nonreligious but rather comparative-theological), with diminishing interest in the nonclinical roots of the theory (biologic, developmental) and a continued interest in linguistic hermeneutic aspects. The "scientific" contribution to psychoanalysis that seems of greatest value to me today is the study and assessment of the clinical process and outcome. Science in related disciplines is of interest to psychoanalysis primarily as the major art form of the twentieth and twenty-first centuries.

WHY I CHOSE THIS PAPER

Robert Michels, M.D.

I have written about psychoanalytic technique, history, sociology, education, and theory, but "Psychoanalysts' Theories" was my first paper that focused on metatheory—the role and function of theory in psychoanalysis. As I have become less and less certain of the validity of psychoanalytic theories, I have become more and more convinced of their importance to our work. In this paper I address that apparent paradox.

PSYCHOANALYSTS' THEORIES

ROBERT MICHELS, M.D.

THE TITLE OF this contribution, "Psychoanalysts' Theories," rather than the more familiar "Psychoanalytic Theories," is deliberate. Psychoanalytic theories are to be found in books, journals, and libraries, and as part of the scholarly dialogue of that small group of psychoanalysts who generate formal theories and speak and write about them. These theories are complicated, confusing, and abstract. They are also represented, although not always with great precision or accuracy, in the minds of all working psychoanalysts, including that majority who would never consider writing a paper on psychoanalytic theory, where they contribute to what I am calling "psychoanalysts' theories." My focus is on these latter theories, which are situated in the minds of practicing psychoanalysts rather than in books or journal articles, and which therefore make a difference to patients. I will discuss their history, their subject matter, and their several functions. As psychoanalysts, we should anticipate that these latent or implicit theories might be quite different from the manifest public ones; that elegance, logic, or consistency might turn out to be only minor virtues in this kind of theory; and that psychoanalysts not only might not know what their implicit theories are, but also might argue vehemently that they are actually something quite different.

I believe that Joseph Sandler (1983) was addressing this same subject, although reaching a different conclusion, when he wrote:

> The fledgling psychoanalyst will bring with him into his consulting room what he has learned from his own analyst, from his supervisors and other teachers, and from his reading. He will carry in his head the theoretical and clinical propositions that he has gathered from these var-

---

"Psychoanalysts' Theories," by Robert Michels, M.D., was first published in *Psychoanalysis on the Move: The Work of Joseph Sandler,* edited by Peter Fonagy, Arnold M. Cooper, and Robert S. Wallerstein (New York: Routledge, 1999), pp. 187–200. Used with permission.

> ious sources, and these propositions will be, for the most part, the official, standard or public ones. The human mind being what it is, he will continue to underestimate the discrepancies and incongruities in the public theories and will learn to move from one part of his theory to another without being aware that he has stepped over a number of spots in this theory that are conceptually weak.
>
> With increasing clinical experience the analyst, as he grows more competent, will preconsciously (descriptively speaking, unconsciously) construct a whole variety of theoretical segments which relate directly to his clinical work. They are the products of unconscious thinking, are very much partial theories, models or schemata, which have the quality of being available in reserve, so to speak, to be called upon whenever necessary. That they may contradict one another is no problem. They coexist happily as long as they are unconscious. They do not appear in consciousness unless they are consonant with what I have called official or public theory, and can be described in suitable words. Such partial structures may in fact represent better (i.e., more useful and appropriate) theories than the official ones, and it is likely that many valuable additions to psychoanalytic theory have come about because conditions have arisen that have allowed preconscious part-theories to come together and emerge in a plausible and psychoanalytically socially acceptable way. (pp 37–38)

In contrast to Professor Sandler, I suggest that we recognize the role and importance of these part-theories. Therefore we can change our rules for psychoanalytic acceptability, rather than wait for part-theories to become acceptable.

HISTORY

At one time, psychoanalysts believed that they should construct scientific theories about the workings of the human mind, particularly the influence of biological factors (i.e., the body, the brain, or the inherited constitutional endowment) on the mind. Their view was that these theories could then be applied to a variety of problems, including the treatment of patients. Freud's earliest explication of psychoanalytic theory fit this mold. However, a number of observers have pointed out that the theories of the mind developed by psychoanalysts were actually byproducts of the clinical situation, abstracted from rather than applied to it. Psychoanalytic theorists, starting with Freud himself, had not studied biological data—brains, bodies, or evolution. Rather they collected experiences in their clinical work and then speculated about biological models that might be consistent with those experiences. Furthermore, critics added that the biological theories that were developed did not serve some of the functions desirable for a good scientific theory; specifically, they did not generate strategies for testing or for possible invalidation and, more generally, they were not very helpful in furthering scientific inquiry. At the same time, although psychoanalysts had developed a rather credible psychological science in their clinical work, they were much less interested in developing it systematically than in elaborating their speculative biological hypotheses.

A first step toward developing theories based on psychoanalytic data was to bring psychoanalysts' speculations closer to their clinical experience. Theorizing shifted from neurobiology and evolution to psychology. Psychoanalytic models of perception, cognition, learning, memory, and personality were developed. The results, however, were only mixed. The new theories were closer to the data generated by the psychoanalytic method, but they often seemed to offer little more than the existing models of academic psychology. They seemed less exciting and less evocative of new clinical insights than were the earlier speculations, and served as perhaps little more than formalizations or tautological restatements of clinical observations. A common complaint was that psychoanalysis had become a complex and dull general psychology rather than an exciting, if unscientific, speculative biology.

The next step involved the redefinition of the subject matter of psychoanalytic theory so that it focused on the events occurring in clinical psychoanalysis that can be studied by the psychoanalytic method, rather than either on biological speculations stemming from those events or on subsequent psychological reformulations of them. However, this change of focus raised new problems. The original biological theories suggested the causes or underlying meanings of the patient's mental experiences and, therefore, the kinds of interpretations an analyst might want to make. The psychological theories that followed attempted to describe and formulate what might be happening in the patient's mind, and, although they might not lead to interpretations, they did help to organize and integrate clinical data. The new clinical theories studied the therapeutic process—what transpired in the consultation room between analyst and patient—but they did not tell the analyst what to say. Analysts could continue to make the same interpretations that analysts have always made, but if they could no longer be grounded in biology and could not yet be grounded in clinical theory, the only justification that remained was a professional tradition. This led to the danger that there would be no way of deciding whether a given interpretation was correct or, perhaps better, whether it was truly psychoanalytic, and—because different analysts interpreted the tradition differently—the field threatened to become chaotic.

Several theories emerged, however, as possible replacements for the original biological theories and as sources of interpretive inspiration.

These emerging theories drew on extra-analytic bodies of knowledge, as well as on clinical psychoanalytic data—knowledge that many believed to be useful in suggesting interpretations in the analytic situation. The most well-known theories were about child development, based in part on the direct observation of children. Others included social or group psychology, anthropology, linguistics, and, more recently, neurobiology.

SUBJECT MATTER

The same issues may be considered from the perspective of the several types of theory rather than from the viewpoint of the history of the development of theory. Such a perspective would recognize that each type of theory can be traced back to the beginnings of psychoanalysis, although from time to time the dominant mode of theorizing may have shifted in the evolution of the discipline. It would also underline the different epistemological status of the various types of theories, rather than their developmental continuity.

There have been at least three distinct types of theories in psychoanalysis: bridging theories, psychological theories, and clinical theories. Because of the recurrent failure to clarify which type is being discussed, there has been considerable confusion about these theories. Both the scientific status and the clinical implications of each type are quite different.

Bridging Theories

Bridging theories attempt to explain mental phenomena by tracing them across some boundary to a domain outside of mental life. There are a variety of different bridging theories, depending on the boundary that is crossed and the subject matter that lies beyond it. Mental life can thus be traced to the brain and its somatic origins, as in Freud's (1895) "Project for a Scientific Psychology," his drive theory, Karl Pribram's writings (1989), or Morton Reiser's monograph (1984). It can be traced to its phylogenetic and evolutionary origins, as in Freud's "Totem and Taboo" (1913), John Bowlby's work (1969), or contemporary ethology. Mental life can also be traced to its developmental protomental origins, as in Freud's "Three Essays on the Theory of Sexuality" (1905), or in the work of Anna Freud, Margaret Mahler, Rene Spitz, David Levy, Robert Emde, Daniel Stern, or any of those who study babies and children to learn about the origins of mental life. It can be traced to its social origins in studies of parent–child, family, and group relations, as Freud did in his papers on the Oedipus complex and group psychology, and as the Sullivanian and object relations theorists have done.

Common to all of these bridging theories is that they draw on knowledge from other fields of observation and other disciplines in order to speculate about mental life. There are two corollaries to this fact. First, bridging theories often provide rich images or metaphors and evocative formulations that can translate mental experience and generate valuable clinical interpretations. Second, these theories themselves cannot possibly be tested in the psychoanalytic situation, because they are based on hypotheses and observations from nonanalytic settings. The clinical interpretations they inspire can be tested and can be shown to be valuable or useless, but such findings neither support nor refute the theories that generated them. Clinical psychoanalysts like these theories; philosophers of science disdain them, viewing them as systems of interpretive metaphor that can neither be validated in the psychoanalytic situation nor lead to a science of psychoanalysis.

It is interesting to note the similarity between psychoanalytic theories that come from other areas—biology, developmental psychology, linguistics, anthropology—and the theories that are brought to psychoanalysts by their patients. Both of these theories serve to limit the domain in which analytic exploration is appropriate. Both our scientific theories and our patients warn us not to go beyond some boundary; that some phenomena cannot be understood simply in terms of the inner world but are determined by forces—biological or social or developmental—that are constraints on that inner world. When a patient presents such a theory, it is always possible that it is "true" (and perhaps it is always a little true). However, any experienced analyst also explores its role as a resistance and, in the process, expects to find not the limits of analyzability but rather the area of most fruitful inquiry. No doubt this experience in the clinical setting is one reason why analysts are often mistrustful of any theory that seems to provide extra-analytic justification for limiting the boundaries of analytic inquiry.

Psychological Theories

The second type of theory is psychological theory. It involves models of mental functioning, rather than suggestions about the origins of mental life. Chapter 7 of "The Interpretation of Dreams" (Freud 1900), parts of "The Ego and the Id" (Freud 1923), and many of Heinz Hartmann's writings exemplify psychological theories. Unlike biological or social or anthropological theories, psychological theories represent what psychoanalysis should be about for those who believe it should be a general psychology. These theories are less likely to suggest metaphors or meanings or to inspire creative clinical interpretations, whereas they are more likely to offer systems for organizing and integrating clinical data. Rather than trying to explain why things happen, they provide guidelines for describing, classifying, and discussing what is happening. They are useful to some clinicians, while others associate them with the dangers of an overly mechanistic and sterile technique. They tend to be far more prominent in the didactic curricula of institutes than in the mental life of analysts at work.

Clinical Theories

The third type, clinical theories, are rooted in the clinical situation. These theories are also psychological, but they are about a very special and restricted area of psychology: what happens in the consultation room. They also can be traced back to Freud's earliest papers, such as "Studies on Hysteria" (Breuer and Freud 1893–1895), but are most prominent in his papers on technique, such as "Analysis Terminable and Interminable" (Freud 1937) or in more recent works by Otto Fenichel, Ralph Greenson, and others. Clinical theories do not provide a general psychology, but rather are about the specific psychology of transference, resistance, alliance, working through, and acting out, as well as similar concepts. They are directly concerned with the analytic situation and often suggest general clinical strategies and hypotheses that can be tested there. However, they seldom suggest the content of specific interpretations or interventions, although they may suggest formal principles for conducting an analysis. They are like the theories of harmony, rhythm, and musicology—vital for dissecting, understanding, and discussing music, but insufficient for composing a symphony.

In recent years, interest in psychoanalytic thinking has shifted from the first, extra-analytic type and even the second, general psychological type to this third, clinical type of theory. This shift has made it more likely that theory and practice can be mutually enriching, and has invited ideas such as those discussed here.

FUNCTION: RELATION OF THEORY TO PRACTICE

Let us shift from an overview of the history of psychoanalytic theory and a consideration of the different types of theories to a discussion of the functions of theories, how they are used, and the roles they play. Although theories are important in teaching, supervision, and research, the place to start is with what interests psychoanalysts most—the role of theory in practice.

Scientific Basis of Practice

Most professions based on scientific knowledge and theory expect the practitioner to learn and master the theory and then apply it to individual problems or cases. Some view psychoanalysis in these terms. For example, Ralph Greenson (1968) said that the analyst "must listen to the material of his patient, permitting his own associative fantasies and memories to have free play as he does so; yet he must scrutinize and expose to his intellectual capacities the insights so obtained" (p. 16). Greenson echoes Fenichel in presenting the image of an analyst oscillating "between the use of empathy and intuition on the one hand and ...theoretical knowledge on the other" (Greenson 1968, p. 16).

Generation of Interpretations

There is a problem, however, when this somewhat restricted version of the traditional view of the role of theory in the science-based professions is applied to psychoanalysis. This problem generates a different view of the relationship between theory and practice. Our instructions to practicing analysts suggest a state of mind that is "free floating" or "evenly hovering," that is open to empathic perception, trial identification, and adaptive regression. But this state of mind is not that of someone applying a complex scientific theory to a body of data. Rather, it is the state of mind of someone using theory as a source of inspiration to extend and enrich a network of associations. The psychoanalyst who knows and uses psychoanalytic theories this way listens to the patient, enriched by an associative context that includes the shared experiences of the entire community of psychoanalysts, past and present, as well as the psychoanalyst's own clinical and personal experience.

Viewed from this perspective, there is little difference between psychoanalytic case histories and psychoanalytic theories, or between psychoanalytic theories and other theories. The only question is: does the theory enrich the experience of the analyst with the patient? Furthermore, there is little concern about compatibility or contradiction among theories. Finally, within this perspective, we do not ask whether psychoanalytic theories are true or false, just as critics do not ask whether works of art are true or false, philosophers of science do not ask whether scientific theories are true or false, and psychoanalysts do not ask whether interpretations are true or false. The critic wants to know what impact a work of art has on the audience and the culture. The philosopher of science wants to know whether a theory fosters scientific inquiry, generates hypotheses, and suggests experiments. The psychoanalyst wants to know whether an interpretation stimulates new material and leads to therapeutic progress. We want to know whether a psychoanalytic theory helps psychoanalysts to analyze, or whether it guides them to new insights and understandings. In each case, the test is not one of truth or falsity, but rather one of assessing the impact of an intervention on an ongoing process (Michels 1983).

However, even this view of theory as a source of inspiration or metaphor rather than as a systematic scientific structure to be applied to the data of the specific clinical situation, may overemphasize the cognitive aspects of psychoanalysis and the primacy of insight. It seems to imply that the most important role of the analyst is to make interpretations. In fact, theory has an additional and often more powerful impact on clinical work, one that generates a third view of the impact of theory on psychoanalytic practice.

Influence on the Analyst's Role

Theories influence the analyst's stance, manner, attitude, and approach to the patient, the analyst's role, and particularly the analyst's perception of that role. The following examples illustrate such influence.

Listening

The first example goes back to the very beginning of psychoanalysis and the core of its meaning. One of the essential aspects of psychoanalysis is that the analyst listen to the patient. One of Freud's first major theoretical formulations was that the patient's words, no matter how fragmented, incoherent, or irrelevant they might seem on the surface, conceal a hidden but important meaning, and, furthermore, that meaning can be deciphered by paying close attention to what is said and how it is said. Whether this theory is "right" or "wrong," whether the analyst ever understands the patient's real meaning, whether the uncoding is correct or fanciful, indeed whether it even makes sense to speak of a "real" meaning, this theory helps to sustain the analyst's attentive and patient listening and thus supports a central feature of the psychoanalytic stance. (The special importance of being listened to by someone who is trying to make sense out of what one is saying may stem from the universal experience of having a parent try to make sense out of the infant's meaningless babbling and, in the process, to transform a psychologically prestructural organism into a communicating social being.) The meanings discovered by psychoanalytic inquiry may be therapeutic, but the experience of being listened to by an attentive, concerned guide in the search for meaning may well be even more therapeutic.

Nonjudgmental Interest

A second essential of psychoanalysis is that, in addition to listening attentively and patiently, the analyst be interested and curious while being neither critical or judgmental. Developing nonjudgmental interest may be even more difficult than listening attentively, because we are all socialized to make judgments about behavior (or own and that of others) and to hold people responsible for what they do. We make exceptions only when we believe persons to be so infantile or helpless or disorganized that they are not in charge of their lives. We know, however, that such an attitude toward a patient, except in psychiatric crises, seriously compromises psychoanalysis. Here again, we have a theory that is helpful. The concept of a dynamic unconscious—of powerful forces that shape behavior and that are at the same time both within the patient and yet outside awareness—supports the paradoxical but crucial belief that the patient should not be judged or held morally culpable, despite being the master of his or her own fate. Once again, the issue is not whether this concept is "true" or "false." (Indeed, the Anglo-American debate on criminal responsibility and the insanity defense has foundered on this essentially meaningless question.) However, regardless of its epistemological status, or whether it ever generates a specific clinical interpretation, this theory comes to our aid by maintaining an essential component of the analytic attitude.

Libido Theory

For a third example, I will consider a more complex theory, one of the oldest, most powerful, and most criticized theories in psychoanalysis: libido theory. Again, my interest is not in whether the theory is true or false, or even in whether it can be tested or falsified, but rather in what difference it makes to a practicing analyst. Libido theory suggests that the analyst should search for patterns based on infantile bodily experiences. Rather than accept the patient's conscious level of discourse as the most critical or significant one, the analyst should constantly attempt to translate or reformulate, to find forbidden, primitive, exciting, and, particularly, naughty meanings in the most mundane statements. This process of reformulation is what makes psychoanalysis seem to outsiders interesting, ridiculous, and disturbing, all at the same time. Analysis requires not only that analysts listen and avoid moral disapproval, but also that they translate and elaborate on their patients' themes. It is not enough for analysts to be friendly, supportive, and receptive; they must also be interesting. True or false, libido theory generates some of the most interesting statements made by psychoanalysts.

Psychic Conflict

A fourth and final example of the theories that guide psychoanalysis is the concept of psychic conflict. Once again, regardless of the scientific status of this concept, it leads the analyst to accept and tolerate—and perhaps even to search for—paradox, ambiguity, and contradiction. Particularly in its more comprehensive formulation as the principle of multiple function, the concept of psychic conflict encourages a continuing openness to new or additional meanings and understandings rather than a search for closure and correct or final answers. This theoretical concept encourages the continuing exploration that is central to the analytic process.

Effects of Alternative Theories

If theories function in part by shaping therapeutic attitudes, then alternative theories may have different impacts. This is true not only because of their differential validity or scientific status, or even the different interpretations they suggest, but also because they encourage different stances.

For example, structural theory focuses on divisions within the patient's mind and encourages the analyst to maintain an active interest in what is being excluded or omitted. Its proponents believe that this examination of what is not said is central to psychoanalysis, in that it sheds light on psychic conflict, repression, and the dynamic unconscious. Its critics fear, however, that structural theory places the analyst in a constantly adversarial or, at best, in a neutral, uninvolved, or unempathic posture *vis-à-vis* the patient, thus encouraging detached observation rather than emotional participation.

Object relations theory emphasizes the internal world, a derivative of the social field, the mental representations of the relationships between the patient and significant others. Just as structural theory reduces mental life to conflicts among components of the mind, object relations theory reduces it to interactions among images of self and others. The critics of object relations theory are concerned that it overemphasizes social and environmental determinants of behavior at the expense of intrapersonal and, particularly, biological ones, and furthermore that it encourages the analyst to be excessively preoccupied with what is going on between patient and analyst rather than within the patient's mind. Its proponents believe that it rehumanizes a psychoanalytic model that had begun to consider people as though they were machines instead of social beings.

Self psychology emphasizes the inherent growth potential of the individual and suggests that other people in the patient's life, including the analyst, are either incorporated as vital substrates for this growth program, helping to nurture and promote it, or that they become irrelevant and even destructive to it. Proponents of the model emphasize the positive, affirmative orientation it encourages, often seeing alternative theories as encouraging an inappropriate focus on problems that are merely symptoms of arrested psychic development. Critics are concerned that self psychology achieves this affirmative stance by colluding with the patient in denying the darker aspects of mental life (e.g., hostility and negative feelings that are more than reactive responses to environmental precipitants), along with disavowed aspects of mental conflict.

Support for the Analyst

Finally, theories operate, quite simply, by comforting the psychoanalyst. This function is in addition to that of organizing knowledge that can be applied to clinical data, their interpretation-generating or metaphoric function suggesting meanings and relationships, and their impact on the general stance, manner, attitude, and approach of the analyst. Psychoanalysis is a difficult profession, and psychoanalysts spend much of their time uncertain—perhaps even confused or bewildered—as they attempt to comprehend amorphous or chaotic experiences that do not always fit into place. The work is lonely, and psychoanalysts crave reassurance, support, and company. Theory can provide that support.

A theory can be seen as a kind of transitional object: it links the psychoanalyst to a teacher or mentor; it provides a sense of security, a reassurance that someone knows and understands; and it gives refuge when the going is difficult. Moreover, as with some other transitional objects, analysts may cling to a particular theory all the more when others ridicule it or try to take it away and replace it with a cleaner, more modern substitute. Old theories, like old teddy bears, are not less beloved because they are torn or perhaps a little smelly.

This comforting function of theory is particularly important for students or novices. It provides a partially illusory safety and reassurance that continues until accumulating personal clinical experience diminishes both its power and the need for its supportive function. When this process goes smoothly, all is well. However, at times the de-idealization of theory precedes the development of personal experience, and the student is prematurely left without adequate support. Many such students become critical of psychoanalysis and turn against it. Other students may elevate theory above clinical experience and never de-idealize it. Such students become followers of psychoanalysis, rather than independent professionals, and they tend to become the favorite targets of attacks by those who do not place theory above clinical experience.

This nonspecific function of theory for psychoanalysts is reminiscent of one of the functions that interpretations play for psychoanalytic patients. Interpretations both comfort and reassure, whether or not the patient understands and uses them. Interpretations, like theories, are evaluated in terms of their impact on the process, and, as with theory, it is of little interest to question whether they are true or false. Both interpretations and theories serve to clarify what is confusing and to provide links between easily observable surface phenomena and deeper structures hidden from direct view. By doing so, both help to bring into awareness those deeper structures (Michels 1983).

In summary, theories are important to analysts' analyzing. They generate rules and guidelines, suggest meanings and interpretations, inform the basic stance and posture of the analyst, and provide comfort and security. The first of these functions, the traditional role of scientific theory in professional practice, may well be the least important.

FUNCTION: RELATION OF THEORY TO TEACHING AND RESEARCH

Psychoanalysts teach, and theories are educational aids. Clinical maxims, such as "analyze the resistance before the content" or "focus on the material associated with the patient's strongest affect," are condensed theories and are frequently used in supervision. However, rather than focusing on theories, good supervision focuses on clinical material: on the patient, the analyst, and the events that transpire between them, or, from time to time, on the reflections of those events in the supervisory process. In general, the supervising psychoanalyst uses theory in much the same ways as does the analyzing psychoanalyst, although the relative emphasis of its several functions differs. The supervisor is far more likely to function in a cognitive mode and to apply theory in a truly scientific way. The supervisor may draw on theory for metaphor and inspiration, although good supervision is more concerned with enhancing the supervisee's sensitivity to meaning and ability to construct metaphors. One's supervisory stance, like one's analytic stance, may be colored by a favorite psychoanalytic theory, but supervision is education, not treatment, so the supervisor's attitude should be informed more by educational than by psychoanalytic theory. Finally, supervisors are further along in their own developmental course and less likely than analysts to need the emotional support provided by theory.

Although theories have a place in the consultation room and the supervisory office, they are most usually found in the curriculum and the classroom. As part of the curriculum, theories play a central role in pedagogy. In fact, they are more central to the classroom teaching of psychoanalysis than most other disciplines because the primary data are hard to come by, and the history of the field is as much a history of theoretical reformulation as it is one of new primary observations. One corollary of this central role is our concern that candidates begin their clinical work before they have had too much classroom instruction, lest their premature and excessive exposure to theory lead to notions or styles inappropriate to the conduct of analysis. There are few other fields that raise such concerns about too much education interfering with practice. Bertram Lewin (1965) has even suggested that theories originate as derivatives of teaching, that they grow out of the teacher's attempt to explain to a student, or, in his words, that "teaching and theorizing coincide and that the business of teaching leads to the production of theories" (p. 138).

Professions based on scientific knowledge involve both teaching and research. To an astonishing extent, psychoanalysis has focused its academic activities on teaching, with the role of research largely replaced by theoretically informed discourse. However, in recent years there has been some interest in activities that are more similar to the scientific research associated with other professions, particularly in the areas of child development and clinical process. Theories are essential for such research: they define problems and make the difference between simply collecting data and developing new knowledge that can have a cumulative impact on the field. Psychoanalytic theories have been productive in stimulating research in other fields, such as developmental psychology, and there is even some suggestion that psychoanalytic theory has, in turn, been enriched by new knowledge from developmental psychology. The more critical question is whether theories have fostered research in psychoanalysis itself. Here the answer is less clear. Systematic research is rare, and the questions it addresses often seem minor. One result is that serious and talented clinicians often have little interest in research. Another is that some of the most creative and original thinkers in the field are skeptical about the future of psychoanalytic research. A major challenge is whether psychoanalysts can develop theories that will stimulate research that might lead to new knowledge in psychoanalysis.

CONCLUSION

Freud (1933, p. 81) said that the "right abstract ideas" produce order and clarity when applied to the raw material of observation. Interpretations in clinical analysis also do this; theories do the same in the scientific study of psychoanalysis. They also enrich the clinical work and codify and crystallize what has been learned. Without theories, the field cannot progress. However, a question that has long troubled psychoanalysis is how to decide which theories are the "right" ones. Validation by some objective test, the strategy in most sciences, has largely eluded psychoanalytic inquiry. The sanction of authority, never very attractive, is no longer even possible, since there is no agreement on the appropriate authority. Theories borrowed from other disciplines are increasingly unsatisfactory, while those stemming from the study of analysis itself are more productive of formal principles than of suggestions for content.

Our best current guide to the content of our clinical interpretations is a tradition that was originally developed on the basis of extra-analytic theorizing but has now largely fallen out of favor. Perhaps our clinical theory again has a guideline to offer, that the right theories are right for the same reasons that right interpretations are right—not because they are true or validated outside of the psychoanalytic process, but because they lead to progress, new material, or new ideas, rather than to stasis and stagnation. Good theories generate problems that lead to better theories, and therefore any theory that remains unchanged fails the test.

REFERENCES

Bowlby J: Attachment and Loss (1969). New York, Basic Books, 1980

Breuer J, Freud S: Studies on hysteria (1893–1895), in The Standard Edition of the Complete Psychological Works of Sigmund Freud [SE], Vol 2. Translated and edited by Strachey J. London, Hogarth Press, 1955, pp 1–311

Freud S: Project for a scientific psychology (1950 [1887–1902]). SE, 1:281–397, 1966

Freud S: The interpretation of dreams (1900). SE, 4–5:1–627, 1953

Freud S: Three essays on the theory of sexuality (1905). SE, 7:123–145, 1953

Freud S: Totem and taboo (1913). SE, 13:1–162, 1953

Freud S: The ego and the id (1923). SE, 19:1–66, 1961

Freud S: New introductory lectures on psycho-analysis (1933). SE, 22:1–182, 1964

Freud S: Analysis terminable and interminable (1937). SE, 23:209–253,1964

Greenson R: The Technique and Practice of Psychoanalysis. New York, International Universities Press, 1968

Lewin BD: Teaching and the beginnings of theory. Int J Psychoanal 46:137–139, 1965

Michels R: The scientific and clinical functions of psychoanalytic theory, in The Future of Psychoanalysis: Essays in Honor of Heinz Kohut. Edited by Goldberg A. New York, International Universities Press, 1983

Pribram K: Psychoanalysis and the natural sciences: the brain-behaviour connection from Freud to the present, in Dimensions of Psychoanalysis. Edited by Sandler J. Madison, CT, International Universities Press, 1989, pp 139–163

Reiser M: Mind, Brain, Body: Toward a Convergence of Psychoanalysis and Neurobiology. New York, Basic Books, 1984

Sandler J: Reflections on some relations between psychoanalytic concepts and psychoanalytic practice. Int J Psychoanal 64:35–45, 1983

19

THOMAS H. OGDEN, M.D.

INTRODUCTION

Thomas Ogden received his B.A. from Amherst College in Massachusetts and his M.D. from Yale University School of Medicine in New Haven, Connecticut, where he also did his psychiatric residency. He served for a year as an Associate Psychiatrist at the Tavistock Clinic in London and did his analytic training at the San Francisco Psychoanalytic Institute in California, where he has remained on the faculty. Dr. Ogden is a Supervising and Personal Analyst at the Psychoanalytic Institute of Northern California. He has for more than 25 years served as Director of the Center for the Advanced Study of the Psychoses and at various times has been a member of the North American Editorial Board of *The International Journal of Psychoanalysis, Psychoanalytic Dialogues,* and *The Bulletin of the Menninger Clinic.* He is a member of the Standing Committee on the Psychoses of the International Psychoanalytical Association and a member of the International Advisory Panel of *The Complete Works of Donald W. Winnicott.*

Dr. Ogden is the author of more than 50 papers in major psychoanalytic journals on topics as varied as "On Psychoanalytic Writing," "On Psychoanalytic Supervision," "Reverie and Metaphor: Some Thoughts On How I Work as a Psychoanalyst," "Listening: Three Frost Poems," "Borges and the Art of Mourning," "The Concept of Interpretive Interaction," "On the Nature of Schizophrenic Conflict," and "On Holding and Containing, Being and Dreaming." He is the author of seven books, and his books and papers have been published in more than 17 languages.

Dr. Ogden's honors include the 2004 *International Journal of Psychoanalysis* Award for the Most Important Paper of the Year, the William C. Menninger Award of the Central Neuropsychiatric Association, and the Seymour L. Lustman Memorial Psychiatric Research Prize.

During the past decade, Ogden's concepts of the analytic third and the analyst's reverie have become increasingly important and widely discussed topics, and he has supplied important new dimensions to the discussions of intersubjectivity and countertransference.

The following is Dr. Ogden's statement concerning the place of his work in American psychoanalysis:

> The papers I wrote in my first 10 years of analytic writing (1974–1984) were papers that both introduced American psychoanalysts to British psychoanalytic thinking—primarily the work of Klein, Winnicott, Fairbairn, and Bion—but also served as a vehicle for the development of my own ideas.
>
> In my 1979 paper "On Projective Identification," and in my books *Projective Identification and Psychotherapeutic Technique* and *The Matrix of the Mind: Object Relations and the Psychoanalytic Dialogue*, I was not simply "explaining" the ideas of Klein, Fairbairn, Winnicott, and Bion to an audience that had almost no familiarity with their work, I was creating my own version of ideas that they introduced. My idea of projective identification was not, and still is not, what a British Kleinian would endorse. I view projective identification as an unconscious intrapsychic/interpersonal process, whereas the London Kleinians (despite the work of Bion and Rosenfeld) still view it almost entirely as an intrapsychic process. Similarly, I have tried to invent anew many of Winnicott's, Fairbairn's, and Bion's ideas. A reviewer of *The Matrix of the Mind* in *The Psychoanalytic Quarterly* complained that he could not tell where Klein's, Winnicott's, and Fairbairn's ideas ended and where mine began. I took it as the highest compliment he could have paid me.
>
> In the years that followed (1984–1989), I wrote about what I refer to as the "autistic-contiguous position," a mode of generating experience that is equally important as, but more primitive than, the paranoid-schizoid and depressive positions. It is an almost entirely sensation-dominated form of experiencing in which there is no inside or outside, only surfaces and perimeters. These contributions made use of the work of Tustin, Bick, and Meltzer as starting points for the development of my own ideas. The papers I wrote during this period were collected in my book *The Primitive Edge of Experience.*
>
> Between 1989 and 2001, an important focus of my thinking and writing was on the place in the analytic process of reverie and the analytic third. During these years I wrote a good deal on how we communicate in the analytic setting (i.e., the way we convey our thoughts and feelings through the effects that we create in our use of language). In other words, style (voice, tone, use of metaphor and so on) on the one hand, and content, on the other, are inseparable. I have explored this by look-

ing closely at the poetry of Frost, Heaney, and Stevens as well as the fictions of Borges. My books *Subjects of Analysis, Reverie and Interpretation: Sensing Something Human,* and *Conversations at the Frontier of Dreaming* present these aspects of my analytic thinking.

My new book, *This Art of Psychoanalysis: Dreaming Undreamt Dreams and Interrupted Cries,* is published in the New Library of Psychoanalysis series. This work builds upon the entirety of my writing up to this point. In the papers collected in this book, I offer a revised conception of the place of dreaming in analytic theory and its role in analytic practice. Following Bion, I view dreaming (which continues both while we are awake and asleep) as synonymous with unconscious psychological work. The aim of psychoanalysis, from this perspective, is to assist the patient in dreaming his or her lived experience more fully.

Central to psychoanalysis, as I conceive of it, is the analyst's participation in dreaming the patient's "undreamt" and "interrupted" dreams. Interrupted dreams (metaphorical nightmares) are emotional experiences with which the patient is able to dream (to do genuine unconscious psychological work) up to a point. However, past a certain point, the patient's dreaming is disrupted—the capacity for dreaming is overwhelmed by the disturbing nature of what is being dreamt. At that point the patient "wakes up," that is, ceases to be able to do unconscious psychological work (e.g., as seen in a child's play disruption). The place at which dreaming ceases is marked by the creation of neurotic and other forms of nonpsychotic symptomatology. By contrast, undreamt dreams are emotional experiences with which the patient is able to do little or no conscious or unconscious psychological work. Undreamable experience is held in split-off states such as pockets of psychosis or in psychosomatic disorders and severe perversions.

For me, the thread running through all of what I have said is that my position in the analytic world has not been that of an advocate of a school of psychoanalysis (or as an adversary of "opposing" schools of psychoanalysis). Neither do I view myself as a "lone voice," because that suggests that I think of myself as a renegade. I would much prefer to describe myself as an independent thinker.

WHY I CHOSE THIS PAPER

Thomas H. Ogden, M.D.

I chose "The Analytic Third: Implications for Psychoanalytic Theory and Technique" for inclusion in this volume because it represents for me not the end of a line of thought but a gathering of thoughts that had their origins in my earliest efforts at analytic writing in the 1970s. The central idea in this paper on the analytic third is the notion that much of the time in the analytic setting it takes two people genuinely to think and to dream. This idea, though implicit in Freud's work, was first articulated by Bion and Rosenfeld in the form of their development of the concept of projective identification as an unconscious, psychological-interpersonal process. That concept provided me a point of entry into my own explorations of the ways in which analyst and analysand participate in thinking thoughts and dreaming dreams that neither person could have done on his or her own.

THE ANALYTIC THIRD

Implications for Psychoanalytic Theory and Technique

THOMAS H. OGDEN, M.D.

THE ANALYTIC THIRD IS a concept that has become for me in the course of the past decade an indispensable part of the theory and technique that I rely on in every analytic session. In the present paper I draw on previous clinical and theoretical contributions (Ogden 1994a, 1994b, 1999), in an effort to gather together in one place a number of elements of my thinking on the subject of the analytic third. As will be discussed, I consider the dialectical movement of individual subjectivity (of the analyst and analysand as separate individuals, each with his or her own unconscious life) and intersubjectivity (the jointly created unconscious life of the analytic pair) to be a central clinical phenomenon of psychoanalysis, one that virtually all clinical analytic thinking attempts to describe in ever more precise and generative terms.

My own conception of analytic intersubjectivity represents an elaboration and extension of Winnicott's (1960) notion that "There is no such thing as an infant [apart from the maternal provision]" (p. 39, fn.). I believe that in an analytic context, there is no such thing as an analysand apart from the relationship with the analyst, and no such thing as an analyst apart from the relationship with the analysand. Winnicott's now famous statement is to my mind intentionally incomplete.

"The Analytic Third: Implications for Psychoanalytic Theory and Technique," by Thomas H. Ogden, M.D., was first published in *The Psychoanalytic Quarterly,* 73(1):167–194, 2004. Slightly adapted and abridged for this publication. Used with permission.

He assumes that it will be understood that the idea that there is no such thing as an infant is playfully hyperbolic and represents one element of a larger paradoxical statement. From another perspective (from the point of view of the other "pole" of the paradox), there is obviously an infant, and a mother, who constitute separate physical and psychological entities. The mother–infant unity coexists in dynamic tension with the mother and infant in their separateness.

In both the relationship of mother and infant and the relationship of analyst and analysand, the task is not to tease apart the elements constituting the relationship in an effort to determine which qualities belong to whom; rather, from the point of view of the interdependence of subject and object, the analytic task involves an attempt to describe the specific nature of the experience of the unconscious interplay of individual subjectivity and intersubjectivity. In Part I of the present paper, I shall attempt to trace in some detail the vicissitudes of the experience of being simultaneously within and outside of the unconscious intersubjectivity of the analyst–analysand that I have termed the *analytic third*[1] (Ogden 1994a). This third subjectivity, the intersubjective analytic third, is a product of a unique dialectic generated by/between the separate subjectivities of analyst and analysand within the analytic setting. It is a subjectivity that seems to take on a life of its own in the interpersonal field between analyst and analysand.

In Part II of this contribution, I will offer a reconsideration of the phenomenon of projective identification and its role in the analytic process by viewing it as a form of the intersubjective analytic third. In projective identification, as I understand it, the individual subjectivities of both analyst and analysand are to a large extent subsumed by a third subject of analysis, an unconscious, co-created one: the *subjugating third.* A successful analytic experience involves a superseding of the third by means of mutual recognition of analyst and analysand as separate subjects and a reappropriation of the (transformed) individual subjectivities of the participants.

---

[1]It is beyond the scope of this paper to offer a comprehensive review of the literature concerning an intersubjective view of the analytic process and the nature of the unconscious interplay of transference and countertransference. See Bion's (1962) and Green's (1975) work concerning the "analytic object" and Barranger's (1993) notion of the "analytic field" for conceptions of unconscious analytic intersubjectivity that overlap with what I call the "analytic third." For thoughtful reviews of the rather large body of literature on the transference-countertransference, see Boyer (1993) and Etchegoyen (1991).

PART I. THE ANALYTIC THIRD IN CLINICAL PRACTICE

I will now present a fragment of an analysis followed by a discussion of the importance of the analyst's attending to the most mundane, everyday aspects of the background workings of his or her mind (which appear to be the analyst's "own stuff" entirely unrelated to the patient). I shall also discuss the analyst's task of using verbal symbols to speak with a voice that has lived within the intersubjective analytic third, has been changed by that experience, and is able to speak from it and about it to the analysand (who has also lived the experience of the third).

Clinical Illustration: The Purloined Letter

In an analytic session with Mr. L, a patient with whom I had been working for about 3 years, I found myself looking at an envelope on the table next to my chair. For the previous week or 10 days, I had been using the envelope to jot down phone numbers retrieved from my answering machine, ideas for classes I was teaching, errands I had to do, and other notes to myself. Although the envelope had been in plain view for over a week, I had not noticed until that moment in the meeting that there was a series of vertical lines in the lower right hand portion of the front of the envelope, markings that seemed to indicate that the letter had been part of a bulk mailing. I was taken aback by a distinct feeling of disappointment. The letter that had arrived in the envelope was from a colleague in Italy who had written to me about a matter that he felt was delicate and should be kept in strictest confidence.

I then looked at the stamps and for the first time noticed two further details. The stamps had not been canceled, and one of them had words on it that, to my surprise, I could read. I saw the words *Wolfgang Amadeus Mozart* and realized after a moment's delay that the words were a name with which I was familiar, and were "the same" in Italian as they were in English.

As I retrieved myself from this reverie, I wondered how this might be related to what was going on at that moment between the patient and me. The effort to make this shift in psychological state felt like the uphill battle of attempting to "fight repression" that I have experienced as I have tried to remember a dream that is slipping away on awakening. In years past, I have put aside such lapses of attention and have endeavored to devote myself to making sense of what the patient was saying since, in returning from such reveries, I am inevitably a bit behind the patient.

I realized I was feeling suspicious about the genuineness of the intimacy that the letter had seemed to convey. My fleeting fantasy that the letter had been part of a bulk mailing reflected a feeling that I had been duped. I felt that I had been naive and gullible, ready to believe that I was being entrusted with a special secret. I had a number of fragmentary associations, including the image of a mail sack full of letters with stamps that had not been canceled, a spider's egg sac, *Charlotte's Web,* Charlotte's message on the cobweb, Templeton the rat, and innocent Wilbur. None of these thoughts seemed to scratch the surface of what was occurring between Mr. L and me: I felt as if I were simply going through the motions of countertransference analysis in a way that seemed forced.

As I listened to Mr. L (the 45-year old director of a large nonprofit agency), I was aware that he was talking in a way that was highly characteristic of him—he sounded weary and hopeless, and yet was doggedly trudging on in his production of "free associations." He had during the entire period of the analysis been struggling mightily to escape the confines of his extreme emotional detachment from himself and from other people. I thought of Mr. L's description of his driving up to the house in which he lives and not being able to feel it was *his* house. When he walked inside, he was greeted by "the woman and four children who lived there," but could not feel they were *his* wife and *his* children. "It's a sense of myself not being in the picture and yet I *am* there. In that second of recognition of not fitting in, it's a feeling of being separate, which is right next to feeling lonely."

I tried out in my own mind the idea that perhaps I felt duped by him and taken in by the apparent sincerity of his effort to talk to me. But this idea rang hollow to me. I was reminded of the frustration in Mr. L's voice as he explained to me again and again that he knew that he must be feeling something, but he did not have a clue as to what it might be.

The patient's dreams were regularly filled with images of paralyzed people, prisoners, and mutes. In a recent dream he had succeeded—after expending an enormous amount of energy—in breaking open a stone and finding hieroglyphics carved into its interior surfaces, like the markings of a fossil. In the dream, his initial joy was extinguished when he realized that he could not understand a single element of the meaning of the hieroglyphics. In the dream, his discovery was momentarily exciting, but ultimately an empty, painfully tantalizing experience that left him in thick despair. Even the feeling of despair was almost immediately obliterated upon awakening, becoming a lifeless set of dream images that he "reported" to me (as opposed to telling me). The dream had become a sterile memory and no longer felt alive as a set of thoughts and feelings.

I considered the idea that my own experience in the hour might be thought of as a form of projective identification in which I was participating in the patient's experience of the despair of being unable to discern and experience an inner life that seemed to lie behind an impenetrable barrier. This formulation made intellectual sense, but felt clichéd and emotionally lacking. I then drifted into a series of narcissistic, competitive thoughts concerning professional matters that began to take on a ruminative quality. These ruminations were unpleasantly interrupted by the realization that my car, which was in a repair shop, would have to be collected before 6:00 P.M. when the shop closed. I would have to be careful to end the last analytic hour of the day precisely at 5:50 if there were to be any chance at all of my getting to the garage before it closed. I had a vivid image in my mind of myself standing in front of the closed garage doors with the traffic roaring in back of me. I felt intense helplessness and rage (as well as some self-pity) about the way in which the owner of the garage had shut his doors precisely at 6:00 P.M. despite the fact that I had been a regular customer for years and he knew full well that I would need my car. In this fantasied experience, there was a profound feeling of desolation and isolation, as well as a palpable, physical sensation of the hardness of the pavement, the stench of the exhaust fumes, and the grittiness of the dirty glass windows of the garage door.

Although I was not fully conscious of it at the time, in retrospect, I can better see that I was quite shaken by this series of feelings and images that had begun with my narcissistic/competitive ruminations and had ended with the fantasies of impersonally terminating the hour of my last patient of the day and then being shut out by the owner of the garage.

As I again returned to listening in a more focused way to Mr. L, I labored to put together the things that he was currently discussing: his wife's immersion in her work and the exhaustion that they both felt at the end of the day, his brother-in-law's financial reversal and impending bankruptcy, an experience while jogging in which the patient was in a near accident with a motorcyclist who was riding recklessly. I could have taken up any one of these images as a symbol of themes that we had previously discussed, including the detachment itself—which seemed to permeate all that the patient was talking about as well as the disconnection I felt both from myself and from Mr. L. However, I decided not to intervene because it felt to me that if I were to try to offer an interpretation at this point, I would only be repeating myself and saying something for the sake of reassuring myself that I had something to say.

The phone in my office had rung earlier in the meeting and the answering machine had clicked twice to record a message before resuming its silent vigil. At the time of the call, I had not consciously thought about who might be calling, but at this point in the hour I checked the clock to see how much longer it would be before I could retrieve the message. I felt relieved to think of the sound of a fresh voice on the answering machine tape. It was not that I imagined finding a specific piece of good news; it was more that I yearned for a crisp, clear voice. There was a sensory component to the fantasy—I could feel a cool breeze wash across my face and enter my lungs, relieving the suffocating stillness of an overheated, unventilated room. I was reminded of the fresh stamps on the envelope—clear, vibrant in their colors, unobscured by the grim, mechanical, indelible scarring of machine-made cancellation marks.

I looked again at the envelope and noticed something about which I had been only subliminally aware all along: my name and address had been typed on a manual typewriter—not a computer, not a mailing label, not even an electric typewriter. I felt almost joyous about the personal quality with which my name was being "spoken." I could almost hear the idiosyncratic irregularities of each typed letter, the inexactness of the line, the way in which each *t* was missing its upper portion above the bar. This felt to me like the accent and inflection of a human voice speaking *to me,* knowing my name.

These thoughts and feelings, as well as the physical sensations associated with these fantasies, brought to mind (and body) something that the patient had said to me months earlier, but had not mentioned subsequently. He had told me that he felt closest to me not when I said things that seemed right, but when I made mistakes, when I got things wrong. It had taken me these months to understand in a fuller way what he had meant when he had said this to me. At this point in the meeting, I began to be able to describe for myself the feelings of desperateness that I had been feeling in my own and the patient's frantic search for something human and personal in our work together. I also began to feel I understood something of the panic, despair, and anger associated with the experience of colliding again and again with something that appears to be human, but feels mechanical and impersonal.

I was reminded of Mr. L's description of his mother as "brain dead." The patient could not remember a single instance of her ever having shown evidence of feeling anger or intense feeling of any sort. She immersed herself in housework and "completely uninspired cooking." Emotional difficulties were consistently met with platitudes. For example, when the patient as a 6-year-old was each night terrified that there were creatures under his bed, Mr. L's mother would tell him, "There's nothing there to be afraid of." This statement became a symbol in the analysis of the discord between the accuracy of the statement on the one hand (there were in fact no creatures under his bed) and the unwillingness/inability of his mother to recognize the inner life of the patient (there was something he was frightened of that she refused to acknowledge, identify with, or even be curious about).

Mr. L's chain of thoughts—which included his commenting on his wife's and his own feelings of exhaustion, his brother-in-law's impending bankruptcy, and the potentially serious or even fatal accident—now struck me as a reflection of the patient's unconscious attempts to talk to me about his inchoate feeling that the analysis was depleted, bankrupt, and dying. He was experiencing the rudiments of a feeling that he and I were not talking to one another in a way that felt alive; instead, I seemed to him unable to be other than mechanical with him just as he was unable to be human with me.

I told the patient that I thought that our time together must feel to him like a joyless, obligatory exercise, something like a factory job where one punches in and out with a time card. I then said that I had the sense that he sometimes felt so hopelessly stifled in the hours with me that it must feel like being suffocated in something that appears to be air, but is actually a vacuum.

Mr. L's voice became louder and full in a way that I had not heard before as he said, "Yes, I sleep with the windows wide open for fear of suffocating during the night. I often wake up terrified that someone is suffocating me, as though they've put a plastic bag over my head." The patient went on to say that when he walked into my consulting room, he regularly felt that the room was too warm and that the air was disturbingly still. He said that it had never once occurred to him to ask me either to turn off the heater at the foot of the couch or to open a window, in large part because he has not been fully aware until now that he had such feelings. He said that it was terribly discouraging to realize how little he allows himself to know about what is going on inside of him, even to the point of not knowing when a room feels too warm.

Mr. L was silent for the remaining 15 minutes of the session. A silence of that length had not previously occurred in the analysis. During that silence, I did not feel pressured to talk. In fact, there was considerable feeling of repose and relief in the respite from what I now viewed as the "anxious mentation" with which he and I had so often filled the hours. I became aware of the tremendous effort that Mr. L and I regularly expended in an effort to keep the analysis from collapsing into despair: I imagined the two of us in the past frantically trying to keep a beach ball in the air, punching it from one to the other. Toward the end of the hour, I became drowsy and had to fight off sleep.

The patient began the next meeting by saying that he had been awakened by a dream early that morning. In the dream he was underwater and could see other people who were completely naked. He noticed that he, too, was naked, but he did not feel self-conscious about it. He was holding his breath and felt panicky that he would drown when he could no longer hold his breath. One of the men, who was obviously breathing underwater without difficulty, told him that it would be okay if he breathed. Mr. L very warily took a breath in the dream, and found that he could breathe. The scene changed, although he was still underwater. He was crying in deep sobs and was feeling profound sadness. A friend whose face he could not make out talked to him. Mr. L said that he felt grateful to the friend for not trying to reassure him or cheer him up.

The patient said that when he awoke from the dream he felt on the verge of tears. He got out of bed because he just wanted to feel what he was feeling although he did not know what he was sad about. Mr. L noticed the beginnings of his familiar attempts to change the feeling of sadness into feelings of anxiety about office business or worry about how much money he had in the bank and other matters with which he distracts himself.

Discussion

The foregoing account was offered not as an example of a watershed in an analysis, but rather in an effort to convey a sense of the unconscious dialectical movement of individual subjectivity and intersubjectivity in the analytic setting. I have attempted to describe something of the way in which my experience as analyst (including the barely perceptible and often extremely mundane background workings of my mind and body) is contextualized by the intersubjective experience created by analyst and analysand. No thought, feeling, or sensation can be considered to be the same as it was or will be outside of the context of the specific (and continually shifting) unconscious intersubjectivity created by analyst and analysand.

I would like to begin the discussion by saying that I am well aware that the form in which I presented the clinical material was a bit odd, in that I gave almost no information of the usual sort about Mr. L until rather late in the presentation. This was done in an effort to convey a sense of the degree to which Mr. L was at times quite absent from my conscious thoughts and feelings. My attention was not at all focused on Mr. L during my periods of reverie. (I use Bion's [1962] term *reverie* to refer not only to those psychological states that clearly reflect the analyst's active receptivity to the unconscious of the analysand, but also to a motley collection of psychological states that seem to reflect the analyst's narcissistic self-absorption, obsessional rumination, daydreaming, sexual fantasizing, bodily sensations, and so on.)

Turning to the details of the clinical material itself as it unfolded, my experience of the envelope (in the context of this analysis) began with my noticing the envelope itself, which, despite the fact that it had been physically present for weeks, came to life at that point as a psychological event, a carrier of psychological meanings, that had not existed prior to that moment. I view these new meanings not simply as a reflection of a lifting of a repression within me; rather, I understand the event as a reflection of the fact that a new subject (the analytic third) was being generated by (between) Mr. L and me, which resulted in the creation of the envelope as an "analytic object" (Bion 1962; Green 1975). When I noticed this new "object" on my table, I was drawn to it in a way that was so completely ego-syntonic as to be an almost completely unselfconscious event for me. I was struck by the machine-made markings on the envelope, which, again, had not been there (for me) to this point: I experienced these markings for the first time in the context of a matrix of meanings having to do with my distress at not feeling spoken to by Mr. L in a way that felt personal to me. The uncancelled stamps were similarly "created" and took their place in the intersubjective experience that was being elaborated. Feelings of estrangement and foreignness mounted to the point that I hardly recognized Mozart's name as a part of a common language.

A detail that requires some explanation is the series of fragmentary associations having to do with *Charlotte's Web*. Although highly personal and idiosyncratic to my own life experience, these thoughts and feelings were also being created anew within the context of the experience of the analytic third. I had consciously known that *Charlotte's Web* was very important to me, but the particular significance of the book was not only repressed, it had also not yet come into being in a way that it would exist in this hour. It was not until weeks after the described meeting that I became aware that this book was originally (and was in the process of becoming) intimately associated with feelings of loneliness. I realized for the first time (in the succeeding weeks) that, as a child, I had read this book several times during a period of intense loneliness and that I had thoroughly identified with Wilbur as a misfit and outcast. I view these largely unconscious associations to *Charlotte's Web* not as a retrieval of a memory that had been repressed, but as the creation of an experience (in and through the unconscious analytic intersubjectivity) that had not previously existed in the form that it was now taking. This conception of analytic intersubjectivity is central to the conception of the analytic process that I am developing: The analytic experience occurs at the cusp of the past and the present and involves a past that is being created anew (for both analyst and analysand) by means of an experience generated between analyst and analysand (i.e., within the analytic third).

Each time my conscious attention shifted from the experience of my own reveries to what the patient was saying and how he was saying it to me and being with me, I was not returning to the same place I had left seconds or minutes earlier; I was in each instance changed by the experience of the reverie, sometimes in only barely perceptible ways. When I refocused my attention on Mr. L after experiencing a series of thoughts and feelings concerning the envelope, I was more receptive to the schizoid quality of Mr. L's experience and to the hollowness of both his and my own attempts to create something together that felt real. I was more keenly aware of the feeling of arbitrariness associated with his sense of his place in his family and the world, as well as the feeling of emptiness associated with my own efforts at being *his* analyst.

I then became involved in a second series of "self-involved" thoughts and feelings (following my only partially satisfactory attempt to conceptualize my own despair and that of the patient in terms of projective identification[2]). My thoughts were interrupted by anxious fantasies and sensations concerning the closing of the garage and my need to end the last analytic hour of the day on time. My car had been in the garage the entire day, but it was only with this patient at precisely this mo-

---

[2]I believe that an aspect of the experience with Mr. L that I am describing can be understood in terms of projective identification, but at the point in the session when the idea occurred to me I was using the concept of projective identification predominantly as an intellectualizing defense.

ment that the car as analytic object was created. The fantasy involving the closing of the garage was created at that moment not by me in isolation, but through my participation in the unconscious intersubjective experience with Mr. L. Thoughts and feelings concerning the car and the garage did not occur in any of my other analytic sessions that day.

In the reverie concerning the closing of the garage and my need to end the last analytic hour of the day on time, the experience of bumping up against immovable, mechanical inhumanness in myself and others was repeated in a variety of forms. Interwoven with the fantasies were sensations of hardness (the pavement, glass, and grit) and suffocation (the exhaust fumes). These fantasies generated in me a sense of anxiety and urgency that was increasingly difficult for me to ignore (although in the past I might well have dismissed these fantasies and sensations as having no significance to the analysis except as an interference to be overcome).

Returning to listening to Mr. L in a focused way, I was still feeling quite confused about what was occurring in the session, and was sorely tempted to say something in order to dissipate my feelings of powerlessness. At this point, an event that had occurred earlier in the hour (the phone call recorded by my answering machine), occurred for the first time as an analytic event (that is, as an event that held meaning within the context of the unconscious intersubjectivity that was being elaborated). The voice recorded on the answering machine tape now held a promise of being the voice of a person who knew me and would speak to me in a personal way. The physical sensations of breathing freely and suffocating were increasingly important carriers of meaning. The envelope became still a different analytic object from the one that it had been earlier in the session: it now held meaning as a representation of an idiosyncratic, personal voice (the hand-typed name and address with an imperfect *t*).

The cumulative effect of these experiences within the analytic third led to the transformation of something the patient had said to me months earlier about feeling closest to me when I made mistakes. The patient's statement took on new meaning, but I think it would be more accurate to say that the (remembered) statement was now a new statement for me, and in this sense was being made for the first time.

I began at this point in the hour to be able to use language to describe for myself something of the experience of confronting an aspect of another person and of myself that felt frighteningly and irrevocably inhuman. A number of themes that Mr. L had been talking about took on a coherence for me that they had not previously held: the themes now seemed to me to converge on the idea that Mr. L was experiencing me and the discourse between us as bankrupt and dying. Again, these familiar themes were now becoming new analytic objects (for me) that I was encountering freshly. I attempted to talk to the patient about my sense of his experience of me and the analysis as mechanical and inhuman. Before I began the intervention, I did not consciously plan to use the imagery of machines (the factory and the time clock) to convey what I had in mind. I was unconsciously drawing on the imagery of my reveries concerning the mechanical (clock-determined) ending of an analytic session and the closing of the garage. I view my "choice" of imagery as a reflection of the way in which I was speaking *from* (not about) my unconscious experience of the analytic third (the unconscious intersubjectivity being created by Mr. L and me). At the same time, I was speaking about the analytic third from a position as analyst outside of it.

I went on in an equally unplanned way to tell the patient of an image of a vacuum chamber (another machine), in which something that appeared to be life-sustaining air was, in fact, emptiness (here I was unconsciously drawing on the sensation-images of the fantasied experience of exhaust-filled air outside the garage and the breath of fresh air associated with the answering machine fantasy[3]). Mr. L's response to my intervention involved a fullness of voice that reflected a fullness of breathing (a fuller giving and taking). His own conscious and unconscious feelings of being foreclosed from all that is human had been experienced in the form of images and sensations of suffocation at the hands of the killing mother/analyst (the plastic bag [breast] that prevented him from being filled with life-sustaining air).

The silence at the end of the session was in itself a new analytic event, and reflected a feeling of repose that stood in marked contrast to images of being violently suffocated in a plastic bag or of feeling disturbingly stifled by still air in my consulting room. There were two additional aspects of my experience during this silence that held significance: first, the fantasy of a beach ball, frantically kept aloft by being punched between Mr. L and me, and second, my feeling of drowsiness. Although I felt quite soothed by the way in which Mr. L and I were able to be silent together (in a combination of despair, exhaustion, and

[3]It was in this indirect way (i.e., in allowing myself to freely draw upon my unconscious experience with the patient in constructing my interventions) that I "told" the patient about my own experience in and of the analytic third. This indirect communication of the countertransference contributes in an important way to the feeling of spontaneity, aliveness, and authenticity of the analytic experience.

hope), there was an element in the experience of the silence (in part reflected in my somnolence) that felt like faraway thunder (which I retrospectively view as warded-off anger).

I shall only briefly comment on the dream with which Mr. L opened the next session. I understand it as simultaneously a response to the previous session and the beginnings of a sharper delineation of an aspect of the transference-countertransference in which Mr. L's fear of the effect of his anger on me, and of his homosexual feelings toward me, were becoming predominant anxieties. (I had had clues about this earlier on that I had been unable to use as analytic objects—e.g., the image and sensation of roaring traffic behind me in my garage reverie.)

In the first part of the dream, the patient was underwater with other naked people, including a man who told him that it would be all right to breathe, despite his fear of drowning. As he breathed, he found it hard to believe he was really able to do so. In the second part of Mr. L's dream, he was sobbing with sadness while a man whose face he could not make out stayed with him, but did not try to cheer him up. I view the dream as in part an expression of Mr. L's feeling that in the previous session, the two of us had together experienced and had begun to better understand something important about his unconscious ("underwater") life, and that I was not afraid of being overwhelmed (drowned) by his feelings of isolation, sadness, and futility, nor was I afraid for him. As a result, he dared to allow himself to be alive (to inhale) what he formerly feared would suffocate him (the vacuum breast/analyst). In addition, there was a suggestion that the patient's experience did not feel entirely real to him, in that in the dream, he found it difficult to believe he was really able to do what he was doing.

In the second portion of Mr. L's dream, he more explicitly represented his enhanced ability to feel his sadness in such a way that he felt less disconnected from himself and from me. The dream seemed to me to be in part an expression of the patient's gratitude to me for not having robbed him of the feelings he was beginning to experience, as I would have done had I interrupted the silence at the end of the previous day's meeting with an interpretation or other form of effort to dissipate—or even transform—his sadness with my words and ideas.

I felt that in addition to the gratitude (mixed with doubt) that Mr. L was experiencing in connection with these events, there were less acknowledged feelings of ambivalence toward me. I was alerted to this possibility in part by my own drowsiness at the end of the previous session, which often reflects my own state of defendedness. The fantasy of punching the beach ball (breast) suggested that it might well be anger that was being warded off. Subsequent events in the analysis led to me to feel increasingly convinced that the facelessness of the man in the second portion of Mr. L's dream was in part an expression of the patient's (maternal transference) anger at me for being so elusive as to be shapeless and nondescript (as he felt himself to be). This idea was borne out in the succeeding years of analysis as Mr. L's anger at me for "being nobody in particular" was directly expressed. In addition, on a more deeply unconscious level, the patient's being invited by the naked man to breathe in the water reflected what I felt to be an intensification of Mr. L's unconscious feeling that I was seducing him into being alive in the room with me, in a way that stirred homosexual anxiety (represented by the naked man's encouraging Mr. L to take the shared fluid into his mouth). I did not interpret the sexual anxiety reflected in the dream until much later in the analysis.

Reverie and the Analytic Third

In the clinical sequence described, it was not simply fortuitous that my mind "wandered" and came to focus on a machine-made set of markings on an envelope covered by scribblings of phone numbers, notes for teaching, and reminders to myself about errands to be done. The envelope itself (in addition to carrying the meanings mentioned above), also represented (what had been) my own private discourse, a private conversation not meant for anyone else. On it were notes in which I was talking to myself about the details of my life. The workings of the analyst's mind during analytic hours in these unselfconscious, "natural" ways are highly personal, private, and embarrassingly mundane aspects of life. It requires great effort to seize this aspect of the personal and the everyday from its unselfreflective area of reverie for the purpose of talking to oneself about the way in which this aspect of experience has been transformed in such a way that it has become a manifestation of the unconscious interplay of analytic subjects. The "personal" (the individually subjective) is never again simply what it had been prior to its creation in the intersubjective analytic third, nor is it entirely different from what it had been.

I believe that a major dimension of the analyst's psychological life in the consulting room with the patient takes the form of reverie concerning the ordinary, everyday details of his own life (that are often of great narcissistic importance to him).[4] I have attempted to demonstrate in this clinical discussion that these reveries are not simply reflections of inattentiveness, narcissistic self-involvement, unresolved emotional conflict, and the like. Rather, this psychological activity represents symbolic and protosymbolic (sensation-based) forms given to the unarticulated (and often not yet felt) experience of the analysand as they are taking form in the unconscious intersubjectivity of the analytic pair (i.e., in the analytic third).

This form of psychological activity is often viewed as something that the analyst must get through, put aside, overcome, and so on, in his effort to be emotionally present with, and attentive to, the analysand. I am suggesting that a view of the analyst's experience that is dismissive of this category of clinical phenomenon leads the analyst to diminish (or ignore) the significance of a great deal (in some instances, the majority) of his experience with the analysand. I feel that a principal factor contributing to the undervaluation of such a large portion of the analytic experience is the fact that such acknowledgment involves a disturbing form of heightened self-consciousness. The analysis of this aspect of the transference-countertransference requires an examination of the way we talk to ourselves and what we talk to ourselves about in a private, relatively undefended psychological state. In this state, the dialectical interplay of consciousness and unconsciousness has been altered in ways that resemble a dream state. In becoming self-conscious in this way, we are tampering with an essential inner sanctuary of privacy, and therefore with one of the cornerstones of our sanity. We are treading on sacred ground, an area of personal isolation in which, to a large extent, we are communicating with subjective objects (Winnicott 1963; see also Ogden 1991). This communication, like the notes to myself on the envelope, is not meant for anyone else, not even for aspects of ourselves that lie outside of this exquisitely private/mundane "cul-de-sac" (Winnicott 1963, p. 184). This realm of transference-countertransference experience is so personal, so ingrained in the character structure of the analyst, that it requires great psychological effort to enter into a discourse with ourselves in a way that is required to recognize that even this aspect of the personal has been altered by our experience in and of the analytic third. If we are to be analysts in a full sense, we must self-consciously attempt to bring even this aspect of ourselves to bear on the analytic process.

Some Additional Comments

Because the analytic third is experienced by analyst and analysand in the context of his or her own personality system, personal history, psy-

---

[4]Here and in the remainder of this paper, male pronouns are used to refer equally to both genders.

chosomatic make-up, and so on, the experience of the third, although jointly created, is not identical for each participant. Moreover, the analytic third is an asymmetrical construction because it is generated in the context of the analytic setting, which is powerfully defined by the relationship of roles of analyst and analysand. As a result, the unconscious experience of the analysand is privileged in a specific way; i.e., it is the past and present experience of the analysand that is taken by the analytic pair as the principal (although not exclusive) subject of analytic discourse. The analyst's experience in and of the analytic third is (primarily) utilized as a vehicle for the understanding of the conscious and unconscious experience of the analysand. (Analyst and analysand are not engaged in a democratic process of mutual analysis.)

The analytic third, though often having a coercive effect that limits the capacity of analyst and analysand to think as separate individuals, may also be of a generative and enriching sort. For instance, experiences in and of the analytic third often generate a quality of intimacy between patient and analyst that has "all the sense of real" (Winnicott 1963, p. 184). Such experiences involve feelings of enlivening humor, camaraderie, playfulness, compassion, healthy flirtatiousness, charm, and so on. These experiences in the analytic third may hold particular importance to the analysis in that they may be the first instances in the patient's life of such healthy, generative forms of object relatedness. More often than not, I defer interpreting meanings of such analytic events until much later in the analysis, if I interpret at all. It is living these experiences as opposed to understanding them that is of primary importance to the analysis.

PART II. PROJECTIVE IDENTIFICATION AND THE SUBJUGATING THIRD

Having discussed in Part I the experience of the analytic third in the clinical setting, I will now address the question of how the concept of the analytic third enriches psychoanalysis at the level of clinical theory. To that end, I shall offer some reflections on the process of projective identification conceptualized as a form of unconscious, intersubjective thirdness. In particular, I shall describe the unconscious interplay of mutual subjugation and mutual recognition that I view as fundamental to projective identification. (For discussions of other forms of the analytic third, see Ogden 1996, 1999.)

The understanding of projective identification that I shall propose is founded on a conception of psychoanalysis as a process in which a variety of forms of intersubjective *thirdness* are generated, which stand in dialectical tension with the analyst and analysand as separate psychological entities. In projective identification, a distinctive form of analytic thirdness is generated that I shall refer to as the *subjugating third,* since this form of intersubjectivity has the effect of subsuming within it, to a very large degree, the individual subjectivities of the participants.

I use the term *projective identification* to refer to a wide range of psychological-interpersonal events, including the earliest forms of mother–infant communication (Bion 1962); unconsciously fantasied, coercive incursions into and occupation of the personality of another person; schizophrenic confusional states (Rosenfeld 1965); and healthy "empathic sharing" (Pick 1985, p. 45).

Projective identification involves the creation of unconscious narratives (symbolized both verbally and nonverbally) that involve the fantasy of evacuating a part of oneself into another person. This fantasied evacuation serves the purpose of either protecting oneself from the dangers posed by an aspect of oneself or of safeguarding a part of oneself by depositing it in another person who is experienced as only partially differentiated from oneself (Klein 1946, 1955; see also Ogden 1979). The aspect of oneself that, in unconscious fantasy, resides in the other person is felt to be altered in the process, and under optimal conditions is imagined to be retrieved in a less toxic or endangered form (Bion 1959). Alternatively, under pathogenic conditions, the reappropriated part may be felt to have been deadened or to have become more persecutory than it had previously been.

Inextricably connected with this set of unconscious fantasies is a set of interpersonal correlates to the fantasies (Bion 1959; Joseph 1987; Racker 1968; Rosenfeld 1971). The interpersonal quality of the psychological event does not follow from the unconscious fantasy; the unconscious fantasy and the interpersonal event are *two aspects of a single psychological event.* Projective identification, conceived of in this way, is by now a widely accepted component of psychoanalytic theory. In what follows, I will offer a reworking—more an elaboration than a revision—of this understanding of projective identification.

The interpersonal facet of projective identification—as I view it from the perspective generated by the concept of the analytic third—involves a transformation of the subjectivity of the "recipient" in such a way that the separate "I-ness" of the other-as-subject is (for a time and to a degree) subverted. In this unconscious interplay of subjectivities, "You [the 'recipient' of the projective identification] are me [the projector] to the extent that I need to make use of you for the purpose of experiencing through you what I cannot experience myself. You are not me to the extent I need to disown an aspect of myself and in fantasy hide myself (disguised as not-me) in you." The recipient of the projective identification becomes a participant in the negation of himself as a separate subject, thus making "psychological room" in himself to be (in unconscious fantasy) occupied (taken over) by the projector.

The projector in the process of projective identification has unconsciously entered into a form of negation of himself as a separate "I" and in so doing has become other-to-himself: he has become, in part, an unconscious being outside of himself (residing in the recipient) who is simultaneously "I" and "not I." The recipient is and is not oneself (the projector) at a distance. The projector in this process is becoming someone other than who he had been to that point. His experience of occupying the recipient is an experience of negating the other as subject and coopting the recipient's subjectivity with his own subjectivity; at the same time, the occupying part of the projector's self is objectified (experienced as a part object) and disowned. The outcome of this mutually negating process is the creation of a third subject, "the subject of projective identification," which is both and neither projector and recipient. Thus, projective identification is a process by which the individual subjectivities of both projector and recipient are being negated in different ways: the projector is disavowing an aspect of himself that he imagines to be evacuated into the recipient while the recipient is participating in a negation of himself by surrendering to (making room for) the disavowed aspect of the subjectivity of the projector.

It does not suffice to say that projective identification simply represents a powerful form of projection or of identification or a summation of the two, since the concepts of projection and identification address only the intrapsychic dimension of experience. Rather, projective identification must be understood in terms of a mutually creating, negating, and preserving dialectic of subjects, each of whom allows himself to be "subjugated" by the other—i.e., negated in such a way as to become, through the other, a third subject (the subject of projective identification).

What is distinctive about projective identification as a form of analytic relatedness is that the analytic intersubjectivity characterizing it is one in which the (asymmetrical) mutual subjugation, which mediates the process of creating a third subjectivity, has the effect of profoundly subverting the experience of analyst and analysand as separate subjects. In the analytic setting, projective identification involves a type of partial collapse of the dialectical movement of subjectivity and intersubjectivity, resulting in the subjugation (of the individual subjectivities of analyst and analysand) by the analytic third. The analytic process, if successful, involves the reappropriation of the individual subjectivities of analyst and analysand, which have been transformed through their experience of (in) the newly created analytic third (the "subject of projective identification").

Projective identification can he thought of as involving a central paradox: the individuals engaged in this form of relatedness unconsciously subjugate themselves to a mutually generated intersubjective third for the purpose of freeing themselves from the limits of whom they had been to that point. In projective identification, analyst and analysand are each limited and enriched; each is stifled and vitalized. The new intersubjective entity that is created, the subjugating analytic third, becomes a vehicle through which thoughts might be thought, feelings might be felt, sensations might be experienced, dreams might be dreamt, which to that point had existed only as potential experiences for each of the individuals participating in this psychological-interpersonal process. In order for psychological growth to occur, there must be a superseding of the subjugating third and the establishment of a new and more generative dialectic of oneness and twoness, similarity and difference, individual subjectivity and intersubjectivity.

Although Klein (1955) focused almost entirely on the experience of psychological depletion involved in projective identification, the work of Bion (1962), Racker (1968), Rosenfeld (1971), and others has demonstrated that projective identification also involves the creation of something potentially larger and more generative than either of the participants (in isolation from one another) is capable of generating. The vitalization or expansion of the individual subject is not exclusively an aspect of the experience of the projector; the "recipient" of a projective identification does not simply experience the event as a form of psychological burden in which he is limited and deadened. In part, this is due to the fact that there is never a recipient who is not simultaneously a projector in a projective identificatory experience. The interplay of subjectivities is never entirely one sided: each person is being negated by the other while being newly created in the unique dialectical tension generated by the two.

The recipient of the projective identification is engaged in a negation (subversion) of his own individuality in part for the unconscious purpose of disrupting the closures underlying the coherence/stagnation of the self. Projective identification offers the recipient the possibility of creating a new form of experience that is other-to-himself and thereby creates conditions for the alteration of the person whom he has been to that point and whom he has experienced himself to be. The recipient is not simply identifying with an other (the projector); he is becoming an other and experiencing (what is becoming) himself through the subjectivity of a newly created other/third/self.

The two subjects entering into a projective identification (albeit involuntarily) each unconsciously attempt to overcome (negate) themselves and in so doing make room for the creation of a novel subjectivity, an experience of I-ness that each individual in isolation could not have created for himself. In one sense, we participate in projective identification (often despite our most strenuous conscious efforts to avoid doing so) in order to create ourselves in and through the other-who-is-not-fully other; at the same time, we unconsciously allow ourselves to serve as the vehicle through which the other (who-is-not-fully other) creates himself as subject through us. In different ways, each of the individuals entering into a projective identification experiences both aspects (both forms of negating and being negated) in this intersubjective event. It does not suffice simply to say that in projective identification, one finds oneself playing a role in someone else's unconscious fantasy (Bion 1959). More fully stated, one finds oneself unconsciously both playing a role in *and* serving as author of someone else's unconscious fantasy.

In projective identification, one unconsciously abrogates a part of one's own separate individuality in order to move beyond the confines of that individuality: one unconsciously subjugates oneself in order to free oneself from oneself. The generative freeing of the individual participants from the subjugating third depends upon 1) the analyst's act of recognizing the individuality of the analysand (e. g., by means of his accurate and empathic understanding and interpretation of the transference-countertransference) and 2) the analysand's recognition of the separate individuality of the analyst (e.g., through the analysand's making use of the analyst's interpretations).

The projector and the recipient of a projective identification are unwitting, unconscious allies in the project of using the resources of their individual subjectivity and their intersubjectivity to escape the solipsism of their own separate psychological existences. Both have circled in the realm of their own internal object relations, from which even the intrapsychic discourse that we call self-analysis can offer little in the way of lasting psychological change when isolated from intersubjective experience. (This is not to say that self-analysis is without value; rather, I believe that it has severe limitations when isolated from intersubjective spheres such as those provided by projective identification.) Human beings have a need as deep as hunger and thirst to establish intersubjective constructions (including projective identifications) in order to find an exit from unending, futile wanderings in their own internal object world. It is in part for this reason that consultation with colleagues and supervisors plays such an important role in the practice of psychoanalysis.

The unconscious intersubjective alliance involved in projective identification may have qualities that feel to the participants like something akin to a kidnapping, blackmailing, seduction, mesmerization, being swept along by the irresistible, frightening lure of an unfolding horror story, and so on. However, the degree of pathology associated with a given projective identificatory experience is not to be measured by the degree of coercion involved in the fantasied subjugation; rather, pathology in projective identificatory experience is a reflection of the degree of inability/unwillingness of the participants to release one another from the subjugation of the third by means of a mutual act of recognition (often mediated by means of interpretation) of the unique and separate individuality of the other and of oneself.

In sum, the concept of projective identification, to my mind, is substantially enriched by viewing it as a form of the intersubjective analytic third. In projective identification, so conceived, there is a partial collapse of the unconscious dialectical movement of individual subjectivity and intersubjectivity, resulting in the co-creation of a subjugating analytic third (within which the individual subjectivities of the participants are to a large degree subsumed). A successful psychoanalytic process involves the superseding of the unconscious third and the reappropriation of the (transformed) subjectivities by the participants as separate (and yet interdependent) individuals. This is achieved through an act of mutual recognition that is often mediated by the analyst's interpretation of the transference-countertransference and the analysand's making genuine psychological use of the analyst's interpretation.

REFERENCES

Barranger M: The mind: from listening to interpretation. Int J Psychoanal 74:15–24, 1993

Bion WR: Group dynamics: a review (1952), in Experiences in Groups. New York, Basic Books, 1959, pp 141–192

Bion WR: Attacks on linking. Int J Psychoanal 40:308–315, 1959

Bion WR: Learning From Experience. New York, Basic Books, 1962

Boyer LB: Countertransference: history and clinical issues, in Master Clinicians on Treating the Regressed Patient, Vol 2. Edited by Boyer LB, Giovacchini PL. Northvale, NJ, Jason Aronson, 1993, pp 1–21

Etchegoyen RH: The Fundamentals of Psychoanalytic Technique. London, Karnac, 1991

Green A: The analyst, symbolization and absence in the analytic setting. (On changes in analytic practice and analytic experience). Int J Psychoanal 56:1–22, 1975

Joseph B: Projective identification: some clinical aspects, in Melanie Klein Today, Vol 1: Mainly Theory. Edited by Spillius E. New York, Routledge, 1987, pp 183–150

Klein M: Notes on some schizoid mechanisms (1946), in Envy and Gratitude and Other Works, 1946–1963. New York, Delacorte, 1975, pp 1–24

Klein M: On identification (1955), in Envy and Gratitude and Other Works 1946–1963. New York, Delacorte, 1975, pp 141–175

Ogden T: On projective identification. Int J Psychoanal 60:357–373, 1979

Ogden T: Some theoretical comments on personal isolation. Psychoanalytic Dialogues: A Journal of Relational Perspectives 1:377–390, 1991

Ogden T: The analytic third: working with intersubjective clinical facts. Int J Psychoanal 75:3–20, 1994a

Ogden T: Projective identification and the subjugating third, in Subjects of Analysis. Northvale, NJ, Jason Aronson, 1994b, pp 97–106

Ogden T: The perverse subject of analysis. J Am Psychoanal Assoc 44:1121–1146, 1996

Ogden T: The analytic third: an overview, in Relational Perspectives in Psychoanalysis: The Emergence of a Tradition. Edited by Mitchell S, Aron L. Hillsdale, NJ, Analytic Press, 1999, pp 487–492

Pick I: Working through in the countertransference (1985), in Melanie Klein Today, Vol 2: Mainly Practice. Edited by Spillius E. London, Routledge, 1988, pp 34–47

Racker H: Transference and Countertransference. New York, International Universities Press, 1968

Rosenfeld H: Psychotic States: A Psycho-Analytic Approach. New York, International Universities Press, 1965

Rosenfeld H: Contribution to the psychopathology of psychotic states: the importance of projective identification in the ego structure and the object relations of the psychotic patient, in Problems of Psychosis. Edited by Doucet P, Laurin C. Amsterdam, Excerpta Medica, 1971, pp 115–128

Winnicott DW: The theory of the parent-infant relationship (1960), in The Maturational Processes and the Facilitating Environment. New York, International Universities Press, 1965, pp 37–55

Winnicott DW: Communicating and not communicating leading to a study of certain opposites (1963), in The Maturational Processes and the Facilitating Environment. New York, International Universities Press, 1965, pp 179–192

20

PAUL H. ORNSTEIN, M.D.

INTRODUCTION

Paul Ornstein received his medical degree in Heidelberg, Germany, after surviving the Holocaust in Hungary. He did his psychiatric training at the University of Cincinnati in Ohio, where he is Professor of Psychiatry (Emeritus) and Professor of Psychoanalysis (Emeritus). He is a graduate of the Chicago Institute for Psychoanalysis, a Training and Supervising Analyst at the Cincinnati Psychoanalytic Institute, and Codirector of the International Center for the Study of Psychoanalytic Self Psychology at the University of Cincinnati. He is currently Lecturer in Psychiatry at Harvard University Medical School (Massachusetts Mental Health Center), is a faculty member of the Psychoanalytic Institute New England East and the Boston Psychoanalytic Institute, and teaches as well at the Massachusetts Institute for Psychoanalysis.

Dr. Ornstein has written on psychoanalytic psychotherapy, the interpretive process in psychoanalysis, and self psychology. He coauthored a book with Michael Balint on focal psychotherapy and edited and introduced the collection of Heinz Kohut's selected writings, *The Search for the Self,* volumes 1–4. Dr. Ornstein has nearly 100 scientific publications to his credit. Both alone and with his wife Anna, he has conducted more than 200 seminars and workshops in most major psychoanalytic training centers in the United States and abroad; the latter included centers in Argentina, Austria, Australia, Canada, Germany, Greece, Hungary, Holland, Israel, Italy, Indonesia (Bali and Yogyakarta), Norway, Peru, Sweden, Switzerland, and Turkey.

Dr. Ornstein is a former member of the editorial boards of *The Journal of the American Psychoanalytic Association* and *Psychoanalytic Inquiry,* is an active member of the editorial board of *Progress in Self Psychology,* and has lectured throughout the psychoanalytic universe. In the last decade, he has been studying the works of Dostoyevski and has presented a number of workshops on that topic at meetings of the American Psychoanalytic Association as well as at annual conferences on the psychoanalytic psychology of the self.

He has said of himself:

> I did a major review of Kohut's work in editing and introducing the first two volumes of his selected papers and another major review of his later work for the last two volumes of his additional selected papers.
>
> My main interest in self psychology involved the treatment process, and it is on this topic that I have written more than a half dozen papers and then quite a number (in addition to some jointly with Anna Ornstein) in which I have expanded, and to a degree made more explicit, what Kohut left unelaborated and then also modified what he left us with. In the areas of "expansion," I have written about empathy and have studied the relationship between theory and practice (also with Anna), as well as the supervisory process and other training issues in psychoanalysis. In my plenary address at the American Psychoanalytic Association in 2002, I have reformulated the nature of the psychoanalytic process, delineating the patient's and the analyst's contributions to the development of an identifiable micro- and macroprocess—regardless of the analyst's preferred guiding theory as an inevitable "natural" evolution.
>
> Together, Anna and I have introduced self psychology over the last 20 years in many countries. We have established a Center for the Study of Self Psychology in Cincinnati and have had 25 visiting clinicians and scholars from abroad to study with us for months at a time, some of them repeatedly returning for supervision for a week or a month annually, even today, in Boston. We have established a similar center with a colleague in Konstanz, Germany, where we have held a marathon clinic conference for a long weekend yearly for over 14 years. Next March will be our 15th consecutive year. We have gone back to Vienna, Rome, and Konstanz to lecture and conduct clinical seminars repeatedly over the years.

WHY I CHOSE THIS PAPER

Paul H. Ornstein, M.D.

There are always multiple reasons (some within, others outside of awareness) for such an important choice as the paper being included in this volume. I shall focus only on some of those reasons of which I am immediately aware.

This paper, "Chronic Rage From Underground," deals with one of the most difficult clinical problems: the understanding and analytic response to rage in the analytic situation, especially when this rage is hidden and cannot be felt by the patient. Yet the patient whose case is presented, Mr. K, insists that his rage is lodged within him, and he would wish to connect to it emotionally so as to feel what he now cannot feel.

In the course of this long and arduous analysis, I learned much that is valid for me across the clinical spectrum. The repeated disruptions of the transference and their repair progressively permitted my participation in this analysis on an ever-deepening level and allowed me to illustrate some generally useful principles of analysis from a self psychological perspective. When such disruptions exposed Mr. K's hidden rage, they presented me with an opportunity to grasp the nature of my participation in triggering the disruptions and offered me a variety of ways for their analytic repair. It was Mr. K, among others, whose analysis taught me how to analyze at greater depth, which turned out to be generally valid in my work. Hence, I have reported about several crucial aspects of this analysis in a number of publications. This paper represents well my analytic work guided by self psychology, and that is the main reason I have selected it for inclusion in the present volume.

CHRONIC RAGE FROM UNDERGROUND

Reflections on Its Structure and Treatment

PAUL H. ORNSTEIN, M.D.

IN HIS *Notes From Underground,*[1] Dostoyevski (1864) presents us with an unparalleled portrayal of his protagonist's chronic rage. This rage resides mostly within, a private inner experience that nevertheless dominates all behavior from its internal hiding place. Only occasionally does the rage burst forth into open, violent, vindictive, and revengeful attacks on those whose real or imagined slights create immense suffering for the protagonist. This suffering (as silent to the external observer as the rage it provokes) is marked by a subjectively painful sense of humiliation and degradation; by pervasive hypochondriacal preoccupations; by a constant elaboration of the most detailed plans for revenge to right even the slightest, but greatly magnified, wrong; and, most significantly, by a whole series of behaviors that we would undoubtedly judge from the outside as self-defeating but that Dostoyevski illuminates from the inside as desperate attempts to regain lost self-regard. All these reactions are embedded in the context of a pervasive sense of superiority and self-importance, which exists side by side with a sense of utter worthlessness and unbearable shame.

---

[1]The literal translation of the original Russian title is, more accurately, "Notes From a Hole in the Floor," i.e., from a mousehole.

"Chronic Rage From Underground: Reflections on Its Structure and Treatment," by Paul H. Ornstein, M.D., was first published in *The Widening Scope of Self-Psychology,* Volume 9, edited by Arnold Goldberg, pp. 143–157.

Dostoyevski lets the fictitious author of *Notes* reveal his agonies in the first person, thereby lending these compulsively honest, often monotonously repetitious, yet courageous and cogent self-revelations a particular urgency and dramatic intensity. This succeeds in drawing the reader inside the whole experience, inside every detail of it. The immediacy of the communication in the first person is so compelling that we cannot emerge from the reading of these notes (or from listening to them on tape as I have recently done) unscathed. A whole gamut of reactions is mobilized in the process, as if we were listening to a patient's free associations. And we can completely extricate ourselves neither from the "underground man's" revelations nor from our own affect-laden reactions to them. We admire him for being able to see so clearly into every nook and cranny of his inner world, but we get frustrated and annoyed that all this power of observation, all this cogent knowledge, is unable to move him out of his self-defeating behavior. We get bored with the repetitiousness of his reacting to such minuscule slights with such huge investments of energy in planning his revenge; we see that it brings him no relief, whether he is able to go through with his revengeful act or not. If he does act, he agonizes over having done it; and if he does not, he ends up in endless recriminations for his cowardliness. There is no escape for him from self-loathing and self-torment. His constant inner dialogue with those who already harmed him in the past and with those who inevitably will in the future takes up every moment of his waking hours and animates his inextinguishable memories of a lifetime of insults and injuries.

Notes From Underground reads as if Dostoyevski were familiar with "Thoughts on Narcissism and Narcissistic Rage" (Kohut 1972). In fact, Dostoyevski has provided us with an independent data base of observations and interpretations that not only buttresses our own but actually fills in many of the details not yet fully articulated in our literature. These "notes" present a remarkably vivid, pertinent microscopic study of the personality structure and experiences of those who suffer from chronic rage.

But my goal here is not an exhaustive analysis of Dostoyevski's *Notes From Underground,* tempting as it would be to offer a comprehensive exploration of it in all its details. I have referred to it here only to set the stage for my brief remarks on some theoretical as well as clinical issues related to the broad topic of aggression and rage.

I shall first reflect briefly on Kohut's fundamental contributions to our understanding and treatment of aggression and narcissistic rage and then introduce a particularly difficult clinical problem in the analysis of a patient of mine, Mr. K, who has been feeling dominated by his chronic, silent rage and revengefulness and has long been presenting me with his own "notes from underground," to which it has often been difficult for me to find a sustained, optimum analytic response.

REFLECTIONS ON KOHUT'S FUNDAMENTAL CONTRIBUTIONS ON AGGRESSION AND RAGE

Kohut's (1972) "Thoughts on Narcissism and Narcissistic Rage" has long been considered one of his most brilliant contributions (see Ornstein and Ornstein 1993). It is a veritable tour de force that further strengthened the core of his clinical and theoretical innovations, presented in *The Analysis of the Self* just one year earlier (Kohut 1971). I have often regretted that he did not extend it to a monograph-length study with more detailed, lengthier clinical illustrations. But even in this relatively brief essay Kohut advanced a number of clinical and theoretical formulations that are to this very day the cornerstones of our approach to aggression and rage—even if some of them (since they were advanced prior to 1977) have to be reformulated or otherwise updated within the framework of an evolving psychology of the self. I need not review here what Kohut said in 1972, but I wish to review some of his key propositions in order to highlight why they are of such fundamental significance and to indicate in what areas they need further empirical validation as well as conceptual clarification.

It is remarkable that although he did not assemble his experiences and ideas about narcissistic rage into a monograph, Kohut did deal rather systematically with this topic: He offered an encompassing classification; he postulated the etiology and pathogenesis of narcissistic rage and of a whole spectrum of related phenomena; and, finally, he outlined the principles of treatment and portrayed the gradual transformation of narcissistic rage into mature aggression. I shall comment in passing on each of these three main areas.

Classification

Kohut constructed a spectrum of rage experiences, starting with fleeting annoyance and anger at one end and culminating in the furor of the catatonic and the grudges of the paranoiac at the other. The spectrum includes additional forms of rage, such as the well-known "catastrophic reaction" of the brain-damaged and its many attenuated variations, as well as the child's reaction to painful injuries, and Kohut left it to further empirical research to delineate still other forms.

Kohut viewed narcissistic rage as just one specific band in this whole spectrum, but because he considered this the best-known among all related phenomena, he designated the entire spectrum as narcissistic rage. This has created some ambiguity and has led to the frequent question, Is all aggression narcissistic rage? Yes, from our current perspective I would say that all destructive aggression is at its roots narcissistic rage—whatever its outward manifestation, however mild or severe, acute or chronic. Kohut (1972) himself wrote that "underlying all these emotional states [within the spectrum] is the uncompromising insistence on the perfection of the idealized selfobject and on the limitless power and knowledge of the grandiose self" (p. 643). This "dynamic essence" of narcissistic rage is common to all experiences within the broad spectrum of rage phenomena, from the mildest and most fleeting to the most persistent and destructive.

Note that Kohut did not construct a spectrum from mature aggression at one end to the most destructive rage at the other, arranging these phenomena on a continuum, the usual analytic approach in portraying drive-related phenomena being to place the normal at one end of a spectrum and the pathological at the other. Instead, in 1972 Kohut properly contrasted narcissistic rage with mature aggression and thereby indicated their separate origins and development. Once he replaced the concept of mature (or nondestructive) aggression with self-assertiveness (or self-assertive ambition), he further sharpened the view that the latter was primary and the former was secondary or reactive and that the two were clearly not within the same developmental line.

Thus, we can reaffirm that it is appropriate to speak of the various forms of rage as all belonging under the umbrella of narcissistic rage and contrast these with self-assertiveness. To label one specific band in the spectrum as well as the whole spectrum itself as narcissistic rage has the advantage of indicating the commonality or fundamental characteristic of all phenomena included in the spectrum. It would be desirable, however, to find an equally evocative but more fitting designation to finally leave behind the now-ambiguous and undesirable term *narcissistic*.[2]

Etiology and Pathogenesis

It is in relation to the etiology and pathogenesis of narcissistic rage and its experiential content that Kohut made his most innovative contributions. While many analysts before him had given up the notion of aggression as a drive and considered it as arising secondarily due to frustration, Kohut specified both the matrix from which the rage arose and the structural and dynamic conditions under which this occurred. He pinpointed various kinds of traumatic injuries to the grandiose self and traumatic obstacles to merger with the idealized parent imago and thus located the propensity for rage within this highly vulnerable, archaic, narcissistic matrix of the personality. In this connection he elaborated in some detail on the experiential content of the various forms of narcissistic rage.

The 1972 essay fits in with and also buttresses the conceptual edifice that Kohut (1971) built in *The Analysis of the Self.* The key point he made is this: It is not the rage as an intensification and unbridled expression of the aggressive drive that is the essence of the pathology; the essence of the pathology is the underlying structural deficiency of the self—its vulnerability and periodic, transient collapse in response to certain types of injury. The implication is clear: We do not achieve a direct transformation of narcissistic rage into healthy self-assertiveness. To the degree that we can restore the structural integrity of the self it will gradually become capable of asserting itself and pursuing its ambition. To

---

[2]In a more comprehensive discussion of our nosology I would draw the analogy between Freud's (1937) assessment of the entire spectrum of psychopathology, from the neuroses at one end through the various personality disorders in the middle to the psychoses at the other end, using the parameter of qualitatively different structural changes in the ego. Freud described the ego in psychoses as characterized by a structural defect, in personality disorders by a structural deformity, and in the neuroses—where the ego was hitherto considered intact—by a structural modification. Each of these ego alterations was then specified. Kohut (1977) did the same when he assessed the entire spectrum of psychopathology using the parameter of qualitatively different structural changes in the self. He described the self in the psychoses as fragmented (never having attained cohesiveness); in the personality disorders as enfeebled and/or fragmentation-prone (but having at one time been cohesive); and, finally, in the neuroses as cohesive (with sufficient stability) but capable—under the impact of traumata during the oedipal phase—of becoming secondarily enfeebled or fragmented. The main point is that each component of the spectrum of psychopathology can profitably be viewed from this perspective as a self disorder at bottom, albeit with qualitative differences in both phenomenology and structure.

In a more thorough reassessment of our nosology the impact of Kohut's (1978) postulate that we need selfobjects from birth to death, i.e., that development proceeds from archaic to mature selfobjects, would also have to be considered. Would then the assumption that the mature selfobject replaces the "object" in our theoretical discourse (Ornstein 1991) further affect our nosology of rage?

the degree that it still suffers from enfeeblement or periodic fragmentation it will continue to show a propensity for rage reactions as a consequence of fragmentation and/or efforts at restitution. In other words, self-assertiveness is a function of the healthy self whereas rage is a function of a vulnerable, structurally deficient self.

Treatment Principles

Psychoanalysts frequently assert that there is only one way to understand psychopathology, namely, analytically—and they have in mind their own preferred psychoanalytic paradigm for this purpose—but that there are many ways to treat the patient. While this may well be a widespread attitude, I see it as a special advantage of Kohut's formulations that his nosology (including etiology and pathogenesis), as well as his dynamic and structural considerations, leads directly to the treatment principles he espoused. There is in his work a closely intertwined connection between theory and practice. Thus, it logically follows from his view of rage that it is the underlying self disorder per se that occupies center stage within the psychoanalytic or psychotherapeutic process via the particular selfobject transference. The interpretive emphasis in the working through is on the disturbances that produce the rage and/or on how the rage is used to prevent further disintegration or to attempt to restore the integrity of the self.[3]

Certain forms of chronic rage, walled off from being experienced by the patient and from reaching direct expression in the transference, present particular difficulties in the treatment process. It is to such a difficulty that I shall now turn with the aid of a brief clinical example.

I hope to illustrate aspects of the nature of the particular self disorder in which the patient's chronic rage was embedded. Along with that I wish to show that the usual effort of focusing on the repair of the various kinds of disruptions of the mirror transference (rather than seeking

---

[3]Critics have claimed that self psychologists do not deal with narcissistic rage interpretively but, instead, bypass it. These critics are superficially accurate in that we pay no direct interpretive attention to tracing the source of the rage to the aggressive drive at various developmental levels (oral, anal, phallic, and oedipal)—if that is what is meant by its analytic interpretation. That our interpretations focus on the surrounding psychopathology and its amelioration—with salutary consequences for decreasing the propensity for rage—has thus far not altered this particular criticism. Nor have the critics acknowledged that this is primarily an empirical question.

direct access to the rage), when successful, regularly diminished the outward manifestations of the hidden rage to a good degree. The patient would behave in a calmer, more integrated fashion but would still bitterly complain about not feeling anything or not really participating in his own inner experiences, and he would again, at the next disruption, feel nothing of his rage. It was only after the discovery of an attitude in myself—a somewhat camouflaged reluctance or reserve vis-à-vis the patient's concrete mirroring needs and demands—that locked in his inability to feel his rage or to participate in any of his own experiences that further progress could be made. The patient sensed this reservation no matter how much I acknowledged the legitimacy of his archaic needs and demands. This discovery and the changes I was able to make in my approach as a result were followed by a slow transformation of the patient's archaic expectations for concrete, overt responses for mirroring into an expectation that I should know precisely and accept without reservation all of his feelings, needs, and demands (and give evidence of this acceptance through my emotional presence with him!). It was only then that a prolonged stalemate began to be resolved.

MR. K'S PERVASIVE, CHRONIC, UNDERGROUND[4] RAGE

In Mr. K's prolonged and arduous analysis his profound and persistent hunger for mirroring appeared to be the central theme. For quite some time, however, this remained hidden and unavailable to our joint analytic scrutiny. No matter what the varied contents of his free associations were, our joint effort at their elucidation was frequently greeted by one of the following remarks, uttered with painful resignation: "That didn't work for me" or "That failed for me completely." Since our understanding appeared to hit the mark just moments before, I was often quite puzzled. "In what way did it not work?" I asked. Mr. K had no immediate response. It took a while to discover that the failure related to the fact that Mr. K secretly expected some sign of explicit appreciation of his considerable interpretive skills, his scrupulous honesty in not holding back anything, or the precision and fearlessness with which he

---

[4]*Underground* symbolically refers here to the hidden, sequestered, or walled-off "depth of his soul," as Mr. K frequently put it. It is where his rage resides and where he cannot get to it. He does not feel the rage; he cannot experience it or connect to it, but he knows it is there.

could describe inner experience, even of the most disturbing kind. It was these that he wished to show off; the actual content was of lesser significance. What we finally understood in this phase of the analysis was that Mr. K cared little about what he alone or we jointly discovered—although he sharply objected to every inaccuracy regarding his subjective experiences that I may have introduced into our analytic conversation. What mattered to him was whether or not he could feel that I truly appreciated what he brought to the session. If he felt that I was not with him in his (often considerably subdued or hidden) excitement but maintained an analytic neutrality, as he viewed it, the failure was disturbing to him and its consequences would last for days or weeks. He would become withdrawn, apathetic, and without energy. He would then speak in a colorless monotone for a while, without his usual vivid imagery and richly expressive metaphors. This would tone me down too, and Mr. K would then rightly point to my "apathy," no matter how slight—and often not even recognized by me until his comment on it or until it dawned on me that he was holding up a mirror to me with his own behavior to express how he experienced me. Nothing was more effective in reestablishing good communication or in repairing the breach in the mirror transference than when I could show him what in my attitude, tone of voice, or behavior he experienced as hurtful to him and would then say that he was portraying this feeling of having been assaulted in his own behavior toward me. This not only made good sense to him, but he also experienced it as an accepting stance on my part. He did not feel criticized for behaving the way he did or feel he was being asked to modify his own behavior—which is how his parents always responded ("You shouldn't feel this way!"). Thus, repair could be established and Mr. K's inner rage would temporarily subside. I say "inner rage" again because he could not *feel* the rage. He only knew that he acted on it because his behavior revealed it to him.

An example will illustrate what I mean. Mr. K started one early morning session with an apathetic demeanor and a long silence. It was difficult to get going and we could make no headway until I realized that his nonparticipation might have been triggered by something that transpired between us. On my way to the waiting room a few minutes earlier I had suddenly realized, with some concern, that I had forgotten to prepare for an important meeting later that day. Preoccupied briefly with this thought, I did not have a receptive smile for Mr. K on encountering him. When I inquired at first in general terms as to what might have triggered his withdrawal, we got nowhere. When I suggested that his gloomy demeanor perhaps reflected how he experienced me on entering the waiting room, he immediately confirmed my assumption. He added that whenever he felt that he was not eagerly met but only "routinely" invited into the office, he rebelled against being there: "If you are not present [emotionally], I won't be either. I will not come out of my rabbit hole into a vacuum, it is dangerous for me." He then elaborated at great length on the poisonous atmosphere at home during his infancy and childhood, and it became clearer how the analytic situation at times inadvertently replicated for him his early environment.

It was henceforth somewhat easier for both of us to discern and deal with disruptions and repair. After we recovered from such an episode, however, the cycle would soon begin again. I admired Mr. K's tenacity and his, in many subtle ways, unextinguished hopefulness in the face of repeated "failures," and I hoped that he would ultimately sense my full appreciation of him and what he was accomplishing in gaining a better sense of the nature of his inner experiences. What I still found myself reluctant to do was to offer him an unrestrained, explicit admiration—at times it seemed he wanted that escalated into outright jubilation—for his, admittedly, great analytic feats of remarkable insightfulness, especially in relation to his ingenious interpretation of his dreams. I was reacting to the fact that there was no carryover from one such apparently successful session to the next. It was as if in each session trust had to be built up again from the beginning.

Only much later did it become clear to me that since I truly admired Mr. K in many ways, I had expected him to discover this without my having to prove it to him at every turn. But before I knew this as explicitly as I am relating it now, my expectation that he should discover it had become a countertransference obstacle in the analytic process. As was usually the case, Mr. K helped me discover it, which ameliorated it somewhat. His frequent bouts of emotional withdrawal—his "defiant nonpresence in the room," as he put it—tipped me off. I could see his withholding and reluctance, expressions of his unforgiving, chronic rage, as a magnified reproduction of what he accurately perceived as some reservation or reluctance on my part to give him the explicit admiration he craved. He once characterized my withholding explicit approval and appreciation for some brilliant work he had done in the session as the same "arrogance [his] father would show under similar circumstances." The word arrogance—as you might imagine—prevented me for a time from seeing its relevance, that is until I could calmly reflect on the fact that I held a certain view as to what was a proper analytic response and to the degree that I held that view, I could not listen to him from his vantage point without reservation. I then no longer bristled at his description of my behavior as arrogance. (If Breuer had refused to follow Anna O's request that he listen to everything she had to say in a particular way, she might rightly have called him arrogant and given up treatment. Where is the limit to the extent to which we have to follow the patient's need [request or demand] for a certain kind of responsiveness in order to enable the analytic process to move forward—and without which it would stagnate? Who can tell? And why is it so difficult to find it?)

Whenever the issue of my "withholding" could be included in the analytic conversation, there were, at least temporarily, some salutary effects. At other times Mr. K insisted that withdrawal and nonpresence constituted a baseline state for him and that this could change only after we established "rapport" (an emotional presence on my part that then—and only then—allowed him to be present) in the session. Only under these conditions could he climb out of his "rabbit hole." Otherwise, he would have to remain emotionally absent.

During some stretches of this period, Mr. K would sense my "presence" only when he felt enough of an appreciation and affirmation from me through my tone of voice (to which he was very sensitive), the amount I talked (the more I did, the more valued and valuable he felt), and the number of "genuine" questions I asked (the greater the number of questions, the more he could feel my participation in his struggle; otherwise, he felt alone with it). The accuracy or correctness of my understanding mattered little, and that rankled me at times, even if only mildly. Mr. K could acknowledge my having hit the nail on the head—"but only intellectually," he would add; something was always missing. Only the absence of appreciation and affirmation was registered and put on the ledger, rarely to be forgotten. Mr. K experienced these episodes as devastating. He could not imagine that my repeated "stupidity" or "callousness" was not a deliberate attempt to foil his efforts, put him in his place, humiliate him, a belief that chronically fed his rage.

What sustained me in the interim, nevertheless, was the fact that while these ruptures were frequent, painful, and lasting, the efforts at repair always yielded significant memories from the past as well as some additional understanding of what was going on in his experiences with me, namely, how I affected him and how he needed to protect himself from feeling "foiled, defeated, and humiliated."

To give you just one telling example from this period: Mr. K would frequently pepper his free associations (whatever the content, to which I was listening attentively) with some hurried, offhanded, "tucked away" remark about a physical sensation he was just having—such as "My anus is tense now" or "There is a cramp in my rear end"—and would then, without stopping, go on with whatever he was talking about. When I would later on recap what he said and try to make sense of it, he would have two strenuous objections. I almost said "violent objections," but this was precisely the problem; he could not feel his rage at me, just as on the many occasions when he spoke of his inordinate rage at his mother and father (for their emotional distance and other more specific hurtful behaviors) he was unable to make contact with the rage on an experiential level by feeling it and owning it. He only "knew" that he was enraged. His first objection was that I was trying to make sense of what he said instead of just registering it and letting him know that I heard it (this is reminiscent of Kohut's Ms. F [Kohut 1971, pp. 283–293]). He wanted me to first ask him what sense he made of it; otherwise, he felt "annihilated" by my comments and felt that I was appropriating his thoughts for my purposes, leaving him with nothing. His second objection was that I did not pick up and reflect his reference to his anal sensations. He felt that this was a deliberate disregard of him and that it meant that I was as repulsed by his anal references as his mother had been in wiping the feces off him in his infancy and childhood, a response that contributed, he believed, to his feeling like a "repulsive little shit" ever since. Furthermore, Mr. K insisted that those few references to his body and its functions were the only real "feeling-communications," that the rest was all unreal (from his left brain) and of little consequence in this analytic endeavor. It was not knowledge that he lacked but an ability to put thoughts and feelings together, or, as he put it, "to experience fully and own what was going on inside of [him]." It was late in this phase of the analysis that I translated his many references to his anal sensations as his relentless efforts at getting connected to his archaic mother. My earlier frequent misses thwarted this development of finally understanding the meaning of the patient's side remarks, whereas my subsequent alertness to them enhanced progress.

Through numerous such incidents we learned that Mr. K was putting himself forward for acceptance and approval in this tentative and cautious way, and that my "nonresponse" to his side remarks about his bodily sensations were therefore understandably devastating to him. It was as if I did not permit feelings to enter our relationship; I was putting obstacles in the way of his establishing "rapport" with me and was thereby keeping him at a distance and preventing him from bringing the 2-year-old walled-off child in him together with the adult.

It was evident from the beginning of the analysis that Mr. K's numerous "dysfunctions" (as he called them)—his inability to attend to trivial household chores, finish important tasks he began to work on, pay his bills on time, and so forth—were almost lifelong behavioral expressions of his rage and revengefulness at his parents, particularly his mother. They were also his defiance vis-à-vis his coercive father and his expressed profound need to extract from his parents, in fantasy, what they never gave him and what he felt he could not go on without. This attitude and behavior led him to an elaborate fantasy, his "symbiotic scenario," in which he had to obtain from the outside what he never received from his parents: a feeling of being valued (and thereby gaining self-regard and a sense of personal dignity and worthwhileness). These became central themes in the transference, and Mr. K's rage became focused around his frustrations in obtaining them in the analytic situation.

I shall now move quickly across a prolonged time span. I recognized that it was not enough to acknowledge the legitimacy of Mr. K's archaic needs in words, no matter how much I believed in the sincerity of my own acceptance of them. The words of acknowledgment had to reflect genuine receptivity to the emergence of these needs in the transference, whatever form they took. This was not always easy to convey. Mr. K had to feel the genuineness of my receptivity, the absence of any reluctance or reservation, in order to experience himself as genuine and to be able to connect to his inner feelings—but not yet to his rage. His expectations in this new phase were clearly articulated by him at the tail end of a prolonged effort to repair a painful disruption. He wanted to feel free to lambaste me and express his rage (even if only in words without feeling), and he wanted me "to accompany [him] into the depth of [his] abyss, without criticism and intolerance for [his] fury." He was confident that if he could feel that I was with him without reservation and without reluctance, he could make contact with whatever he would find there.

Mr. K found an apt metaphor to help me accompany him on this journey into his "underground": he wanted to pull up to the screen of the analysis all that he saw there and have me witness it, accept it, and thereby help him detoxify it. He did not want me to *do* anything about it except to perfectly reflect his inner experiences. Such a reflection, he believed, would make them real for him, with a good chance that he would then be able to own them with feeling and then, hopefully, let go of them. After what we had been through before, this was an easier task to follow, I thought. And for a while it was. But the demand for perfect attunement still leads to painful disruptive episodes. Occasionally, Mr. K reflects on the fact that he is now able to feel "somewhat better connected" to me and hence also to his own inner self.

CONCLUDING REMARKS

Among the many lessons I have learned from my work with Mr. K and have illustrated in this chapter, several stand out as of fundamental importance. Although Mr. K undoubtedly suffered from lifelong "dysfunctions" (see also Ornstein 1987, p. 91), he began his second analysis with me with a certain intensity of hope that he could overcome them. In spite of the fact that he built around himself a "defensive wall of apparent tranquility…maintained with the aid of social isolation, detachment, and fantasied superiority" (Kohut 1972, p. 646), he began on the couch as if this wall did not exist. Only after the first major disruption of his quickly developing mirror transference did it seem to have been brought visibly into play. Mr. K's fear of becoming retraumatized kept him behind his wall, with repeated, subtle (indeed, to me often barely recognizable) forays outside his wall to extract the appreciation and validation he felt I was deliberately withholding. When I would inadvertently miss these efforts—rather than notice, explicitly welcome, and admire them—Mr. K felt justified in retreating again.

It would be an easy way out to say simply that at that point in the analysis Mr. K's transference "clicked in" and we were dealing with the inevitable. While this is true, this does not permit us the proper "reparative" focus. It is more important for the treatment process to center on those elements of the current precipitants for the disruptions that are truly unwelcome intrusions into the treatment process, some of which can and should be remedied by the analyst. These intrusions may be classified as countertransference phenomena, inadequate understanding of the nature of the patient's subjective experience, or incorrect application of existing theory and treatment principles. The term *failure* in describing analytic interventions that lead to severe disruptions has become very unpopular—to the detriment of progress in the theory of treatment and in refining the analyst's proper responsiveness.

The question of how to deal with persistent demands for the concrete satisfaction of various archaic mirroring needs—the question, in other words, of whether the self-psychologically informed analyst should actually mirror his patients or not—is a frequent one, and the available answers are not always clear-cut. Mr. K provided me with some additional guidelines, worthy of further empirical study. A less reserved response to his initial demands for mirroring (of the sort that Kohut acceded to with Ms. F?) might well have prevented the escalation of these demands to the point of a transference-countertransference stalemate. A tonally expressed emotional receptivity on my part—which I thought was there from the beginning but which he experienced as missing—might well have led us much earlier to the point where Mr. K could accept me as a validating witness to his experiences rather than as someone concretely fitting in with his archaic "symbiotic scenario," a function with which I obviously had some difficulty.

The manifestations of Mr. K's chronic rage, as would be expected, fluctuated very much in accordance with whether he felt my "receptive and willing presence" or not. They were clearly secondary to disruptive experiences in the transference and were both consequences of these disruptions as well as relentless retaliations for them. Simultaneously, they were also efforts to get reconnected to me and to attempt to extract penance: "I need a dignity payment from you, because you defeated me and humiliated me," he said. At least in words, if not yet in feeling, at the point where my narrative ends Mr. K is able to express his fury unsparingly. Nothing appears to ameliorate his rage, however, more consistently than "establishing rapport," his phrase for getting emotionally reconnected to me.

POSTSCRIPT

In comparing the protagonist of Dostoyevski's novel and Mr. K, there is one striking observation that immediately attracts the attention of the clinician: both are highly expressive in words, images, and metaphors, and both have an extraordinary degree and quality of insight—without this being a leverage for change.

The man from underground is deeply locked into a chronic, repetitive cycle of behavior and experiences that constantly validate his negative self-assessment, a situation that only reinforces his rage and revengefulness. He strives to improve his situation and relationships, but he cannot elicit the desired responses from his environment that would, it may seem to the reader, make internal change possible. He is on the verge of reaching out to others on a few occasions, but these end disastrously. The man's narrative ends abruptly with this sentence: "I've had enough of writing these *Notes From Underground.*" Dostoyevski appends the following remarks: "Actually the notes of this lover of paradoxes do not end here. He couldn't resist and went on writing. But we are of the opinion that one might just as well stop here" (p. 203), indicating that there has been no movement thus far and there will be none.

Mr. K, on the other hand, struggles with establishing a different kind of relationship from his previous ones in the treatment situation. He rightly expects that the therapist's responsiveness will make a difference. If that responsiveness catalyzes Mr. K's ability to connect to his inner feelings, to undo his internal polarization (as he describes it), and if his feelings from underground then emerge into an analytic milieu of safety and are greeted with acceptance rather than being recoiled from (even if ever so mildly), a process of change may be initiated that predominant emphasis on insight cannot achieve.

REFERENCES

Dostoyevski F: Notes From Underground (1864). New translation with afterword by Andrew MacAndrew. New York, Penguin, 1961

Freud S: Analysis terminable and interminable (1937), in The Standard Edition of the Complete Psychological Works of Sigmund Freud, Vol 23. Translated and edited by Strachey J. London, Hogarth Press, 1964, pp 216–253

Kohut H: The Analysis of the Self. New York, International Universities Press, 1971

Kohut H: Thoughts on narcissism and narcissistic rage (1972), in The Search for the Self, Vol 2. Edited by Ornstein PH. New York, International Universities Press, 1978, pp 615–658

Kohut H: The Restoration of the Self. New York, International Universities Press, 1977

Kohut H: Reflections on advances in self psychology (1978), in Advances in Self Psychology. Edited by Goldberg A. New York, International Universities Press, 1980, pp 473–554

Ornstein PH: On self-state dreams in the psychoanalytic treatment process, in The Interpretation of Dreams in Clinical Work. Edited by Rothstein A. Madison, CT, International Universities Press, 1987, pp 87–104

Ornstein PH: Why self psychology is not an object relations theory: clinical and theoretical considerations, in The Evolution of Self Psychology. Progress in Self Psychology, Vol 7. Edited by Goldberg A. Hillsdale, NJ, Analytic Press, 1991, pp 17–29

Ornstein PH, Ornstein A: Assertiveness, anger, rage, and destructive aggression: a perspective from the treatment process, in Rage, Power, and Aggression. Edited by Glick RA, Roose SP. New Haven, CT, Yale University Press, 1993

21

ETHEL SPECTOR PERSON, M.D.

INTRODUCTION

Ethel Person is a graduate of the University of Chicago, New York University College of Medicine, and the Columbia University Center for Psychoanalytic Training and Research in New York, where she is a Training and Supervising Psychoanalyst. She holds the positions of Professor of Clinical Psychiatry, College of Physicians and Surgeons, Columbia University, and Geographic Rule Supervising Analyst at the Greater Kansas City Psychoanalytic Institute. From 1981 to 1991, she was Director of the Columbia Center, and she has at various times served as a Fellow on the Board of Professional Standards of the American Psychoanalytic Association, Program Committee, North American Vice President of the International Psychoanalytical Association (IPA), and Founding Editor of the IPA newsletter. She has been on the editorial boards of *The Journal of the American Psychoanalytic Association, The International Journal of Psychoanalysis, Partisan Review,* and *Studies in Gender and Sexuality,* to mention but a few. She is the recipient of many honors, including the George E. Daniels Merit Award of the Association for Psychoanalytic Medicine, the Mount Airy Foundation Gold Medal Award for Distinction and Excellence in Psychiatry, the Sigmund Freud Award of the American Society of Psychoanalytic Physicians, and the Award for Distinguished and Meritorious Service to the IPA. She has held numerous visiting professorships around the world and has given an extraordinary number of keynote and plenary lectures.

Dr. Person is the author of four books that have been powerfully influential both within psychoanalysis and among the general public. They are *Dreams of Love and Fateful Encounters: The Power of Romantic Passion, By Force of Fantasy: How We Make Our Lives, The Sexual Century: Selected Papers on Sex and Gender,* and *Feeling Strong: The Achievement of Authentic Power.* She, along with Arnold Cooper and Glen Gabbard, edited *The American Psychiatric Publishing Textbook of Psychoanalysis.*

She says of the trajectory of her career:

> I went to medical school to become a psychoanalyst, a decision that I arrived at as a college student at the University of Chicago, where I first discovered Freud. The psychiatrists and psychoanalysts with whom I have trained have been pivotal in shaping my career. I was fortunate in my mentors. My first psychiatric mentor was Alexander Thomas when I was a medical student at New York University. Alex had a commonsense approach but also a bent toward research. My major influences in analytic training at the Columbia University Center for Psychoanalytic Training and Research were Abram Kardiner and Lionel Ovesey. My work overlaps with theirs in several ways, certainly in terms of the cultural perspective, emphasizing differences not only between eras and locales, but also between men and women. I also see myself in line with Kardiner and Ovesey as a researcher. I never did the kind of research one generally thinks of as research, but I went outside my office to find background on what I could learn about sex and gender. The sexologist Harry Benjamin put me in touch with the sexual networks I wanted to explore. By totally restricting oneself to observing insights from patients, one sometimes gets depth, but not breadth, and both are important in thinking through specific issues.
>
> Arnold Cooper and Will Gaylin, my two supervisors, were both extremely intelligent and kind, and I learned a great deal from them. My career was also shaped by two previous directors of the Columbia Psychoanalytic Center, John Weber and George Goldman, who wanted me as the Director of the Columbia Psychoanalytic Center to follow Weber. Arnold Cooper and Joe Sandler pulled me into the IPA. I have also profited intellectually through my participation in a long-term study group composed of academic women with whom I met for several years to discuss women's issues. All of this is by way of saying I was lucky to be surrounded by first-rate people and first-rate minds and nurtured in the early parts of my career.
>
> One of the major intellectual impacts on my thinking came out of my close friendship with the political scientist Hans Morgenthau, who was both brilliant and proved courageous in his opposition to the Vietnam War, a decision that cost him the possibility of being appointed Secretary of State. It was through him that I became interested in how power and powerlessness shape our lives. As most analysts, I have also learned from my patients about courage, diversity, the range of gifts people may have, and the will to change.
>
> I have written primarily about sex, gender, love, fantasy, and power.

As a theorist, I place myself somewhere between object relations and a cultural perspective based on a healthy respect for what is inborn, which I see not as restricted to drive, but also encompassing temperament, gifts, talent, etc. Like Lionel Ovesey, I have remained averse to those who "suck it out of their thumbs" and conclude too much on the basis of too little research. Psychoanalysis has been a good career choice for me. We are all lucky when we enjoy our work.

WHY I CHOSE THIS PAPER

Ethel Spector Person, M.D.

I chose "Knowledge and Authority: The Godfather Fantasy" for inclusion in this volume because it was my first coherent paper on the necessity of theorizing power in psychoanalytic theory. There are references to power in the psychoanalytic literature, particularly recently, but they relate primarily to issues of sex and gender.

My aim in the paper was to put power into a theoretical framework that was psychoanalytical and that addressed the impact on the individual of the hierarchical structures in which we all reside.

The transference model emphasizes our early-life reliance on parental strength and authority to counter our legitimate feelings of weakness and vulnerability. What it leaves out is any acknowledgement of the new anxieties generated through life. These anxieties are not exclusively related to early life feelings of weakness and vulnerability, but also to our fears of death and oblivion. To counter these fears, we attempt to establish transcendent meaning in our lives.

My argument is that it is impossible to grasp the full thrust of our psychological need, either to seize the godhead or to participate in transcendent-oriented groups simply by looking backward to the fears and terrors of childhood. The history of the world is the history of groups that compete not only for natural resources, trade advantages, or priority, but also for transcendent meaning that confers significance on life. This paper is about obedience to ideology, on the one hand, and resistance to authority, on the other. I argue that both provide a major engine for the historical change and upheavals that punctuate the human journey. I believe this is one of my more original papers and touches on topics that have not been adequately theorized within psychoanalysis.

KNOWLEDGE AND AUTHORITY

The Godfather Fantasy

ETHEL SPECTOR PERSON, M.D.

PSYCHOANALYTIC THEORY, the foundation of our contemporary insight into individual psychology, has had much less to say about the individual in relation to the rest of the world—as either a shaper of that world or a product of it. In its failure to consider the individual's integration into the larger social world or, conversely, the impact of the social world on the individual psyche, psychoanalytic theory is in the tradition of several millennia of Western thought, which has long cherished the belief that the psyche is fundamentally ahistorical. The sociologist Richard Sennett (1980) describes the ahistorical position succinctly: "The human being was a creature placed in the circumstances of history but not essentially a product of those circumstances" (p. 6).

That position went unchallenged until nineteenth-century social psychologists, building on the earlier work of the Italian philosopher Giambattista Vico, radically upended the ahistorical viewpoint. Unfortunately, psychoanalytic interest lagged behind. Recently, however, psychoanalysts, while still primarily interested in personal history, have begun to acknowledge the broader historical perspective, in particular as regards the way social arrangements and beliefs impact on sex and gender (Chodorow 1994; Haynal et al. 1983; Kernberg 1985; Person 1995, 1999; Roustang 1976). Another intellectual task that we have only

---

"Knowledge and Authority: The Godfather Fantasy," by Ethel Spector Person, M.D., was first published in *The Journal of the American Psychoanalytic Association*, 49:1133–1155, 2001. Abridged for this publication. Used with permission.

begun to undertake with any seriousness is to do the reverse kind of analysis: to explain how certain psychological propensities that appear to be hardwired and thus immune to effects of history may nonetheless turn out to be *agents* of history. Freud himself began this task.

It is the role the often conflicted impulses of obedience and rebellion play in our lives—and in the world beyond our personal lives—that I will be discussing. Both obedience and rebellion are critical to individual development. When elaborated into submission to authority or resistance to or cooptation of authority, they may also act as part of the engine of historical change.

Our very sense of autonomy, what I call personal power—or true *self*-government—may be born in our natural resistance to external authority. This innate psychological propensity figures at the beginning of Judeo-Christian religion. It is symbolically depicted in the story of Adam and Eve's disobedience of God. For Erich Fromm (1964), this story highlights "disobedience [as] the condition for man's self-awareness, for his capacity to choose, and thus... this first act of disobedience is man's first step toward freedom" (pp. 19–20). It is only because of his expulsion from the Garden of Eden that man is able to make his own history.

The Adam and Eve story can be read as a mythic version of the plot line by which each of us emerges from the embeddedness of early life. Horner (1989) describes the way resistance to authority emerges in early development: "if one is to become a grown-up in a world of grown-ups, sooner or later there must be an 'overthrow' of parental authority, with a resultant change in the locus of security, direction, decision-making, and the taking of responsibility" (pp. 84–85). This "overthrow" is not necessarily rebellious in its intent, or so I would maintain. It originates as a function of an innate drive to self-initiated action, to the expression of power.

As I define it, power is a desire/drive, a motivational force, as important in our lives as sex, bonding, or aggression. The impulse fueling power, though innate, is shaped by learning and experience. In earliest life, we act instinctively rather than volitionally—we suck a nipple, grasp a bottle, cry in discomfort. Among psychoanalysts and psychologists this "instinct" goes by many names—life force, *élan vital.* Horner calls it intrinsic power, the power of the self (p. 14). Winnicott (1950) calls it aggression (pp. 84–99). Shulman (1987) distinguishes between the infant's preintentional force and the later appearance of will, in which his awareness of his own agency is paramount (p. 68). Like Shulman, I believe the power drive is initially hardwired and only later takes on the quality of intentionality. Yet our earliest instinctual form of self-assertion or self-will is the kernel of the power drive or power motive.

Self-will is easily observable in the relationship of children to their parents. From infancy on, the baby's natural desire to have its own way inevitably meets opposition from the parents, resulting in a clash of wills. Beginning toward the end of the first year of life and accelerating during the second year, the baby begins to develop a new set of skills and abilities that often brings the project of self-assertion—"I can do it myself"—into immediate conflict with his parents. The "terrible twos" are good evidence of our natural resistance to power in the service of self-expression. While parents may view this period as a disagreeable time of negativity, the child's ebullience of will, as manifested in the insistence on "no" or "yes," is necessarily correlated with his crystallization of oneself as an autonomous being (Spitz 1957). The toddler's mastery of these two words—no and yes—and eagerness to stand by the judgments so rendered, is at once a major leap toward the formation of an independent sense of self and, often enough, the beginning of an overt power struggle with the parents. One might say that in developing the self, the baby becomes a political animal.

Resistance to power, one of the basic dialectics of power, is evident not only in the relationship of the growing child to its parents but also in the almost inevitable resistance of people to imperatives handed down from others, as is evident in the political arena. The economist and political theorist John Kenneth Galbraith (1983) believes that a resistance to power "is as integral a part of the phenomenon of power as its exercise itself" (p. 72). Were there no innate human propensity to resist power, we would all be subject to those most versed in its exercise, and tyrants would prevail.

Yet there is an opposing impulse to our natural resistance to authority: we may experience a sometimes desperate temptation to surrender to it. Drawing on Freud, the sociologist Philip Rieff (1961) suggests that because love is related to the "parental fact of domination," it follows that "power is the father of love, and in love one follows the paternal example of power, in a relation that must include a superior and a subordinate." Moreover, he argues that whereas Christianity proclaimed the ultimate authority to be the source of love, "Freud discovered the love of authority" (p. 168). Because children see their parents as their "Gods of Survival" (Gaylin 1979, p. 32), in whose power resides their safety, their sustenance, and their pride, they are sometimes reluctant to recognize any sign of weakness in their parents and may fail to express any counter will. Freud's genius allowed him to see the infant's helplessness but also see beyond it and grasp that there is an active love of the power of the Other.

Resist/submit; point/counterpoint. These conflicting predilections often coexist in us side by side. They permeate the power balances we establish in our personal relationships. While in some relationships we are primarily submissive and in others primarily dominant, in most intimate relationships our place on the dominant/submissive axis is constantly shifting. But turn us loose in a group and dominance and submissiveness stop being merely antagonists in an internal conflict. Resistance to power and obedience, together, propel us into group life. A predilection for both allows us to integrate into a hierarchical structure, whether familial, religious, corporate, or even psychoanalytic.

Power matters to us even above and beyond any instinctual endowment to assert ourselves, as Freud understood, because of our feelings of powerlessness (Freud 1927, pp. 17–18, 23–24). In addition to our learning to manage interpersonal relationships, in addition to achieving some measure of real autonomy (in terms of writing our life story), in addition to putting behind us such political tragedies as marred our infancy and early childhood, we have profound existential dilemmas to confront and make our peace with however we can. Such personal power as we can individually muster is seldom adequate to assuage our deepest existential anxieties or to gratify our need for establishing some overarching sense of larger meaning in our lives. Many of us seek to counter these needs by seeking one or another form of transcendence. But in seeking transcendence we inevitably make use of our innate disposition to both submission and resistance to authority.

Let me tentatively propose that there are three strategies that we invoke as we try to reconcile our need for transcendence while being inextricably tied to fundamental motives of resistance and submission: 1) we seek to seize for ourselves the power of the gods; 2) we seek to nestle in the protective embrace of one or another god; or 3) we seek to clothe a mere mortal in the cloak of godly power. This third strategy, with a nod to Mario Puzo, I call the godfather fantasy. The secular counterpart to the first two, it encompasses the conflictual impulses of rebellion and obedience. That is, in invoking this fantasy, we may aspire to become a godfather figure in our own right, or we may seek instead to procure for ourselves the protection of one or another godfather. Or we may seek both.

STRATEGY 1: SEIZING THE GODHEAD

While people in all eras have sought the power of the gods, in classical antiquity people lived more familiarly with their gods than we do. In the myths of antiquity, men danced with the gods, fought with them, and were made love to by them. As a consequence, there were some among the ancients who were half god, half man. They were the imaginative link that first gave voice to man's dream of possessing the godhead.

The ambivalent project of seeking the godhead runs through classical mythology. In Greek myths, the hero is flawed not just by his failures but by his very aspirations. Many of our basic myths, some as ancient as recorded history, depict our envy-inspired struggle to wrest power from the gods—for example, Prometheus's theft of fire from Zeus.

Prometheus was a lesser god, the son of a Titan and Titaness. Zeus enlisted Prometheus to provide gifts to all earth's creatures, with the exception of one precious gift—the eternal fire, sacred to the gods alone. Prometheus was sympathetic to humans, who, unlike the other animals, was helpless in the natural world. Disobeying Zeus's command, he stole the fire to give it to man. Aeschylus, in *Prometheus Bound,* tells of Prometheus's other gifts to man—writing, divination, and "dark and riddling" knowledge—gifts that gave men powers far beyond their human limitations (Aeschylus 458 B.C., p. 45). In a rage, Zeus condemned Prometheus to eternal punishment for his act of hubris.

The drama critic Walter Kerr (1967) points out that to be the hero of a classical tragedy, a man generally had to have something of a god in him (p. 93). The whole genre, he writes, is an exploration of the possibilities of human freedom. He goes on to say that "at the heart of classical tragedy, feeding it energy, stands godlike man, passionately desiring a state of affairs more perfect than any that now exists" (p. 107).

For Kerr, man's freedom means that man must "follow where freedom leads, without foreknowledge, without any sort of certainty, prepared only for discovery and ready for surprise.... in Man's mind freedom exists in his godlike capacity for manufacturing the symbols of language and mathematics which Prometheus is so proud to have handed down" (p. 122). Such knowledge and the powers that flow from it, Kerr argues, freed man to move among the stars and to name things that he could not actually see, while his memory extended his powers so as to seem to him he might command the cosmos (p. 122).

However, such knowledge of the stars can so overheat the imagination as to exact a heavy price. Cecil Rhodes, the British-born diamond magnate, South African statesman, and financier who changed the map of Africa, wistfully bemoaned "these stars that you see overhead at night, these vast worlds which we can never reach. I would annex the planets if I could. I often think of that. It makes me sad to see them so clear and so far away" (quoted in Morgenthau 1946, pp. 192–193). While it might appear that Rhodes understood the natural limitation to human power, nonetheless it was his overweening ambition that ultimately undid him. While prime minister of the Cape Colony, he organized a conspiracy to overthrow the Transvaal government. As a consequence, he was forced to resign and became the symbol incarnate of the overreaching and scheming British capitalist, a victim of his own boundless ambition. Aside from his mixed legacy in Africa, he is probably best known as a man passionately devoted to knowledge, who in his will endowed the fabled Rhodes scholarships.

Knowledge is two-edged. While it can serve as a bulwark against total obeisance to external authority, it can also so ignite our grandiosity that it seduces us into potentially destructive acts. Freedom to know gives us the illusion that we have the power to command what will transpire.

One of the characters in André Malraux's novel *Man's Fate* (1934) meditates on power: "What fascinates them in this idea, you see, is not real power, it is the illusion of being able to do exactly as they please. The king's power is the power to govern, isn't it? But man has no urge to govern: he has an urge to compel.... To be more than a man, in a world of men. To escape man's fate.... Not powerful: all-powerful. The visionary disease, of which the will to power is only the intellectual justification, is the will to god-head: every man dreams of being god" (p. 228). As Malraux's character so aptly intuits when he speaks of "man's fate," what man is seeking when he seizes the godhead is his own right—as messiah, ruler, or tyrant—to escape mortality. For absolute rulers, the power to decree death or to grant life must reinforce that sense of power over mortality, which is the ultimate power. It is also, of course, ultimately illusory. The political theorist Hans Morgenthau observed that those who persist in trying to achieve transcendence through personal power, who seek the godhead through total conquest, are inevitably destroyed, as illustrated by the fate of all world conquerors from Alexander to Hitler, and as symbolically rendered in the legends of Icarus and Faust (pp. 192–193).

STRATEGY 2: SUBMISSION TO GOD

While aspirants to the godhead are not restricted to classical antiquity (witness the popularity of the Faust legend), still and all, a seismic transformation appears to have occurred in the Christian era in the way most men regarded themselves. While the Greeks believed that they—excluding, of course, slaves and women—partook of the nature of the gods and aspired to freedom, Christianity posited man as created by

God but "not born of him" (Kerr 1967, p. 97). Many of us, unable or unwilling to claim the godhead in our own right, seek safety and salvation through allegiance and obedience to a deity, or to the deity's purported representatives on earth. Through religion we seek transcendence, in which the longing to be one with the cosmos, to put aside individual ambitions, offers the hope of transcendence. The submergence of the self into religion and obedience to God creates meaning in our lives.

To preserve the ideal of God, we must acknowledge our own inadequacy and our sins, thus the saying "It is better to be a sinner in a world with God than to live in a godless world." The exact opposite of expressing hubris, of aspiring to the godhead, the Christian ideal calls for humility and obedience. We see in these two strategies versions of the two tendencies I spoke of earlier: one to resist and to assert the self, the other to submit. It is as if transcendence can be had by taking one or the other to an ultimate limit while excluding the opposite tendency.

A more complex and darker vision of transcendence, in which both tendencies are present, is to be found in "The Legend of the Grand Inquisitor" in *The Brothers Karamazov* (Dostoyevsky 1880). The legend that Ivan Karamazov recounts to his brother Alyosha is at once a story of corrupted power as seen in the actions of the Grand Inquisitor, who aspired to the godhead, and a portrait of the ordinary Christian's psychology of obedience, of servility. Who better to write this tale than Dostoyevsky, a man who struggled for most of his life with opposing impulses of submission and rebellion (Rahv 1949, p. 167) and who better to appreciate it than Freud, who regarded *The Brothers Karamazov* as "the most magnificent novel ever written"? (1928, p. 177).

Fifteen centuries after the Crucifixion, according to the "poema" Ivan recites, Christ reappears in Seville at the time of the Inquisition—for Dostoyevsky the very epitome of all the evils to be found in the West. It is a weekend when the Cardinal, the Grand Inquisitor himself, has had several hundred heretics burned to death. Appearing in human form, just as he had looked 15 centuries earlier, Christ is recognized and welcomed by the people. He raises a girl from the dead at the very moment the Inquisitor appears on the scene. Witnessing the miracle, the Inquisitor orders Christ's arrest and incarcerates Him in "a murky vaulted prison" of the Holy Inquisition (Dostoyevsky 1880, p. 287). The submissive crowd, despite the spiritual glow they feel in the presence of Christ, makes no protest.

The night before Christ is to be burned at the stake, he is visited by the Inquisitor, "an old man, of almost ninety, tall and straight, with a withered face and sunken eyes, in which, however, there is still a fiery, spark-like gleam" (p. 287). "Why have you come to get in our way?" he asks Christ, and then launches into a terrible indictment of Christ, delivered in the service of a shameless rationalization of the Church's abuse of power.

The Grand Inquisitor accuses Christ of having failed his flock 15 centuries earlier when he resisted Satan's three temptations, as recounted in Matthew. It was in the name of freedom that Christ refused to succumb to the first temptation in the desert, that of changing stones into bread. This the Grand Inquisitor believes was his first error. His second error was his refusal to leap from the pinnacle of the temple; his third, his rejection of Satan's offer to give him unimagined worldly power.

Men cannot believe when guided by their hearts alone, the Grand Inquisitor argues; they need to be convinced of the necessity of worship. Because Christ believed that man should not be moved by miracles, he allowed himself to be crucified like a thief: "You desired that man's love should be free, that he should follow you freely, enticed and captivated by you. Here again you overestimated men" (p. 293). How, he asks, could Christ, who placed such a great moral burden on man's shoulders by offering him freedom, claim to love man?

The Grand Inquisitor understands all too well the psychological longings that give rise to man's obedience. Had Christ turned stones into loaves, the Inquisitor argues, he would have provided an answer to man's age-old anguished question: "Before whom should one bow down?" (p. 292). He goes further: "man seeks to bow down before that which is already beyond dispute, so far beyond dispute that all human beings will instantly agree to a universal bowing-down before it.... For the sake of a universal bowing-down they have destroyed one another with the sword.... You knew, you could not fail to know that peculiar secret of human nature, but you rejected the only absolute banner that was offered to you and that would have compelled man to bow down before you without dispute—the banner of earthly bread, and you rejected it in the name of freedom and the bread of heaven.... But only he can take mastery of people's freedom who is able to set their consciences at rest" (p. 292). Here, as several commentators have noted, Dostoevsky seems to anticipate the totalitarian movements of the twentieth century in which what people seemed to long for is "an indisputable, general, and consensual ant-heap" (p. 296).

The Grand Inquisitor, an atheist who acknowledges his allegiance to Satan, accepts the inevitability and the legitimacy of the three temptations that Christ rejected. He improves on Christ's model of Christianity by basing it on miracles, mystery, and authority, which the political scientist Dennis Dalton (1998) construes as the metaphorical counterparts to economic power, psychological power, and political power.

The Inquisitor tells Christ that on the very next morning he will burn him at the stake. Christ, who has not spoken a single word throughout the Inquisitor's entire soliloquy, approaches the Inquisitor and kisses his "bloodless, ninety-year-old lips." The old man shivers, opens the door and says, "Go and do not come back…do not come back at all…ever…ever!" (p. 302). "The kiss burns within his heart," but he does not change his mind (p. 302). His commitment to temporal power prevails over the power of his belief. He accepts Satan's wisdom.

STRATEGY 3: THE GODFATHER FANTASY

Albert Camus (1957) believed that "for anyone who is alone, without God and without a master, the weight of days is dreadful. Hence one must choose a master, God being out of style" (p. 133). Exactly so with the Godfather. If we can't have a God let us have the compelling master with his own share of mystery, miracles and authority. The fascination so many of us have with the Godfather novel and its progeny (sequels, films, copycats) is evident in their overwhelming commercial success.

That success is in part the result of two interlocking fantasies embedded in the plot line. For a few, the godfather fantasy is about becoming the Godfather, procuring for oneself a secular version of the godhead. For many more the fantasy is about seeking vicarious power through a connection to one or another mortal—a godfather or godmother, a titan of industry, a mentor, a totalitarian leader—whom they imbue with the mystique of power and to whom they pledge obeisance. For them the fantasy is primarily about securing riches, knowledge, and vicarious authority in the here and now through attachment to a powerful godfather figure. Sometimes this figure is objectively powerful enough and possesses a sufficiently strong and cogent world-view that he draws to himself an extended group, who come to share his ideology to the extent that they pledge obeisance to him.

Such a figure is Mario Puzo's fictional Don Corleone. Head of a Mafia family, Don Corleone ruthlessly rules over a vast and vicious crime empire; he uses his power not only for the huge financial rewards it brings, but also for the protection it affords for both his blood family and his crime "family." But of what does the Godfather's power consist? Of the same stuff as the Grand Inquisitor's, I would argue: miracle, mystery, and authority, or put another way, his power lies in our need for him to be powerful.

For those who may raise an eyebrow at my segue from the Grand

Inquisitor to the Godfather, let me note a connection between *The Brothers Karamazov* and Puzo that I happened upon only recently. Mario Puzo confesses that he was deeply influenced by Dostoyevsky's novel. In his 1997 preface to a new edition of his novel *The Fortunate Pilgrim* (Puzo 1964), he writes, "All young writers dream of immortality—that hundreds of years in the future the new generations will read their books and find their lives changed, as my life was after reading *The Brothers Karamazov* at the age of 15. I vowed I would never write a word that was not absolutely true to myself and I felt I had achieved that in *The Fortunate Pilgrim*" (p. xi). That book, 10 years in the writing, received splendid reviews but was a commercial failure. Only after that experience did Puzo embark on *The Godfather,* the purpose of which was to gain money and fame. Yet commercial as its intent may have been, what Puzo renders in *The Godfather* is a secular version of the themes that run through "The Legend of the Grand Inquisitor."

Like the Grand Inquisitor, Don Corleone produces small miracles to secure the adherence of his flock, some of whom he might call upon later for one or another small service.

> Don Vito Corleone was a man to whom everybody came for help, and never were they disappointed. He made no empty promises, nor the craven excuse that his hands were tied by more powerful forces in the world than himself. It was not necessary that he be your friend, it was not even important that you had no means with which to repay him. Only one thing was required. That you, you yourself, proclaim your friendship. And then, no matter how poor or powerless the supplicant, Don Corleone would take that man's troubles to his heart. And he would let nothing stand in the way to a solution of that man's woe. His reward? Friendship, the respectful title of "Don" and sometimes the more affectionate salutation of "Godfather." (Puzo 1969, p. 14)

For those who came under his protective wing, the Don's gratification of their humble requests was nothing less than miraculous, stones turned into bread—sometimes a kind of economic power, sometimes political power.

Like the Grand Inquisitor, the Godfather is simultaneously the center of knowledge and political power. Between the head of the family, Don Corleone, who dictates policy, and the men who actually carry out his orders, there are three levels of political operatives. At the top is the Consigliere. As Puzo tells us, "The Don gave his orders only to the *Consigliere*.... In that way nothing could be traced to the top. Unless the *Consigliere* turned traitor.... But no *Consigliere* had ever betrayed a Don.... There was no future in it" (p. 50). Under the Consigliere are two sub-bosses, who in turn control the foot soldiers.

The internal organization of the family must be cemented by ancillary power. Don Corleone's enforcer, Luca Brasi, is described as "one of the great blocks that supported the Don's power structure" (p. 25). Luca "did not fear the police, he did not fear society, he did not fear God, he did not fear Hell, he did not fear or love his fellow man but he had elected, he had *chosen* to fear and love Don Corleone" (p. 25). In his portrait of Luca, Puzo provides one of his many astute psychological observations. Even such a man so fearless, so cold-blooded a killer as Luca had to find someone to whom he could subordinate himself (p. 41).

The Don also goes outside his organization to enlist political power through payoffs to police, judges, and even senators At his daughter's wedding a United States Senator calls to apologize for not personally attending, but says he had no alternative since FBI agents were taking down the license numbers of those inside. Of course, it was by way of a message from the Don, well-informed by his insiders at the FBI, that the Senator had been warned not to come.

The Don also wields psychological power, perhaps the most chilling of all. A prime example of his mastery of this kind of power appears in the story of his confrontation with a powerful movie producer, Jack Woltz. Woltz had refused the Don's request to give a plum role to singer and movie star Johnny Fontane (a character widely believed to be based on Frank Sinatra). The Godfather sends his Consigliere to negotiate. Woltz greets Hagen courteously, but kisses him off. When Hagen proposes that Don Corleone could help Woltz with some small problems, Woltz responds, "All right, you smooth son of a bitch, let me lay it on the line for you and your boss, whoever he is. Johnny Fontane never gets that movie. I don't care how many guinea mafia goombas come out of the woodwork" (p. 56). As his final display of power, he adds that J. Edgar Hoover is one of his personal friends.

Unflappable, Hagen responds that Don Corleone knows about Woltz's friendship with Hoover and respects him for it, after which he takes his leave. Woltz cannot imagine that Don Corleone has the power to threaten him in any serious way. As many of you will remember from the film if not the novel, Woltz wakes up one morning to find the severed head of his beloved prize horse Khartoum on the pillow next to him: "Woltz was not a stupid man, he was merely an extremely egotistical one. He had mistaken the power he wielded in his world to be more potent than the power of Don Corleone. He had merely needed some proof that this was not true. He understood this message" (p. 69). This psychological power is akin to the kind of power displayed in the Inquisitor's act of burning heretics at the stake.

Different as they may appear to be, the Catholic Church at the time of the Inquisition and the Mafia as it grew in the United States resemble each other in the techniques they used to keep their subjects in thrall. Through their respective versions of miracles, mystery, and authority, they both wielded (and in the case of the Mafia continue to wield) economic, psychological, and political power. This is the modus vivendi of all hierarchical forms of power.

Let me step back a moment. What I am saying is that the godfather fantasy is so compelling not just because we have a wish to dominate and command but because we have a wish to attach ourselves to power through submissiveness and obedience. The godfather fantasy allows us to imagine a world in which both tendencies can be lived out to the hilt, directly and vicariously.

DISCUSSION

What is the evidence that most of us have some propensity to obedience? Our compliance in ceding autonomy to authority is demonstrated in one of the most brilliant, and perhaps immoral, psychological research studies ever performed. Dr. Stanley Milgram, then a member of the Yale University Department of Psychology, designed a series of studies whose express purpose was to examine the degree to which the average person would obey authority even if ordered to cause severe pain to others (Milgram 1974, p. 166). Milgram constructed a kind of psychological psychodrama in which there were three players: the lead investigator, the teacher, and the student. The lead investigator, the designated authority, wore a lab coat and told the volunteers that the purpose of the experiment was to further the cause of education and that they were to act as the teachers. But the putative subjects of the experiment, the students, were, unbeknown to the volunteers, part of the research team, actors hired to play the role of subjects. While the purpose of the experiment as presented to the volunteers was to discover whether punishing a student for wrong answers facilitated the learning process, its real purpose was to determine the degree to which the volunteers would obey authority even when they knew they were inflicting pain on someone else.

The volunteers in the role as teacher were asked to punish the students each time they gave an erroneous answer by administering a series of electric shocks of increasing magnitude. In reality, the shock generator delivered no shock. But the teachers believed they were delivering real shocks, and they experienced the students' cries of pain and pleas for mercy as real. The actor students had been instructed to increase their cries according to the voltage, from mild grunts at the lower levels to loud cries and pleas to be released at 150 volts. Most of the teachers—the real experimental subjects—displayed symptoms of stress and distress, objected to the barbarity of the experiment, and begged the investigator to stop it. Yet over 60% participated in the experiment all the way up to the 450-volt upper limit.

Milgram designed further experiments to test the hypothesis advanced by some critics that the cruelty of the "teachers" must originate in repressed aggressive impulses. He gave the teachers the opportunity to shock the students at any level of their own choice. Given this opportunity, almost all the teachers administered the lowest shocks possible. Milgram concluded that if destructive impulses were really pressing for release, and the teachers could justify their use of high shock levels in the cause of science, they would have taken the opportunity to make the students suffer. Yet there was "little if any tendency on the part of the subjects to do this" (p. 167).

Why did the subjects obey? Most of them rationalized their behavior as useful to society. Milgram proposed that the suppression or disappearance of one's own sense of responsibility was the most far-reaching consequence of submission to authority. He argued that "when individuals enter a condition of hierarchical control, the mechanism which ordinarily regulates individual impulses is suppressed and ceded to the higher-level component" (p. 131).

Such submissiveness in a hierarchical situation can be observed even among groups portrayed as extremely individualistic and macho. An airplane's cockpit crew is a small, highly structured group whose effectiveness as a crew is affected by any number of socio-psychological, personality, and group interactional variables (Foushee and Helmreich 1988, p. 193). Researchers H. Clayton Foushee and Robert Helmreich reported that two kinds of breakdown can occur in communication, the first the result too little cohesion within the group, the second the result of too much (p. 195). The phrase "too much cohesion" is a gloss on the submissiveness of one of the crew. The researcher Eugene Tarnow (2000) independently identified excessive obedience on the part of a copilot as problematic and concluded that a captain's "excessive need to maintain control in conjunction with his copilot's lack of assertiveness ... may lead to a crisis in the air" (Tarnow 2000, p. 112). He was able to pinpoint submissiveness as the cause of several crashes. Too often, a subordinate in a hierarchy will feel shame or pride depending on how well he carries out the authority's demands, even if he deplores the action required of him.

We should take note. We are accustomed to thinking that someone's will to power can get out of hand and lead to disaster, but the converse is also true. The will to submission can also get out of hand and lead to destruction. We kill more people in the name of ideological causes run amok than we destroy by virtue of thwarted passion, personal vendettas, criminality, or greed.

The impulse to cede independence of action to an authority, whether the Grand Inquisitor, the Godfather, the Professor, or the Commander, widespread as it is, requires psychological exploration. Two different frames of reference can be invoked to explain, at least in part, this impulse. The first emphasizes our dependency and sense of powerlessness in early life, the second, our sense of powerlessness in the face of death and the need for transcendent meaning as an antidote.

Freud (1921) turned toward an exploration of man's "thirst for obedience" and the nature of the group mind in *Group Psychology and the Analysis of the Ego*. He proposed that "in the individual's mental life someone else is invariably involved, as a model, as an object, as a helper, as an opponent; and so from the very first individual psychology, in this extended but entirely justifiable sense of the word, is at the same time social psychology as well" (p. 69). He had previously explored the psychological meaning of hypnosis in terms of erotic submission and used this insight to explain the patient's transference to the psychoanalyst. He saw both phenomena as evidence that people have a craving for direction and authority originating in earliest life; this craving is assuaged by an erotic tie to, and identification, first with a father and, later, with a chief of one sort or another. Freud believed the longing for a father, behind whom lurked a primal father, explained the "uncanny and coercive characteristics of group formations" (p. 127). The chief is a "dangerous personality, toward whom only a passive-masochistic attitude is possible, to whom one's will has to be surrendered" (p. 127). This is because the individual has "an extreme passion for authority" and "wishes to be governed by unrestricted force" (p. 127). These wishes arise out of unconscious erotic longings: "a group is held together by a power of some kind: and to what power would this feat be better ascribed than to Eros, which holds together everything in the world" (p. 92).

Many psychoanalysts have concurred with Freud that the individual's propensity for self-subordination and surrender to a leader is yet another manifestation of the many phenomena that can be understood as later-life manifestations of the charismatic overvaluation of parental power so necessary when one is young and truly powerless. The leader-follower relationship, whether expressed in hero-worship, in the mentor/protégé relationship, in transference, or in any of its other forms, is indeed partly—but never wholly—inspired by the longing for an antidote to the weakness and helplessness of childhood.

How does the transfer from parent to the larger world take place? Freud showed how the longing for parental authority invariably undergoes an internal metamorphosis. The family romance is the means through which a child disillusioned with his or her own parents can construct an imaginary mother and father, who are the "real" parents. Children daydream, for example, that they have been adopted or abducted from their "real" parents, people who generally are infinitely superior to the everyday false parents with whom they unhappily find themselves. Thus, the child has a built-in escape clause that allows issues of submission and domination to be moved outside the immediate relationship with the parents and into the wider world.

The source of family romance fantasies is twofold: children are angry at their parents for what they see as unjust restrictions or they become disillusioned with their belief in their parents as all-powerful. Either way the issue is power. Withdrawing idealization from these unsatisfactory parents and transferring it to the longed-parents of their imagination, children create for themselves a set of fantasied parents—generally, though not inevitably, noble, rich, or famous—who not only love them unconditionally but who are powerful in the external world and can have a significant impact on it.

Although children often transfer power to a parent surrogate, they may also seize it for themselves. Bruno Bettelheim (1976) argues that the family romance is essential to the development of personal authority, insofar as the transformation of the good mother into an evil stepmother provides an impetus to develop a separate self. He may overstate the case, as there appears to be an instinctual component to the quest for autonomy. But Bettelheim correctly emphasizes that a major impetus in the family romance is to "develop initiative and self-determination" (p. 274).

A premier example of a family romance fantasy is embedded in the text of the recently published Harry Potter novels (Rowling 1998, 1999a, 1999b, 2000) and bears out Bettelheim's insight that such fantasies serve to promote a sense of self-determination and personal power. Harry is an orphan whose mother and Wizard father were killed by the archwizard, the villain Voldemort, when Harry was just a baby. As a consequence, Harry was sent to live with an aunt and uncle, the Dursleys. They are "Muggles," who have no magical powers and who hate and fear Wizards. They dote on their son, Dudley, and are ashamed of Harry's Wizard blood. Harry is treated unfairly, systematically deprived while Dudley is consistently overindulged.

Harry suffers through 10 miserable years of neglect and abuse before the Wizards send for him. Hagrid, a giant, accompanies him to the Hogwarts School of Witchcraft and Wizardry, a magical world parallel to but invisible to the world of the Muggles. It is at Hogwarts that Harry first discovers the extent of his powers and ultimately becomes the instrument for undoing a vast conspiracy, masterminded by Voldemort, against the good Wizards. Harry displays all the characteristics requisite to becoming a kind of godfather, albeit a benevolent one.

The Grand Inquisitor's flock, Corleone's crime family, and the group of Wizards to which Harry Potter belongs are all fictional renditions of groups that form a closed community united by a shared mentality, bolstered by miracles, mystery and authority.

While Freud brilliantly elaborated the group mind in *Group Psychology,* what he omitted was not just the urgent need so many of us have to unite with others but to do so in an "ant-heap" of shared belief. Such a need for ideology takes us beyond Eros. The function of the group mind—as distinct from the function of transference—is to provide a transcendent meaning to life. The transference model correctly emphasizes our early life reliance on parental strength and authority to counter our legitimate feelings of weakness and vulnerability. What it leaves out is any acknowledgment of the new anxieties generated throughout life. These anxieties do not originate in early-life feelings of vulnerability but are related to our ultimate fate, to our fears of death and oblivion. To counter these fears, we attempt to establish transcendent meaning in our lives. A few of us develop overweening ambitions and counter our death anxiety by striving for immortality in our achievements, sometimes creative and artistic, sometimes in an attempt to seize the godhead in our own right. More often, however, such fears are countered in the context of allying ourselves with an already existing transcendent project. A transcendent group encompasses a shared credo, a belief system and a corollary code of behavior. Sometimes such an ideology consists of promises of immortality, sometimes of more secular goals. Participation in the group mind assuages the fear of meaninglessness, not the terrors of childhood.

The transcendent function of the group mind is achieved through vicarious participation in the godhead: short of the promise of eternal life one may still be part of a chosen people or a master race, a descendant of Allah or of the Sun God, a follower of Mohammed or Buddha, or a warrior in one of the great conquering armies of history. Joint submission to a group leader or a group ideal is often facilitated by the invocation of an outside enemy—Christ for the church hierarchy in Dostoevsky's rendition of the Inquisition, rival Mafioso for Corleone,

Voldemort for Harry Potter and the good Wizards. What is at stake is affiliation with an elite group that confers real or symbolic survival. In the contemporary world, science offers the hope of a new approach for participating in the godhead. As a result of our newfound technological wizardry and the dream of vastly extending the duration of life, we flatter ourselves that our control of the physical world will be without limits. If a meteor hits Earth, we will climb into our spaceships and flee to a faraway galaxy. If our body parts wear out, we look forward to replacement parts à la the Bionic Man.

What shatters transcendent groups? Sometimes they fall prey to outside enemies. But sometimes they are victims to internal dissent, to the natural resistance invoked in response to power and particularly to its abuse. Such resistance to authority can set a limit to the indefinite perpetuation of any one ideology and, in the process, can sometimes create a new ideology or faith. We find this kind of resistance in the back-to-Jesus movements, themselves generally organized around one or another charismatic. Here the faithful find cause for resistance in the hierarchical structure of official churches, which interpose a layer between God and the individual.

Resentment of and resistance to authority were pivotal, too, in the birth of the Mafia. Only when Michael Corleone, Don Corleone's idealistic youngest son, tries to separate from his father's world, only to have a rival Mafioso's attempted murder of his father abruptly bring him back, does he become aware of "the roots from which his father grew." Through the voice of Michael Corleone, Puzo shares with us the history of the birth of the Mafia:

> The word "Mafia" had originally meant place of refuge. Then it became the name for the secret organization that sprang up to fight against the rulers who crushed the country and its people for centuries. Sicily was a land that had been more cruelly raped than any other in history. The Inquisition had tortured rich and poor alike. The landowning barons and the princes of the Catholic Church exercised absolute power over the shepherds and farmers. The police were the instruments of their power and so identified with them that to be called a policeman is the foulest insult one Sicilian can hurl at another.
>
> Faced with the savagery of this absolute power, the suffering people learned never to betray their anger and their hatred for fear of being crushed.... They learned that society was their enemy and so when they sought redress for their wrongs they went to the rebel underground, the Mafia. And the Mafia cemented its power by originating the law of silence.... *Omerta* became the religion of the people. (Puzo 1978, p. 324).

We cannot grasp the full power of our psychological need either to seize the godhead or to participate in transcendent-oriented groups simply by looking backwards to the fears and terrors of childhood. The history of the world is the history of groups that compete not only for natural resources, trade advantages, or priority in the balance of power, but also for a transcendent meaning that confers significance on life. Authority that attaches to nationalistic fervor or religious belief attains compliance because its precepts are accepted as legitimate or true and this because they are cloaked in a shared belief system in the form of ideology (Stoessinger 1961, p. 26). Because ideology rationalizes and legitimates power, it transforms power into authority, thus diminishing the amount of power necessary to attain compliance. This is the meaning of the Grand Inquisitor's insistence that people long for "an indisputable unanimous ant-heap" that ratifies a belief system and in doing so gives meaning to life. Thus is produced an apparently endless cycle of devout causes, each of them protected by an honor guard ready to die in its defense. Stability is threatened either internally, through resistance to authority, or externally, through the clash of two incompatible ideologies. Taken together, resistance to authority and obedience to ideology provide a major engine for the historical changes and upheavals that punctuate the human journey.

REFERENCES

Aeschylus: Prometheus Bound (ca. 458 B.C.), in Great Books of the Western World, Vol 5. Edited by Hutchins RM. Chicago, IL, Encyclopedia Britannica, 1952, pp 40–51

Bettelheim B: The Uses of Enchantment: the Meaning and Importance of Fairy Tales. New York, Alfred A Knopf, 1976

Camus A: The Fall. New York, Alfred A Knopf, 1957

Chodorow N: Femininities, Masculinities, Sexualities: Freud and Beyond. Lexington, University of Kentucky Press, 1994

Dalton D: Dostoevsky's grand inquisitor, in Power Over People: Classical and Modern Political Theory. Great Courses on Tape, Part II. The Teaching Company, 1998

Dostoyevsky F: The legend of the Grand Inquisitor, in The Brothers Karamazov (1880). Translated by McDuff D. London, Penguin, 1993, pp 283–304

Foushee HC, Helmreich RL: Group interaction and flight crew performance, in Human Factors in Aviation. Edited by Wiener EL, Nagel DC. New York, Academic Press, 1988, pp 189–227

Freud S: Group psychology and the analysis of the ego (1921), in The Standard Edition of the Complete Psychological Works of Sigmund Freud [SE], Vol 18. Translated and edited by Strachey J. London, Hogarth Press, 1955, pp 67–143

Freud S: The future of an illusion (1927). SE, 21:1–56, 1961
Freud S: Dostoevsky and parricide (1928). SE, 21:177–194, 1961
Fromm E: Escape from Freedom (1941). New York, Owl Books, 1994
Fromm E: The Heart of Man: Its Genius for Good and Evil. New York, Harper & Row, 1964
Galbraith JK: The Anatomy of Power. Boston, Houghton Mifflin, 1983
Gaylin W: Feelings: Our Vital Signs. New York, Harper & Row, 1979
Haynal A, Molnar M, De Puymége G: Fanaticism: A Historical and Psychoanalytical Study. Translated by Koseoglu LB. New York, Schocken, 1983
Horner A: The Wish for Power and the Fear of Having It (1989). Northvale, NJ, Jason Aronson, 1995
Kernberg O: Internal World and External Reality (1980). New York, Jason Aronson, 1985
Kerr W: Tragedy and Comedy. New York, Simon and Schuster, 1967
Malraux A: Man's Fate (1934). New York, Vintage, 1969
Milgram S: Obedience to Authority. New York, Harper & Row, 1974
Morgenthau H: Scientific Man vs. Power Politics. Chicago, IL, University of Chicago Press, 1946
Person E: By Force of Fantasy: How We Make Our Lives. New York, Basic Books, 1995
Person E: The Sexual Century. New Haven, CT, Yale University Press, 1999
Puzo M: The Fortunate Pilgrim (1964). New York, Ballantine, 1977
Puzo M: The Godfather (1969). New York, Penguin, 1978
Rahv P: The legend of the Grand Inquisitor (1949), in The Myth and the Powerhouse: Essays on Literature and Ideas. New York, Noonday Press, 1966, pp 144–174
Rieff P: Freud, The Mind of the Moralist. New York, Doubleday, 1961
Roustang F: Dire Mastery: Discipleship from Freud to Lacan (1976). Translated by Lukacher N. Washington, DC, American Psychiatric Press, 1982
Rowling JK: Harry Potter and the Sorcerer's Stone (1997). New York, Scholastic, 1998
Rowling JK: Harry Potter and the Chamber of Secrets. New York, Scholastic, 1999a
Rowling JK: Harry Potter and the Prisoner of Azkaban. New York, Scholastic, 1999b
Rowling JK: Harry Potter and the Goblet of Fire. New York, Scholastic, 2000
Sennett R: Authority. New York, Alfred A Knopf, 1980
Sexton JB, Thomas EJ, Helmreich RL: Error, stress, and teamwork in medicine and aviation: cross sectional surveys. BMJ 320(7237):745–749, 2000
Shulman ME: On the problem of the id in psychoanalytic theory. Int J Psychoanal 68:171–173, 1987
Spitz RA: No and Yes: On the Genesis of Human Communication. New York, International Universities Press, 1957
Stoessinger JG: The Might of Nations: World Politics in Our Time. New York, Random House, 1961

Tarnow E: Self-destructive obedience in the airplane cockpit and the concept of obedience optimization, in Obedience to Authority: Current Perspectives on the Milgram Paradigm. Edited by Blass T. Hillsdale, NJ, Lawrence Erlbaum, 2000, pp 111–123

Winnicott DW: Aggression in relation to emotional development (1950), in Collected Papers: Through Paediatrics to Psycho-Analysis. Edited by Winnicott C, Sheperd R, Davis M. London, Tavistock, 1984, pp 204–218

22

FRED PINE, PH.D.

INTRODUCTION

Fred Pine is a graduate of the College of the City of New York, received his Ph.D. in Clinical Psychology from Harvard University in Cambridge, Massachusetts, and did his psychoanalytic training at the New York Psychoanalytic Institute. He worked as a postdoctoral fellow and member of the research staff with Robert R. Holt and George S. Klein at New York University, was a visiting researcher at the Hampstead Centre for the Psychoanalytic Study and Treatment of Children (now the Anna Freud Centre) in England, and conducted longitudinal studies of child development as an Associate Professor at the Downstate Medical Center in New York. He is currently Emeritus Professor of the Department of Psychiatry, Albert Einstein College of Medicine in New York, Visiting Professor at the New York University Postdoctoral Program in Psychotherapy and Psychoanalysis, and a Training and Supervising Analyst of the New York Freudian Society. He has been a member of the editorial boards of *Psychoanalysis and Contemporary Thought*, *Psychoanalytic Psychology*, *Bulletin of the Menninger Clinic*, and *The American Journal of Psychotherapy*. He is on the faculty of the Columbia Psychoanalytic Center in New York.

Dr. Pine is the author of more than 75 papers. These cover a range that includes studies in infant and child development; clinical discussions of diagnostic issues in children and adults as well as of aspects of psychoanalytic technique and process; critical discussions of the development of ideas in psychoanalysis; and basic theory. His books include *Drive, Ego,*

Object and Self: A Synthesis for Clinical Work; The Psychological Birth of the Human Infant: Symbiosis and Individuation (in collaboration with M.S. Mahler and A. Bergman); *Developmental Theory and Clinical Process;* and *Diversity and Direction in Psychoanalytic Technique,* now in its second edition.

Some of Dr. Pine's many honors and awards include a Research Career Development Award of the National Institute of Mental Health, President of the Division of Psychoanalysis of the American Psychological Association, the Distinguished Scientific Contribution Award of the Division of Psychoanalysis of the American Psychological Association, and Hartmann Scholar of the New York Psychoanalytic Institute. His many honorary lectures include the Hartmann Lecture of the New York Psychoanalytic Institute, the Distinguished Psychoanalyst Lecture of the University of Texas Health Sciences Center, Dallas, the Lou and Harlan Crank Lecture of the Topeka Psychoanalytic Institute, and the Maurice Friend Lecture in Child Psychoanalysis of the Psychoanalytic Association of New York.

Pine has said of himself:

> My role in today's psychoanalytic scene: I think I am a creative integrator and rationalist, the latter in the sense of writing clearly without recourse to authority, mystification, or ideology. I like to think of myself as writing in the intersection of developmental theory and psychoanalytic clinical theory, a form of thinking that underlies my integrative approaches to multiple models. Though this involves extensive theorizing, central to my approach is an anchoring in recognizable details, clinical and developmental, just as we anchor a psychoanalysis in details. I believe that is why my writings are widely appreciated and utilized.

WHY I CHOSE THIS PAPER

Fred Pine, Ph.D.

"The Four Psychologies of Psychoanalysis and Their Place in Clinical Work" was the first of a series of writings attempting an integrative approach to diverse psychoanalytic models. I chose it for this volume because it seems to have the widest appeal of my several writings. Clearly, because many oppose its ideas while many find them clinically invaluable, it has struck a controversial chord among contemporary analysts.

This paper was my first relatively full effort in a journal publication to provide an integrative view of psychoanalytic theories in an era of multiple models. It is published here in its original form, although I have added numerous modifications, additions, and clinical illustrations in subsequent publications (see Pine 1989, 1990, 2003). In this introductory note I want only to orient the reader by specifying two points.

First, in my title and in the text I attempt maximally to *differentiate* psychological processes and theories regarding drives, ego function, internalized object relations, and subjective experiences of self. With the perspective of time, I can see that I did that to highlight the breadth of current theories and the quite different forms of understanding they make possible. But today I would emphasize *integration.* The several theories are attempts to represent issues that every person confronts in the course of development, all of which leave psychic residues (often troubling ones) that become interlocked in every individual's mental functioning. All four "psychologies," I propose, are part of a single psychoanalytic theory of mind.

Second, in this paper, written after object relations and self theories became prominent in psychoanalytic writings (adding to Freud's focus on instinctual drives), I engage these diverse theories of *mind.* Although I discuss their clinical relevance, I do not take clinical process and technique as my subject matter. But in the years since first publication of this article, the "two-person" aspects of the psychoanalytic process have become central in the literature, including ideas regarding enactment, intersubjectivity, induced states, and positive use of countertransference experience. However, I see no need to alter my views on theories of mind. Today I would say that the psychological issues captured by the terms *drive, ego, object relations,* and *self* are expressed not only on the traditional "stages" on which the psychoanalytic action was seen to be taking place (i.e., free association, transference, the dream, and the reported and remembered life) but additionally on the various two-person "stages" just listed. And in reverse, the psychic issues that are played out on any stage, from the dream and free association to induced states and enactments, will still turn out to be those of drives, ego function, internalized object relations, and self experience. One would expect theories of mind and of clinical process to interdigitate, as indeed they do.

With these orienting comments, this 1988 paper stands as is.

REFERENCES

Pine F: Motivation, personality organization, and the four psychologies of psychoanalysis. J Am Psychoanal Assoc 37:27–60, 1989

Pine F: Drive, Ego, Object, and Self: A Synthesis for Clinical Work. New York, Basic Books, 1990

Pine F: Diversity and Direction in Psychoanalytic Technique. New York, Other Press, 2003

THE FOUR PSYCHOLOGIES OF PSYCHOANALYSIS AND THEIR PLACE IN CLINICAL WORK

FRED PINE, PH.D.

PSYCHOANALYSIS HAS PRODUCED what I shall refer to as "four psychologies"—the psychologies of drive, ego, object relations, and self. Each takes a somewhat different perspective on human psychological functioning, emphasizing somewhat different phenomena. While the four certainly overlap, each adds something new to our theoretical understanding, and each has significant relevance in the clinical situation. My aim in this paper is to highlight that relevance. Earlier (Pine 1985) I attempted to give a developmental integration of the four psychologies, a picture of how each may find its place in the psychology of the individual during the course of development. Here I shall focus on clinical implications—in particular, for the concept of evenly hovering attention and for an understanding of the mutative effects of psychoanalysis. While the four psychologies are more or less familiar, counterposing them to one another highlights some problems and potentialities in clinical technique.

Before addressing the relation of these four psychologies to the larger theoretical systems of which they are a part, let me give a brief sketch of each of the four. These sketches are of necessity simplified in order to allow me to get on to the main task of this paper, their application to the clinical situation.

"The Four Psychologies of Psychoanalysis and Their Place in Clinical Work," by Fred Pine, Ph.D., was first published in *The Journal of the American Psychoanalytic Association*, 36:571–596, 1988.

THE FOUR PSYCHOLOGIES

From the standpoint of the psychology of drive, the individual is seen in terms of the vicissitudes of, and struggles with, lasting urges, forged in the crucible of early bodily and family experience, and taking shape as wishes that are embodied in actions and in conscious and unconscious fantasies. Because many of these wishes come to be experienced as unacceptable and dangerous, psychic life is seen as organized around conflict and its resolution—signified by anxiety, guilt, aspects of shame, inhibition, symptom formation, and pathological character traits. In Freud's original work, the theoretical underpinnings of these ideas lay in views of instinctual drive and epigenetically unfolding psychosexual stages. But at the experiential level of human functioning, the focus is on wish and urge, defense against them, and conflict (cf. Holt 1976; Klein 1976).

From the standpoint of the psychology of the ego, the individual is seen in terms of capacities for adaptation, reality testing, and defense, and their use in the clinical situation and in life at large to deal with the inner world of urges, affects, and fantasies, and the outer world of reality demands. Developmentally, the capacities for adaptation, reality testing, and defense are seen as slowly attained and expanding over time. While historically the major ego concepts developed as an outgrowth of drive-conflict psychology and remain intimately tied to it via conceptions of defense against drive, Hartmann's work (1939) introduced a significant emphasis on adaptation to the average expectable environment, as well. A developmental conception of ego functioning allows also for significant emphasis on a concept of "ego defect." That is, since adults (and older children) have capacities for adaptation, reality testing, and defense that infants do not have, we have to assume that these developed in between. Anything that develops can develop poorly or in aberrant ways; developmental failures in the domain of adaptive capacities can be viewed as "ego defects," e.g., affect intolerance and flooding, unreliable delay and control over impulses, failure to obtain object constancy. Such "defects" are not unrelated to conflict; conflict may have been contributory to their going wrong developmentally, and they will in any case enter into the individual's fantasy life and self-experience, and hence become elements in conflict and take on multiple functions (Waelder 1930). But I believe they can also usefully (from a working clinical standpoint) be seen as defects—adaptational incapacities or faulted capacities.

From the standpoint of the psychology of object relations, the individual is seen in terms of an internal drama, derived from early childhood, that is carried around within as memory (conscious or unconscious) and in which the individual enacts one or more or all of the roles (Sandler and Rosenblatt 1962). These internal images, loosely based on childhood experiences, also put their stamp on new experience, so that these in turn are assimilated to the old dramas rather than experienced fully in their contemporary form. These internal dramas are understood to be formed out of experiences with the primary objects of childhood, but are not seen as veridical representations of those relationships. The object relation *as experienced* by the child is what is laid down in memory and repeated, and this experience is a function of the affect and wishes active in the child at the moment of the experience. Thus, illustratively and hypothetically, the "same" quietly pensive and inactive mother will be experienced as a depriver by the hungry child, but perhaps as comfortingly "in tune" by the child who is itself contentedly playing alone. Significant for the clinical relevance of object relations psychology is the tendency to repeat these old family dramas, a repetition propelled by efforts after attachment or after mastery or both.

From the standpoint of the psychology of self-experience, the individual is seen in terms of the ongoing subjective state, particularly around issues of boundaries, continuity, and esteem, and his or her reactions to imbalances in that subjective state (Sandler 1960). I deliberately refer to "self-experience" rather than "the self" not only to bypass problems of conceptualization and reification regarding "the self," but also to remain at the level of subjective experience. But notably, the domain of "self" in the current literature is organized not only around subjective state per se, but around particular features of that subjective state. Thus, degree of differentiation of self from other has a central place, and here I refer to the sense of separateness, of boundaries (Mahler et al. 1975; Pine 1979), or contrariwise, of loss or absence of boundaries. Additionally, stemming from Kohut's work (1977), the degree of wholeness/fragmentation, continuity/discontinuity, or esteem of the self is also seen as central. It is doubtless no accident that both of these areas have to do with the relation of self to other, whether via differentiation from the "dual-unity" (Mahler 1972), or the contemporary selfobject serving functions for the self (Kohut 1977), or the actual historical (mirroring and ideal-forming) functions served by the parent for the child. These all have the ring of connection to those early stages in the development of the self that Stern (1985) refers to as "self with other." And they remind us of Spitz's (1957) earlier description of the development of the "I" inherently in relation to the "non-I" and, later, of the self in relation to the object. Thus, what I shall work with as the domain of the psychology of self-experience is subjective experience specifically around feelings of self-definition in relation to the object.

In listing these as four (conceptually separable, but not separate) psychologies, I do not mean to suggest that psychoanalysis has heretofore ignored any of these several points of view. While the drive and ego perspective on individual functioning were more formally part of Freud's *theory*, psychoanalytic *practice* clearly deals with them all. Early object relations and their repetition are significant parts of the working stuff of an analysis, and the ongoing subjective state is always a touchstone for the in-session work. All four are by now well established in aspects of the psychoanalytic literature. I describe them as four psychologies to highlight differences in their perspective because I believe they each generate different questions regarding the clinical work, and alert us to different facets of the processes of change. My aim here is pragmatic; it is useful to grant each of the four psychologies a place in our minds, as I hope to show.

Before pursuing that aim, however, I wish to clarify three further points regarding conceptual aspects of these four psychologies as I shall use them. First, each has been addressed within larger theoretical systems—e.g., the self psychology of Kohut (1977), the object relations theory of Fairbairn (1941), the ego psychology of Hartmann (1939), and the drive psychology of Freud (e.g., 1905). But it is *not* these larger theoretical systems to which I refer when I refer to "psychologies." Rather, I refer back to the clinical phenomena from which those several theories evolved. Earlier (Pine 1985—see especially Chapter 5) I referred to these as *personal* psychologies rather than *theoretical* psychologies. Second, are these truly separate psychologies or are they simply differing perspectives on the phenomena? Though I cannot develop the argument in full here, I believe there is a basis in the development of the individual for thinking of them *both* ways. Early on, there are moments in the life of the infant where one or another psychology dominates experience (Pine 1985) and, later on, some individuals achieve personalities organized primarily in one or another way (Pine 1989); in this sense they are separate psychologies. But there is also no doubt that in innumerable less extreme instances of human psychic functioning, they are blended and are best seen as perspectives on experience. Third, are these seen as an exhaustive list of the human psychologies? In particular, I have been asked, what of a psychology of superego? or of interpersonal relations? For now, it makes most sense to me to see superego as a significant part of both the object relations psychology (with respect to identification) and the drive psychology (with particular respect to aggressive drive). And I see interpersonal relations not as a separate psychology, but as one of the domains (the other being the intrapsychic) where the other four are played out.

To return now to the place of the four psychologies in clinical work.

Evenly Hovering Attention

Psychoanalytic technique proper came into being when Freud gave up forced association techniques and hypnosis and substituted open-ended listening, listening with "evenly hovering attention" (Freud 1912) to the content of the patient's associations. Provided that we listen with evenly hovering attention, uncommitted to any specific expectations regarding what is going on in a particular treatment hour, waiting to allow the clinical material to take whatever unique shape it will, we are constantly surprised—delightedly and profoundly—by the seemingly endless variability in the functioning of the human mind. But in spite of these continually renewed lessons of the indispensability of open-mindedness, strong counterpressures work within us in the opposite direction. It is the natural tendency of mind to make sense of things, to make order out of disorder, to seek closure and certainty. Sitting with a patient, listening to the often mystifying flow of associations, the treating clinician's mind will quite naturally "find" ordering principles, "red threads" weaving through the content, "meanings."

Indeed we count on this tendency of mind in our clinical work. Freud's guideline of evenly hovering attention for the listening clinician only makes sense if we recognize its counterpart: the sense-making, meaning-finding, ordering tendencies of the human mind. Freud's idea was, of course, to allow meaning to emerge rather than to be imposed by preformed notions. The clinician's mind is never blank. It is filled with personal history, one's own analysis, the general background of what has been learned from all previous patients, the prior clinical history with this particular patient, and general theory. The intent of evenly hovering attention is not to produce blank minds, but uncommitted ones—minds receptive to the organization of this particular content from this particular patient in this particular hour in ways true to its potentially unique offering.

Total uncommittedness is an impossibility, and the prime source of the interruption of evenly hovering attention is Freud's monumental theoretical achievement itself. The creation of psychoanalytic theory, with its view of human functioning as organized around drives and conflict, itself creates basic expectations and assumptions about the potential meanings of the contents of an analytic hour. Thus, while we may approximate evenly hovering attention—that is, uncommitted listening—in relation to the particular contents of a particular hour, ordinarily we have in mind a general set of theoretical constructs which dictate what the *potential* meanings are in what we are hearing. Uncommitted listening to this particular hour generally occurs in the context of broader theoretical commitments regarding a conception of personality development, organization, and its unfolding in the treatment situation. This is a profound limitation on truly even-handed or uncommitted listening.

To highlight this issue in another way, let me perhaps overstate a certain paradox: As scientists, psychoanalytic clinicians work under a self-expectation to be true to the phenomena, to be servants to the data, to be reporters of the observed. This presses in the direction of open-mindedness. But as professionals, psychoanalytic clinicians work under a self-expectation to be knowledgeable, to be expert in a body of knowledge they can apply in the relief of psychic distress. Patients come to us, and pay us, to be experts, not scientists. This presses in the direction of closure.

To date, and not without struggle, psychoanalysis has produced, out of the tension between open-mindedness and closure, the four psychologies that I have already outlined—ways of ordering the data of lives. These have evolved from the listening process—one or another analyst selectively attuned to one or another aspect of clinical phenomena. Though "evenly hovering attention" means that we hold all of this to the side as we allow the red threads of particular hours to show through, theoretical commitments, taken-for-granted views regarding development and pathology, can profoundly dictate the range of potential meanings to which we are receptive. Tendencies to organize the material along lines of conflict, of narcissistic transferences, of oedipal pathology, or of preoedipal pathology flow from theoretical commitments and not only from open-ended listening. Different theories lead us to approach the clinical hour with different questions (silently) in mind. And these can affect what we come to understand, how we phrase interpretations, and ultimately the entire conduct, and presumably the outcome, of an analysis. What are some of these theory-derived questions?

They are numerous; and I believe they are productive, not restrictive, when they are held in *back* of our minds—as *potential* ways of thinking of the associative content and its accompanying affect. The task of analytic listening remains that of suspension between knowledge of human functioning and open-ended ignorance of how a particular hour in a particular patient will come to be best understood.

The drive psychology, as analysts have worked with it since its beginnings with Freud, alerts us always to ask (silently, in nonverbalized ways even to ourselves, but always in the background, guiding our listening): What wish is being expressed? What is the relation of the wish to consciousness? What is the fantasy, and how does it reflect a compromise between wish and defense and reality? How is the wish being defended against? How effective/adaptive is the defense? Can the particular anxiety seen be traced to this or that wish, ineffectively defended against, and can the particular guilt seen be understood in terms of the operation of conscience in relation to this or that wish? Similarly for symptoms and inhibitions: How do they reflect compromise formations between wish, and defense, and conscience, and the patient's historical realities? Likewise for character: How have particular urges been transformed and meshed with defensive styles so as to contribute to characteristic and ordinarily ego-syntonic modes of function? And related questions influence our historical-reconstructive-formulative view: What early under- or overgratifications of particular drives (and their related wishes) have occurred, producing early fixations and tendencies to regression? Is there any evidence for genetically greater drive strength in one or another area, or for early trauma that provoked increased activity around particular drives—either the genetic or traumatic factors possibly accounting for resistance to change? The questions apply powerfully to the ongoing clinical work—notably Freud's defining features of psychoanalysis—transference and resistance, for the transference is understood ultimately in terms of the press of drives for satisfaction, now playing themselves out on the person of the analyst. And resistance is understood in terms of the automatic, unconsciously working counterpressures against the entry of conflictual drive derivatives into consciousness. So the question: Which drive, and how defended against? applies here as well.

The array of questions is long, and years of psychoanalytic work have demonstrated their fruitfulness. In classical psychoanalytic theory, the sexual urges (in their broad sense, as expanded by Freud) have remained first in importance in formulations regarding human drives, with aggression being a major second. And the questions, those listed and other related ones that could be added, seem at times (and in some patients) to provide us with entry into all we need to know about the person with whom we are working.

But is this really so? Is it true that such questions lead us to all we now know and need to know about human function? Of course not. I doubt that any clinical psychoanalysis is fully organized around conceptions of drives and their workings. Among drive theorists (historically and, to some degree still) there is a tendency to formulate published cases in these terms, and this probably accurately represents much of the work, but such formulations partly reflect the available conceptual tools and partly social convention and social conformity pressure among analysts. Clearly other questions, stemming from different theoretical bases, can be formulated.

Some of those deriving from the psychology of the ego, particularly those related to defense, seem almost indistinguishable from some of those from the psychology of drive—being the other side of the same coin. We may ask: What defenses are operative against the drives, and how effective (rigid, flexible, reliably available or not) are they? But even here the questions extend beyond drive psychology, with our questions now potentially expanding to: How are affects being defended against (A. Freud 1936), and how is relatedness itself being defended against (Modell 1984)? But the questions stimulated by our psychology of the ego, and particularly of its development, go well beyond questions of defense. They include a whole set of questions of the kind: What tools of adaptation have failed to develop or have developed aberrantly—for example, tension maintenance, the capacity for delay, object constancy, concern for others, the socialization of urge? The list could go on and on. Within recent analytic writings such questions have been subsumed within the larger question: To what degree do we think of such things in terms of deficit or in terms of conflict? The question, largely stimulated by Kohut's (1977) formulations regarding deficits in early selfobject relations that produce deficiencies in the self-experience, is too either-or and too bounded by experience with analyzable (even marginally analyzable) patients. Certainly when we recognize (as discussed above) that the infant is not born with his adult tools for adaptation fully in place, we also recognize that they have to develop—and therefore can develop poorly or well, whether or not they are also involved in and even stunted as a result of conflict. Psychoanalysis as a general psychology has to recognize pathology beyond the range of the analyzable, and there concepts of deficit in ego function are indispensable and unavoidable. But I believe such questions to be relevant to most analyses as well, to varying degrees.

The psychology of object relations produces yet other questions to ask of the clinical data, yet other perspectives on the history of the individual and the workings of pathology. Object relations theory is not a single theory, and the questions within these theories that I find most useful, sitting somewhere in the back of my mind as I do clinical work, include: What old object relationship is being repeated? Which of the roles in the object relationship is the patient enacting—his or her own, or that of the other, or both? Is the patient behaving like the person that:

He was? He wished to be in the parents' eyes? They wanted him to be? They were? He wished they were? And what early passive experiences are being repeated actively? Such questions are based on the idea that all significant early relationships get repeated in action later on, either out of efforts to repeat pleasure experiences or to master traumatic ones. And the "pleasure experiences" obviously need not be "pleasurable" in "objective" terms (i.e., you or I might not think of them as pleasurable), but they are the carriers of the relationship with the parents of childhood, and however good or bad those experiences may have been, they are experiences with the only parents the patient has had, and so reflect forms of attachment and familiarity, and thus safety, no matter what pain they may also include. Thus the questions can be reframed to ask such things as: Do these behaviors repeat earlier experiences with the parents and thus serve to hold on to those relationships? Or are they efforts to master old traumatizing relationships by repeating them actively with others? And then there are historically based questions: To what degree are these relations, as carried in memory, enacted in identification, or repeated in action—to what degree are they veridical renditions of what happened in childhood? Presumably they are never fully veridical. In any event, we shall never really know (Spence 1982), but (and here the drive and ego psychologies interweave with that of object relations) they presumably reflect the *experienced* object relation, that experience determined by the drive state or ego state of the patient at the moment of the relational event. Thus, once again, it is *that* experience that is laid down as memory, not anything that can be called an "objective" event in its own right. There is no objective event in this sense, only subjective experience, and yet the sorting out of personal history, of its realities and its subjectivities, can, I believe, be exceptionally useful to the patient in analysis.

Last, let us consider questions for the clinical situation stimulated by the psychology of the self. As noted already, I neither subscribe to nor reject the specific formulations advanced by Kohut (1977) and others under the name "self psychology." Rather, I refer to generic features of the human situation variously addressed by different contributors. Among the questions I find useful (again as questions sitting in the back of my mind—that is, as potential modes of conceptualizing the clinical data or addressing the actual patient) are those having to do with boundaries, integration, and esteem: How stable a sense of differentiated self-boundaries is present? How much are fantasies of merger, enactments of merger, or panics regarding loss of boundaries a factor in the clinical situation? How do the differentiated boundaries stand up in relation to the stresses of living? How much is derealization or depersonalization a part of the picture? Also: To what extent is discontinuity of the self- experience present? Does it feel subjectively (to the analyst) that one is with the same patient each session or is there a subjective sense of discontinuity? To what extent does the patient experience himself or herself as the center of action in his or her own life, or as the "cause" of that life? Further: What is the ongoing sense of self-value, of esteem? What pathological efforts to right imbalances in that subjective state of self are present—grandiosity, denial, flights into activity, disdain of others?

Each of the four psychologies has a somewhat different conception of humankind and our essential tasks. Drive psychology emphasizes the taming, socialization, and gratification of drives. Ego psychology emphasizes the development of defense with respect to the internal world, adaptation with respect to the external world, and reality testing with respect to both. Object relations theory focuses on the task of simultaneously carrying within us (through identification and internalized object relations) the record of the history of our significant relationships—which is essential to our humanness and is a basis for social living—and, on the other hand, of freeing ourselves from the absolute constraints of those relationships so that new experiences can be greeted, within limits, as new and responded to on their own, and contemporary, terms. And psychologies of the self focus on the diverse tasks of forming a differentiated and whole sense of self (both in contradistinction to and in relation to the other), of establishing the self as a center of initiative and as the owner of one's inner life, and of developing an ongoing sense of subjective worth. "Evenly hovering attention" will be most even-handed when attention allows for the organization of the session content in these diverse ways.

MUTATIVE FACTORS IN TREATMENT

Just as the four psychologies can enrich our concept of evenly hovering attention, so too can they enrich our understanding of the mutative factors in psychoanalysis. By alerting us to different aspects of mind, they alert us to a wider range of therapeutic happenings. I shall, in what follows, address these in terms of each of the four psychologies first for verbal interventions and insight, and then for relational effects of the treatment. This division itself implicitly reflects the various psychologies—for the power of insight is embedded in a theory of the ego, of cognition and learning and affect transformation, and the power of relationships is embedded in both the theory of object relations and the self, the latter seen as taking shape in relation to the other (Kohut 1977; Mahler 1972; Spitz 1957). What follows will be a sample of issues in the psychology of change, meant to illustrate the utility of a view from the position of the four psychologies.

Verbal Interventions

The series of questions generated by the four psychologies, just outlined, are themselves central to an understanding of the place of verbal intervention in the treatment process. To be effective, such an intervention must be in some sense "true"—i.e., it must touch the patient's experience so that he or she can resonate with it. To do this, I believe, requires interpreting at different times within one or another of the varying conceptual frameworks of the several psychologies.

Regarding the psychology of drive, I am of course in the familiar center of classical psychoanalytic technique, and shall be brief. Making the unconscious conscious, and "where id was there shall ego be" (Freud 1933) have reference to the interpretation of unconscious conflict, powered by conscience, utilizing ineffective or rigid defenses, and operative against unacceptable urges or wishes. The therapist's task is interpretation, with the aim of gradually producing modification of conflict, conscience, and inflexible modes of defense, all permitting reorganization to take place with greater success in the patient's acceptance of thoughts and urges, in conflict resolution, affect tolerance, displacement, and sublimation. Especially when the analytic process is stuck in some way, or on those occasions when complexly interwoven material has come together within the confines of a single hour (see Kris's [1956] "good analytic hour"), the power of interpretation of unconscious conflict—its power to move the process forward—is truly impressive.

With regard to the psychology of internalized object relations, where early experiences are seen to be repeated in part because of the stress associated with them (repetition in efforts after mastery) and in part because of the pleasure associated with them (repetition in efforts after gratification), the therapist's task is, once again, interpretation, with the aim of freeing the patient to meet new experience as *new,* without absorbing it into the old drama of historically based object relations. Transference, which can be understood in terms of the continuing pressure of urges to be expressed, played out on the person of the analyst, can equally be conceptualized as the tendency to repeat old internalized object relations. Here, too, the power of interpretation to bring about a sudden new perspective on what is going on in an analysis (in the transference) or in the patient's life outside, and to move the process forward, is compellingly clear.

In both the regions of drive and of internalized object relations—that is, with respect both to unconscious wishes and to unconsciously compelled repetitions of old object relations—interpretation brings the power of the patient's cognitive apparatus to bear and permits the patient to see and to change habitual ways. If this were all there were to it, however, analyses would be a lot shorter than they are. Seeing and *believing*, seeing and *remembering*, or seeing and *changing* are clearly not coincident with one another, and the patient's attachment to the old wishes and/or relationships is not easily renounced, and so analysis as we know it, with continual discovery, rediscovery, and working through, is the expectable mode. That this takes place within a powerful relationship is altogether what gives it the chance of being more than just words. It is the immediacy of interpretation in the transference that makes it *real*, and the intensity of the patient-analyst relationship that makes it *matter*.

Still, it is clear that interpretation does not always lead to change. Freud's (1916) concepts of "adhesion of libido" and "resistance of the id" (Freud 1926) essentially merely gave recognition to the fact of nonchange—when fact it was—without really clarifying anything. And Eissler's (1953) concept of "parameters" essentially legitimized what analysts were learning that good technique required—namely doing different kinds of things at times.

So, with this in mind, and turning to the regions of self and ego pathology, the situation regarding interpretation can be seen to be different. Though lines cannot be sharply drawn and there are no either-ors in this work, still an "interpretation" of a *defect* in ego function or a *deficiency* in self-experience does not in itself lead to a useful "now I see" experience.[1] The relational aspects of the analytic encounter may play an important role here, but I will come to that later. For now, let me stay with aspects of verbal intervention and their impact. What makes interpretation potentially mutative with an unconscious urge or wish and the anxieties and defenses associated with it is that the conflict dates from the childhood era where it might have seemed to make sense (e.g.,

---

[1]A *deficiency* is like not having enough money in the bank; the *input* from caretakers has been insufficient in kind to produce a good self-experience. A *defect* is like something being broken. Whether through genetic factors, early illness (see Pine 1986), parental inputs, or intrapsychic conflict, some tool of ego function fails to develop or develops aberrantly.

the threat of castration for certain wishes) but can be judged differently in light of adult reality. The mutative potential of interpretation of repetitions of old internalized object relations similarly rests on the presumption that, today, having a life separate from the parents of childhood, the patient can be different. But interpretations that make the patient see, for example, deficiencies in the subjective self-experience (low esteem, shaky boundaries, discontinuity) pose the danger of rubbing salt in wounds or of eliminating hope and merely causing pain.

In areas of primary deficiency, verbalization may have a significant mutative potential when it comes in the form of description, explanation, and reconstruction—especially within the overall "holding" context of the analytic relationship (Modell 1984). The aim is to help the patient become familiar with these inner states, to bring them into the sphere of verbalization and shared understanding, and to help understand how they came about in the family history. My experience is that this gradually enables the patient to better bear the pain of such states by becoming familiar with their quality, triggering events, course, and source (though it does not eliminate the pain) which in turn permits bearing (sustaining) them rather than acting upon them. But in other regions of self-disturbance, interpretation certainly has a role—and it shades over into what I am calling description or explanation or reconstruction. To draw here on illustrations I have given elsewhere (Pine 1985): "You got frightened when I used the word 'we' because it made you feel I was invading you as it used to be with your mother"; or "your parents' failure to respond to you made you lose touch with who you were, so when I don't greet you as you come in you can't believe that you and I are the same two people who worked together yesterday"; or "you're showing me what your parents thought of themselves and of you by behaving in such a way as to advertise how worthless you are"; or "succeeding at school made you feel like a person, separate from others, and so you rushed back with failure to get your parents and me reinvolved with you."

In relation to the psychology of ego function, much of what we work with in a psychoanalysis with a reasonably intact patient is clinically inseparable from interpretive work on drive and conflict. The whole area of rigid, malfunctional, ineffective, and outdated defense is at the core of such interpretive work and is familiar enough. However, the area of ego defect—that is, the faulty initial development of basic tools of functioning, requires comment exactly parallel to that of defect in the self-experience. Interpretive interventions often produce helplessness, depression, or narcissistic mortification. Yet, as with deficiencies in the self-experience, to describe, explain the workings of, and reconstruct the origins of such defects can be a positive step in the treatment that, at the minimum, permits the patient to feel recognized, understood, not alone with the defect, and gradually to come to some terms with it; these are essentially reconstructions, which the *patient* receives educatively.

Let me assert a number of points regarding verbal intervention and change before continuing. 1) Interpretation, bringing consciousness and the power of the cognitive apparatus to bear on inner life, is a powerful mutative factor in psychoanalysis; 2) it is most effective in an intense patient-analyst relationship where every communication from the analyst *matters* to the patient; 3) it is ordinarily most powerful when linked to the transference, where it is most immediate and real; 4) (and this is a more distinctive part of my argument) it (interpretation) is most effective when it is most "true" (and "true" here means touching the patient's experience so that he or she resonates with what has been said), and this requires working with shifting theoretical models—in our current language, models of drive, ego, object relations, and self; 5) in areas of defect—notably regarding aspects of the faulty development of self experience or of functional tools of adaptation—interpretation can at times produce painful confirmation without therapeutic impact, though other modes of verbalization—describing, explaining, reconstructing—can produce familiarity, some degree of acceptance, a capacity to bear, and modest change as well.

Until now, in discussing both the concept of evenly hovering attention and the verbal interventions the analyst makes, I have been attempting to show how the analyst's behavior can be productively influenced by having conceptions of each of the four psychologies in the back of his or her mind. Schafer (1983), in his emphasis on diverse psychoanalytic narratives, and Jacobson (1983), in his explicit use of structural theory and representational world theory (in an analysis of the psychoanalytic encounter) are recent forebears of this kind of effort—though each in quite different ways.

Relational Aspects of the Therapeutic Encounter

Here, I shall use the four psychologies more as conceptual tools to analyze a process that simply happens under the special circumstances of a clinical psychoanalysis.

Patients use the relationship with us, and experience us, in ways that foster the analysis, support resistance, feel to them like condemnation, punishment, or humiliation on the one hand, or love, praise, and special attention and guidance on the other. Much of this eventually becomes clear and is itself subjected to analysis if all goes well. But after what is conflictful, and in that sense "noisy" and noticeable, enters the analysis and is gradually pared away, there remain other ways in which we are functional in the psychic lives of patients—ways that are relatively conflict-free—that contribute to the mutative power of the analytic encounter.

From the standpoint of the psychology of drive: the *absence of condemnation* that accompanies the analyst's inquiries, observations, and interpretations with respect to wishes the patient regards as taboo, can gradually lead to modification of conscience, as Strachey (1934) pointed out long ago. Additionally, that the analyst continually *survives,* in the sense of not being drawn into reciprocal sexual fantasy or behavior and not retaliating with rage or rejection in the face of the patient's rage, provides a model for the patient to follow. The situation is as Winnicott (1963) described in the infant-mother relationship: the mother who repeatedly survives the infant's destructiveness enables the infant to learn that its destructiveness will not destroy, can be safely (gradually) "owned," and can be expressed even toward loved ones. The patient in analysis, both through repeated talking of wish and fantasy regarding both sexuality and rage, and through observation of the analyst's matter-of-fact response, learns that "nothing happens"—no action, no seduction, no condemnation, no retaliation—just survival, going on with life. While, to be sure, at times this leads to disappointment, further provocation, fantasied condemnation, or wished-for action, as analysis of all of these continues, what remains is survival. Life goes on, now with formerly taboo wishes more fully owned.

From the standpoint of the psychology of object relations, one core feature of an analysis is its provision of a new, "corrective," object relationship for the patient, one that can gradually enter into the world of internalized object relations. I do not say this with instructional intent; I am not suggesting that the analyst "should be" this way or that—nice, helpful, or what have you. What I am saying is that the analyst, with his or her sustained attention, concern, noncondemnation, and persistent efforts to understand, is different from the internalized parent of childhood. It has long been recognized that the child analyst is a "new object," not only a transference object to the child patient; I do not believe this ever fully disappears, even for adult patients (Loewald 1960). And, as I do not say instructionally that analysis provides a new, corrective, object relationship, so do I not say it naively. If the patient steadily experienced it that way, something of the necessary storm and stress of the analytic relationship would surely be missing. Rather, what is new and corrective is that the patient can continually rediscover, following analysis of transference distortion and following mutual recovery from analyst errors and empathic failures, that the analyst remains basically well-intentioned and concerned. The work generally moves in that direction over time. If the patient, nearing termination, is unable to view the analyst with reasonably consistent trust, and with a sense that he or she has been able to be helpful and clarifying at least some of the time, surely we would feel that something has not gone well.

A second object relational component of the analytic encounter with mutative effect is what Loewald (1960) has addressed in his discussion of the disintegrative and integrative experiences of an analysis. The free-associative process (and the couch, and the analyst's silence and interpretations) continually lead to mini-disintegrative experiences; the analyst's intervention (or, sometimes, mere presence) permits new integrations to occur, and, through these, progressive mastery. But it is precisely the background object relation with the analyst, on the model of the parent-child relation, that permits these integrations to occur.

From the standpoint of the psychology of the self—still looking at effects carried by the patient-analyst relationship in itself—we come to Kohut's (1971, 1977) work, which is most explicit on the subject. Not only does he point out that the patient's experience of feeling "mirrored," empathically understood, by the analyst and/or idealizing the analyst—can in part compensate for deficient experiences in the patient's childhood that have contributed to a lack of esteem and well-being in the self-experience, but he cautions against interpreting these experiences too early out of the analyst's ultimately countertransferential discomfort that he or she is not being sufficiently "analytic," that is, is allowing the idealization or the patient's pleasure in feeling mirrored. His point is that, while interpretation (or, in my terms earlier—description, explanation, and reconstruction) has a significant place, so too, and especially in deficit states, does *experiencing*.

Beyond these specific "narcissistic" transferences, as Kohut called them earlier on (1971), it is my impression that all patients take something of that sort from the analytic encounter. Though it is often slow in coming (because so much of the therapeutic dialogue pertains to the patient's self-perceived "badness"), generally the patient slowly comes to feel valued by the therapist—valued enough to be worked with in the face of perceived "badness" and valued enough for the analyst to be reliably there, attentive, and working in sessions day in and day out, year in and year out. Certainly that impacts at least in small ways on self-esteem. (I have also been impressed by the direct experiential aspect of boundary formation when that is at issue.)

From the standpoint of the psychology of the ego, I shall mention only some of the more general relational impacts on ego function that are inherent in the psychoanalytic encounter. Once again, I refer to Loewald's (1960) paper, wherein he addresses the function of speech as it works for the patient:

> Once the patient is able to speak, nondefensively, from the true level of regression which he has been helped to reach by analysis of defenses, he himself, by putting his experiences into words, begins to use language creatively, that is, begins to create insight. The patient, by speaking to the analyst, attempts to reach the analyst as a representative of higher stages of ego-reality organization, and thus may be said to create insight for himself in the process of 1anguage-communication with the analyst as such a representative. (p. 26)

The very act of putting experience into words, motivated as it is by the effort to "reach the analyst" and communicate, gives form to (often) previously unformed experience and is part of a movement of such experience to higher levels of ego organization.

I would add that the analyst's silence is crucial here. The analyst's silence and the patient's recumbent posture and free-associative task not only create the conditions for a certain kind of *passivity* in the patient—wherein experience will flow, unscreened, sometimes regressively—but can be seen as creating the conditions for a certain kind of patient *activity*—giving shape to experience in the absence of any external shaping demands, putting things into words, and ultimately being both experiencer and observer of inner life.

I have made no attempt to be complete in describing potentially mutative effects of the relational aspect of the analytic encounter, but I have tried to show how the perspective of each of the four psychologies alerts us to aspects of those effects. They are largely *inherent* in the process; they do not require us to do anything special. They simply happen between people and, in analysis, they happen in ways that are functional (and malfunctional) in multiple ways for the patient. As the malfunctional, the pathological, uses of the relationship the patient makes are pared away by interpretation, more functional uses of the relationship, serving growth, remain—often not noticed because largely conflict-free and not verbalized, though equally often recognized verbally between analyst and analysand as part of the total process.

In sum, then, I have tried in this section to conceptualize the mutative factors in psychoanalysis in a broad way. While interpretation in the transference can be most dramatic in its mutative potential, it is certainly not the whole of what takes place in an analysis. Overall I have suggested that, in the context of an intense and intimate relationship where things *matter* for the patient, both interpretation (and other verbal interventions) and relational factors, have important mutative effects. I have used the four theories current on the psychoanalytic scene today as vehicles to explore the mutative potential of the psychoanalytic encounter. I have tried, also, to make the following points: 1) Interpretation (even interpretation in the transference, and well timed) has its major mutative potential when (to put it simplistically) it is "right"—that is, when it touches on something experientially (not necessarily consciously) valid in the patient—and to do that we have to interpret, varyingly, in the languages of each of the four psychologies—more in this one than that one for different patients, more of this one now and that one at another time in any single patient. 2) The patient finds meanings in the relationship itself, also along lines we can conceptualize in terms of the four psychologies; this happens because processes active in patients (in each of these domains) find and recruit meanings that "work" for inner life. When we are aware of and interpret found meanings that are problematic in terms of the patient's pathology, when we pare them away, we still leave the patient with found meanings that work for the patient in nonpathological ways, that foster change and renewed development.

CONCLUDING REMARKS

If one were stranded on a desert isle, it would probably be better to find there a set of tools than say, a finished house. The house would indeed provide shelter from the start, but the tools could be used flexibly in innumerable ways—including the building of a house—to enhance the capacity to get along. I view what I have called the four psychologies of psychoanalysis as just such tools to be used flexibly when "stranded" in the position of analytic listener. They do not provide, at the start, a finished house—a theoretical structure—but they are, I find, immensely useful to help one "get along" in doing analysis. I have tried to illustrate some of their clinical utility herein.

But is it legitimate to think of them as four psychologies of *psychoanalysis?* Is this such a hodge-podge that it no longer deserves that name? I do not think so. I believe that each of the four, and especially the four taken together, require just such a complex and multifaceted view of human functioning as only psychoanalysis provides; and I see them as consistent with the core of psychoanalysis, even in its traditional form. Separately and jointly, the four psychologies share the assumptions of *psychic determinism,* of *unconscious mental functioning,* and of (for want of a better term) the *primary process*—that aspect of thinking based on symbol and metaphor, on "irrational" connection among ideas, which does not heed the rules of reality and socialized communication. Only by following the premises underlying this triad of psychic phenomena can we find our way to the place of the phenomena of each of the four psychologies in the lives of our patients. Furthermore, the four psychologies all work with core psychoanalytic assumptions which state that individual character is shaped by *early, bodily based,* and *object-related* experiences, all organized in *interconnected* (both *multiply functional* and *conflictual*) ways. The bodily based experiences of drive and gratification, of apparatus and function, are among the contents thus organized, as are the object-tied experiences involved in drive gratification, the learning of modes of psychological functioning, the creation and growth of the self-experience, and the shaping of the representational world (Sandler and Rosenblatt 1962). They are indeed four psychologies *of psychoanalysis,* and as such they find places in each psychoanalytic treatment within the traditional boundaries of quiet listening, work with resistance and transference, and the clinical triad of neutrality, abstinence, and relative anonymity. But they do not simply fit into the traditional confines of psychoanalysis. Rather, they require us to see psychoanalysis not only as a psychology of *conflict,* but also of *repetition* and of *development,* the latter with all the attendant delays and aberrations inherent in any developmental process. The use of the four psychologies in clinical work, I believe, provides a fuller approximation to the phenomena of human development and clinical psychoanalysis than any one or two alone—and they are responsive to the clinical material that cultural changes and changing psychopathology in contemporary patients bring our way.

REFERENCES

Eissler KR: The effect of the structure of the ego on psychoanalytic technique. J Am Psychoanal Assoc 1:104–143, 1953

Fairbairn WRD: A revised psychopathology of the psychoses and psychoneuroses. Int J Psychoanal 22:250–279, 1941

Freud A: The Ego and the Mechanisms of Defense (1936). Writings, Vol 2. New York, International Universities Press, 1966

Freud S: Three essays on the theory of sexuality (1905), in The Standard Edition of the Complete Psychological Works of Sigmund Freud [SE], Vol 7. Translated and edited by Strachey J. London, Hogarth Press, 1953, pp 159–168

Freud S: Recommendations to physicians practicing psychoanalysis (1912). SE, 12:109–120, 1958

Freud S: Introductory lectures on psychoanalysis (1916). SE, 16, 1963
Freud S: Inhibitions, symptoms, and anxiety (1926). SE, 20:77–175, 1959
Freud S: New introductory lectures on psychoanalysis (1933). SE, 22:1–182, 1964
Hartmann H: Ego Psychology and the Problem of Adaptation (1939). New York, International Universities Press, 1958
Holt RR: Drive or wish? A reconsideration of the psychoanalytic theory of motivation (1976), in Psychology Versus Metapsychology: Psychoanalytic Essays in Memory of G.S. Klein. Edited by Gill MM, Holzman PS. Psychol Issues Monogr 36. New York, International Universities Press, 1976, pp 158–197
Jacobson JG: The structural theory and the representational world (1983). Psychoanal Q 52:514–542, 1983
Klein GS: Psychoanalytic Theory: An Exploration of Essentials. New York, International Universities Press, 1976
Kohut H: The Analysis of the Self. New York, International Universities Press, 1971
Kohut H: The Restoration of the Self. New York, International Universities Press, 1977
Kris E: On some vicissitudes of insight in psychoanalysis (1956), in Selected Papers. New Haven, CT, Yale University Press, 1975, pp 252–271
Loewald HW: On the therapeutic action of psychoanalysis. Int J Psychoanal 41:16–33, 1960
Mahler MS: On the first three subphases of the separation-individuation process. Int J Psychoanal 53:333–338, 1972
Mahler MS, Pine F, Bergman A: The Psychological Birth of the Human Infant. New York, Basic Books, 1975
Modell A: Psychoanalysis in a New Context. New York, International Universities Press, 1984
Pine F: On the pathology of the separation-individuation process as manifested in later clinical work: an attempt at delineation. Int J Psychoanal 60:225–242, 1979
Pine F: Developmental Theory and Clinical Process. New Haven, CT, Yale University Press, 1985
Pine F: On the development of the "borderline-child-to-be." Am J Orthopsychiatry 56:450–457, 1986
Pine F: Motivation, personality organization, and the four psychologies of psychoanalysis. J Am Psychoanal Assoc 37:31–64, 1989
Sandler J: The background of safety. Int J Psychoanal 41:352–356, 1960
Sandler J, Rosenblatt B: The concept of the representational world. Psychoanal Study Child 17:128–145, 1962
Schafer R: The Analytic Attitude. New York, Basic Books, 1983
Spence DP: Narrative Truth and Historical Truth: Meaning and Interpretation in Psychoanalysis. New York, WW Norton, 1982
Spitz RA: No and Yes. New York, International Universities Press, 1957
Stern DN: The Interpersonal World of the Infant. New York, Basic Books, 1985

Strachey J: The nature of the therapeutic action of psychoanalysis. Int J Psychoanal 15:127–159, 1934

Waelder R: The principle of multiple function: observations on overdetermination (1930), in Psychoanalysis: Observation, Theory, Application: Selected Papers of Robert Waelder. Edited by Guttman SA. New York, International Universities Press, 1998, pp 68–83

Winnicott DW: The development of the capacity for concern (1963), in The Maturational Processes and the Facilitating Environment. New York, International Universities Press, 1965, pp 73–82

23

OWEN RENIK, M.D.

INTRODUCTION

Owen Renik is a graduate of Columbia College and the State University of New York at Syracuse Medical School. He did his residency in the Department of Psychiatry of Mount Zion Hospital, San Francisco, and his analytic training at the San Francisco Psychoanalytic Institute. Dr. Renik has been an active teacher and researcher and participated in the Psychotherapy Research Project with Drs. Joseph Weiss and Harold Sampson. He was Associate Chief of the Department of Psychiatry, Mount Zion Hospital, and Associate Clinical Professor in Psychiatry, University of California, San Francisco. He is a Training and Supervising Analyst at the San Francisco Psychoanalytic Institute and is on the Faculty of the Colorado Society for Psychology and Psychoanalysis and of the Karen Horney Institute. Among his many significant positions at the International Psychoanalytical Association have been Chair of the International Association of Scientific Secretaries, Chair of the North American Program Committee, and Chair of the North American New Groups Committee. At the American Psychoanalytic Association he has been Chair of the Program Committee, Secretary of the Board of Professional Standards, and member of the Committee on Psychoanalytic Education.

Dr. Renik has been Editor-in-Chief of *The Psychoanalytic Quarterly*, Associate Editor of *The Journal of the American Psychoanalytic Association*, and on many editorial boards, including *Psychoanalytic Inquiry, Critical Issues in Psychoanalysis*, and *The American Psychoanalyst*. He is the author of nearly 100 publications and has been particularly interested in investigating the dogma and shibboleths of psychoanalytic practice and technique. He has been a leader in pointing up the authoritarian and dogmatic aspects of traditional analytic neutrality and anonymity and the nature of scientific discourse in psychoanalysis.

He has said of himself:

> I see my place in contemporary psychoanalysis as someone who selectively values some long-standing concepts and principles, but considers uncritical acceptance of received wisdom to be the bane of our field. Because I grew up within and eventually held positions of responsibility within the establishment, I tend to be heard differently than those colleagues who question traditional analytic thinking from a position of having been excluded.

WHY I CHOSE THIS PAPER

Owen Renik, M.D.

As with many colleagues, I was motivated to become a psychoanalyst out of therapeutic zeal, a zeal that arose from efforts on my part toward self-cure as well as toward the satisfaction of childhood wishes to have been able to help loved ones in pain. Psychoanalysis appealed to me because it seemed to offer the best available way to understand and treat emotional distress. Therefore, I have never been much interested in theoretical constructs unless they can be directly applied to advantage in work with patients.

I'm particularly fond of this paper, "Playing One's Cards Face Up in Analysis," because it is completely clinically oriented. It certainly has theoretical referents: what I discuss represents the convergence of several lines of thought that interested me very much over the years, concerning the irreducible subjectivity of the analyst's participation in treatment, the misconceived technical ideals of analytic anonymity and neutrality, conceptions of reality and reality testing, and the importance of therapeutic benefit as an outcome criterion for judging clinical analytic work. But my ideas on those theoretical subjects were sufficiently developed that I could bring them together and translate them into a set of specific, practical recommendations for the conduct of clinical analysis. It was satisfying to feel able to go beyond a critique of existing principles and to propose another approach. I tried to illustrate that approach in detail with case examples, and to anticipate and address at least some of the common questions and objections with which I had become familiar through many discussions with colleagues about the problem of self-disclosure.

PLAYING ONE'S CARDS FACE UP IN ANALYSIS

An Approach to the Problem of Self-Disclosure

OWEN RENIK, M.D.

I THINK WE CAN SAY that there is by now significant consensus among contemporary analysts concerning at least some aspects of the problem of self-disclosure. It's widely agreed that we need to re-think what we even *mean* by an analyst's self-disclosure, given that everything an analyst does is self-disclosing somehow or other, and given as well that every purposeful effort by an analyst at self-disclosure is likely to obscure some things about the analyst while it reveals others (e.g., Greenberg 1995; Renik 1995; Singer 1977). At the same time, it's widely agreed that intentional self-disclosure by an analyst, however we conceptualize it, is an important element of clinical method (Miletic 1998). Clearly, we need to develop ways of thinking systematically about what, when, and how an analyst optimally discloses; but generalizations concerning this subject always elicit concern. No one wants to lose sight of the importance of taking into account case-specific factors and judgments particular to the clinical moment (e.g., Aron 1991; Cooper 1998; Rosenbloom 1998).

Analysts overall are reluctant to unequivocally endorse self-disclosure (Moroda 1997). Nonetheless, my own experience has been that clinical

---

"Playing One's Cards Face Up in Analysis: An Approach to the Problem of Self-Disclosure," by Owen Renik, M.D., was first published in © The Psychoanalytic Quarterly, 1999. *The Psychoanalytic Quarterly*, Volume 68, Number 4, pages 521–539. Used with permission.

work benefits when the analyst takes a stance from which self-disclosure, rather than anonymity, is the norm. When I analyze, I try as best I can to play my cards face up: that is to say, I'm consistently willing to make my own views—especially my own experience of clinical events, including my participation in them—explicitly available to the patient. I find that it is crucial for an analyst to have what Frank (1997) calls "an attitude of willingness to be known by the patient" (p. 309). This attitude toward self-disclosure directly contradicts not only the longstanding, traditional technical principle of analytic anonymity, but the more contemporary idea that it is helpful for the analyst to be "selective" about self-disclosure, thereby maintaining a "relative anonymity" (e.g., Jacobs 1999).

I mean to propose that playing one's cards face up in analysis is a useful overall policy, a general principle that best directs an analyst's conduct in the clinical situation. Commitment to this policy can be difficult and requires discipline. An analyst's personal values—tensions between the analyst's narcissistic and altruistic interests, for example—are fundamentally and decisively implicated in the effort to play one's cards face up. Ehrenberg (1995, 1996) speaks directly to this aspect of analytic self-disclosure when she discusses it in relation to the analyst's emotional availability and vulnerability. Often, what is at stake for the analyst in describing his or her own experience is exposure to a kind of explicit, unameliorated scrutiny by the patient that can be most distressing. A willingness to self-disclose, in these moments, involves a choice for the patient's welfare over the analyst's comfort.

However, while there are ethical aspects to decisions concerning self-disclosure, the main virtues of playing one's cards face up in analysis are practical. The attitude toward self-disclosure that I want to discuss is consistent with any number of trends in contemporary analytic thinking that take the analyst off a pedestal and permit the patient to claim greater authority, thus expanding the patient's functioning in the treatment situation. More and more, we have been leveling the clinical analytic playing field; and an important part of this process has been the discovery that explicit communication by an analyst of his or her experience is crucial to the sort of cooperation between analyst and patient that permits honest and open-minded clinical investigation. As Gerson (1996) puts it, "By allowing the patient access to himself or herself as a subject in the analysis, the analyst reveals a process of knowing rather than a known product" (p. 642).

Some colleagues have understood these developments to stem from a *Zeitgeist*—a movement toward greater democracy in the culture at large, a postmodern turn in intellectual life (e.g., Bader 1998). I don't agree. Over the years, there has been an evolution toward less self-importance and more candid self-exposure by analysts, and we fail to appreciate its significance if we dismiss it as determined by political aims or academic fashion. We have every reason to think that it has been motivated by immediate, pragmatic considerations: analysts have been learning how to establish a more collaborative treatment relationship with their patients because it yields better clinical results. My impression, which I would like to discuss and illustrate in some detail, is that playing one's cards face up is a more effective clinical practice than the deliberate pursuit of even relative anonymity.

NEGOTIATING SELF-DISCLOSURE

Of course, questions have been raised about the utility of purposeful self-disclosure by an analyst. One often-expressed, understandable concern is that too much emphasis on the merits of the analyst's self-disclosure disposes to an intrusive clinical approach (e.g., Mitchell 1997). Actually, I don't think the problem of intrusiveness by an analyst is specific to the activity of self-disclosure. Any aspect of an analyst's method (whether it arises from the analyst's preferred theory, the analyst's character, or, very likely, both), whatever its virtues, will also have the liability of impinging upon the patient's freedom one way or another, and constraining analytic investigation. The only safeguard against intrusion by an analyst, I believe, is for the analyst to remain open to input from the patient about his or her technique. Certainly, a policy that directs the analyst toward self-disclosure has to be accompanied by a willingness on the analyst's part to pay careful attention to his or her decisions concerning self-disclosure and to deal with them collaboratively within the treatment relationship. The following still holds for me.

> I would say that an analyst should try to articulate and communicate everything that, *in the analyst's view,* will help the patient understand where the analyst thinks he or she is coming from and plans to go with the patient.... I emphasize *in the analyst's view* because, clearly, patient and analyst may disagree about what it is useful for an analyst to disclose, in which case the matter becomes open for consideration—neither the analyst's nor the patient's view being privileged *a priori*....
>
> By acknowledging that an analyst's judgments concerning what constitutes relevant...disclosure on his or her part are subjective, we indicate a role for the patient as constructive critic of those judgments. This is a reciprocal of the analyst's familiar role as critic of the patient's self-disclosure. We know that when a patient tries to say everything that

> comes to mind, an analyst is able to point out things the patient overlooked. Similarly, when an analyst tries to make his or her analytic activity as comprehensible as possible, a patient is able to point out things the analyst overlooked. (Renik 1995, pp. 485–488)

In my observation, self-disclosure by an analyst does not lead to undue focus of attention upon the analyst at the patient's expense. In fact, just the opposite is the case: the more an analyst acknowledges and is willing to discuss his or her personal presence in the treatment situation, the less room the analyst takes up and the more he or she leaves for the patient. A reticent analyst looms large, occupying center stage as a mysterious object of interest. The patient remains very well aware of being engaged in an encounter with another individual human being; and the patient's need to know the analyst's intentions, assumptions, values—the patient's need to know about the person with whom he or she is actually dealing—does not go away, even if the analyst deems it irrelevant to exploration of so-called "psychic reality" (see Renik 1998). I think we are all familiar with how a game of "Guess What's on My Mind" tends to be initiated when an analyst tries to remain even relatively anonymous. Too many patients have wasted too much time playing that game. My experience has been that, ironically, self-disclosure helps an analyst *avoid* becoming an intrusion. Here is an example.

Anne

In her analysis, Anne repeatedly seemed to need to relinquish critical thoughts about her husband when they arose, turning to self-doubt instead. Growing up, Anne had experienced her mother as loving, but quite controlling and intolerant of independence, let alone contradiction from her children. Anne and I discussed the possibility that her difficulty in feeling critical of her husband might connect to a sense of danger that she had learned in relation to her mother.

Anne was a TV journalist whose career was really starting to take off. One day, she described how her husband had seemed conspicuously uninterested when she was telling him, with great excitement, about a story she was working on. Anne considered that her husband might be threatened by her success; but after a time, she decided instead that there must have been something about the way she had been talking to her husband that turned him off.

After listening to her account, I said, "I'm confused. What gives you the impression that your way of talking turned your husband off?" Anne responded, with slight irritation, "I don't think you're confused, Owen. I think you have a view of what's going on. Why don't you just say what you think?" Well, of course, Anne was right. I wasn't really confused. My hypothesis was that Anne had once more felt the need to criticize herself instead of her husband. However, I didn't know for sure that Anne was abdicating her critical capacities, and I expressed myself inconclusively because I wanted to leave room for the possibility that in this instance she might actually have been perceiving something about herself that warranted her self-criticism. I explained this to Anne.

She considered. "That makes sense," she said. "I can understand where you were coming from. But why didn't you just explain your concerns? Instead, you presented yourself as confused, and that wasn't really true—not to mention that it goes against your policy, which you've explained to me, of making your thinking explicit so that we can discuss it if we need to. Not that it's such a big deal, but why did you bullshit like that?"

Good question, I thought, and said as much to Anne. I told her what came to my mind. I was aware of not wanting to seem controlling like Anne's mother. The kind of presumptuousness that Anne felt she got from her mother was something I particularly dislike, so I was taking pains to be sure Anne experienced me differently. As the hour ended, I was thinking out loud in this vein in response to Anne's question.

The next day Anne began by saying how useful the previous session had been. She was curious about my personal reasons for reacting as I did; but the really interesting thing to her, the more she thought about it, was that I had been, in a way, intimidated by her—sufficiently concerned about her disapproval to even misrepresent myself a bit. She had never considered that I might be worried about her opinion of me. She always thought of me as completely self-confident and self-sufficient. She thought of her husband in the same way, but revising her view of me made her question her view of him too. Last evening she told her husband what had happened in her analysis and asked him whether he worried about having her approval. He told her he did. For example, he said, when she talked about her work, he was very reluctant to say anything because she frequently seemed to think that he was leaping to conclusions about what she was telling him.

So, Anne pointed out to me, there *was* something she did that made other people back off from her. In that sense, she had been right the day before when she had distrusted the idea that her husband was too competitive to be interested in her work, and had wondered instead whether something about her way of talking to her husband had been the problem. Similarly, Anne went on, whatever my susceptibilities were, she realized that she had played a role in my becoming so careful with her that I pretended to be confused when I wasn't. Anne continued to elaborate how useful it had been for her to recognize that she could inadvertently intimidate other people by communicating her exaggerated sensitivities. She and her husband had gone on to have a very long talk about it last night, and afterward they'd made love more intimately and passionately than they had in years. Sexually, too, Anne felt, she'd been shutting her husband down without realizing it. Obviously, she concluded, she was too ready to assume that the people she cared about would treat her the way her mother had, and this expectation was having unintended, destructive effects in her personal relationships.

Discussion

To begin with, I hope I have illustrated what I mean by playing one's cards face up in analysis. At a couple of points during the session, Anne asked me, essentially, what I thought I was doing: first when she challenged my statement that I was confused; then, after I explained my understanding of why I'd said that I was confused, when she pressed me to explain my motivation for misrepresenting my state of mind. Each time Anne asked for my view of what I was up to, I gave it to her. I didn't decline to answer her questions, or even defer answering them, suggesting that Anne reflect upon her reasons for asking me what I thought I was doing. Instead, I responded to her inquiry as a constructive request for information that would be useful for her to consider, and we took it from there. Clearly, I was not striving for even relative anonymity. On the contrary, my aim was to be as explicit as possible about my own view of my participation in events.

Although I talked quite a bit about my own experience of events, there was no evidence that Anne experienced me as intrusive. Actually, she and I collaborated on the nature and extent of my self-disclosure. Sometimes Anne asked me to say more about what was on my mind; at other times, she was explicit about feeling that it was not useful for her to inquire further about my thinking. Anne established her own need to know, and it seemed to work out very well. She certainly did a lot of profitable self-investigation, much of which could be described as transference analysis.

I find that I am able, by and large, to establish an atmosphere in which my patients feel free to ask me to say more if they think I need to explain myself further, or to say less, if they think I'm talking too much; an atmosphere in which I, in turn, can inquire into a patient's motivation if the patient appears to me either excessively interested in hearing from me, or conspicuously incurious about my ideas. Anne and I operated in such an atmosphere, and in my opinion, it is a sine qua non for honest, unfettered, and consequential analytic inquiry. Needless to say, there are times when collaboration about the analyst's self-disclosure is hard to achieve, and when this happens, the reasons for it are invariably worth understanding. It has been my experience, however, that my willingness to self-disclose elicits in my patients neither an insatiable curiosity about me, nor a wish to learn my opinions so that they can be taken as received wisdom. My impression is that in general, patients do not want to be intruded upon, and are happy to collaborate with their analysts to avoid being intruded upon, given the chance.

In this respect, the interchange with Anne that I've described has to be understood in the context of the history of her analysis. I intend my vignette to portray not only a particular clinical moment, illustrative of a policy of playing one's cards face up in analysis, but the effect of operating on the basis of that policy over time. Anne obviously felt quite free to confront me with her observations and inferences about my participation because from previous experience with me, she anticipated that if she did, she would get an accounting from me, and we would continue to discuss what we were doing—as each of us saw it—as long as that seemed useful. Had I been less forthcoming all along in her treatment, I doubt that Anne would have been as able to inquire into my view of my own activity as she was in the hours I've reported.

AUTHORIZING THE PATIENT AS COLLABORATOR

It should go without saying that an analyst's view of his or her own participation in clinical events is irreducibly subjective. I think Greenberg (1995) sums up the situation perfectly when he says: "I am not necessarily in a privileged position to know, much less to reveal, everything that I think and feel" (p. 197). An analyst cannot reliably give an accurate, complete account of his or her participation in clinical events. Therefore, the point of an analyst's willingness to self-disclose is not that it provides the patient with an accurate, complete account of the analyst's activity. (For example, I was unable to explain myself very satisfactorily to Anne, as she was quick to point out!) *Rather, the benefit of an analyst's willingness to self-disclose is that it establishes the analyst's fallible view of his or her own participation in the analysis as an appropriate subject for collaborative investigation—something analyst and patient can and should talk about explicitly together.* This makes it possible for the patient to open up analytic opportunities by calling to the analyst's attention aspects of the analyst's functioning of which the analyst would otherwise not be aware. Anne's inquiry into my claim to be confused is an excellent instance in point.

Precisely for this reason, colleagues influenced by Sullivan and the interpersonalist school have for years been advocating the virtues of actively soliciting the patient's observations about the analyst's personal functioning within the treatment relationship (e.g., Aron 1991). However, they have tended not to recommend that the analyst respond with reciprocal self-disclosure to the patient's input. The assumption has been that an analyst's "self-revelation can foreclose full exploration of the patient's observations and his reactions to them" (Greenberg 1991, p. 70).

My clinical experience has led me to a very different conclusion. I have found that when a patient makes a pointed comment or inquiry about an analyst, if the analyst does not respond by giving his or her own view about what the patient is bringing up, if the analyst is unwilling to pursue an explicit exchange of views with the patient, as needed, then the patient concludes that the analyst is not really interested in receiving active consultation. When a patient calls an analyst's attention to aspects of his or her participation in treatment that the patient feels are significant, even problematic, and the analyst, instead of saying what he or she thinks about the patient's observations, encourages the patient toward further self-reflection, the patient learns that offering his or her observations will not be interpersonally consequential, and the patient becomes much less interested and willing to offer them. I find that when an analyst does not operate according to an ethic of self-disclosure, the analyst, despite claims to the contrary, discourages free confrontation and questioning by the patient. The analyst's unwillingness to make his or her own views available conveys to the patient that the analyst wishes to protect him- or herself by avoiding scrutiny. Usually the patient complies.

A willingness to self-disclose on the analyst's part facilitates self-disclosure by the patient, and therefore productive dialectical interchange between analyst and patient is maximized. When, on the other hand, an analyst refrains from making his or her own views fully available, for whatever ostensible reason, the patient eventually responds in kind and dialectical interchange between patient and analyst is constrained. It takes a second analysis for the patient to fully say what he or she thought about the first analyst, and a third analysis to say what he or she thought about the second analyst, and so on. In order for a patient to want to volunteer his or her interpretations of an analyst's experience (Hoffman 1983), the patient needs to have responses to his or her interpretations from the analyst.

I should note that by emphasizing the patient's role as a consultant to the analyst, I am diminishing neither the importance of the analyst's self-analysis nor the utility of obtaining consultation from colleagues. Both of these practices have been highly recommended and much discussed in our literature, with good reason. However, even if we regard the analyst's self-analysis as a central, ongoing aspect of clinical work, we can acknowledge its limitations. There is significant truth, after all, to the old joke that the problem with self-analysis is the countertransference. Consultation with colleagues, too, while it is a valuable resource, is not a cure-all. An analyst only seeks consultation when he or she feels it is needed, and even the shrewdest consultant cannot proceed very far beyond what the treating analyst presents. The patient, however, is in a position to offer uniquely informed, in-the-moment consultation, even if the analyst has not identified a need for it. Had Anne not picked up on my claim to be confused, for example, I would never have noted it, let alone thought that it was worth looking into.

SELF-DISCLOSURE AND THE ANALYST'S STYLE

My own style as a person, and therefore as an analyst, is toward the active, exhibitionistic rather than the reserved end of the spectrum. All things being equal, I usually prefer to mix it up with a patient and field the consequences rather than risk missing out on an opportunity for productive interchange. By suggesting that the analyst play his or her cards face up, however, I am not rationalizing my personal style or elevating it into a technical principle. Willingness to self-disclose, as a policy, can and should apply across the individual styles of various analysts. In fact, whatever an analyst's particular style, by playing his or her cards face up, the analyst increases the probability that he or she will receive consultation concerning his or her personal style from a patient—which is exactly what an analyst is most likely to need, inasmuch as it is our personal styles that generate our blind spots.

When Anne inquired into my way of expressing myself, eventually exposing a subtle hypocrisy on my part, she was analyzing a component of my personal style. Even more salient was the patient who said to me, explaining how she felt I was getting in her way, "You know, Owen, I think you believe it's important for an analyst to be open and non-authoritarian, that you try to be that way with me, and that it has been very helpful overall. But besides that, I think you have a personal stake in not being seen as domineering and unfair, so that when I see you that way, rightly or wrongly, you're quick to react and to try to sort it out; and that gets in the way of you being able to listen to me sometimes. So, ironically, you can wind up doing the very thing you're trying to avoid" (Renik 1998, p. 572). There I was, the analyst hoisted by his own petard: the atmosphere created by me playing my cards face up permitted my patient to constructively criticize me for a tendency on my part to explain myself too much! Thus, a disconcerting but exemplary consultation from a patient, which illustrates that a policy of willingness to self-disclose does not direct the analyst to talk about him- or herself all the time, but instead permits collaboration between analyst and patient concerning how much and what the analyst says about him- or herself.

Apropos this last example of the benefits of an analyst's willingness to self-disclose, I'd like to consider the relation between playing one's cards face up in analysis and idealization of the analyst by the patient. When an analyst adopts a posture of anonymity, it invites idealization of the analyst by the patient, posing an important obstacle to analytic work (see Renik 1995). On the other hand, an analyst's willingness to self-disclose obviously does not prevent idealization of the analyst by the patient, since it is at least as easy for an analyst to be idealized for being open, candid, or forthcoming as for any other reason. (There's a well-known story that makes the point. It's about the old Jewish man who gazed at himself in the mirror and mused, "You know, I'm not very good-looking; and I'm not very smart; and I'm not very rich; but boy, am I humble!") Furthermore, we know that idealization of the analyst by the patient is a crucial, useful phase in certain analyses—perhaps, to some degree, in all analyses—so that for an analyst to be intolerant of being idealized can be as much of a problem as for an analyst to require being idealized. I want to emphasize, therefore, that although I think we should not systematically *encourage* idealization of the analyst by the patient via a stance of analytic anonymity, the purpose of playing one's cards face up in analysis is not to *discourage* idealization of the analyst by the patient. Rather, *the purpose of an analyst playing his or her cards face up is to facilitate examination and revision, when necessary, of the analyst's modus operandi, whatever it is*—whether, for example, the analyst is too impatient with being idealized, or too eager to be idealized.

FORMS OF SELF-DISCLOSURE

In speaking of playing one's cards face up in analysis, I am referring to a consistent policy of willingness on the analyst's part to self-disclose. I mean to contrast playing one's cards face up with notions of selective self-disclosure (see, e.g., Jacobs 1999) which direct the analyst to consider non-disclosure his or her default position and self-disclosure an exceptional activity. I want to make clear, however, that an analyst's systematic willingness to self-disclose does not prevent the analyst from taking into account case-specific factors and judgments relevant to a particular clinical moment. Case-specific factors and judgments relevant to a particular clinical moment never militate *against* self-disclosure; they determine the *form* of an analyst's self-disclosure. The problem is not *whether* to self-disclose, but *how* to self-disclose.

Sometimes, playing one's cards face up in particular clinical circumstances seems a relatively straightforward matter. For example, when I awoke one morning, bone-tired with a very sore throat, I immediately telephoned Anne, who was my first patient of the day. "I'm sorry for the short notice," I said, "but I'm going to have to cancel our appointment today. It's nothing serious. I think I've got that 24-hour virus that's been going around, so I hope to be in tomorrow." Anne thanked me for calling and wished me a speedy recovery.

Now, it is very rare that I cancel an hour on short notice, and I thought it likely Anne would worry if I didn't explain the reasons for my cancellation. I'm sure some colleagues would argue that by reassuring Anne, I foreclosed a useful opportunity for her to investigate her fantasies about my cancellation—for example, fantasies expressing hostile wishes toward me. I don't think so. In my view, had I cancelled without explanation, it would have been a contrived and mysterious act. Anne's reaction to such unnatural behavior would have afforded her little opportunity to investigate her manner of participation in ordinary human relationships.

Actually, we did meet the next day, and Anne began her hour by reporting a dream from the night before, following my cancellation. The dream was that she was lying on a couch, reading a book by Faulkner. Her first association to the dream was the title of one of Faulkner's novels, *As I Lay Dying;* and it made her remember that after my call, she'd had the thought that maybe I was sicker than I realized. Anne was embarrassed to recall thinking that because she felt it reflected her childish anger at me for not keeping our appointment. She was dying to see me, and I should drop dead for canceling! Clearly, my reassurance did not prevent Anne from entertaining a hostile fantasy. I would suggest that, in fact, having had my explanation for the cancellation available to her facilitated Anne's recognition that imagining me gravely ill was an expression of her own anger. If she had been left in the dark about why I cancelled, she could have more easily chalked up her *As I Lay Dying* dream to realistic concerns.

There are times, on the other hand, when the direction indicated by a policy of playing one's cards face up is not self-evident. One summer day, Anne walked into my office wearing a short dress made of thin, silky material that clung to her body, revealing every curve to advantage. Did a willingness to self-disclose direct me to tell her what was on my mind? Of course not. For an analyst to play his or her cards face up doesn't mean that the analyst free-associates. What it means is that the analyst does not keep his or her thoughts private *as a matter of analytic principle.* When an analyst chooses not to say something to a patient, the choice is made on the same basis as it would be in any conversation: What is the purpose of the communication? Is it likely to be understood as intended? I could not see that anything helpful would be achieved by telling Anne that I was turned on to her; in fact, I could imagine some negative consequences. I decided to keep my sexual feelings to myself for the same kinds of reasons that would lead me not to express sexual feelings stimulated by, let's say, my teenage daughter or one of her friends.

Now, as it happened, things became more complex when Anne, obviously aware that she had made an impression, asked coyly as she entered my office, "Like the dress?" I said simply, "You look terrific." She smiled and thanked me. During the hour, her thoughts returned a number of times to my appreciation of her as a woman and my apparent comfort in acknowledging it. Various implications that this interaction had for her came to mind, especially in relation to what she had experienced as her father's rigid defenses against the anxiety stirred up in him when she began to mature sexually.

I chose to respond to Anne's flirtatious inquiry with a direct, but circumscribed description of my response to her. It seemed to work out very well. Of course, other ways of handling the situation might have worked out equally well or better. My point is only that while playing one's cards face up means that the analyst makes every effort to render his or her experience available to the patient, the particular way an analyst chooses to communicate his or her experience is determined by ordinary, pragmatic considerations. There was nothing specifically psychoanalytic about the aims and concerns that led me to limit as I did what I disclosed to Anne. I agree with Fitzpatrick's (1999) summary of the issues involved in dealing with the erotic aspects of the treatment relationship:

> While dangers of exploitation and overstimulation from disclosure of sexual and loving feelings by the analyst are well known, they may be counterposed by less obvious but equally strong dangers of confusion and seductiveness when the subject of the analyst's feelings remains taboo. We need a way of discussing these vital responses to our patients that will be neither exploitive nor withholding, but clarifying. (p. 124)

THE ANALYST'S SELF-DISCLOSURE AND COLLABORATION WITHIN THE TREATMENT RELATIONSHIP

Elsewhere (Renik 1998) I have discussed what I see as the disadvantages of various versions of the concept of a special, psychoanalytical reality. I think it is of the utmost importance that we acknowledge that the clinical psychoanalytic situation is ordinarily real. What the analytic treatment relationship can be, within ordinary reality, however, is extraordinarily candid. That requires courage on the part of both participants. In order to be candid, a patient needs candor from his or her analyst.

Of what does an analyst's candor consist? As I mentioned at the beginning of these remarks, inasmuch as an analyst's activity is always determined in part by unconscious motivations, the concept of self-disclosure by an analyst is problematic. No matter how hard an analyst tries to play his or her cards face up, some cards will remain face down—and the analyst cannot know which ones, or how many. In other words, an analyst's effort to play his or her cards face up does not provide the patient with a reliable account of the analyst's activities. What I've suggested, however, is that an analyst's willingness to engage in self-disclosure does establish ground rules that make for a more truly collaborative, mutually candid interchange between analyst and patient about the treatment relationship than can take place when the analyst pursues a policy of even relative analytic anonymity.

I realize that a radical policy of willingness to self-disclose goes against long-standing, even currently prevailing, views in our field. I submit that self-disclosure by the analyst is an issue about which we can benefit from consultation from our patients—perhaps an issue about which we are *especially* in need of consultation from our patients. Most of all, I would say that we should be interested in the judgment of those patients who come to us simply to be healed, without any ambition to become analysts themselves. For example, Anatole Broyard (1992), fiction writer and essayist, in his extraordinary memoir entitled *Intoxicated by My Illness,* described what he wanted in the way of an interchange with his doctor. Broyard was reflecting upon the healing relationship in general, but I think what he had to say applies very well to clinical psychoanalysis in particular.

> While he inevitably feels superior to me because he is the doctor and I am the patient, I would like him to know that I feel superior to him, too, that he is my patient also and that I have my diagnosis of him. There should be a place where our respective superiorities can meet and frolic together. (p. 45)

Does this sound like the kind of treatment relationship that is facilitated by cautious self-expression on an analyst's part, designed to preserve a degree of anonymity? I don't think so. Broyard goes on to make the following recommendation:

> In responding to [the patient], the doctor may save himself. But first he must become a student again; he must dissect the cadaver of his professional persona; he must see that his silence and neutrality are *unnatural.* (p. 57)

My impression is that Broyard speaks eloquently and cogently for most patients, and I think we are obliged to take what he has to say very seriously. If we believe, as Hoffman (1983) suggests, that the patient is a legitimate interpreter of the analyst's experience, then we need to listen to and respect the thinking not only of the patients we treat, but of those (the overwhelming majority) whose objections to clinical analysis are such that they do not come to analysts for treatment.

According to the popular view, an effective therapist is candid and forthcoming—like the ones we see in *Ordinary People* or *Good Will Hunting*. I agree with the popular view, the naïve idealization that characterizes movie portrayals of psychotherapists notwithstanding. It seems to me that we are justified in recommending to analysts a policy of playing one's cards face up because, as a general rule, self-disclosure by an analyst is in the patient's best interest; and, in my opinion, the burden of proof is on an analyst who chooses to adopt a stance of even relative anonymity to show that the analyst is not protecting him- or herself at the patient's expense. When an analyst is consistently willing to self-disclose, the patient is more fully authorized as a collaborator in the clinical work. The patient's active participation may require the analyst to endure a measure of disconcerting exposure, but the analyst may also discover that he or she is no longer practicing an impossible profession.

REFERENCES

Aron L: The patient's experience of the analyst's subjectivity. Psychoanalytic Dialogues 1:29–51, 1991

Bader MJ: Post-modern epistemology: the problem of validation and the retreat from therapeutics in psychoanalysis. Psychoanalytic Dialogues 8:1–32, 1998

Broyard A: Intoxicated by My Illness. New York, Fawcett Columbine, 1992

Cooper SH: Countertransference disclosure and the conceptualization of analytic technique. Psychoanal Q 67:128–156, 1998

Ehrenberg DB: Self-disclosure: therapeutic tool or indulgence? Contemp Psychoanal 31:213–229, 1995

Ehrenberg DB: The analyst's emotional availability and vulnerability. Contemp Psychoanal 32:275–286, 1996

Fitzpatrick K: Terms of endearment in clinical analysis. Psychoanal Q 68:119–125, 1999

Frank KA: The role of the analyst's inadvertent self-revelations. Psychoanalytic Dialogues 7:281–314, 1997

Gerson S: Neutrality, resistance, and self-disclosure in an intersubjective psychoanalysis. Psychoanalytic Dialogues 6:623–646, 1996

Greenberg J: Countertransference and reality. Psychoanalytic Dialogues 1:52–73, 1991

Greenberg J: Self-disclosure: is it psychoanalytic? Contemp Psychoanal 31:193–205, 1995

Hoffman IZ: The patient as interpreter of the analyst's experience. Contemp Psychoanal 19:389–422, 1983

Jacobs T: On the question of self-disclosure by the analyst: error or advance in technique? Psychoanal Q 68:159–183, 1999

Maroda KJ: On the reluctance to sanction self-disclosure: commentary on Kenneth A. Frank's paper. Psychoanalytic Dialogues 7:323–326, 1997

Miletic MJ: Rethinking self-disclosure: an example of the clinical utility of the analyst's self-disclosing activities. Psychoanalytic Inquiry 18:580–600, 1998

Mitchell S: To quibble. Psychoanalytic Dialogues 7:319–322, 1997

Renik O: The ideal of the anonymous analyst and the problem of self-disclosure. Psychoanal Q 64:466–495, 1995

Renik O: The perils of neutrality. Psychoanal Q 65:495–517, 1996

Renik O: Getting real in analysis. Psychoanal Q 67:566–593, 1998

Rosenbloom S: The complexities and pitfalls of working with the countertransference. Psychoanal Q 67:256–275, 1998

Singer E: The fiction of anonymity, in The Human Dimension in Psychoanalysis. Edited by Frank KA. New York, Grune & Stratton, 1977, pp 181–192

24

ROY SCHAFER, PH.D.

INTRODUCTION

Roy Schafer is a graduate of City College of New York. He received his Ph.D. from Clark University in Worcester, Massachusetts, and graduated from the Western New England Institute for Psychoanalysis in New Haven, Connecticut, where he was later appointed Training and Supervising Analyst. He has, at various times, served as Chief of the Adult Testing Section of the Menninger Clinic, and later at the Austen Riggs Center, Chief Clinical Psychologist at Yale University School of Medicine in New Haven, Connecticut, and has held the positions of Clinical Professor at Yale University and Professor of Psychology and Psychiatry at Cornell University Medical College in New York. He has been President of the Western New England Psychoanalytic Society, Vice President of the International Psychoanalytical Association, and Training and Supervising Analyst at the Columbia University Center for Psychoanalytic Training and Research in New York.

Dr. Schafer has served on numerous editorial boards, including *The Journal of the American Psychoanalytic Association, The International Journal of Psychoanalytic Psychotherapy, The Bulletin of the Menninger Clinic, Psychological Issues, The International Journal of Psychoanalysis,* and *Psychoanalysis and Contemporary Thought.*

Dr. Schafer's many honors include the first Freud Memorial Professor and Lecturer, University College, London, the Sandor Rado Lecturer, Columbia University Center for Psychoanalytic Training and Research, the Freud Anniversary Lecturer of the New York Psychoanalytic Institute, the American Psychological Association Division of Psychoanalysis Award for Contributions in Psychoanalysis, the Edith Weigert Lecture of the Washington School of Psychiatry, the George E. Daniels Merit Award of the Association for Psychoanalytic Medicine, the Heinz Hartmann Lecture of the New York Psychoanalytic Society and Institute, and the Mary S. Sigourney Award for Contributions to the Field of Psychoanalysis.

Dr. Schafer is the author of more than 100 papers on topics ranging from psychological testing procedures to generative empathy in the treatment setting, the loving and beloved superego in Freud's structural theory, and, most recently, caring and coercive aspects of the psychoanalytic situation. He is the author of 12 books, including *Psychoanalytic Interpretation in Rorschach Testing, Projective Testing and Psychoanalysis, Aspects of Internalization, A New Language for Psychoanalysis, The Analytic Attitude, Retelling a Life: Narration and Dialogue in Psychoanalysis, The Contemporary Kleinians of London, Bad Feelings: Selected Psychoanalytic Essays, Tradition and Change in Psychoanalysis,* and *Insight and Interpretation: The Essential Tools of Psychoanalysis.*

Dr. Schafer has played an extraordinary role in the development of psychoanalysis in America. He is closely associated with David Rapaport in establishing the core elements of Freudian theory. His book on Rorschach testing has been a classic in that field. He has an enduring interest in philosophy and the humanities, and he has examined the clinical activity of the psychoanalyst with a fresh eye, as little as possible influenced by the metapsychology that held sway until the current era of pluralism. His elaboration of hermeneutic ideas has been crucial in constructing contemporary psychoanalysis. His effort was never to overturn existing theory but rather to achieve a fuller understanding of the clinical roots of psychoanalytic concepts and the technical problems that arise in the course of any analysis. He has played a key role in making bridges to feminist studies and critiques of psychoanalysis, as well as to the humanities and historical and philosophical studies. More recently, he has been instrumental in the evolution of Kleinian thought into a portion of the mainstream of American psychoanalytic thinking.

WHY I CHOSE THIS PAPER

Roy Schafer, Ph.D.

I chose "Narration in the Psychoanalytic Dialogue" for inclusion in this volume because it marked a special turning point—not the only such point, but one that fully opened up and legitimized the possibility of telling about psychoanalysis in America in a variety of systemic and thorough ways. It has also helped build a bridge to the humanities and historical studies that, as I see it, hadn't yet been near completion, "applied analysis" not being a two-way bridge to my mind. To say more would require a full essay—not appropriate here.

NARRATION IN THE PSYCHOANALYTIC DIALOGUE

Psychoanalytic Theories as Narratives

ROY SCHAFER, PH.D.

FREUD ESTABLISHED A TRADITION within which psychoanalysis is understood as an essentialist and positivist natural science. One need not be bound by this scientific commitment, however; the individual and general accounts and interpretations Freud gave of his case material can be read in another way. In this reading, psychoanalysis is an interpretive discipline whose practitioners aim to develop a particular kind of systematic account of human action. We can say, then, either that Freud was developing a set of principles for participating in, understanding, and explaining the dialogue between psychoanalyst and analysand or that he was establishing a set of codes to generate psychoanalytic meaning, recognizing this meaning in each instance to be only one of a number of kinds of meaning that might be generated.

Psychoanalytic theorists of different persuasions have employed different interpretive principles or codes—one might say different narrative structures—to develop their ways of doing analysis and telling about it. These narrative structures present or imply two coordinated accounts: one, of the beginning, the course, and the ending of human development; the other, of the course of the psychoanalytic dialogue. Far from being secondary narratives about data, these structures provide primary narratives that establish what is to count as data. Once in-

---

"Narration in the Psychoanalytic Dialogue: Psychoanalytic Theories as Narratives," by Roy Schafer, Ph.D., was first published in *Critical Inquiry,* 7(1):29–53, 1980.

stalled as leading narrative structures, they are taken as certain in order to develop coherent accounts of lives and technical practices.

It makes sense, and it may be a useful project, to present psychoanalysis in narrational terms. In order to carry through this project, one must, first of all, accept the proposition that there are no objective, autonomous, or pure psychoanalytic data which, as Freud was fond of saying, compel one to draw certain conclusions. Specifically, there is no single, necessary, definitive account of a life history and psychopathology, of biological and social influences on personality, or of the psychoanalytic method and its results. What have been presented as the plain empirical data and techniques of psychoanalysis are inseparable from the investigator's precritical and interrelated assumptions concerning the origins, coherence, totality, and intelligibility of personal action. The data and techniques exist as such by virtue of two sets of practices that embody these assumptions; first, a set of *practices of naming and interrelating* that is systematic insofar as it conforms to the initial assumptions; and second, a set of *technical practices* that is systematic insofar as it elicits and shapes phenomena that can be ordered in terms of these assumptions. No version of psychoanalysis has ever come close to being codified to this extent. The approach to such codification requires that the data of psychoanalysis be unfailingly regarded as constituted rather than simply encountered. The sharp split between subject and object must be systematically rejected.

In his formal theorizing, Freud used two primary narrative structures, and he often urged that they be taken as provisional rather than as final truths. But Freud was not always consistent in this regard, sometimes presenting dogmatically on one page what he had presented tentatively on another. One of his primary narrative structures begins with the infant and young child as a beast, otherwise known as the id, and ends with the beast domesticated, tamed by frustration in the course of development in a civilization hostile to its nature. Even though this taming leaves each person with two regulatory structures, the ego and the superego, the protagonist remains in part a beast, the carrier of the indestructible id. The filling in of this narrative structure tells of a lifelong transition. If the innate potential for symbolization is there, and if all goes well, one moves from a condition of frightened and irrational helplessness, lack of self-definition, and domination by fluid or mobile instinctual drives toward a condition of stability, mastery, adaptability, self-definition, rationality, and security. If all does not go well, the inadequately tamed beast must be accommodated by the formation of pathological structures, such as symptoms and perversions.

Freud did not invent this beast, and the admixture of Darwinism in his account only gave it the appearance of having been established in a positivist scientific manner. The basic story is ancient; it has been told in many ways over the centuries, and it pervades what we consider refined common sense.

Refined common sense structures the history of human thought about human action. It takes into account the emotional, wishful, fantasy-ridden features of action, its adaptive and utilitarian aspects, and the influence on it of the subject's early experiencing of intimate formative relationships and of the world at large. The repositories of common sense include mythology, folk wisdom, colloquial sayings, jokes, and literature, among other cultural products, and, as Freud showed repeatedly, there are relatively few significant psychoanalytic propositions that are not stated or implied by these products (Schafer 1977). Refined common sense serves as the source of the precritical assumptions from which the psychoanalytic narrative structures are derived, and these structures dictate conceptual and technical practices.

But common sense is not fixed. The common sense presented in proverbs and maxims, for example, is replete with internal tension and ambiguity. Most generalizations have countergeneralizations (A penny saved is a penny earned, but one may be penny wise and pound foolish; one should look before one leaps, but he who hesitates is lost; and so on). And just as common sense may be used to reaffirm traditional orientations and conservative values (Rome wasn't built in a day), it may also be used to sanction a challenge to tradition (A new broom sweeps clean) or endorse an ironic stance (The more things change, the more they remain the same). Since generalizations of this sort allow much latitude in their application, recourse to the authority of common sense is an endless source of controversy over accounts of human action. Still, common sense is our storehouse of narrative structures, and it remains the source of intelligibility and certainty in human affairs. Controversy itself would make no sense unless the conventions of common sense were being observed by those engaged in controversy.

For Freud, the old story of the beast was indispensable, and he used it well. His tale of human development, suffering, defeat, and triumph was extraordinarily illuminating in its psychological content, scientifically respectable in its conceptualization and formalization, dramatically gripping in its metaphorical elaboration, and beneficial in his work with his analysands. Because this archetypal story has been mythologically enshrined in the metaphoric language that all of us have learned to think and live by, it is more than appealing to have it authorized and apparently confirmed by psychological science. At the same time, however, it is threatening to be told persuasively how much it is the beast that pervades, empowers, or at least necessitates our most civilized achievements. Except when moralizing about others, human beings do not wish to think consciously of having bestial origins, continuities, and destinies, and so they develop defenses and allow themselves to think only of certain aspects of their "natures." Through his uncompromising effort to establish a systematic psychoanalytic narrative in these terms, Freud exposed this paradoxical attitude toward his fateful story of human lives.

Freud's other primary narrative structure is based on Newtonian physics as transmitted through the physiological and neuroanatomical laboratories of the nineteenth century. This account presents psychoanalysis as the study of the mind viewed as a machine—in Freud's words, as a mental apparatus. This machine is characterized by inertia; it does not work unless it is moved by force. It works as a closed system; that is, its amount of energy is fixed, with the result that storing or expending energy in one respect decreases the energy available for other operations. Thus on purely quantitative grounds, love of others limits what is available for self-love, and love of the opposite sex limits what is available for love of the same sex. The machine has mechanisms, such as the automatically operating mechanisms of defense and various other checks and balances.

In the beginning, the forces that move the machine are primarily the brute organism's instinctual drives. Here the tale of the mental apparatus borrows from the tale of the brute organism and consequently becomes narratively incoherent: the mechanical mind is now said to behave like a creature with a soul—seeking, reacting, and developing. The tale continues with increasing incoherence.

To sketch this increasing incoherence: in the beginning, the mental apparatus is primitive owing to its lack of structure and differentiated function. Over the course of time, the apparatus develops itself in response to experience and along lines laid down by its inherent nature; it becomes complex, moving on toward an ending in which, through that part of it called the ego, it can set its own aims and take over and desexualize or neutralize energies from the id. At the same time, the ego takes account of the requirements of the id, the superego, external reality, and its own internal structural problems, and it works out compromises and syntheses of remarkable complexity. When nothing untoward happens during this development, the machine functions stably and efficiently; otherwise, it is a defective apparatus, most likely weak in its ego, superego, or both. A defective apparatus cannot perform some of the functions for which it is intended, and it performs some others unreliably, inefficiently, and maladaptively, using up or wastefully discharging precious psychic energy in the process. Its effective operation depends on its mechanisms' success in restricting the influence of the archaic heritage of infancy. This machine is dedicated to preserving its own structure; it guarantees its own continuity by serving as a bulwark against primal chaos, and changes itself only under dire necessity. This mechanistic account accords well with the ideology of the Industrial Revolution. We still tend to view the body in general and the nervous system in particular as marvelous machines, and traditional metapsychologists still ask us to view the mind in the same way.

Both of Freud's primary narrative structures assume the thoroughgoing determinism of evolutionary necessity and of Newtonian forces. No room is left for freedom and responsibility. Those actions that appear to be free and responsible must be worked into the deterministic narrative of the beast, the machine, or the incoherent mingling of the two. Freedom is a myth of conscious thought.

Freud insisted on these two narrative structures as the core of what he called his metapsychology, and he regarded them as indispensable. But, as I said at the outset, Freud can be read in other ways. One can construct a Freud who is a humanistic existentialist, a man of tragic and ironic vision (Schafer 1970), and one can construct a Freud who is an investigator laying the foundation for a conception of psychoanalysis as an interpretative study of human action (Schafer 1976, 1978). Although we can derive these alternative readings from statements made explicitly by Freud when, as a man and a clinician, he took distance from his official account, we do not require their authority to execute this project; and these alternative readings are not discredited by quotations from Freud to the opposite effect.

That Freud's beast and machine are indeed narrative structures and are not dictated by the data is shown by the fact that other psychoanalysts have developed their own accounts, each with a more or less different beginning, course, and ending. Melanie Klein, for example, gives an account of the child or adult as being in some stage of recovery from a rageful infantile psychosis at the breast (Klein 1948; Segal 1964). Her story starts with a universal yet pathological infantile condition that oscillates between paranoid and melancholic positions. For her, our lives begin in madness, which includes taking in the madness of others, and we continue to be more or less mad though we may be helped by fortuitous circumstances or by analysis. Certain segments of common speech, for example, the metaphors of the witch, the poisonous attitude, and the people who get under your skin or suck out your guts, or the common recognition that we can all be "crazy" under certain circumstances, all support this account that emphasizes unconscious infantile fantasies of persecution, possession, and devastation.

To bypass many other more or less useful narratives that over the years have been proposed in the name of psychoanalysis, we currently have one developed by Heinz Kohut (1971, 1977). Kohut tells of a child driven in almost instinctlike fashion to actualize a cohesive self. The child is more or less hampered or damaged in the process by the empathic failures of caretakers in its intimate environment. Its growth efforts are consequently impeded by reactive and consoling grandiose fantasies, defensive splitting and repression, and affective "disintegration products" that experientially seem to act like Freud's drives or else to take the form of depressive, hypochondriacal, perverse, or addictive symptoms. In truth, however, these pathological signs are, according to Kohut, bits and pieces of the shattered self striving to protect itself, heal itself, and continue its growth. The ending in Kohut's story is for each person a point on a continuum that ranges from a frail, rageful, and poverty-stricken self to one that is healthy, happy, and wise.

For the most part, Kohut remained aware that he was developing a narrative structure. He went so far as to invoke a principle of complementarity, arguing that psychoanalysis needs and can tolerate a second story, namely, Freud's traditional tripartite psychic structure (id, ego, superego). On Kohut's account, this narrative of psychic structure is needed in order to give an adequate account of phases of development subsequent to the achievement, in the early years of life, of a cohesive self or a healthy narcissism. This recourse to an analogy with the complementarity theory of physics fails to dispel the impression one may gain of narrative incoherence. The problem is, however, not fatal: I am inclined to think that complementarity will be dropped from Kohut's account once it becomes clear how to develop the tale of the embattled self into a comprehensive and continuous narrative—or once it becomes professionally acceptable to do so (see also Schafer 1980a).

NARRATION IN THE PSYCHOANALYTIC DIALOGUE

We are forever telling stories about ourselves. In telling these self-stories *to others* we may, for most purposes, be said to be performing straightforward narrative actions. In saying that we also tell them *to ourselves*, however, we are enclosing one story within another. This is the story that there is a self to tell something to, a someone else serving as audience who is oneself or one's self. When the stories we tell others about ourselves concern these other selves of ours, when we say, for example,

"I am not master of myself," we are again enclosing one story within another. On this view, the self is a telling. From time to time and from person to person, this telling varies in the degree to which it is unified, stable, and acceptable to informed observers as reliable and valid.

Additionally, we are forever telling stories about others. These others, too, may be viewed as figures or other selves constituted by narrative actions. Other people are constructed in the telling about them; more exactly, we narrate others just as we narrate selves. The other person, like the self, is not something one has or encounters as such but an existence one tells. Consequently, telling "others" about "ourselves" is doubly narrative.

Often the stories we tell about ourselves are life historical or autobiographical; we locate them in the past. For example, one might say, "Until I was 15, I was proud of my father" or "I had a totally miserable childhood." These histories are present tellings. The same may be said of the histories we attribute to others. We change many aspects of these histories of self and others as we change, for better or worse, the implied or stated questions to which they are the answers. Personal development may be characterized as change in the questions it is urgent or essential to answer. As a project in personal development, personal analysis changes the leading questions that one addresses to the tale of one's life and the lives of important others.

People going through psychoanalysis—analysands—tell the analyst about themselves and others in the past and present. In making interpretations, the analyst retells these stories. In the retelling, certain features are accentuated while others are placed in parentheses; certain features are related to others in new ways or for the first time; some features are developed further, perhaps at great length. This retelling is done along psychoanalytic lines. What constitutes a specifically psychoanalytic retelling is a topic I shall take up later.

The analyst's retellings progressively influence the what and how of the stories told by analysands. The analyst establishes new, though often contested or resisted, questions that amount to regulated narrative possibilities. The end product of this interweaving of texts is a radically new, jointly authored work or way of working. One might say that in the course of analysis, there develops a cluster of more or less coordinated new narrations, each corresponding to periods of intensive analytic work on certain leading questions. Generally, these narrations focus neither on the past, plain and simple, nor on events currently taking place outside the psychoanalytic situation. They focus much more on the place and modification of these tales within the psychoanalytic dialogue. Specifically, the narrations are considered under the aspect of transference and resisting as these are identified and analyzed at different times in relation to different questions. The psychoanalytic dialogue is characterized most of all by its organization in terms of the here and now of the psychoanalytic relationship. It is fundamentally a dialogue concerning the present moment of transference and resisting.

But transference and resisting themselves may be viewed as narrative structures. Like all other narrative structures, they prescribe a point of view from which to tell about the events of analysis in a regulated and therefore coherent fashion. The events themselves are constituted only through one or another systematic account of them. Moreover, the analysis of resisting may be told in terms of transference and vice versa.

In the traditional transference narration, one tells how the analysand is repetitively reliving or reexperiencing the past in the present relationship with the analyst. It is said that there occurs a regression within the transference to the infantile neurosis or neurotic matrix, which then lies exposed to the analyst's view. This is, however, a poor account. It tells of life history as static, archival, linear, reversible, and literally retrievable. Epistemologically, this story is highly problematic. Another and, I suggest, better account tells of change of action along certain lines; it emphasizes new experiencing and new remembering of the past that unconsciously has never become the past. More and more, the alleged past must be experienced consciously as a mutual interpenetration of the past and present, both being viewed in psychoanalytically organized and coordinated terms. If analysis is a matter of moving in a direction, it is a moving forward into new modes of constructing experience. On this account, one must retell the story of regression to the infantile neurosis within the transference; for even though much of its matter may be defined in terms of the present version of the past, the so-called regression is necessarily a progression. Transference, far from being a time machine by which one may travel back to see what one has been made out of, is a clarification of certain constituents of one's present psychoanalytic actions. This clarification is achieved through the circular and coordinated study of past and present.

The technical and experiential construction of personal analyses in the terms of transference and resisting has been found to be therapeutically useful. But now it must be added that viewing psychoanalysis as a therapy itself manifests a narrative choice. This choice dictates that the story of the dialogue and the events to which it gives rise be told in terms of a doctor's curing a patient's disease. From the inception of psychoanalysis, professional and ideological factors have favored this kind of account, though there are some signs today that the sickness narrative is on its way to becoming obsolete. Here I want only to emphasize that there are a number of other ways to tell what the two people in the analytic situation are doing. Each of these ways either cultivates and accentuates or neglects and minimizes certain potential features of the analysis; none is exact and comprehensive in every way. For example, psychoanalysis as therapy tells the story from the standpoint of consciousness: consciously, but only consciously, the analysand presents his or her problems as alien interferences with the good life, that is, as symptoms in the making of which he or she has had no hand; or the analyst defines as symptomatic the problems the analyst consciously wishes to emphasize; or both. In many cases, this narrative facilitates undertaking the analysis; at the same time, a price is paid, at least for some time, by this initial and perhaps unavoidable collusion to justify analysis on these highly defensive and conscious grounds of patienthood.

My own attempt to remain noncommittal in this respect by speaking of analyst and analysand rather than therapist and patient is itself inexact in at least three ways. First, it does not take into account the analyst's also being subject to analysis through his or her necessarily continuous scrutiny of countertransferences. Second, during the analysis, the analysand's self is retold as constituted by a large, fragmented, and fluid cast of characters. Not only are aspects of the self seen to incorporate aspects of others, they are also unconsciously imagined as having retained some or all of the essence of these others; that is, the self-constituents are experienced as introjects or incomplete identifications, indeed sometimes as shadowy presences of indeterminate location and origin (Schafer 1968, Chapters 4 and 5). The problematic and incoherent self that is consciously told at the beginning of the analysis is sorted out, so far as possible, into that which has retained otherness to a high degree and that which has not. A similar sorting out of the constituents of others' selves is also accomplished; here the concept of projecting aspects of the self into others plays an important role. The upshot is that what the analysand initially tells as self and others undergoes considerable revision once the initial consciously constructed account has been worked over analytically. A third inexactness in my choice of terminology is that the division into analyst and analysand does not provide for the increasing extent to which the analysand becomes coanalyst of his or her own problems and, in certain respects, those of the analyst, too. The analysand, that is, becomes coauthor of the analysis as he or she becomes a more daring and reliable narrator. Here I touch on yet another topic to take up later, that of the unreliable narrator: this topic takes in analyst as well as analysand, for ideally both of them do change during analysis, if to different degrees, and it leads into questions of how, in the post-positivist scheme of things, we are to understand validity in analytic interpretation.

If we are forever telling stories about ourselves and others and to ourselves and others, it must be added that people do more than tell: like authors, they also show. As there is no hard-and-fast-line between telling and showing, either in literary narrative or in psychoanalysis, the competent psychoanalyst deals with telling as a form of showing and with showing as a form of telling. Everything in analysis is both communication and demonstration (cf. Booth 1961).

Perhaps the simplest instances of analytic showing are those nonverbal behaviors or expressive movements that include bodily rigidity, lateness to or absence from scheduled sessions, and mumbling. The analyst, using whatever he or she already knows or has prepared the way for, interprets these showings and weaves them into one of the narrations of the analysis: for example, "Your lying stiffly on the couch shows that you're identifying yourself with your dead father"; or, "Your mumbling shows how afraid you are to be heard as an independent voice on this subject." Beyond comments of this sort, however, the analyst takes these showings as communications and on this basis may say (and here I expand these improvised interpretations), "You are conveying that you feel like a corpse in relation to me, putting your life into me and playing your dead father in relation to me; you picture me now as yourself confronted by this corpse, impressing on me that I am to feel your grief for you." Or the analyst might say, "By your mumbling you are letting me know how frightened you are to assert your own views to me just in case I might feel as threatened by such presumption as your mother once felt and might retaliate as she did by being scornful and turning her back on you." In these interpretive retellings, the analyst is no longer controlled by the imaginary line between telling and showing.

Acting out as a form of remembering is a good case in point (Freud 1914). For example, by anxiously engaging in an affair with an older married man, a young woman in analysis is said to be remembering, through acting out, an infantile oedipal wish to seduce or be sexually loved and impregnated by her father, now represented by the analyst. In one way, this acting out is showing; in another way, it is telling by a displaced showing. Once it has been retold as remembering through acting out, it may serve as a narrative context that facilitates further direct remembering and further understanding of the analytic relationship.

The competent analyst is not lulled by the dramatic rendition of life historical content into hearing this content in a simple, contextless, time-bound manner. Situated in the present, the analyst takes the telling also as a showing, noting, for example, when that content is introduced, for it might be a way of forestalling the emotional experiencing of the immediate transference relationship; noting also how that content is being told, for it might be told flatly, histrionically, in a masochistically self-pitying or a grandiosely triumphant way; noting further the storyline that is being followed and many other narrative features as well. The analyst also attends to cues that the analysand, consciously or unconsciously, may be an unreliable narrator, highlighting the persecutory actions of others and minimizing the analysand's seduction of the persecutor to persecute; slanting the story in order to block out significant periods in his or her life history or to elicit pity or admiration; glossing over, by silence and euphemism, what the analysand fears will cast him or her in an unfavorable light or sometimes in too favorable a light, as when termination of analysis is in the air, and, out of a sense of danger, one feels compelled to tell and show that one is still "a sick patient." All of which is to say that the analyst takes the telling as performance as well as content. The analyst has only tellings and showings to interpret, that is, to retell along psychoanalytic lines.

What does it mean to say "along psychoanalytic lines"? Earlier I mentioned that more than one kind of psychoanalysis is practiced in this world, and so I will just summarize what conforms to my own practice, namely, the storylines that characterize Freudian retellings. The analyst slowly and patiently develops an emphasis on infantile or archaic modes of sexual and aggressive action (action being understood broadly to take in wishing, believing, perceiving, remembering, fantasizing, behaving emotionally, and other such activities that, in traditional theories of action, have been split off from motor action and discussed separately as thought, motivation, and feeling). The analyst wants to study and redescribe all of these activities from the standpoint of such questions as "What is the analysand doing?" "Why now?" "Why in this way?" and "What does this have to do with me and what the analysand fears might develop between us sexually and aggressively?"

Repeatedly the analysand's stories (experiences, memories, symptoms, selves) go through a series of transformations until finally they can be retold not only as sexual and aggressive modes of action but also as defensive measures adopted (within modes of response commonly called anxiety, guilt, shame, and depression) to disguise, displace, deemphasize, compromise, and otherwise refrain from boldly and openly taking the actions in question. The analyst uses multiple points of view (wishful, defensive, moral, ideal, and adaptive) and expects that significant features of the analysand's life can be understood only after employing all of these points of view in working out contextual redescriptions or interpretations of actions. Single constituents are likely to require a complex definition; for example, sexual and aggressive wishing are often simultaneously ascribable to one and the same personal problem or symptom along with moral condemnation of "self" on both grounds.

The Freudian analyst also progressively organizes this retelling around bodily zones, modes, and substances, particularly the mouth, anus, and genitalia; and in conjunction with these zones, the modes of swallowing and spitting out, retaining and expelling, intruding and enclosing, and the concrete conceptions of words, feelings, ideas, and events as food, feces, urine, semen, babies, and so on. All of these constituents are given roles in the infantile drama of family life, a drama that is organized around births, losses, illnesses, abuse and neglect, the parents' real and imagined conflicts and sexuality, gender differences, sibling relations, and so on. It is essential that the infantile drama, thus conceived, be shown to be repetitively introduced by the analysand into the analytic dialogue, however subtly this has been done, and this is what is accomplished in the interpretive retelling of transference and resisting.

DRIVES, FREE ASSOCIATION, RESISTANCE, AND REALITY TESTING

To illustrate and further develop my thesis on narration in the psychoanalytic dialogue, I shall next take up four concepts that are used repeatedly in narrations concerning this dialogue: drives, free association, resistance, and reality testing.

Drives

Drives appear to be incontrovertible facts of human nature. Even the most casual introspection delivers up a picture of the passive self being driven by internal forces. It might therefore seem perfectly justified to distinguish being driven from wishing, in that wishing seems clearly to be a case of personal action. The distinction is, however, untenable. It takes conscious and conventional testimony of drivenness as the last or natural word on the subject; but to take it that way is to ignore the proposition that introspection is itself a form of constructed experience based on a specific narration of mind.

The introspection narrative tells that each person is a container of experience fashioned by an independently operating mind, and that by the use of mental eyes located outside this container, the person may look in and see what is going on (cf. Ryle 1943). The introspection narrative has been extensively elaborated through a spatial rendering of mental activity, perhaps most of all through the language of internalization and externalization. This spatial language includes: inner world, inwardly, internalize, projection, deep down, levels, layers, and the like (Schafer 1972). Thus the introspector stands outside his or her mind, thinking—with what? A second mind? We have no unassailable answer. The introspection narrative tells us that far from constructing or creating out lives, we witness them. It thereby sets drastic limits on discourse about human activity and responsibility. The uncritical and pervasive use of this narrative form in daily life and in psychological theories shows how appealing it is to disclaim responsibility in this way.

The drive narrative depends on this introspection narrative and so is appealing in the same way. It appeals in other ways as well. As I mentioned earlier, the drive narrative tells the partly moralistic and partly Darwinian-scientific tale that at heart we are all animals, and it sets definite guidelines for all the tales we tell about ourselves and others. By following these guidelines, we fulfill two very important functions, albeit often painfully and irrationally. We simultaneously derogate ourselves (which we do for all kinds of reasons), and we disclaim responsibility for our actions. Because these functions are being served, many people find it difficult to accept the proposition that drive is a narrative structure, that is, an optional way of telling the story of human lives.

Consider, for example, a man regarding a woman lustfully. One might say, "He wishes more than anything else to take her to bed"; or one might say, "His sexual drive is overwhelming and she is its object." The wishing narrative does not preclude the recognition that physiological processes may be correlated with such urgent wishing, though it also leaves room for the fact that this correlation does not always hold. In case the physiological correlates are present, the wishing narrative also provides for the man's noticing these stimuli in the first place, for his having to give meaning to them, for his selecting just that woman, and for his organizing the situation in terms of heterosexual intercourse specifically. From our present point of view, the chief point to emphasize is that the wishing narrative allows one to raise the question, in analytic work as in everyday life, why the subject tells himself that he is passive in relation to a drive rather than that he is a sexual agent, someone who lusts after a specific woman.

A similar case for wishful action may be made in the case of aggression. In one version or theory, aggression is a drive that requires discharge in rages, assaults, vituperation, or something of that sort. In another version, aggression is an activity or mode of action that is given many forms by agents who variously wish to attack, destroy, hurt, or assert and in each case to do so for reasons and in contexts that may be ascertained by an observer. The observer may, of course, be the agent himself or herself.

In the course of analysis, the analysand comes to construct narratives of personal agency ever more readily, independently, convincingly, and securely, particularly in those contexts that have to do with crucially maladaptive experiences of drivenness. The important questions to be answered in the analysis concern personal agency, and the important answers reallocate the attributions of activity and passivity. Passivity also comes into question because, as in the case of unconscious infantile guilt reactions (so-called superego guilt), agency may be ascribed to the self irrationally (for example, blame of the "self" for the accidental death of a parent).

Free Association

The fundamental rule of psychoanalysis is conveyed through the instruction to associate freely and to hold back nothing that comes to mind. This conception is controlled by the previously mentioned narrative of the introspected mind. One is to tell about thinking and feeling in passive terms; it is to be a tale of the mind's running itself, of thoughts and feelings coming and going, of thoughts and feelings pushed forward by drives or by forces or structures opposing them. Again, the analysand is to be witness to his or her own mind. The psychoanalytic models for this narration are Freud's "mental apparatus" and "brute organism."

If, however, one chooses the narrative option of the analysand as agent, that is, as thinker and constructor of emotional action, the fundamental rule will be understood differently and in a way that accords much better with the analyst's subsequent interpretive activity. According to this second narrative structure, the instruction establishes the following guidelines: "Let's see what you will do if you just tell me everything you think and feel without my giving you any starting point, any direction or plan, any criteria of selection, coherence, or decorum. You are to continue in this way with no formal beginning, no formal middle or development, and no formal ending except as you introduce these narrative devices. And let's see what sense we can make of what you do under these conditions. That is to say, let's see how we can retell it in a way that allows you to understand the origins, meanings, and significance of your present difficulties and to do so in a way that makes change conceivable and attainable."

Once the analysand starts the telling, the analyst listens and interprets in two interrelated ways. First, the analyst retells what is told from the standpoint of its content, that is, its thematic coherence. For example, the analysand may be alluding repeatedly to envious attitudes while consciously portraying these attitudes as disinterested, objective criticism. By introducing the theme of envy, the analyst, from the special point of view on analytic narration, identifies the kind of narrative that is being developed. (Of course, one does not have to be an analyst to recognize envy in disguise; but this only illustrates my point that analytic narration is not sharply set off from refined common sense.) The specific content then becomes merely illustrative of an unrecognized and probably disavowed set of attitudes that are held by the analysand, who is shown to be an unreliable narrator in respect to the consciously constructed account. Ultimately, the unreliability itself must be interpreted and woven into the dialogue as an aspect of resisting.

The analysand's narrative, then, is placed in a larger context, its coherence and significance are increased, and its utility for the analytic work is defined. The analyst has not listened in the ordinary way. Serving as an *analytic* reteller, he or she does not, indeed, cannot coherently, respond in the ordinary way. Listening in the ordinary way, as in countertransference, results in analytic incoherence; then the analyst's retellings themselves become unreliable and fashioned too much after the analyst's own "life story."

In the second mode of listening and interpreting, the analyst focuses on the action of telling itself. Telling is treated as an object of description rather than, as the analysand wishes, an indifferent or transparent medium for imparting information or thematic content. The analyst has something to say about the how, when, and why of the telling. For example, the analyst may tell that the analysand has been circling around a disturbing feeling of alienation from the analyst, the narration's circumstantial nature being intended to guarantee an interpersonally remote, emotionally arid session; and if it is envy that is in question, the analyst may tell that the analysand is trying to spoil the analyst's envied competence by presenting an opaque account of the matter at hand.

In this way, the analyst defines the complex rules that the analysand is following in seeming to "free associate" (Schafer 1978, lecture 2). There are rules of various kinds for alienated discourse, for envious discourse, and so on, some very general and well known to common sense and some very specialized or individual and requiring careful definition in the individual case, but which must still, ultimately, be in accord with common sense. The analyst treats free association as neither free nor associative, for within the strategy of analyzing narrative actions, it is not an unregulated or passive performance.

The analysand consciously experiences many phenomena in the passive mode: unexpected intrusions or unexpected trains of thought, irrelevant or shameful feelings, incoherent changes of subject, blocking and helpless withholdings of thoughts, and imperative revisions of raw content. The analysand consciously regards all of these as unintentional violations of the rules he or she consciously professes to be following or wishes to believe are being followed. But what is to the analysand flawed or helpless performance is not that to the analyst. In analysis, free associating is a no-fault activity. What is consciously unexpected or incomprehensible is seen rather as the analysand's having unconsciously introduced more complex rules to govern the narrative being developed: the analysand may have become uneasy with what is portrayed as the drift of thought and sensed that he or she was heading into danger, or perhaps the tale now being insistently foregrounded is a useful diversion from another and more troubling tale. In the interest of being "a good patient," the analysand may even insist on developing narratives in primitive terms, for instance, in terms of ruthless revenge or infantile sexual practices, when at that moment a more subjectively distressing but analytically useful account of the actions in question would have to be given in terms of assertiveness, or fun-lovingness, or ordinary sentimentality. Whatever the case may be, a new account is called for, a more complex account, one in which the analysand is portrayed as more or less unconsciously taking several parts at once—hero, victim, dodger, and stranger. These parts are not best understood as autonomous subselves having their say ("multiple selves" is itself only a narrative structure that begs the question); rather, each of these parts is one of the regulative narrative structures that one person, the analysand, has adopted and used simultaneously with the other, whether in combination, opposition, or apparent incoherence. The analyst says, in effect, "What I hear you saying is…" or "In other words, it's a matter of…," and this is to say that a narrative is now being retold along analytic lines as *the only narrative it makes good enough sense to construct at that time.*

Resistance

Resistance can be retold so as to make it appear in an altogether different light; furthermore, it can be retold in more than one way. Before I show how this is so, I should synopsize Freud's account of resistance (see, for example, Freud 1912). For Freud, "*the* resistance," as he called it, is an autonomous force analogous to the censorship in the psychology of dreams. The term refers to the many forms taken by the analysand's opposition to the analyst. The resistance, Freud said, accompanies the analysis every step of the way, and technically nothing is more important than to ferret it out and analyze it. The resistance is often sly, hidden, secretive, obdurate, and so on. In the terms of Freud's theory of psychic structure, there is a split in the analysand's ego; the rational ego wants to go forward while the defensive ego wants to preserve the irrational status quo. The analysand's ego fears change toward health through self-understanding, viewing that course as too dangerous or too mortifying to bear. These accounts of resistance establish narrative structures of several pairs of antagonists in the analytic situation: one part of the ego against another, the ego against the id, the analysand against the analyst, and the analyst against the resistance. The conflict centers on noncompliance with the fundamental rule of free association, a rule that in every case can be observed by the analysand only in a highly irregular and incomplete fashion. Presenting the resistance as a force in the mind, much like a drive, further defines the form of the analytic narration. Resistance is presented as animistic or anthropomorphic, a motivated natural force that the subject experiences passively.

How does the story of resistance get to be retold during an analysis? In one retelling, resistance transforms into an account of transference, both positive and negative. Positive transference is resistance attempting to transform the analysis into some repetitive version of a conflictual infantile love relationship on the basis of which one may legitimately abandon the procedures and goals of analysis itself. In the case of negative transference, the analyst is, for example, seen irrationally and often unconsciously as an authoritarian parent to be defied. Through a series of transformations, and with reference to various clues produced by the analysand, the opposition is retold by the analyst as an enactment of the oral, anal, and phallic struggles of infancy and childhood, that is, as a refusal to be fed or weaned or else as a biting; or as a refusal to defecate in the right place and at the right time, resorting instead to constipated withholding or diarrheic expelling of associations, feelings, and memories; or as furtive masturbation, primal scene voyeurism and exhibitionism, defensive or seductive changes of the self's gender, and so on. Thus the distinction between the analysis of resistance and the analysis of transference, far from being the empirical matter it is usually said to be, is a matter of narrative choice. Told in terms of transference, resistance becomes disclaimed repetitive activity rather than passive experience. And it is as activity that it takes its most intelligible, coherent, and modifiable place in the developing life-historical contexts. Resis*tance* becomes resist*ing*.

There is another, entirely affirmative way to retell the story of resistance. In this account, the analysand is portrayed as doing something on his or her behalf, something that makes sense unconsciously though it may not yet be understood empathically by the analyst. The analyst may then press confrontations and interpretations on the analysand at the wrong time, in the wrong way, and with the wrong content. Kohut's account of narcissistic rage in response to such interventions presents the analysand as protecting a fragile self against further disintegration in response to the analyst's empathically deficient interventions. Or the analysand may be protecting the analyst against his or her own anticipated ruthless, destructive, or at least permanently alienating form of love. Matters of personal pride and honor may be involved. In one instance, the analysand's resisting was understood as a form of self-abortion and in another instance as a refusal to be forced into what was taken to be a phallic role.

Whatever the case and whatever the manifestly oppositional attitude, the analysand is portrayed as engaged in a project of preservation, even enhancement, of self or analyst or both. The project is one that the analysand at that moment rightly refuses to abandon despite what may be the misguided efforts of the analyst to narrate the analysis along other lines. In this affirmative narration of resisting, the analyst may be an uncomprehending brute or an unwitting saboteur. One young woman's spontaneously defiant insistence on persistently excoriating her parents had to be retold analytically in two main ways: as a turning away from the unbearable horror of her imagined inner world and as a firm assertion on her part that the problem resided in the family as a system and not merely in her infantile fantasies and wishes. On the one hand, there was a crucial strategy of self-prevention implied in her apparent resisting: as she said at one point, "If I let myself appreciate myself and see what, against all odds, I've become, it would break my heart." On the other hand, there was the analysand's search for the self-affirming truth of parental madness. To have thought of her strident analytic activity simply as resisting would have been to start telling the wrong kind of psychoanalytic story about it.

A third way to retell the story of resisting radically questions the analysand's use of ability and inability words. It is developed along the following lines. "Resistance" seems to go against the analysand's wishes and resolutions. The analysand pleads inability: for example, "Something stops me from coming out with it," or "My inhibitions are too strong for me to make the first move," or "I can't associate anything with that dream." The narrative structure of inability in such respects is culturally so well established that it seems to be merely an objective expression of the natural order of things. Yet it may be counted as another aspect of the analysand as unconsciously unreliable narrator. In the first example (not coming out with it), the retelling might be developed along these lines: "You *don't* come out with it, and you *don't* yet understand why you *don't* act on your resolution to do so." In the third example (inability to associate), it might be developed like this: "You *don't* think of anything that seems to you to be relevant or acceptable, anything that meets your rules of coherence, good sense, or good manners, and you dismiss what you *do* think of."

In giving these examples, I am not presenting actual or recommended analytic interventions so much as I am making their logic plain. In practice, these interventions are typically developed in ways that are tactful, tentative, circuitous, and fragmentary. For a long time, perhaps, the "don't" element is only implied in order to limit the analysand's mishearing description as criticism and demand; *exhortation* has no place in the analyst's interventions. Nor am I suggesting that the analyst's initial descriptions are the decisive words on any important subject. They are only the first words on the subject in that they begin to establish the ground rules for another kind of story to be told and so of another kind of experience to construct. These are the rules of action language and the reclaiming of disclaimed action.

Choosing action as the suitable narrative language allows the analyst to begin to retell many inability narrations as disclaimings of action. In order to analyze resistance—now to be designated as resist*ing*—one must take many narrations presented by analysands in terms of *can* and *can't* and retell them in terms of *do* and *don't* and sometimes *will* and *won't*. Usually, the analysand is disclaiming the action unconsciously. That this is so does not make the disclaiming (defense, resistance) any the less an action; nor does it make what is being disclaimed any the less an action. In analytic narration, one is not governed by the ordinary conventions that link action to conscious intent.

So often, the analyst, after first hearing "I can't tell you" or "I can't think about that," goes on to establish through close and sustained consideration of free associations the reasons why the analysand does not or will not tell or think about whatever it is that is troublesome. It may be that the action in question would be humiliating, frightening, or apparently incoherent and therefore too mad to be tolerated. It may be that unconsciously the not telling or not thinking is an act of anal retention or oedipal defiance that is being presented as innocent helplessness. It may be that an important connection between two events has never before been defined, so that the analysand, lacking a suitable narrative structure, simply does not take up the two in one consciously constructed context; connections and contexts might come into existence only through the analyst's interpretive activity. Interpretation may also give the reasons why the context and connections never have been developed. In all such instances, it is no longer ability that is in question; it is the proper designation of a ruled performance.

The same narrative treatments of action and inaction are common in daily life. One hears, "I couldn't control myself," "I can't concentrate on my studies," "I can't love him," and so on. Implicit in these narrations, as in the resisting narrations, is the disclaiming of the activity in what is being told. This disclaiming is accomplished by taking recourse to the terms of uncontrollable, impersonal forces. These accounts, too, may be retold analytically. For instance, after some analysis, "I can't concentrate on my studies" may become the following (synopsized) narrative: "I don't concentrate on what I resolve to work on. I think of other things instead. I think of girls, of my dead father, of all the failures of my life. These are the things that really matter to me, and I rebel against the idea that I should set them aside and just get through the reading like a machine. It's like shitting on demand. Additionally, by not working, I don't risk experiencing either frightening grandiose feelings if I succeed or the shame of mediocrity if I just pass. On top of which, really getting into the work is sexually exciting; it feels something like sexual peeping to read, as I must, between the lines, and it feels wrong to do that." Retold in this way, "I can't concentrate on my studies" becomes "I don't concentrate for certain reasons, some or all of which I did not dare to realize before now. I told myself I was trying to concentrate and couldn't when actually I was doing other things instead and doing them for other reasons." The narrative has changed from the consciously constructed one of helplessness and failure, designed to protect the consciously distressing status quo, to a narrative of unconsciously designed activity in another kind of reality. The new story, told now by a more reliable narrator, is a story of personal action, and as such it may serve as a basis for change.

Nothing in the immediately preceding account implies that for narrative purposes, *inability* words or, for that matter, *necessity* words are narratively ruled totally out of the analytic court. Rather, these words are now found to be useful and appropriate in far more restricted sets of circumstances than before. These sets of circumstances include unusual physical and mental ability and training and also one's inevitable confrontations with the forceful independent actions of others and with impersonal events in the world. Yet even these necessities become analytically relevant only in terms of how the analysand takes them. In any case, necessity (or happening) does not include mental forces and structures that reduce a person to impotence; much impotence is enacted rather than imposed (Schafer 1978, lecture 5).

Reality Testing

Traditionally, the official psychoanalytic conception of reality has been straightforwardly positivistic. Reality is "out there" or "in there" in the inner world, existing as a knowable, certifiable essence. At least for the analytic observer, the subject and object are clearly distinct. Reality is encountered and recognized innocently. In part it simply forces itself on one, in part it is discovered or uncovered by search and reason free of theory. Consequently, reality testing amounts simply to undertaking to establish what is, on the one hand, real, true, objective and, on the other hand, unreal, false, subjective. On this understanding, one may conclude, for example, that *x* is fantasy (psychical reality) and *y* is fact (external reality); that mother was not only loving as had always been thought but also hateful; that the situation is serious but not hopeless or vice versa; and so on.

But this positivistic telling is only one way of giving or arriving at an account of the subject in the world, and it is incoherent with respect to the epistemological assumptions inherent in psychoanalytic inquiry, that is, those assumptions that limit us always to dealing only with *versions* of reality. The account I am recommending necessarily limits one to constructing some version or some vision of the subject in the world. One defines situations and invests events with multiple meanings. These meanings are more or less adequately responsive to different questions that the narrator, who may be the subject or someone else, wants to answer; they are also responsive to the rules of context that the narrator intends to follow and to the level of abstraction that he or she wishes to maintain. Sometimes, for example, an assertive action of a certain kind in a certain situation may with equal warrant be described as sadistic *and* masochistic, regressive *and* adaptive. In this account, reality is always mediated by narration. Far from being innocently encountered or discovered, it is created in a regulated fashion.

The rules regulating the creation of reality may be conventional, in which case no questions are likely to be raised about the world and how we know it; if needed, consensual validation will be readily obtained. But things can be otherwise. Once certain rules are defined, they may prove to violate convention in a way that is incoherent or at least not understandable at a given moment. In this case, the place of these rules requires further investigation and interpretation. Those rules that inform truly original ideas may necessitate revision of accepted ideas about the rules that "must" be followed and the kind of reality that it is desirable or interesting to construct. Freud showed his genius by developing his highly particularized "overdetermined" accounts of the idiosyncratic systems of rules followed in dreams, neuroses, perversions, psychoses, and normal sexual development.

One may say that *psychoanalytic interpretation tells about a second reality.* In this reality, events or phenomena are viewed from the standpoint of repetitive re-creation of infantile, family-centered situations bearing on sex, aggression, and other such matters. Only superficially does the analytic construction of this second reality seem to be crudely reductive; it is crudely reductive only when it is performed presumptuously or stupidly, as when the analyst says, "This is what you are *really* doing." The competent analyst says in effect, "Let me show you over the course of the analysis another reality, commonsensical elements of which are already, though incoherently and eclectically, included in what you now call reality. We shall be looking at you and others in your life, past and present, in a special light, and we shall come to understand our analytic project and our relationship in this light, too. This second reality is as real as any other. In many ways it is more coherent and inclusive and more open to your activity than the reality you now vouch for and try to make do with. On this basis, it also makes the possibility of change clearer and more or less realizable, and so it may open for you a way out of your present difficulties."

From the acceptance of this new account, there follows a systematic project of constructing a psychoanalytic reality in which one retells the past and the present, the infantile and the adult, the imagined and the so-called real, and the analytic relationship and all other significant relationships. One retells all this in terms that are increasingly focused and coordinated in psychoanalytic terms of action. One achieves a narrative redescription of reality. This retelling is adapted to the clinical context and relationship, the purpose of which is to understand anew the life and the problems in question. The analysand joins in the retelling (redescribing, reinterpreting, recontextualizing, and reducing) as the analysis progresses. The second reality becomes a joint enterprise and a joint experience. And if anyone emerges as a crude reductionist it is the analysand, viewed now as having unconsciously reduced too many events simply to infantile sexual and aggressive narratives.

At this point we may return once more to the question of the unreliable narrator, for it bears on the large question of validity of interpretation. To speak of the unreliable narrator, one must have some conception of a reliable narrator, that is, of validity; and yet the trend of my argument suggests that there is no single definitive account to be achieved. Validity, it seems, can only be achieved within a system that is viewed as such and that appears, after careful consideration, to have the virtues of coherence, consistency, comprehensiveness, and common sense. This is the system that establishes the second reality in psychoanalysis. The analysand is helped to become a reliable narrator in this second reality which is centered on transference and resisting. A point of view is maintained and employed that both establishes a maximum of reliability and intelligibility of the kind required and confirms, hermeneutically, that achievement.

THE NORMATIVE LIFE HISTORY

Psychoanalytic researchers have always aimed to develop a normative, continuous psychoanalytic life history that begins with day one, to be used by the psychoanalyst as a guide for participating in the analytic dialogue. Freud set this pattern by laying out the psychosexual stages and defining the instinctual vicissitudes, the stage of narcissism, phase-specific orientations and conflicts (oral, anal, etc.), the origins and consolidation of the ego and superego, and other such developmental periods, problems, and achievements. Yet it is safe to say that in the main, his life histories take shape around the time of the Oedipus complex, that is, the time between the ages of 2 and 5. In his account, earlier times remain shadowy prehistory or surmised constitutional influences, not too accessible to subjective experience or verification.

Today the field of psychoanalysis is dominated by competing theories about these earlier, shadowy phases of mental development. These now include the phase of autism, symbiosis, and separation-individuation; the phase of basic trust and mistrust; the phase of pure narcissism, in which there are no objects which are not primarily part of the self; the mirror phase; and variations on the Kleinian paranoid-schizoid and depressive phases or "positions" of infancy. For the most part, these phases are defined and detailed by what are called constructions or reconstructions, that is, surmises based on memories, symbolic readings, and subjective phenomena encountered in the analysis of adults, though some direct observation of children has also been employed. These surmises concern the nature of the beginning of subjective experience and the formative impact of the environment on that experience, an impact which is estimated variously by different theorists. In all, a concerted attempt is being made to go back so far in the individual's subjective history as to eliminate its prehistory altogether.

These projects are, for the most part, conceived and presented as fact-finding. On the assumption that there is no other way to understand the present, it is considered essential to determine what in fact it was like way back when. Whatever its internal differences, this entire program is held to have heuristic as well as therapeutic value. It is not my present intention to dispute this claim. I do, however, think that from a methodological standpoint this program has been incorrectly conceived.

The claim that these normative life historical projects are simply fact-finding expeditions is, as I argued earlier, highly problematic. At the very outset, each such expedition is prepared for what is to be found: it has its maps and compasses, its conceptual supplies, and its probable destination. This preparedness (which contradicts the empiricists' pretensions of innocence) amounts to a narrative plan, form, or set of rules. The sequential life historical narration that is then developed is no more than a second-order retelling of clinical analysis. But this retelling confusingly deletes reference to the history of the analytic dialogue. It treats that dialogue as though—to change my metaphor—it is merely the shovel used to dig up history and so is of no account, except perhaps in manuals on the technique of digging up true chronologies. The theorists have therefore committed themselves to the narrative form of the case history, which is a simplified form of traditional biography.

Is there a narrative form that is methodologically more adequate to the psychoanalytic occasion? I believe there is. It is a story that begins in the middle, which is the present: the beginning is the beginning of the analysis. The present is not the autobiographical present, which at the outset comprises what are called the analysand's presenting problems or initial complaints together with some present account of the past; the reliability and usefulness of both of these constituents of the autobiographical present remain to be determined during the analysis. Once the analysis is under way, the autobiographical present is found to be no clear point in time at all. One does not even know how properly to conceive that present; more and more it seems to be both a repetitive, crisis-perpetuating misremembering of the past and a way of living defensively with respect to a future which is, in the most disruptive way, imagined fearfully and irrationally on the model of the past.

It soon becomes evident that, interpretively, one is working in a temporal circle. One works backward from what is told about the autobiographical present in order to define, refine, correct, organize, and complete an analytically coherent and useful account of the past, and one works forward from various tellings of the past to constitute that present and that anticipated future which are most important to explain. Under the provisional and dubious assumption that past, present, and future are separable, each segment of time is used to set up a series of questions about the others and to answer the questions addressed to it by the others. And all of these accounts keep changing as the analytic dialogue continues. Freud's major case studies follow this narrative form. His report on the Rat Man (1909) is a good case in point; one has only to compare his notes on the case with his official report on it to see what different tales he told and could have told about this man, that is, *about his work with this man.*

I said that the analytic life history is a second-order history. The first-order history is that of the analytic dialogue. This history is more like a set of histories that have been told from multiple perspectives over the course of the analysis and that do not actually lend themselves to one seamless retelling; I shall refer to it as one history, nevertheless, inasmuch as analysts typically present it in that way. This history is situated in the present; it is always and necessarily a present account of the meanings and uses of the dialogue to date or, in other words, of transference and resisting. The account of the origins and transformations of the life being studied is shaped, extended, and limited by what it is narratively necessary to emphasize and to assume in order to explain the turns in this dialogue. The analysand's stories of early childhood, adolescence, and other critical periods of life get to be retold in a way that both summarizes and justifies what the analyst requires in order to do the kind of psychoanalytic work that is being done.

The primary narrative problem of the analyst is, then, not how to tell a normative chronological life history; rather, it is how to tell the several histories of each analysis. From this vantage point, the event with which to start the model analytic narration is not the first occasion of thought—Freud's wish-fulfilling hallucination of the absent breast; instead, one should start from a narrative account of the psychoanalyst's retelling of something told by an analysand and the analysand's response to that narrative transformation. In the narration of this moment of dialogue lies the structure of the analytic past, present, and future. It is from this beginning that the accounts of early infantile development are constructed. Those traditional developmental accounts, over which analysts have labored so hard, may now be seen in a new light: less as positivistic sets of factual findings about mental development and more as hermeneutically filled-in narrative structures. The narrative structures that have been adopted control the telling of the events of the analysis, including the many tellings and retellings of the analysand's life history. The time is always present. The event is always an ongoing dialogue.

REFERENCES

Booth W: The Rhetoric of Fiction. Chicago, University of Chicago Press, 1961

Freud S: Notes upon a case of obsessional neurosis (1909), in The Standard Edition of the Complete Psychological Works of Sigmund Freud [SE], Vol 10. Translated and edited by Strachey J. London, Hogarth Press, 1955, pp 153–318

Freud S: The dynamics of transference (1912). SE, 12:97–108, 1958

Freud S: Remembering, repeating and working-through (further recommendations on the technique of psycho-analysis II) (1914). SE, 12:147–156, 1958

Klein M: Contributions to Psycho-Analysis 1921–1945: Developments in Child and Adult Psycho-Analysis (1948). New York, McGraw-Hill, 1964

Kohut H: The Analysis of the Self: A Systematic Approach to the Psychoanalytic Treatment of Narcissistic Personality Disorders. New York, International Universities Press, 1971

Kohut H: The Restoration of the Self. New York, International Universities Press, 1977

Ryle G: The Concept of Mind (1943). New York, Barnes & Noble, 1965

Schafer R: Aspects of Internalization. New York, International Universities Press, 1968

Schafer R: The psychoanalytic vision of reality (1970), in A New Language for Psychoanalysis. New Haven, CT, Yale University Press, 1976, pp 22–56

Schafer R: Internalization: process or fantasy? (1972), in A New Language for Psychoanalysis. New Haven, CT, Yale University Press, 1976, pp 155–178

Schafer R: A New Language for Psychoanalysis. New Haven, CT, Yale University Press, 1976

Schafer R: Psychoanalysis and common sense. The Listener, 10 November 1977, pp 609–610

Schafer R: Language and Insight: The Sigmund Freud Memorial Lectures 1975–1976. University College London. New Haven, CT, Yale University Press, 1978

Schafer R: Action language and the psychology of the self. Annual of Psychoanalysis 8:83–92, 1980

Segal H: Introduction to the Work of Melanie Klein. New York, Basic Books, 1964

25

EVELYNE ALBRECHT SCHWABER, M.D.

INTRODUCTION

Evelyne Schwaber is a graduate of Radcliffe College in Cambridge, Massachusetts, Albert Einstein College of Medicine in New York, and the Boston Psychoanalytic Society and Institute, where she is on the faculty. She is a Training and Supervising Analyst at the Psychoanalytic Institute of New England, East, in Needham, Massachusetts, and has been a faculty member of the Massachusetts Institute for Psychoanalysis, the Minnesota Psychoanalytic Institute, and Honorary Member of the Pittsburgh Psychoanalytic Society.

Dr. Schwaber is an award-winning author of more than 60 publications on aspects of clinical listening, and her work has been translated into several foreign languages. She has taught and lectured in Canada, Europe, South America, Australia, and Israel. Her honors include, among others, Freud Memorial Lecturer at the University of London, Visiting Analyst at the University of Rome and the Rome Psychoanalytic Society, the Consortium of Nine Psychoanalytic Institutes in Germany, the Brazilian Psychoanalytic Societies of Rio de Janeiro and São Paulo, the Uruguayan Psychoanalytic Association, the University of Sydney, Australia, the Annual Meeting of the Psychoanalytic Study Group in Frankfurt, Germany, and the Fiftieth Anniversary of the Lou Andreas Salomé Institut in Goettingen. She is Consulting Editor to *Psychoanalytic Inquiry*, Contributing Editor to *The Journal of Clinical Psychoanalysis*, and Past Member of the Editorial Board of *The Israel Psychoanalytic Journal*.

Dr. Schwaber has said of herself:

When I was a candidate at the Boston Psychoanalytic Institute in the late 1960s, senior trainees and faculty members presented clinical material at our seminars, offering what often seemed to me brilliant and amazing interpretations. Amazing, in that they apparently could see hidden meaning that never would have occurred to me. At first in awe of what I was yet to learn, I came to feel quite disheartened; I didn't feel I had the capacity to recognize so profoundly—as my senior colleagues could, and as many of my peers were striving towards—the elusive workings of "the unconscious." How did they know it?

With my first supervised case, my patient's depersonalizing symptomatology seemed to erupt so alarmingly, and randomly, on the couch, that my supervisor suggested I "educate her ego," that is, help her see that what she claimed to experience was imaginary or fantasy; her sense of reality needed to be strengthened. My next supervisor, for my second case, helped me locate the inherent legitimacy in what the patient was saying, the patient's perspective. He didn't explicitly put it this way, but he somehow seemed to address the logic in the patient's description of his experience and perceptions, even of me—it made sense—whereas I, assuming distortion, had been looking for hidden meaning. Finding this way of working—of listening—more natural and less magical, I decided to try to listen to my first patient in this mode. A remarkable shift occurred. I began to see, as could the patient as well, how the appearance of a symptom or state of depersonalization would occur in particular moments which we could elucidate—often, though not necessarily, bearing on some perception of me as not listening, perhaps as judging, presuming, or simply not getting it. Symptomatic eruptions seemed to occur less randomly and with lessened frequency as the patient's vantage point was more profoundly located. Pathways opened to previously hidden recesses, as what was heretofore unconscious came to view. Memories spontaneously emerged as we could see in greater depth the legitimacy—inherently so—in her experience of me and in my evocation or recreation of figures past. No longer struggling to infer meaning in what wasn't said—or subtly to correct presumed distortions—I could attend more closely to what was in words, or affect—as could she.

Both supervisors, highly regarded classical analysts of similar theoretical persuasion, taught me different ways of listening, each of which held distinct clinical impact. I began to recognize that how one listens transcends the theory espoused. In time, I came to see that grappling with this distinction must entail a profound shift in outlook.

Heinz Kohut's writings on narcissism were becoming quite influential in those years, if also increasingly controversial. Reading of his work with Miss F (Kohut 1968), I was struck particularly by Kohut's description of his attempt to go beyond his predetermined theoretical stance, thereby to listen—attending to her verbal *and nonverbal* communications—to something else she was conveying. It was the *moment of discovery* that intrigued me. Listening to her, rather than persisting with his theory-based inferences, he learned how he had been recreating the responses of her depressive mother and of her competitive brother. Thus entering a further domain of her psychic experience, he was led in turn to the discovery of another realm of transference. This shift in stance resonated for me with Freud's early clinical discoveries in which he allowed himself to hear things his patients were communicating that transcended his prior assumptions. It is such capacity to go beyond our prior assumptions or to detour from pathways on which we've entered, towards a *moment of discovery,* which I have been trying to "bottle."

As the theory of self psychology took hold, I found that it too, as did other theoretical preferences, often became a guidepost preempting sustained attendance to the patient's communications, particularly if these were not consonant with the direction undertaken or perhaps with the analyst's own view of him- or herself (see Schwaber 1987, 1996). It seemed to me that there were larger clinical and theoretical implications here regarding the use of theory, which have been central to the focus of my work. Among the ramifications I had noted was the frequent omission in our literature of clinical material that included the verbal and nonverbal exchange between patient and analyst—rather than simply the dynamic and theoretical formulations—as though the analytic dialogue itself was not considered essential to our understanding or to the illumination of the clinical data (Schwaber 1986; see also Klumpner and Frank 1991). By and large, this mode of reporting has, fortunately, since receded.

I have further shared my view that despite the increasing acknowledgment of our ever-present subjectivity and our participatory input, there remains the sense that we are not reckoning with the notion that we, as analysts, have only our own version of it; the patient may have another, still to be learned. "We are not Subjective with a capital *S*" (Schwaber 1998). Another example of the concerns I have expressed has to do with the Kleinian notion of "projective identification," which we do not hear conceptualized as holding psychic equivalency for analyst as well as patient. If, that is, the countertransference bears evidence of the analyst's projective identification, then it ought to follow that the transference too suggests the analyst unconsciously evoking these responses in the patient. For if we are to locate a resonance of commonality, which I believe to be essential in seeking the perspective of the patient, as well as for theoretical consistency, any psychic mechanism must find its way on either side of the couch (Schwaber 2005). A more recent example is reflected in the direction posited in the heightened interest in the clinical implications for the understanding of procedural or *implicit* memory. The view that such mnemonic forms remain indelibly so again risks bypassing open-ended collaborative inquiry into nonverbal cues—as state shifts—and which, I have found, *can* be explicitly elucidated and *can* indeed offer entrée to newly discovered memory paths (as noted in the following paper).

I am often asked about my own theoretical predilection. I consider myself a traditional analyst. I view Freud's theory of psychic reality, with the transference at its helm, as our anchor, offering a fundamental legitimacy to the patient's inner experience as a data base for inquiry.

> I have described my view of the discovery of transference, the participation of the observer intrinsic to the field observed, as marking the entry of depth-psychological observation into the scientific era of relativity (Schwaber 1985). In its paradigmatic significance for our understanding of reality, unique to each one of us as well as holding a collective resonance, it has changed the way we see the world. Grappling within ourselves with this difficult shift offers the propitious, if humbling, chance to recognize, paradoxical as it may seem, that the truth for each of us is but our own, whereas the other's truth is one we can yet find within ourselves, if we but seek it. And so I write of our "struggle to listen" and its "lingering paradoxes."

WHY I CHOSE THIS PAPER

Evelyne Albrecht Schwaber, M.D.

I have been writing about differing aspects of psychoanalytic listening—conceptual, clinical, historical, scientific, philosophical—for some three decades. It has been, for me, an ongoing evolutionary and continuously self-corrective process, each paper prompted by my learning something I had not before known or quite recognized even when on some level I had known it. I choose, thereby, my most recently published paper, "The Struggle to Listen," for inclusion in this volume, to reflect, however transient and limited, my most recent understanding. My hope is that there may be more you will see that I have not.

I am honored to have this work included here.

REFERENCES

Klumpner G, Frank A: On methods of reporting clinical material. J Am Psychoanal Assoc 39:537–551, 1991

Kohut H: The psychoanalytic treatment of narcissistic personality disorders. Psychoanal Study Child 23:86–113, 1968

Schwaber EA (ed): The Transference in Psychotherapy: Clinical Management. New York, International Universities Press, 1985

Schwaber EA: Reconstruction and perceptual experience: further thoughts on psychoanalytic listening. J Am Psychoanal Assoc 34:911–932, 1986

Schwaber EA: Models of the mind and data-gathering in clinical work. Psychoanalytic Inquiry 7:261–275, 1987

Schwaber EA: The conceptualization and communication of clinical facts in psychoanalysis: a discussion. Int J Psychoanal 77:235–253, 1996

Schwaber EA: The non-verbal dimension in psychoanalysis: "state" and its clinical vicissitudes. Int J Psychoanal 79:667–679, 1998

Schwaber EA: On: projective identification and consciousness alteration (letter). Int J Psychoanal 86:900–901, 2005

THE STRUGGLE TO LISTEN

Continuing Reflections, Lingering Paradoxes, and Some Thoughts on Recovery of Memory

EVELYNE ALBRECHT SCHWABER, M.D.

I do not know which to prefer,
The beauty of inflections
Or the beauty of innuendoes,
The blackbird whistling
Or just after.

—*Wallace Stevens,*
"Thirteen Ways of Looking at a Blackbird"

TO WHICH DO WE LISTEN—inflections, innuendoes, tone, words—or after? What happens after?

How do we listen? As the verse suggests, there are subtleties in the distinctions we make, the preferences to which we adhere. It is a truism—such preferences are inevitable. We come with what we believe and have learned to see and regard. It cannot be another way. But how do we then use what we prefer—to see more or turn aside—to open or close paths? How might we seek the answer, poised for the possibility of chagrin it may evoke in us? And what of preferences we had not recognized in ourselves, unseen assumptions—how do we discover them

---

"The Struggle to Listen: Continuing Reflections, Lingering Paradoxes, and Some Thoughts on Recovery of Memory," by Evelyne Albrecht Schwaber, M.D., was first published in *The Journal of the American Psychoanalytic Association,* 53:789–810, 2005.

without turning defensively to theory-based rationalizations ("The patient put those feelings into me," "The patient is in the grips of an unconscious fantasy")? It is my contention that grappling with such questions as we listen will vitally enhance illumination on nuance (inflections, innuendoes, "whistling") with meanings and history that may otherwise remain hidden or be simply left behind, lingering in the realm of what is yet unconscious, or not conscious.

Please join me as I review a series of differing, perhaps commonplace clinical moments—some fragments, some a bit longer, from the work of others and from my own—in the effort to sustain our reflection on these matters. My hope is that these brief glances will convey a cumulative message.

CLINICAL MATERIAL

At a workshop, an analyst cited an exchange in the opening of a session. Her patient said, "I feel really sad but I'm not sure why."

"Do you have to feel sure?" the analyst responded.

"No, I guess not," the patient answered, "but...(he pauses) and yesterday I had the feeling I'm all alone.... I'm not sure what I was saying."

"Does it feel you need to know?" the analyst asked.

The patient is silent for a time, before dialogue then resumes.

What just happened? The analyst, as we see, attending sensitively to these nonverbal cues, offers a heightened glimpse of the sequence in process. Seemingly, with each question the patient slowed down more—first a pause, then becoming unsure what he was saying, and then, silence.

I asked her how she meant her questions to be—a suggestion, however gently put, or simply an effort to learn more? "A suggestion," she answered, now reflecting on this distinction, "to help the patient feel he doesn't have to be so certain, that it's all right not to." A benign aspiration, it would seem; yet, perhaps paradoxically, he appeared here to become more, rather than less, hesitant.

We might wonder: did this preference on the analyst's part, this attempt to guide or suggest how the patient might better feel, however subtly conveyed, lead her away from remarking on the progression of pauses, from inquiring open-endedly, without herself knowing, "what just happened"? To be sure, the patient may not have had an answer, possibly having not even noticed; but invited to observe, without suggestion of meaning, he can reflect in a time of affective proximity without having to infer from a more distant time frame (Busch 1999, 2003a;

Gray 1994). Perhaps he felt his sadness bypassed, or that he wasn't abiding by the analyst's implicit preference; perhaps he wanted to slow down and felt better for it—or something neither he nor we may have yet considered, but if asked, might come forward, having otherwise gone unnoted, or unremembered, outside the realm of conscious awareness.

This is, of course, just a brief exchange between analyst and patient, and between analyst and me, a clinical fragment removed from larger context; there is much more data we do not have that might have led the analyst to knowingly choose at this moment not to ask, "What just now happened?" To ponder that choice—to ask or not—it would need first to be recognized.

Whatever the words expressed, however we phrase our question or other intervention, there is a fundamental difference between listening in an attempt to guide the patient, Socratic fashion, to chart a direction we may prefer, or to see psychic meaning we believe we already see, and listening to learn what we don't *yet* know, to linger with a nuance that might not fit our course, that might indeed reveal to us that we were not listening, despite its espousal, in this latter, open-ended effort. It may seem that I again speak a truism, for our effort is surely to listen in order to learn. But in subtle or not so subtle ways, often unwitting and unrecognized, we veer away from such an underlying outlook and so move to the epistemologically mistaken notion that we can see meaning unconscious to the patient.

This is not simply an endemic dilemma confined to our own discipline or our own time. "All over the world," Milan Kundera (1980) has written, "people prefer to judge rather than understand, to answer rather than ask" (p. 237).[1]

Recounting a session one day, an analyst told of her patient having said to her, "It felt like you didn't understand." Some moments later, reflecting the patient's words back, the analyst commented, "You felt I wouldn't understand."

"Wouldn't," or "didn't"? The distinction went unnoted, the patient's perception thereby unacknowledged—perhaps a defensive rationale, transference as distortion assumed. (We don't know.) But with

[1]The Italian philosopher Giambattista Vico, in 1744, had similar words: "It is another property of the human mind that whenever men can form no idea of distant and unknown things, they judge them by what is familiar and at hand. This axiom points to the inexhaustible source of all the errors about the principles of humanity that have been adopted by entire nations and by all the scholars" (p. 60; cited in Corradi Fiumara 1990, from Vico 1968).

the analyst's change in wording from the declarative to the conditional, the question "How, or what, did I seem not to understand?" is bypassed.

Consider this once oft-cited statement by Martin Stein (1966): "We need not tell our patients they have misjudged a life situation, nor do we as a rule give in to the temptation to correct a misapprehension of some analytic event. Instead, we attempt to correct, by analysis, those distortions of self-observation which become evident in the analytic situation" (p. 276).

The analyst, as the one who "knows" what is correct, what distorted or misapprehended, is to employ proper (or perhaps "neutral") technique and thereby guide the patient to "what is familiar and at hand" (Vico). In recent years, this notion of analyst as authority on knowledge or truth has been more actively challenged on epistemological and philosophical grounds. As I have persistently argued, however, despite this challenge and the concomitant theoretical shifts taking place, the impact on our basic outlook on how we listen remains clouded and warrants continuing reflection.

In this spirit, let me reflect anew on an occurrence with a patient of mine of which I wrote some years back (Schwaber 1995b). An affable, good-looking single man, Mr. L was uncertain which of two women he preferred. He had a way of recounting, in a somewhat obsessive manner, a kind of "checklist" of their attributes. From his descriptions, I had the impression that Chris was someone who seemed to have much more depth than Sara, who sounded in contrast, though fuller-breasted, rather empty-headed. I noticed I had a preference for Chris and was pleased when his attachment to Sara waned a bit, so took great caution to keep my feelings aside and not let them impinge on my "proper analytic" stance, in keeping with the words of Stein.

As the summer approached, Mr. L spoke of plans to spend time with his extended family, including two latency-age girl cousins of whom he was very fond. He told me a dream: "I went into this place where I saw T-shirts in a bin. I went to get one and it said Jill and Cindy, my cousins' names. I picked it up and there were two of them like that. I went to get one and it seemed big, but the woman behind the counter said it was too small; they won't fit."

In his associations, he spoke more of his cousins. There was an element expressed in the dream I had not quite followed (manifestly), and so, trying to clarify, I asked him, "How did the woman know the T-shirts didn't fit? Were your cousins with you?"

"No," he said, "they weren't. She just spoke with authority, that they'd be too small."

"You just took her word as fact then," I now observed.

"Yeah," he responded, as though only now seeing this; "she just sort of said, 'These will never fit.'"

That seemed to have been the end of that, I noted, commenting, as I now saw, that the very manner in which he told me the dream content had a similar message, as though it was a fact that the T-shirts didn't fit, rather than just the woman saying so.

"Yeah!" He was struck by this observation. "If you would like to carry the metaphor even further...," he went on—

"If *I* would like to?" I asked.

He laughed, in apparent recognition of his experience here, though I hadn't yet quite taken in that communication of his view of me. "My mother worked for a while in a clothing store; though she was a buyer, she sometimes worked in sales." I hadn't known of that. "She never approved of my taste in clothes, or women," he elaborated, remembering *now*, as memories newly emerged, how quick his mother was to squelch him. "Yeah," he thought further; "like the woman in the dream, just squelched, without my even noticing, a spontaneous original idea of mine. Here were these two T-shirts with their names on them; I had thought, 'What a coincidence! Like a diamond in the rough.'"

As he went on, I was struck by the dream's imagery: "The woman behind the counter, squelching something without your even noticing... Me too?" I then asked, the question just occurring to me (without foregone assumptions about the answer).

He reflected: "Only to the extent that I think when I spoke of Sara, and listed negatives about her, you didn't say, 'There's the checklist again, with the negatives.' You kind of accepted them, but with Chris, when I did that, you'd point out my being defensive."

"Oh!" I felt. Not wanting my hidden preference to affect our work, I had tried especially hard to listen, quietly and unobtrusively, when he spoke of Sara's faults. I felt secure in the knowledge that I had put my own feelings about her aside, preserving my analytic neutrality. Mr. L experienced my silence differently. I had become for him, as we now learned—and as I now could see about myself, which I had not before—the all-knowing, squelching woman (Schwaber 1995b, pp. 561–562).

A striking metaphor: two T-shirts for two prepubertal girls decreed nonfitting by the mysteriously knowing woman behind.

In hindsight, we might call this an enactment, of the very notion that I felt I knew which was the better choice of woman, evoked perhaps by the way he presented them to me—*though attribution of unconscious motive on his part for such evocation in me can be only speculative.* We would have to pursue this line of inquiry to learn more of his experience and whether there had been such hidden inclination.

Trying to bypass any hint of suggestion, I had commented, I believed unprejudicially, on his seeming defenses. I was found out, as we tend to be, though his experience of me, of my preference, was not at first in Mr. L's awareness. I learned this—*we* learned this—when I shifted my stance, asking, now without suggestive intent, to clarify what I had not understood—as an element of the manifest content of his dream, or whether I too had been squelching something. Feeling recognized, he began to sense an old familiarity in his experience and perceptions, recovering memories and defensive modes previously unnoted or buried. What had been unconscious was discerned, not by leaps of inference about potential meaning, but as a discovery arising from shared observation and inquiry. (I underscore, what *had been* unconscious, for, as I've written [Schwaber 1996], it can only be known, by us or by the patient, in past tense.) For Mr. L, history was spontaneously emerging, following upon recognition: *recognition as the mode of therapeutic action.*

Again I've presented only a fragment of the clinical process. Had I shared additional material, you might have seen evidence sooner of the patient's emerging transference experience of me that at the time had eluded me. You might have recognized the imposition of my perspective, when I had not. But I share with you my *moment of discovery*—learning from him—and the shift in my listening toward that aim, which enabled it.

If we attempt to disguise, as I had in this case, what we inwardly feel or believe, perhaps in the hope that the patient may eventually come on his own to see what we think we already see, we unilaterally relinquish a basic position of collaboration, and simply pay lip service to the notion that the analyst does not hold the authority on knowledge of the patient's psychic world. Further, such an unacknowledged stance may impose on the patient a sense of uncertainty about what he perceives. I think rather that if we have such an idea that we feel should not be made explicit but ought nonetheless guide, that self-awareness, however elusively felt, can serve as a red flag for us to reflect further on what might be stirring that keeps us at distance.[2] In the case of Mr. L, I did not heed that caution.

---

[2]This may seem reminiscent of Isakower's (1957) supervisory caution: "if you wouldn't tell this to the patient, it may be better even for yourself not to entertain the thought" (p. 190; see Schwaber 1995a, p. 276 n).

To be sure, if we have a concern about something we believe may be vital regarding the patient's outer life (e.g., a particular physical symptom being ignored, or some other potential of risk in action, or perhaps an occurrence that seems to us to interfere with the clinical effort), to choose to say so directly is quite another matter. Not disguised under the rubric of so-called "proper" analytic technique (perhaps hidden within an interpretation), such an intervention is not inherently at odds with the outlook of which I speak. It still leaves room to listen without presupposition to the patient's experience and response, that is, to remain open to possibilities of meaning—to say again—*that may not otherwise have occurred to us.* While we cannot be arbiters of the truth in inner meaning—*though surely we can offer our views on it, recognizing them as simply that: our views*—regarding outer reality we do assume a different responsibility (a distinction I underscore).

Let me go on to another example, a brief segment from a session shared at a workshop. The patient presented had planned some months earlier to be leaving treatment for a work-related move. In the session he said, "Thinking why I missed two days last week. I was furious with you. I tried to end this. Got no support from you. I'm really angry. I tried to quit. Then, came the time. I told you I had to. A good reason. Or, regardless of whether it is, I told you. Now the time is going to come and I'm not going to feel any better. I told you, this is what I want and I didn't get support. I told you and you didn't agree with the decision. Damn! I told you and you didn't take me seriously. I asked for help and you didn't give it to me."

"Obviously, you're really angry at me, "the analyst responded. "I've let you down. Almost like I've tricked you. I didn't take you seriously, didn't help you, and you have no hope that anything helpful can happen." The patient agreed.

The analyst here is reflecting back to the patient what she'd heard him say. I then asked her, not knowing, "When you said what you did, did you get it?" She was struck by this question. "No," she said, stirred, in becoming aware that she hadn't really "gotten" it. She had responded to her patient with what seemed attentive, empathic technique, but without fully locating—resonating with—the rationale, the inherent legitimacy of his experience of her. To gain that, to learn how, for example, she "didn't take [him] seriously" and so didn't help, she would have had to extend her inquiry. (A patient of mine would tell me, in such occurrences, "You're just positioning, Dr. Schwaber.")

Here, as in the other examples, I asked the analyst in order to learn what I didn't yet know of what she had in mind. Thus, in these didactic instances as in the clinical, pondering the question (naively asked) prompted a deeper awareness—of assumptions made, nuances skipped over—that how one listens transcends theoretical preference. "Getting it" will call up something of one's own affective recognition of the feeling and perception the patient conveys—in this case, that the analyst did not take him seriously. "Getting it" may require a more sustained exploration of the meaning of apparent discrepancies, cognitive leaps, affect shifts, or other defenses—phenomena that can be mutually observed and perhaps still to be understood, not by assumption or by "positioning." Thus we enlarge our awareness of dimensions left out, possibly outside the verbal realm, uncovering what may be an old, familiar sense of not having been "taken seriously." Some patients may communicate their conflicted concerns primarily through affect; others may directly say, "It feels like you don't get it." "How so? What don't I get?" we might then wonder (and from this inquiry both analyst and patient—and, I would add, student and teacher[3]—may have much to learn).

We may see, listening in order to "get it" is not a passive stance. The extent of our activity may vary, but, as I have tried to convey, I share my thoughts and questions close to "real time." Waiting, while I silently think my thoughts, for what I deem a more optimal moment, would once again put me in the lonely place, and perhaps mistaken, of the "knower." Nor does this outlook inherently lead to more activity. This is not a quantitative matter. I do not speak of more questions, or necessarily interrupting the associative stream—which of course can be interrupted by our silence too—but of our intent behind them. Asking to seek an answer (not as a technical ploy—as to keep the flow of thoughts going or to guide their direction) can enhance our subsequent understanding, obviating the need for another question. Rather than divert us to the intellectual, such inquiry may allow us access to a more closely observed, affectively nuanced terrain (and to a more profound affective resonance).[4]

---

[3]Schindelheim (1995) has written of having felt left behind, unseen by his supervisor, whose attendance seemed primarily focused on his patient, until such cues came to light that allowed him to share this occurrence for them both to see. (I was that supervisor.)

[4]To be sure, in raising questions or making observations that occur to us, but not necessarily to the patient, there is always some element of guidance inherent in the effort to learn. I do not suggest what would be a spurious polarity (between guiding and learning) but again highlight the outlook informing our intervention.

At another workshop, a session was presented in which a patient began the hour remaining quiet for several minutes, a familiar opening. Then she said, "I was thinking...you must get bored when I come here and don't say anything."

"How come I'd be bored?" the analyst asked.

"Don't know...maybe you're used to it...maybe...I wonder...if it makes you feel like you're not helping me."

"You worry you're hurting me and your analysis when you're quiet," the analyst responded.

The patient went on, "Today, I didn't want to come," and the session then continued.

Did she perceive the analyst as bored, or did she assume he must be? If she felt it, on what basis? If she assumed rather than perceived, on what basis also? The analyst asks, "How come I'd be bored?"—an apt question. She responds, wondering if her quiet makes him feel he's not helping her. Why, one could then ask, would that bore or hurt him? Would it be on his account, some sense of injury to his own person, or on hers? Whatever else might underlie the psychic issues evoking the quiet, they may be deeply interwoven with her view of the rationale, the motive, for his response—i.e., is he felt to be fundamentally *for* her?

I recall a patient who told me she worries I'll be hurt if she's sad so much of the time.

"It would hurt my feelings?" I asked, just now considering this (and recognizing that she may have felt some affective resonance in my response to her sadness). "You mean I would be hurt on my own account, not for you?"

"That idea [that it would be for me] never even occurred to me," she said, sounding stirred; "besides, it would be presumptuous."

A new direction opened that felt deeply meaningful to her about her lifelong sense of herself and of others' vulnerability and expectations in relation to her; that is, whose feelings were hurt if she was sad? On whose account did that seem? Again, whatever the "familiar" trajectory (Vico) of conflict-laden or defensive dimensions in her worry about hurting me, this idea—*for her—that had never occurred to her,* and that I hadn't known was absent when I asked, deepened and contextualized their elucidation. Nonverbal memory (Schwaber 1998), not quite repressed though newly recognized—a profound view of an unsafe or unloving world—was coming forward.[5]

---

[5]This core sense of a lack of underlying unconditional acceptance is regrettably, I have found, a not uncommon feeling.

A LONGER EXAMPLE: MR. A

> I am beginning to recognize the objectivity of the world.... The absolute nature of things is independent of my senses (which are all I have to perceive with) and what I perceive is an image in my own psyche. All very fine. Not too hard to formulate and accept intellectually. But to *know* it; to bring it into daily life—that's the problem. And it would be real humility, not just the mock-modesty that generally passes for humility. (Davies 1972, p. 269)

Some patients, with whom we may be familiar, want us to be the ones who know; they may feel they do not. How then are we to listen to learn, not to lead? In a broader sense, their quest marks the paradox in our psychoanalytically informed venture—to listen, recognizing we do not know, in order to come to know.

Let me share segments of a longer example, to highlight a dimension of my struggle with yet another clinical dilemma along these lines of knowing or not.

Mr. A, when I saw him, was a married professional man, an architect in his early thirties, engaging and largely good-humored in his manner of relating. He was remarkably intelligent, high-achieving and imaginative in his many work endeavors, in which he felt quite confident. But in ordinary social interaction and, as we saw, in the analysis, in striking contrast, Mr. A felt himself to be "clueless." As he put it, he just doesn't "get" it. He doesn't understand psychic process, he doesn't understand irrational thinking, nor does he understand defense. He doesn't "get" that there were multiple levels of complexity about his past or in human relatedness, that these are not one-dimensional, linear matters. Difficulties in his marriage had led him to seek help.

Mr. A's mother had escaped as a teenager from the fires of the Holocaust; his maternal grandparents did not survive. In the U.S., his mother married a like-minded American businessman, whose own history was filled with tragedy as well. Both parents had changed religion, relinquishing their Jewish identity before they'd met. As a child, Mr. A was not told of any of this background, nor did he recall conscious curiosity. In his late teens, his mother became visibly (and avowedly) depressed. Sometime while in college, he received a call that she had committed suicide.

Mr. A came by his unawareness seemingly naturally—by that I mean, consistent with his family's style. It did not appear as "pseudo-denseness." Having felt secure in his mother's underlying love and support (and to an extent his father's as well), he was raised with manifest care. It was, however, an ambience without consideration given to feelings, but to solving the rational and pragmatic and performing the required tasks. Mr. A identifies with the character of the butler, Stevens (played by Anthony Hopkins), in the movie *Remains of the Day,* "who didn't say, or even sense, what was in his heart."

(Early in the analysis he had a dream of gremlins in the basement of a strange house, possibly haunted, ones he hadn't noticed before—"weird and slimy"—and a little gremlin keeper who would explain them. My office was in the basement.)

Mr. A seems to pull for my help, for me to give him a "clue." I am tempted to show him the workings of his mind, to point to some apparently "obvious" defensiveness in his stream of associations, or in the detached way he recounts his poignant history, to help him see where his feelings "really" lie. Subtly, without my quite being aware of it, I become a teacher. He comes along, seeming to "get it." Indeed, his expressed transference to me is as to a "teacher." I begin to notice he doesn't look at me when leaving at the hour's end.

In ensuing sessions, he tells me he feels as though he's fallen short—his mind not making the connections or responding as it "should have," unable to do what he "ought to" in analysis. But this was not a constant sense; there were ebbs and flows to this sensation.

I pondered his look away. When I asked about it in a succeeding hour, my question didn't open any observable paths; on the contrary, it may have left him feeling there was something else he didn't "get." Nonetheless, the turn in his glance seemed a clue to what I might not otherwise have noted—an inner voice not being heard, possibly going underground.

A pragmatist, Mr. A spoke often of his style of making "policy decisions," a detached, determined mode of deciding on a course of action between differing options. In one hour, as he tried to select one of several competing thoughts about which to speak, he said, dryly, noting his difficulty, "I don't understand the idea of just letting random thoughts in that aren't related or relevant. There'd be no point, no sense would be made of them; it would be all different tracks."

"It's all one you," I offered, adding another, if seemingly to me apparent view.

"Hmmm...," he responded, lingeringly; "it's like a fundamental recognition that I exist, as me, rather than as a series of operations. It would be comforting to feel satisfied with me, that I'm not just defined by my actions." He sounded notably moved. "Anyway..." He paused. (We had become familiar with his use of this word to convey retreat.) "When I say "anyway" I'm going back to a topic, like getting back on track."

"And away," I noted, "from where you had just been, after I'd said,

'It's all one you.'" (Repeating that phrase, I was perhaps responding to the pull for me when he starts to veer off again. It brought him back.)

"I feel so inarticulate," he said; "there's something in that phrase that's both comforting and respectful, of a being in its own right, which I don't think I am, even of myself. I don't recognize myself except by what I do; there's something very powerful in that notion."

With newfound feeling, Mr. A observed in the ensuing hour, "It seems I'm closer to something that matters to me." I felt that too. At the session's end, he looked directly at me.[6]

Thus, it was in first noting Mr. A's departing look away, which also heightened my awareness of an added affective detachment in his tone, that I began to appreciate these vicissitudes of our interaction—whether (as teacher) "clueing" him in to what I know or think I do, or trying to learn more profoundly what it is like to feel as a series of "different tracks," to feel "without a clue." (In the former instance, I am responding from the position of being in my own shoes, acted upon by him and having to provide something; in the latter, from how it feels to be the seeker.) Indeed, it was out of this latter effort that I came to recognize that the idea of its being "all one him" had somehow been absent.

In an ensuing hour, coming to a familiar standstill—"I don't know where else to go with this"—I could see more clearly and speak to him of the power in "your search for me to clue you in." This very recognition then allowed a deeper elucidation of the issues stirring heightening such a quest at a given moment. What I am reflecting may now seem self-evident, yet the inward turn in me from trying to help him "get it" to trying to "get" him myself felt notable. I might before have commented on something as analytically benign, for example, as pointing to the moment stirring the defense, or the apparent conflict behind it, or made some other seemingly germane intervention. But again, the analysis of defense and conflict is not at issue here; my intent is. As with the analyst's response to my question in the earlier example, "To what end did you ask about your patient's need for certainty—to learn more or suggest (how better to feel)?" I began to recognize that for me as well, it

---

[6]We may note that I've illustrated my offer of a view that went beyond what the patient had himself seen, and that, unforeseen by me, touched him. Again, though perhaps paradoxical, this is not a contradiction of the outlook I propose. My comment, which affectively resonated within him, arose from my *return* to a sustained search for *his* truth, thereby remaining open to learning from whatever response he might then have. I believe he felt that.

would be in order to suggest, to lead Mr. A to "where else to go with this," stepping aside from learning more profoundly about this "not knowing" state. No surprise—our manifest words themselves may not tell the tale.

"I feel I don't have a real tether," he said another time; "I look to K [his wife] to offer that, to my secretary too.... They have a much better sense of how one reacts." How easy to be drawn into that—my words silently, perhaps not consciously to him, offering a tether. We might then consider, interventions deriving from any espoused theoretical perspective could serve that purpose, *unbeknown to both analyst and patient,* remaining so if the factors stirring his search—the sense of "clueless," fear of losing the track, not knowing how to ask or what to think—and the feelings behind it were left aside, bypassed in the inclination to suggest or leap to inference about inner meaning.

Thus, we could see, Mr. A had great difficulty allowing his imagination simply to wander. Sometimes he braced himself to ask direct questions of me: Where did I get a certain picture in my waiting room? Do I read the magazines there? Do they reflect my politics? Where do I go when I go away? Was I afraid, as he was, of the potential for nuclear disaster? Other times, fearing being "impolite" or in some way "off," and that I would not provide an explicit answer, he squelched such questions, permitting himself no stated imaginings, fantasies, scarcely recalling his dreams. Besides, he felt "clueless" as to how to go about such mental roaming.

"I want so much to learn answers to questions I don't even know to ask," he said one day (perhaps also an hysterical defense, but if so, with its own profound complexity). "But politeness is essential, and I don't want to be inappropriate." It's a "thought etiquette," he later reflected, beginning to glean having felt a kind of "thought control" in growing up (which apparently included even commonplace sexual matters, not just historical ones).

"Wanting to know even what to ask, and not daring to; it's a fine line making you uneasy," I commented.

"It's more than uneasy; it's just sort of a desperate situation," he responded.

We might heed the evocative distinction between my adjective, "uneasy" (more pallid), and his, "desperate" (perhaps harder for me to take in).

Incrementally (in our reflections on his often detached tone), Mr. A came to see, to sense, the distance he keeps from feelings of desperation, which he first noted in himself after his mother's death when he set about, as a deliberate "policy," to push them aside to be able to go on with the demands of his life. ("Anyway," he said.) "Basically, around the time of my mom's death, I became oblivious to things"—mundane matters such as dates and schedules—to an extent far beyond his earlier "not knowing." But in the course of our work together, he began to recognize how throughout his life he had detoured away from affectively graphic words, toning them down euphemistically, without even noticing it. "Weird," "ridiculous," replaced "terror," "tragic"—words he could not bear to say. Protecting him from the full force of his despair, anger, and other intense feelings, and from what he later came to see, the dark undercurrent in which he grew up, "clueless" could protect me from its force as well—as his looking to me to "teach" would allow me distance from it. Itself a desperate state, it was a kind of leitmotif—defensive while also defining, protective yet shameful.

A mode of survival and of being: "clueless" about his family's history, religious identity, the fate of his grandparents, the sadness and rage buried beneath the activity in the home, about how to speak of sexuality or of other feelings he did not know—clueless because one should not or dare not ask, either mother or father (who was apparently even more mute about his traumatic past in the U.S.). Nobody actually said not to speak of these things; he just knew it. Noting that, paradoxically, he was not clueless.[7] In *Memory Effects: The Holocaust and the Art of Secondary Witnessing,* Dora Apel (2002) cites the words of an artist son of survivors: "The most important event of my life occurred before I was born" (p. 11; cited in Lipton 2003, p. 101). Mr. A didn't know of that event, or other events that occurred before he was born; or, rather, he didn't know that he might have known, or not. "I was feeling set adrift from my own history," he said one day, during the time of a newly noted Jewish holiday.

One hour, before a summer separation, he saw more clearly his difficulty lingering with any feelings about it. "It's not permanent," he tells of reminding himself. "'Don't complain,' I was taught; 'and by the way, you're more fortunate than most.' All those rules I got from my mom. She never said it; I just got it. Feelings didn't have a place [he was recognizing this more clearly]; it was just what I should be doing.... Won-

---

[7]In his teens, he found himself drawn to reading John Hersey's *The Wall,* a powerful book about the Warsaw ghetto—written not as a factual account, but as a novel. He spoke with no one about it. When I later shared this report with him, he corrected me on this point; it was in fourth or fifth grade that he'd read the book—a time, he felt, that a child would ordinarily be more likely to talk of it.

dering sometimes if people at work are truly interested in me, as me, or just for what I can produce....With you, I do sense a caring, an acceptance.... It's a kind of painful thing; I can't take advantage of that [now]. I need a cue—to be appropriate. I'm unable to rid myself of my own judgments, even if I don't see you as judging. [And we knew how much more pronounced his own judgments when he sees me as judging].... With my mother, I incorporated her values as my own."

He had come upon a more profound and painful awareness of his isolated state—in its immediacy—his difficulty allowing our connection, that is, our separation, to matter (for ultimately, as we could hear, he had not been sure he matters, for himself). "Some of this has to do with the fear of attachment, doesn't it?" I asked. "Yeah!" he exclaimed, shifting affectively closer (as though perhaps he'd gotten his cue). "I was probably most attached to my mom. After giving me all those messages, then splitting on me—that's not a model I'd want to replicate."

The hour was up, the interruption on its way. Afraid of attachment—of trusting it—afraid of memory, yet exquisitely "clued in" to his mother's silent rules and judgments, terrified of feeling loss, yet perhaps tenuously holding on to me, Mr. A, now looking back at me, was on his way to "getting it." Perhaps so, too, was I—though for us both, a struggle always to recur.[8]

SOME THOUGHTS ON RECOVERY OF MEMORY

> If to remember is to provide the disembodied "wound" with a psychic residence then to remember other people's memories is to be wounded by their wounds. More precisely, to let the traces of other people's struggles, passions, past, resonate within one's own past and present, and destabilize them. (Silverman 1996, p. 189)

And yet, there is also the search. In a foreword to A.R. Luria's (1972) *The Man With a Shattered World,* the Russian neuropsychologist's powerful case history of a man relentlessly seeking his memory, lost from a bullet wound to his brain, Oliver Sacks (1987) writes that "perhaps there is a universal here which applies to us all, the lesson also taught by Socrates, Freud, Proust—that a life, a human life, is not a life until it

---

[8]A reviewer of this paper noted, tellingly, I believe, "So the answer to the question you keep raising with different analysts and with yourself, 'Did you get it?' doesn't have a final answer. But it certainly is a question to keep asking."

is examined; that it is not a life until it is truly remembered and appropriated; and that such remembrance is not something passive, but active, the active and creative construction of one's life, the finding and telling of the true story of one's life" (p. xvii).

(One day, finding them, allowing himself to remember his memories of the emotional isolation of his childhood, Mr. A said, "I was thinking today. It takes quite an open heart to regard people with the tenderness to not judge. That thought came to me of what you've provided me. I feel an appreciation for that." This idea—acceptance without judgment of all that he feels [echoing my "It's all one you"]—was novel to him; he hadn't before quite thought of it.[9])

Thus, to say again, what may appear on some level as a defense may also have a central life-affirming element, basic to one's self-definition, adding to the strength and vitality of the hold on it (see Valenstein 1973). Recognizing this dimension may tellingly shift our response in our countertransference. When we try to guide, to dissuade, to get the patient to see what we believe we already see, we may more likely feel a sense of struggle with the patient, who may in turn appear as resistant (which he is, of course), however this is expressed. But rather than simply look for an alternative technical approach, we can draw on this sensation within ourselves (of some contention, or of feeling demanded upon) as a call to notice that we may have been trying to move the patient in our direction, toward our assumption of meaning (while he may have something else to tell us). However this sensation may be evoked by his way of being with us, nothing eases our countertransference dilemma as can seeing it as a vital clue that we may have left our patient's shoes, his vantage point, and then finding our way back, affectively, to seeking its deep-rooted legitimacy (Schwaber 1992a, 1992b). Mr. A's cluelessness, his detached, defensive style, his inability to keep track of schedules, wanting me to provide a guidepost to how things work, all distanced me, even if drawing me in as "tether" (for which response in *me* I cannot presume unconscious motive on *his* part), until I found my way back to trying to listen for what I don't yet know. (That he may be reluctant to connect need not mean that on some level he *wants* to keep me from doing so.) I may not have been entirely aware of my sense of distance; often only on subsequent reflection could I recognize that I

[9]Take Doi (1989, 1993) refers to this feeling as *amae.* In a personal communication Doi notes that Mr. A's remark that he feels my caring as a "kind of painful thing" describes a pivotal accompaniment of *amae.*

wanted him to see—perhaps relinquish the defense—what I was pointing out. Noting his look away, hearing his sense of failure here, I was helped toward that recognition.

These responses are, of course, the reflections of his transference, the reality we seek of his ways of perceiving, experiencing, and interpreting the world—or me. Among the most profoundly encompassing of Freud's discoveries, transference illuminates the paradox in our search for one's individual truth. It is not simply put or projected onto us, who know a truth the patient does not; it is not distorted, nor distinguished as more real if it coincides with our own awareness of our behavior or experience. Mr. L's sense of me as the controlling mother telling him which woman to choose was no more real because I could recognize my participation in evoking it than was Mr. A's experience of me as eliciting in him the feeling of being a failure. That it hadn't been seen by me may just mean I have to try harder to "get it," to not "position." Surely, assumptions about us can be made that don't match our own, as with the woman to whom it hadn't occurred that I might be hurt by her sadness on *her* account; left unexamined, however, such assumptions may suggest our complicity.

Something in our way of being may evoke the sense or *anlage* of an early relationship, an ambience or imagining surrounding it (I may be a fairy godmother, other times a witch). To hear that allows the possibility of locating a resonance of experience or perception that might have been nondeclaratively imprinted (that is, not having been explicitly known). We are reminiscent, we stir reminiscence (as Breuer and Freud [1893] remarked of hysterical suffering), and whether unconscious or bound in implicit memory, its roots may yet be sought.[10]

Trying to stay with what is mutually, affectively observable may perhaps seem at odds with the search for what is unseen or unconscious. Rather, we move more closely to the unseen inhibitions of the associative flow, often so reflexive that neither analyst nor patient

---

[10]I enter the terrain here of the forms of memory and its recovery. There has been much recent attention to this subject, a detailed consideration of which is beyond the scope of this paper, including a debate in the literature regarding the possibility and/or necessity of recovery of repressed memory (Blum 2003a, 2003b; Fonagy 2003). I do share Busch's concern that "the mind, with its dynamic structures that serve multiple functions, is not easily categorized. It seems a daunting task to ascertain whether a complex series of thoughts or feelings…represents an unformulated experience or one…kept at an earlier level of thinking because of conflict" (Blum 2003b, p. 25 n).

thinks to note it (something of the core of one's being unsealed). "When you understand the way my mind works without saying it should work another way, that lets me experience more about how my mind works.... the shame, terror, even chaos," a patient told me.

Another paradox: By inferring what *may* be unconscious, we can elude its more profound discovery.

It is, then, not simply the repression of represented content per se to which I refer when I speak of phenomena that have lain untended, but of the "not conscious" as well—"implicit memory," also called "non-declarative" or "procedural" memory, psychic experience and process that have in a patient's history remained outside explicit awareness.[11] Though some have argued differently (e.g., Davis 2001; Fonagy 1999, 2003; Stern et al. 1998), I believe there is much in such memory and experience, that in our struggle to listen is ultimately knowable (Schwaber 1998). Certainly there are basic questions to consider regarding the dynamic implications in the recovery of experience that has lain outside explicit memory, and only now, in analysis, to enter consciousness. How might the capacity for language bear on that? Are there brain pathways laid down that mark the arrival of awareness? If so, are we uncovering old paths or laying down new ones? How might our understanding of how unconscious processes emerge into view relate to these matters? (I am not speaking of co-constructing new narratives, but of finding what has been "there," however nascent—recognizing, of course, its transience and elusive nature.)[12]

In the case of Mr. L (the man with the T-shirt dream), as the analysis proceeded he became calmer, less obsessive or agitated in his feelings about different women. The anxious dilemma in his question of whom to choose receded with the advent of a calmer state. There was a history to this state, *only uncovered in the analysis,* as we began to note its shifts and vicissitudes. His experience of my calm (the movements within it) evoked his; more important, however, observing this in the moment's immediacy prompted a newfound recognition of his mother's anxious state as a central ambience of his growing up. Did that appear as a memory that had been repressed out of feelings too threatening, or had it

---

[11] In the realm of literature regarding the Holocaust, L. Langer speaks of the "deep memory" of war experience, living beside "common" or narrative memory (cited in Apel 2002, p. 94).

[12] Gerald Edelman (2004) has noted, as paraphrased by Edward Rothstein in the *New York Times* (March 27, 2004), "No brain event happens the same way twice. Even memory is always a variant—a recreation, never a repetition."

never entered his awareness in the first place?

Similarly, was Mr. A's cluelessness evoked by his fear of granting knowledge that he on some level had (and repressed), or had he never quite known it? Did my other patient repress an unchallenged notion of a mother hurting for herself, on her own account, for the child's sadness, or was the posed alternative—hurting for the child's sake—newly recognized? How do the answers here bear on the question of making what is unconscious conscious?

CONCLUDING REMARKS

While striving to listen to learn may seem to be a truism, something we expect of ourselves, what I try to illustrate in this mosaic of clinical moments is the difficulty, perhaps affective disinclination in assuming this perspective—for analyst and patient. This is not a squishy-soft, "niceynice" approach covering over angry or harsher feelings, but one facilitating their emergence and more subtle recognition. Hard as it may be to find our way into another's ways of seeing and experiencing the world, it is surely demanding on the patient to observe and reflect on phenomena that otherwise may pass fleetingly by, or perhaps that he or she may prefer to let pass by.

So to come back, at the end, to the beginning (in the words of T. S. Eliot, perhaps "to know the place for the first time"), I do not suggest that in our effort to listen without preemptive knowing we can create a memory- or desire-free state in ourselves, let alone become theory-free, even if we were to try. Nor should we. We may still prefer the blackbird's inflections to its innuendoes, its whistling to just after. There still may be thirteen ways of looking. We will always draw on theories we espouse, agendas, inferences, preferences we hold, simply our ways of seeing the world. It cannot be otherwise. But that doesn't change the fact that the patient may respond to those ways, may inform us with his own cues (as a look away) about our "desire"—which may have been unknown to himself as well as to us—and about its impact, if we grapple with what I believe to be a fundamental psychoanalytic, philosophical, and scientific notion: that our inferences are only ours—hypotheses, our preferences, just that—ours. Theory can be used to broaden our scope or to narrow it. It can take on a capital T in moments of helplessness or heightened uncertainty, perhaps a need to bring order to what may feel disordered, or to keep distance. I am advocating this ongoing struggle, to bear the "vulnerability" which the philosopher-psychoanalyst Corradi Fiumara (1990) has described, the "real humility" of which Davies speaks, the "open heart" to which Mr. L referred, and gain the closeness and pleasure to learn of such moments. We will hear more nuance (as will our patient), find our own resonance more deeply, as we go beyond our presupposed paths.

In a piece in *The New Yorker,* "The Mind's Eye: What the Blind See," Oliver Sacks (2003) tells of a blind woman traveling with companions who could see. "Sighted people enjoy traveling with me," she said. "I ask them questions, then they look, and see things they wouldn't otherwise. Too often people with sight don't see anything! It's a reciprocal process—we enrich each other's worlds" (p. 55).

I believe that in our struggle to listen, we can enrich each other's worlds.

REFERENCES

Apel D: Memory Effects: The Holocaust and the Art of Secondary Witnessing. New Brunswick, NJ, Rutgers University Press, 2002

Blum HP: Repression, transference, and reconstruction. Int J Psychoanal 84:497–503, 2003a

Blum HP: Response to Peter Fonagy. Int J Psychoanal 84:509–513, 2003b

Breuer J, Freud S: On the psychical mechanism of hysterical phenomena: preliminary communication (1893), in The Standard Edition of the Complete Psychological Works of Sigmund Freud, Vol 2. Translated and edited by Strachey J. London, Hogarth Press, 1955, pp 3–17

Busch F: Rethinking Clinical Technique. Northvale, NJ, Jason Aronson, 1999

Busch F: Back to the future. Psychoanal Q 72:201–215, 2003a

Busch F: Telling stories. J Am Psychoanal Assoc 51:25–42, 2003b

Corradi Fiumara G: The Other Side of Language: A Philosophy of Listening. London, Routledge, 1990

Davies R: The Manticore (1972). New York, Penguin, 1976

Davis JT: Revising psychoanalytic interpretations of the past: an examination of declarative and non-declarative memory processes. Int J Psychoanal 82:449–462, 2001

Doi T: The concept of *amae* and its psychoanalytic implications. Int J Psychoanal 16:349–354, 1989

Doi T: *Amae* and transference love, in On Freud's "Observations on Transference-love." Edited by Person E, Hagelin A, Fonagy P. New Haven, CT, Yale University Press, 1993, pp 165–171

Edelman GM: Interview by Edward Rothstein. New York Times, March 27, 2004

Fonagy P: Memory and therapeutic action. Int J Psychoanal 80:215–223, 1999

Fonagy P: Rejoinder to Harold Blum. Int J Psychoanal 84:503–509, 2003

Gray P: The Ego and Analysis of Defense. Northvale, NJ, Jason Aronson, 1994

Isakower O: Preliminary thoughts on the analysing instrument (1957). J Clin Psychoanal 1:184–194, 1992

Kundera M: Afterword: a talk with the author, by Philip Roth, in The Book of Laughter and Forgetting. New York, Penguin, 1980, pp 229–237

Lipton E: Irrepressible. artjournal, Summer 2003, pp 100–102

Luria AR: The Man With a Shattered World (1972). Cambridge, MA, Harvard University Press, 1987

Sacks O: Foreword, in The Man with a Shattered World, by Luria AR. Cambridge, MA, Harvard University Press, 1987, pp vii–xviii

Sacks O: The mind's eye: what the blind see. The New Yorker, July 28, 2003, pp 48–59

Schindelheim J: Learning to learn, learning to teach. Psychoanalytic Inquiry 15:153–168, 1995

Schwaber EA: Countertransference: the analyst's retreat from the patient's vantage point. Int J Psychoanal 73:349–361, 1992a

Schwaber EA: Psychoanalytic theory and its relation to clinical work. J Am Psychoanal Assoc 40:1039–1057, 1992b

Schwaber EA: The psychoanalyst's mind: from listening to interpretation: a clinical report. Int J Psychoanal 76:271–281, 1995a

Schwaber EA: Toward a definition of the term and concept of interaction. Int J Psychoanal 76:557–564, 1995b

Schwaber EA: The conceptualization and communication of clinical facts in psychoanalysis: a discussion. Int J Psychoanal 77:235–253, 1996

Schwaber EA: The non-verbal dimension in psychoanalysis: "state" and its clinical vicissitudes. Int J Psychoanal 79:667–679, 1998

Silverman K: The Threshold of the Visible World. New York, Routledge, 1996

Stein MH: Self-observation, reality, and the superego, in Psychoanalysis: A General Psychology. Essays in Honor of Heinz Hartmann. Edited by Loewenstein RM, Newman LM, Schur M, Solnit AJ. New York, International Universities Press, 1966, pp 275–297

Stern DN, Sander LW, Nahum JP, Harrison AM, Lyons-Ruth K, Morgan AC, Bruschweiler-Stern N, Tronick EZ: Non-interpretive mechanisms in psychoanalytic therapy: the something more than interpretation. Int J Psychoanal 79:903–921, 1998

Valenstein A: On attachment to painful feelings and the negative therapeutic reaction. Psychoanal Study Child 28:365–392, 1973

Vico G: The New Science of Giambattista Vico. Translated by Bergin IG, Fisch MH. Ithaca, NY, Cornell University Press, 1968

26

THEODORE SHAPIRO, M.D.

INTRODUCTION

Theodore Shapiro graduated from Wesleyan University in Middletown, Connecticut, and Cornell University Medical College, New York, and did his residency at Bellevue Hospital Center. Since 1976, he has been Professor of Psychiatry and Director of Child and Adolescent Psychiatry at the Weill Cornell Medical College of New York Presbyterian Hospital. He did his analytic training at the New York Psychoanalytic Institute, where he is a Training and Supervising Analyst. He has throughout his career combined a full-time academic position with research in child disorders and major contributions to psychoanalysis.

To mention but a few of the positions he has held, he has been on the Program Committee of the American Psychoanalytic Association, Chairman of the Committee on Governance of the American Academy of Child and Adolescent Psychiatry, member of the Child Committee of the Group for the Advancement of Psychiatry, and Chair of the Program Committee of the International Psychoanalytic Association.

Dr. Shapiro has been on numerous editorial boards, and he was the Editor of *The Journal of the American Psychoanalytic Association* (*JAPA*) from 1984 to 1993. As Editor, he instituted significant changes in the direction of the journal toward research and innovative ideas. His work has been widely recognized, and some of his awards include the Wolf C. Hulse Memorial Award of the New York Council on Child Psychiatry, Teacher of the Year Award of the Payne Whitney Clinic, Sandor Rado Lecturer, the A.A. Brill Lecture, the Heinz Hartman Memorial

Lecture of the New York Psychoanalytic Institute, and the keynote address of the Boston meeting of the American Psychoanalytic Association. He is the author of more than 200 papers and reviews and the very important book *Clinical Psycholinguistics.*

He has said of himself:

> My initial introduction to psychoanalysis was rather late. It came during my residency in psychiatry, where John Frosch, then editor of *JAPA,* was my teacher. He introduced me to Freud's thought from a historical perspective. I found the excitement of discovery in that approach. Moreover, the discoveries resonated with my own autobiography. The notion of layers of meaning, the process of self-discovery, and the tendency toward self-deception all rang true. Also, my former philosophical preoccupation with the problem of appearance and reality and the way we represent our worlds in symbols and words—the semiotics of it all—took on a new significance, and later I joined Victor Rosen in the New York Psychoanalytic Institute's Linguistic Study Group, which I later had the pleasure to shepherd until it died. That experience permitted me to write and publish a now out-of-print book, *Clinical Psycholinguistics,* which I still use to teach a course in psychoanalysis and linguistics. Herein lies my claim to a contribution: I tried to introduce my psychoanalytic colleagues to the ferment in linguistics—Chomsky and syntax, Searle and speech acts, Saussure and semiotics.
>
> I thought that Freud's major contribution to the science of meaning and the problems of representation in symptoms, dreams, and words overlapped with what linguists were studying in a rather desiccated form, stripped of human affect. Freud's linguistics was also striking and not labeled as such—"The Antithetical Meaning of Primal Words," "On Negation," "The Psychopathology of Everyday Life," "Screen Memories," etc. The need for a cross-disciplinary foray seemed warranted because it would update our thinking and our theories and also it might offer a new route to Freudian rationalism rather than Lacan's remystification, which had taken hold in so many quarters. I produced a series of papers on linguistic themes ranging from an explication of the role of naming in our treatments (Shapiro 1970) to a more recent discussion of the role of language as a modulator in the development of ego control and civility from kindergarten to negotiating a contract (Shapiro 2004).
>
> Another passion has been development of the mind and the mediating role of language. The forms of fantasy, pre- and unconscious, that become possible with the development of inner speech are many. Freud's catalog of what Erikson coyly named "the tragedies and comedies that occur about the body orifices" can be better understood from the vantage of developmental achievements in linguistic competence. Thus I believed strongly that our view of development had to be infused with more knowledge about how we represent conflicts and pain and defense progressively through the life cycle and how we fall into neuroses because we are stuck in a developmental warp, because we were once helpless and dependent.

So, to summarize, I hope I have brought a developmental and modern view of language and symbolic function to psychoanalysis. I cannot omit the vital and significant privilege of editing JAPA for 10 years as a significant contribution. In that role I tried my best to encourage a broader array of ideas to flourish in a free community of scholarly exchange. The psychoanalytic community responded with an expanded array of writings for peer review. If I can offer a somewhat grandiose finale to the things I believe I contributed, it was to open our field up to a wider interaction with border disciplines and to publish empirical research related to our field. I tried to maintain a focus on psychoanalysis as a science of understanding the self, the mind, and its symbolic propensities that needs our professional aid as demystifiers and interpreters.

WHY I CHOSE THIS PAPER

Theodore Shapiro, M.D.

Having first published "On Reminiscences" in 1993, I am pleasantly surprised and also chagrined that the issues that I addressed then remain relevant to our current psychoanalytic preoccupations. The surprise stems from the fact that my recent writings are a continuation of the themes I addressed then, and the chagrin concerns the fear of stagnation. Have we been mired in themes that represent too little forward movement?

The continuities in my thought indicate an interest in integration among disciplines. I continue to write about the interplay between linguistics and neuroscience in relation to psychoanalysis. This paper is replete with references to past presentations and later expositions. Concerns with interpretation and naming (and with mastery) are in a direct line from a paper with that title (Shapiro 1970). The relative relationship between memory and meaning as a bridge to the neurosciences is clearly in play and has been expanded in a recent paper, "Use Your Words!" (Shapiro 2004). Similarly, I continue to be suspicious of the hermeneutic stance and the two-person psychology position, and in favor of maintaining a modicum of objectivity. These themes persist in my understanding of what psychoanalysis is today and what it was when Freud introduced the idea. I paraphrase Whitehead, referring to Plato, by saying that psychoanalysis is a series of footnotes to Freud. I clearly do not mean that we accept all that he wrote. Instead, I contend that the scope of his work should be encompassed in this postmodern world rather than diminished and narrowed only to the therapeutic encounter in its various forms. More study of the "science" is required, rather than a romanticizing of our work as an art or a creative activity. Freud sought to demystify common events—I frown on remystification.

I fear that we face stagnation and diminished progress because, in my belief, the hermeneutic turn and the constructivist and two-person psychology approaches are too narrow and restrict theory building. They prolong our discourse in "the particular" and "the performative" aspects of the analytic session, leading to a heterologous series of records of analyses without expanding theory. This has taken root in a world in which some continue to try to study, analyze, and understand the therapeutic process and the tropes the human mind uses to construct narratives based on unconscious constellations that lead to human repetition and distress.

On a rereading, this paper strikingly sums up my thoughts on the potential breadth of the Freudian enterprise. I hope it is a stimulus to forward looking. It indicates that psychoanalysts could be inclusive, considering the body and the mind, the drives and the role of remembering, the developmental origins of thought and patterned interactions, the objective study of the subjective mental constellations, and, most psychoanalytically salient, the unconscious determinants of behavior.

REFERENCES

Shapiro T: Interpretation and naming. J Am Psychoanal Assoc 18:399–421, 1970

Shapiro T: Use your words! J Am Psychoanal Assoc 52:331–353, 2004

ON REMINISCENCES

THEODORE SHAPIRO, M.D.

FREUD'S EARLIEST FORMULATION ABOUT psychoneuroses was, "Hysterics suffer mainly from reminiscences" (Breuer and Freud 1895, p. 7). This notion soon became the shibboleth for all neuroses. He could as well have said that neurotics suffer from difficulties in remembering, or from repression or motivated forgetting. All of these represent two sides of the same coin (Erdelyi 1990), but he specifically focused on reminiscences because he believed in the traumatic effect of certain early experiences and because he believed his patients' tales about episodes of sexual assault that reached back into middle childhood—no earlier than 8 years of age in the cases cited in *Studies on Hysteria* (Breuer and Freud 1895).

Psychoanalysis, since that time, has taken a turn that might be paraphrased in parallel form—that *neurotics suffer from narratives.* It is said that these narratives do not permit us to reach for reminiscences as etiologic agents. Those who espouse this view recommend instead an approach to analysis that has been compared to interpretations of texts (Spence 1982, 1987, 1988). Schafer (1988) writes: "interpretation of texts, especially Freud's texts, is interminable. Readings of written texts are necessarily interpretive, and the same applies to what can be called readings of texts patients present verbally and nonverbally in the course of analysis" (p. 296). This view has contributed to the shift in the

---

Presented on April 2, 1991, as the Rado Lecture of the Columbia Psychoanalytic Clinic, New York, and on April 5, 1991, as the Prager Lecture of George Washington University, Washington, DC.

focus to the here-and-now relational frame between analyst and patient. I shall argue that to simply nod to this or similar hermeneutic formulations without reconsidering issues of *how we remember* is not only unwise, but renders our existing theories and models of mind useless, and will, if logically and consistently applied, lead to the abandonment of certain key concepts which I believe hold psychoanalytic theory together. While we may remember imperfectly, we do remember. I shall argue that the psychoanalytic dependence on concepts of repression, defense, splitting, transference, and construction are in fact logically irrelevant in a hermeneutic scheme, and also that recent nonpsychoanalytic advances in understanding of the role of memory in the human mind and brain are relevant to psychoanalysis. But first I shall follow a path of inquiry about Freud's discoveries as they apply, and then reach for the larger issues.

Freud listened to his patients' tales about seductions, but also recorded an early graphic note about a hypnotized patient in his autobiography in 1925: "As she woke up on one occasion, she threw her arms around my neck. The unexpected entrance of a servant relieved us from a painful discussion, but from that time onwards there was a tacit understanding between us that the hypnotic treatment should be discontinued. *I was modest enough not to attribute the event to my irresistible personal attraction, and I felt that I had now grasped the nature of the mysterious element that was at work behind hypnotism*" (Freud 1925, p. 27; italics added). The moment he asserted, "this has little to do with me," Freud opened the door to a new view of a treatment variable that would ultimately evolve into the concept of transference (G. Makari, 1991, unpublished). Earlier in that same paragraph, Freud noted, "the personal emotional relation between doctor and patient was after all stronger than the whole cathartic process, and it was precisely that factor which escaped every effort at control." Thus, actions performed in the present became *current empirical reference points derived from prior relationships.* Current interactions became emblematic of how patients present their past experiences with others. Experiences described in *Studies on Hysteria* include dissociation of affect, giving up hypnotic suggestion for voluntary expanded narratives, and the invocation of repression or motivated forgetting as a way of keeping unpleasant past events or ideas defensively away. Thus, forgetting was dynamically motivated.

Over the next years, with the establishment of the concept of psychic reality and growing attention to the intrapsychic variables of thought formation, Freud began to narrow his field of interest, and his theories were correspondingly directed to *the way the mind works.* He developed a series of models to illuminate pathology, and then normality as well, that included the proposition that childhood was important to adulthood, that the ills of adulthood ranging from perversion through foreplay to neurosis were all related to polymorphous perverse infantile sexuality and the reformulation of experience under the sway of the Oedipus complex. That is, the early stages of wish formation came to be structured around the loving and hating attitudes around the two initial caretakers. and mental operations and fantasies were well structured by nuclear conflict resolution (Shapiro 1977, 1986). These structures in turn occupy a central role in the enactments in transference and recovery of memory as derived from the free-associational process. Thus, Freud posited universal tendencies that were more or less influenced by actuality. Clearly there was not a one-to-one correspondence between stimulus and response, past and present, memory and recall. What we analyze is current experience in terms of the past. We describe the anachronistic intrusions of structured past experiences on current problems, and we point to the prestructured behavior as the basis of current attitudes, behaviors, and conflicts. We study the symbolic representations and transformations of intentions, wishes, and drive components as they conflictedly enter and color surface behavior under the sway of mental agencies. As Anna Freud (1936) noted, we never see the drives in their pure form; we only see their derivatives as filtered through the ego. Later she added that we do not study events, but repercussion of events on the mind.

Insofar as we are doomed by the empirical limitations of our senses to observe surface behavior, it is certainly plausible and possible to derive any variety of theory that would account for the various experiences and interactions, but in order to maintain a coherent and usable theory, we have to posit a small number of deeper memorial organizations which are transformed and amply describe the substructures of surface behaviors. This model links us to other twentieth-century schools of structural thought (Shapiro 1991). Ego psychology depends on the experiential past to account for that which is idiosyncratic and unique in the meaning of behavior, as well as the universals. The distinction used in anthropology between the ideographic and nomothetic clearly coheres with this idea (Barratt 1990). Spence (1986) also calls for moving from the specific (idiographic) to the general (nomothetic) in his argument that we must present our data in a manner that is logical and not rhetorical, so that others may be "independently convinced" (p. 20). At a conference on remembering, he offered: "Subtle transformations in the 'repeated' memory may allow for the emergence of new material" (p. 320), and later, "Memory [in computers] is unchanging... and uninfluenced by use. That clearly is not the way human memory is organized" (p. 321). At that same conference. Fivush (1988) stated, regarding autobiographical memories: "[It] is not simply memories of previously experienced events: it is memory of the self engaging in these activities" (p. 277). Moreover, object-relations theory is highly dependent on how the past is rerendered by the mind in accord with the interactions between wishes arising during development of infants interacting with their parents. Even Spence, and others too, within and outside of psychoanalysis show continuing interest in the past. Nonetheless, by arguing from the extremes of any position, we can tease apart the themes that add to our knowledge and discard those notions that prevent progress or create confusion.

Curiously, while some ferment still exists in academic psychology regarding memory studies, the last 15 or 20 years of psychoanalysis has seen a major shift in focus away from these prior considerations of how we remember. Instead of continuous reworking of the theory of the mind, we currently seem to be focusing on technical issues about the process of understanding patients. This shift has been instructive and in many ways revitalizing, because we had become too involved in small-minded metapsychological issues. These recent technical concerns have led to analysts becoming interested in interactional and process variables that include the countertransference-transference continuum (Jacobs 1986); analyst-patient fit (Kantrowitz et al. 1989); and recasting of the meaning of neutrality formerly seen as an inappropriate imposition of positivistic science (Hoffer 1985; Shapiro 1984). The unique vantage point of the analyst who observes with rapt empathic attention, and finally, explorations of the way in which hermeneutic or interpretive procedures apply to analysis as they do to texts cover our journal pages (see Schafer 1985; Spence 1982, 1986). The general shift in attention is to the narratives that patients tell in the here and now. The encouragement to listen in order to perceive the current, psychic reality is expressed in Schwaber's (1983) rendering of the road to discovery. Gray's (1992) close appraisal of the surface is an ego-psychological adaptation to this view. The analyst's actions also have become the object of scrutiny because they influence the patient's perceptions (Jacobs 1986). In fairness to the fullness of their positions, Schafer, Schwaber, Gray, and Jacobs are not simply hermeneutic in their view as they acknowledge some capacity to discover the past in the present, but their emphasis is on placing greater import on the here and now. In contrast, we can point to Kohut's (1977) view of how the breaks in empathy in the here and now reveal an almost untransformed past interaction representing a reverse tendency, rendering the present as the past unchanged. This represents a reverse trend from the hermeneutic premise.

Otherwise, there seems to be an ambient despair in the psychoanalytic community concerning our capacity to capture the past. Indeed, Masson's *Assault on Truth* (1984) and *Final Analysis* (1990), though largely ignored by "official psychoanalysis," seem to have driven some even more resistantly to hermeneutic barricades. There was some small response in a panel of the American Psychoanalytic Association in 1985 and certain book reviews as well, but otherwise, most analysts have turned away from consideration of his argumentative assault.

The strong form of the hermeneutic argument asserts there is no possibility of verification of past experience because the analyst is struck in the present with his patient and does not probe into the environment or have access to external documentation about *what happened.* The data are filtered through 20 to 40 years of experience. Freud's archeological metaphor of the potsherd and the reconstructions around it are dismissed as pertaining to analogies to historical truth which bear little congruence to narrative truth (Spence 1982). Even as this stance is espoused by some, psychoanalysis is further prodded and challenged by philosophers of science such as Grunbaum (1985). Because we call psychoanalysis a science, we are challenged to demonstrate the possibility of verification from within. The battle cry has become "internal probity fails!" Hermeneutic scholars are not ruffled by such assaults, since they lay no claim to verifiability: they admit only to multiple readings of texts. They dismiss science in this instance with growl words such as *scientism* and *positivism.* Kohutians return to the nineteenth-century refuge of *Geisteswissenschaft* and empathy as a way to beg off the challenge of how to describe the appropriate scientific vantage of analysis.

Thus far, I have laid out the existing arguments as I see them, and reiterated that if we accept the hermeneutic view unexamined, we certainly will also have to accept that we no longer suffer from reminiscences, but rather from narratives, and that we are at risk because the narratives seem so arbitrary since they obey gestaltist-like rules of closure and parsimony which only create coherent stories designed to persuade as if there were no memory, no reminiscence, no traumas, no actual past, no primary maternal bosom or cradle experience, no rage at siblings, no childhood and no polymorphous perverse infantile paradise to rediscover. Concepts such as transference lose their meaning since this idea has no referential significance without accepting that something is transferred, falsely connected, displaced, misapplied to a current circumstance that belongs to attitudes and stances toward earlier objects and memories. These are the metaphors of current reference. Moreover, the attribution of polymorphous perverse infantile sexuality invoked to explain perversion, neurosis, and foreplay (Freud 1905) has little significance in helping us to understand the diverse practices available for man's sexual activity or for that matter to the ubiquitous repugnance toward some of these activities. In addition, the developmental and genetic notions of psychoanalysis should probably pass in the wind as useless, archaic formulations fit for the history shelves as dusty curiosities from an earlier time. While we explore these ideas intramurally, explorers in other sciences are making much of memory and reminiscence in causal proposals. Some psychoanalytic thinkers (Edelson 1985) also are trying to salvage causal propositions for psychoanalysts. Let me catalogue but a few of the nonpsychoanalytic trends that run counter to the antimemory tendencies indicated:

Psychiatry has recently revived post-traumatic stress disorder as an observable entity deriving from verified stressors in the real world. The idea of stress psychology is so central to our modern thought because there are psychophysiological biologically based responses to such states and there is epidemiological evidence that stress is associated with falling ill. Terr (1991) shows prospectively that observed trauma in childhood leads to play which is easily recognized years later as representational of the traumatic events. She even anecdotally records external evidence of an early sexual trauma from the preverbal period being represented in later life. Her frame of reference is clearly psychoanalytic. Pynoos and others (Nader et al. 1990) have managed to show a dose response curve with respect to traumatic effect. Children who were closer to the traumatic event of a sniper peppering a schoolyard with bullets, killing some peers, experienced guilt and other posttraumatic effects. Friendship with the children killed added to strain for those who were not at school. They too experienced guilt. Similarly, Holocaust survivors attest to the role of memory in later suffering (Moskovitz 1985). How can we not attend to these discoveries, especially since it was a prehermeneutic psychoanalytic model that has given rise to the propositions that led to the studies.

Developmental psychologists (Bretherton et al. 1990; M.J. Ward et al. 1990, unpublished) learned that the strange situation paradigm measuring security of attachment employed between 12 and 18 months could be well predicted by taking careful histories from the mother even before the children were born. The agreement has been so good prospectively that developmental psychologists now look retrospectively at adult women subjects' structured narratives relating to their early experience with their mothers, and use the derived results of this careful inquiry with mother to measure the early security of attachment (Main et al. 1985). This is a further extension of Bowlby's (1969) idea that we deal with our children in terms of "working models" of mother-infant interaction, and that these models can be verified in life. Thus, again we are treated to a hypothesis that it may be sufficient to work with or examine a psychological content rather than an external behavior because they are so well correlated.

Primate deprivation research (Suomi et al. 1972), similarly, attests to the effect of early life experience on later behavior. Lack of mothering in young chimps does not have the same effect as in geese following the ethologist Konrad Z. Lorenz because he was seen first. Rather, we see effects at the distance over time with a shift from the specific domain of insult. Isolated or poorly mothered male chimps are later not able to perform mounting postures when sexual contact is prompted by female chimps in estrous. Indeed, we would have no immunology, molecular biology, or genetics, but for concepts analogous to memory as organized in biological systems. In fact, we are stamped by most insistent systems of memory, lock-and-key, by the arrangements of nuclear peptides in DNA molecules. Moreover, Kandel and his coworkers (1979) have shown specific permanent biochemical changes in the nerve endings of sea slugs by virtue of introduction of actual external stimuli.

All of these propositions lead to causal statements that can be studied scientifically, while at the same time, we back off at the accusations of "no probity from within" and embed ourselves in questions of technique and a misapplied version of deconstructionism. I believe that the recent indulgence in studying technique stems in part from disappointment with our ability to elaborate propositions that would be useful in the scientific realm. We seem to be shrinking from our responsibilities rather than accepting them as challenges.

My particular rationale for considering this area arises from prior studies of the abiding effect of language on human experience, and the proposal that we must understand the formative role of language in both theory building and interpreting. If we do so we may track, predict, and apprehend the symbolic exchange between patient and analyst in a manner that may even provide a better understanding of how the mind works. How that exchange permits inclusion of the past as an essential element in current behavior remains as crucial to us as it was to Freud. What the analyst does when he designates or interprets has been very much in the minds of analysts as a factor that fosters change during treatment. I used a language framework when I suggested that an interpretation is an act of naming (Shapiro 1970). The essential notion is that unconscious fantasies are placed in the realm of ego control by turning them into language. We *discover* by naming, and at the same time, we mimic a developmental process that teases apart wishes from the past and their derivatives in current form when we designate the enemy as an unconscious conflictual pattern. It also helps us to understand the presumed displacements to current issues from earlier objects and earlier events.

I toyed with the notion that naming may be creating, but would like to disavow that now, although it is an idea that has been taken up by others more seriously in recent years. For example, Schafer (1977) has written that every interpretation is a new creation since what is being interpreted and said may never have been said in words: "interpretation creates new meanings or new actions" (p. 419). Spence (1982) takes a rather bold contrary step by suggesting that the process of verbalization distorts experience by being expressed. This seems to me to foster an antirational notion that experience is unrepresentable. These assertions permit us to avoid the problem of probity, as Grunbaum (1985) suggests. Namely, we increasingly emphasize the intrapsychic, the method and technique of extracting ideas, and show decreasing interest in determining that what we do bears any relation to the effect of past events on the mind's later representations. Grossman and Stewart (1976) wrote about how we can go wrong in the interpretive process if we treat our formulations as "theoretical clichés" (p. 210). They entreat that interpretations must permit patients to use language as references to experience—they note, "It [interpretation of penis envy] is incorrect as a clinical interpretation because it forces a theoretical impersonal form onto the material" (p. 210). They encourage, instead, a personalized referential system to raise verbal proposals to conviction. This is but one instance of language distorting, but it is surely ill-thought usage and careless jargon that leads to distortion. Having teased apart some of these matters, let us look to Freud for a moment with respect to his position on how the mind integrates memories.

I propose that, from the outset, Freud understood and believed in narrative formation as a feature of memory, but not at the expense of actuality. As early as 1899, in his paper on "Screen Memories," he proposed that there were two species of memory (Freud 1899). He quoted a paper by V. and C. Henri (1897) that indicated that vivid memories were not simply the recovery of facts of the historical past, but they were constructed and reconstructed repeatedly during life in order to signify a composite of events that had become meaningful to the individual. The Henris' discovery that there are continuous and isolated early memories parallels other contemporary ideas as well. For example, William James stated: "All human thinking is essentially of two kinds—reasoning on the one hand, and narrative, descriptive, contemplative thinking on the other—that is to say only what every reader's experience will corroborate" (quoted by Bruner [1986]). Freud cited Jessen (1855) in *The Interpretation of Dreams:* "Total forgetfulness is not serious: but partial forgetfulness is treacherous. For if we then proceed to give an account of what we have forgotten, we are liable to fill in from our imagination the incoherent and disjointed fragments furnished by memory.... We unwillingly become creative artists" (Freud 1900, p. 47n). These fragments within analysis have special significance. Freud used the metaphor of the sham that lies near the gold in order to indicate that what we remember in screen memories, for example, are only signifiers of something "much deeper," more meaningful and potentially much more painful. Indeed, the need to hide arises because of the anticipated pain of direct expression. And he discussed these as "works of fiction" which made one wonder about their genuineness. He ends his 1899 tract with the idea that we have memories *about*, not *from* childhood.

Toward the end of his life, Freud (1937) approached the issue of reconstruction. He indicated that the analyst as a reconstructor is only using small bits of data in order to build a story around which a patient organizes experience of the world. Thus, from the beginning of his career to the end, he shared much with the "psychological constructivists." He did not believe wholeheartedly in the truth of events as remembered, or in their simple isomorphic representation of the past. Nor did he continue to espouse actual traumas the sole etiology of hysteria. Kris (1962) in his classic paper on "The Recovery of Childhood Memories," notes, "the model of hysteria had lost its paramount importance [p. 55].... We are misled if we believe that we are, except in rare instances, able to find 'the events' of the afternoon on the staircase where the seduction happened" (p. 73). Arlow (1969) writes, "This constant intermingling of fantasy and perception helps make it clear why memory is so unreliable, especially memories from childhood" (p. 37). Blum (1980) writes, "Analysts would no longer be seduced by memories" (p. 40). At the academic Conference on Autobiographical Memory cited earlier, Neisser (Neisser and Winograd 1988) spoke about the conference as it would be remembered later.

> The events I have been considering are (or were) all real. They are not figments of my imagination, or yours; they are not hypothetical constructs or intervening variables; they are not codes or mental representations or schemata or scripts. In describing them, I am referring to something that actually happened. Of course, my description is not the only one possible: different people may see the same situation quite differently....
>
> [W]e perceive and remember events at many levels of analysis. We remember conferences, talks, and sentences: lasting personal relationships, special evenings, and pregnant moments; graduate school years,

> particular seminars, memorable remarks. The organization of autobiographical memory evidently parallels the hierarchical organization of the remembered events themselves. (p. 363)

And yet, Spence and others consider Freud and his followers to have been in error arguing that they used narrative truth as though it were historical truth. Why this particular misreading of Freud and mainstream ego psychologists by those who suggest that the only truth is in a reading? Perhaps some are belaboring the earliest hysteria model of recovered events blindly. I think that insofar as they do, they also are likely to use the concept object as though it were a person, and to concretize the psychoanalytic process as though the dyad of analyst and analysand do not work together in the inquiry. Certainly Masson has damned us for not listening enough for the truth of events as reported—that in turn would be akin to a mindless return to the psychology of sensation, as though perception were not a complex organizing enterprise.

It is a failing in our critiques of each other that we pick the worst of our theories and use them as the norm, turning them into whipping boys for our own, sometime new, ideas. I tend toward the same error, for I think this pendular sway to the here and now and the real interaction have been oversold as the significant determinants of behavior. This warrants as strong an argument as can he mustered to alert the reader to the other pole. It does, however, provide a defensive response that I address a straw man. If I can turn attention to the strongest form of the hermeneutic position, I can better address its flaws. I must also apologize to those who argue more nuanced and less militant positions. I would like to offer that remembering, repeating, and working through are still the central signposts of our work and in need of renewal and reminder.

Loewald (1986) suggests epigraphically, "the patient instead of having a past is his past." He also invokes stored interactions without stored objects; this has a ring of truth. It has face validity. The question for us as analysts is not whether the past is there, but how the analyst works with what is here in order to discover how the symbolic process over time organizes the earlier experiences. What experiences attain valence and how do we represent our findings to the patient in such manner that he achieves conviction? We assume that the patient represents his past to the analyst in every interaction with the analyst. We could not work if we did not believe this.

It is the use of language and an understanding of that form of symbolic representation of actions that permit us to tease apart *what* in the presentation relates to the past and *how* it is to be integrated in the present. In short, it is naive to expect that the past will rerepresent itself simply—that there has been no experiential mediation between event and theme. As the analyst turns into words that which may never have been spoken, some (Schafer 1977; Stern 1983) suggest that this is a creative moment. They disavow that this is a moment of discovery or *a description* of that which is now understood. If what the analyst says does not *coincide* with something that is already there to be *described*, then we might as well throw away our claim that we describe anything with our words—we become poets of the couch. The meaning of a symbol is not only embedded in the symbol, but in the symbol maker, and involves understanding how the symbol is used. The vehicle of presentation, however, may be in an enactment in the transference or in what recent philosophers of language describe as *performatives* (Austin 1962) or speech acts (Searle 1969). These in turn are related to what the new cognitive psychologists designate as procedural memories instead of declarative memories (Clyman 1991). We not only remember in words, do things with words—we perform acts and create interactions that have an effect beyond the meaning of what we have to say. There is an intention that gives force to the acts as well as the words. The intention may be to seduce or to convince, but it may also be to inform, and informing encompasses describing. These are types of naming.

Even prior to these newer formal conceptions, the developmental psychologist Carl Buehler suggested that the appeal comes to supersede the expressive function of language. Loewenstein (1956), referring to psychoanalysis, wrote that ultimately the appeal gives way to the propositional function as a mature form of informing. It is the job of the analyst to discover the rules of how memories are embedded in the discourse. As such, remembering is structured by categorical verbal usage, by classes of interactions, by words and by performatives. They are turned from idiosyncratic personal systems to generalized verbal descriptions (from ideographic to nomothetic propositions—from etic to emic forms).

Each time we listen we also look for redundant themes. Thematic categories become more important than surface particulars. In play therapy, the child patient "tells" us using cars, using crayons, using clay. The same story is expressed in different communicative vehicles, but they pertain to the same category of reference. They signify something that demands expression that is there beyond the vehicle of representation. Similarly, classes of interaction apply to repetitious remembered habitual past interactions with a person. The patient in a resistant phase who uses every excuse not to come, will also use every excuse not to say, or every excuse to be obtuse or chatter on, indifferent to the communicative function of words. The passive patient may leave all the work for the analyst—may not make any formulations himself, may obey the rule of free association as though there were no observing ego, and does not change in the least.

Remembering in words is just one specie of remembering. Even Freud reminds us of that. The words used, while they have a common code designation, also have an idiosyncratic significance as they refer to more personal experiences and usage. I have noted that among the various words for excrement, some are stronger as elicitors of affects such as shock or disgust, just as baby words used for feces could bring a blush to anyone's cheeks. Just think of your affective response as you say aloud publicly: excrement, stool, shit, poop, doodoo.

And then finally, among the performatives, there is the forcefulness of words as actions. The meaning of the word is not only in what the word itself means, but in the context of expression, where words do things. The bride saying "I do" performs an act of union (Austin 1962). A patient saying "I had the thought that" is not only isolating thought from himself, but performing an act for the analyst suggesting that he is embarrassed to lay claim to those thoughts. "I see red" may describe an observation, but, "Each time he speaks I see red" evokes a new meaning because of the new verbal context.

The context of an analysis is unique, but it is also in a continuum with other dialogues from the past. It is a two-person circumstance with special features that permits the individual not to focus so much on the responsiveness of the analyst. It is a dialogue in which patients can project the inquiry and the interaction onto the analyst. Freud (1915) suggested that the rhetorical force of the development of love is the context in which interpretations are accepted. He recognized that this is seductive to truth. Those feelings—and their illocutionary force—can distort the degree to which the patient accepts what the analyst says. But if that is all there is, and no rational remembering is elicited, it seems to me that an analysis would ultimately falter and be hobbled, because it would remain too distant from the influences of the patient's past experiences, and the patient's assent would serve only as a surrender to a powerful guru. Freud said, when the young woman threw her arms around his neck, he could not assume he had an "irresistible personal attraction." Surely, we do not intend to be so seductive. Surely our training is designed to diminish some of the narcissism that revels only in admiration. Surely the pain involved in the analytic procedure must have some hope of greater truth than an unrequited love affair with a shrink. Moreover, we are aware of those regressive pulls and are cautious to bring our patients back to reality. Freud gave up hypnosis on those grounds. Screen memories certainly are an example of distorted memories that constitute constructed narratives. With great conviction, the patient retells the remembered, often vivid, story and then proceeds to learn by elemental association that what he thought was true is only true in the sense that the memory is constructed to represent an unconscious fantasy.

The patient says, "Aha," "That fits...." "That makes sense." The memory begins to lose its poignancy as specified, and even the patient begins to lose his conviction that it all happened the way in which he had thought it happened. In order to disavow there has to be a reciprocal alternative avowal that has been discovered for reason's sake.

The conflation of rigid categories is reordered, and disparate associations fall into new places that make better sense to the observing ego. Some of these ideas could be illuminated by case material so that the context of discovery could be discussed and the process of how the recovery of memories would become explicit as we examine the idiom of presentation. Psychoanalysis has added a motivational hitch to simple storage models. Although we tacitly use the same episodic, semantic, or procedural declarative niches of academic psychology, we believe that patients rearrange nature in accord with motives, just as perception depends on prior experience. Memory, again, is not simply like sensation, i.e., passive reception—a camera, a tape recorder.

This is a case that was partially exploited in another presentation (Shapiro 1974). I shall use it to explore the significance of the patient's representations and interactions in order to determine the effect of past on present: it seems much like other cases, but it provides a clue to a transferential experience that helped illuminate *a false memory,* and aided the patient to access a bit of historic storage that was isolated and possibly repressed, and then presented with current distortions. Notice I write false memory, as though I know the true memory. This knowledge derives from the improbability of the stated memory. The case also reveals that the analyst is always working with the stuff of the past. If not, our work would be of another sort.

> A man in his late twenties sought treatment because of difficulties in settling down in a relationship, chronic depression, and low self-esteem. He had recently broken a relationship with a woman that had lasted for some years, because he could not commit himself to marriage. He reported a vivid memory from early childhood a number of times. He was standing in the back yard with three or four boys and one girl, designated as Cindy, who was a "bad girl." They were all urinating over a fence, and Cindy beat the boys in the distance of her stream. This reported contest was not doubted as to the possibility of its occurrence. It

was a memory indeed, a vivid memory as far as our patient was concerned. It was attributed to the fourth year of his life. Perhaps, not surprisingly to an analytic audience, this man had an abiding anxiety about impotence; he reported, as well, multiple dreams and fantasies of phallic women. The latter, too, we recognize as constructs, since hermaphroditism is a rare occurrence and rarely observed by 4-year-olds. We are always making judgments about the truth of statements. Thus, we are always testing our patients' reports for truth against known standards.

Some years into the analysis, the patient related a fantasy. I had told him that I was about to go away for a brief period of time. Knowing that I was affiliated with a university, he created a mental situation in which he could undo his feelings of dependency and inequality and growing gratitude. He had the fantasy that I was to go to a hospital as a consultant, and that I was to be a discussant at a Grand Rounds, which experience he knew about from an early hospitalization. He would help me. He associated to an event designated as a memory. When he was 12 years old, he was in a hospital for observation, and ultimately was subjected to surgery. He was wheeled before a group for presentation. He was frightened. No one examined him, but he remembered a cold and ugly atmosphere; he felt humiliated by the exposure to the onlookers—a group of physicians. He then reported a current image of his girlfriend, squatting on a tile bathroom floor, partially clothed. The tile reminded him of children on the ward in the hospital where he was a patient. He then recalled a girl squatting on a bedpan, but rejected that as uncertain; but there was a burned girl at the far end of the ward whose image became vivid. She had a large curved tin thing over her body, like a tent that prevented covers from touching her burned legs. He quickly had the idea, this time an intrusive fantasy, that she was promiscuous, "She was a wild type—one that you could play doctor with." He remembered always being frightened to do that when invited as a boy. The girl under the tent asked if he would like to see her burns, and she lifted the covers as he peered. He remembered seeing her genitals instead, and only incidentally noted the burns. He felt both revolted and curious. He quickly associated to being reprimanded by the nurse because he was sitting at the edge of the bed of another little girl who had had an appendectomy. He then shifted to the present and thought that his new girlfriend was like all those other dirty little girls. It was a terrible way to describe her, but he realized there was excitement brewing even in the midst of his anxiety, as he remembered and thought anew of the girl who would urinate with the boys. This led back to remembering the "pissing contest" at 4 that had been isolated from its roots of formation years before.

Later on, we were able to confront the issue of the unlikelihood of that memory. For the first time, he could entertain the notion that it was a constructed mental image that embodied and expressed his fear of women. His frequent current impotence was due to anxiety about fantasied castration called up by images of controlling, forceful, and assertive women which derive from even earlier views of his mother and aunt.

Let us return to this brief sequence of analytic work and look for the *memory work* in these representations. Certainly the memory of the little girl beating the boys in a "pissing contest" is incongruous given what we know about the nature of the anatomical differences between the sexes and the capacity for projecting a stream.

The analytic query is why this man needs such a construct. What is its use in the context of his life and in the need to report it to me with such blind faith? The answer may be found, I believe, in the impact of real experience on the immature mind, and in the telescoping of time sequences under the sway of developing mental complexes that utilize new experience in the service of old, well-fused cognitive emotional constellations. This patient's anxieties are redundantly stated in the fact that he has to make up for his sense of defect in his recurrent dreams of phallic women. Or the false memory then could alleviate the anxiety he felt in entertaining the notion that women are not like men, and when they become categorized as manlike in their assertiveness, they frighten. I shall not belabor the contributory relationship to his parents because these data are redundant with the rhetorical need he had to convince me of the dangers he experienced. Historical truth lies in the replay of his experience of an actuality that is restructured to personal purpose. *The external observer may not have seen it as he did. But the external viewer also could not have heard the truth about his experienced world as the analyst did.*

In the current situation of the analysis, he was very eager to come with me to exhibit himself. He looked at accompanying me to the meeting as an opportunity to be my equal. He would show that we was "okay" or better, he and I would be okay together or even that I needed him, and not he, me. The passive-dependent arm of the idea was reversed in the fantasy. He also made up for his apprehension about loss by coming with me. The fantasy further stated he had no warrant to fear being alone and abandoned as I went off. He also might deal with the anger he felt toward me in leaving him by showing me how necessary he was for my performance. Curiously enough, again it is in exhibiting his prowess and his centrality to my being that we see a parallel structure in the complementary pair—woman and phallus, analyst and patient, man and woman, independent hermaphrodite.

We must remember also that there were a number of historically accurate elements in his presentation which somehow reinforced the possibility for the variety of memories he presented. It is unlikely that he concocted the burn tent—it is too close to the reality of devices used in hospitals. It is unlikely that he did not go to the hospital, especially since he bore a scar of the surgery performed. It is likely that he also was presented at Rounds, since his was an unusual case. None of those are important in and of themselves, as historically accurate facts, but they are important insofar as he then incorporated them into a unified narrative that is presented for interpretation of what is being represented.

The transferential moment of my departure, moreover, was no random issue in the recovery of the past. It was a cue to the unconscious; it prodded memory. Mind well, I use the word "represented," not "created." Here Freud has given future generations of analysts a leg up on prior notions about what memory *does* record. Memory records the affectively laden information in codes that analysts must decipher by applying the knowledge gained about transformation of unconscious derivatives in interaction with ego defenses for adaptive purposes. Analysts use words to link the past to the present. They use words also to change enactments into categorical understanding that provides the patient with a verbal grasp of how he uses the past in the present to achieve miscarried aims—how the patient anachronistically replays events that have signifying effects on his current life. This, too, is the stuff of transference. The analysand is in a laboratory of life in the relationship with the analyst. If it is simply a creation of the transference relationship that is to be described, and it has no relation to the past, or better, if the past has no role in its creation, then what are we analyzing, except the here and now? Again, we suffer from reminiscences, and these are not arbitrary creations of the here and now designed to create coherence.

Edelson (1985) remarks that hermeneutics is characterized by subjectivity, the pursuit of meaning, complexity, and uniqueness. Scientific inquiry, on the other hand, is characterized by objectivity, causal notions, abstraction, and generalization. I believe that the search for truth in representation of the past is not equal to the continuous or repeated rereading of a text that is the hermeneutic objective, because an analysis is not a static event to be interpreted and reinterpreted or deconstructed. An analysis employs a means by which a patient can reiterate the significant constellations of his psychological organization in symbolic representations that the analyst then discovers and puts into words so that they can be used in order to understand the motives for current behavior and later applied to redundant reaction patterns.

Narrative appeal and persuasion have been used to support constructivist elements in memory, but leave out the obvious referential significance of how the past impinges on the present. There is a parsimony in remembering which permits constructs such as Luborsky's (1984) core conflictual relationship constellations, or Kris's (1956) personal myth. These are the deep structures that dictate behavior and thought in the individual, and these are the elements to be uncovered in the analysis. They prestructure behavior. They have causal impact as well, because these elements are drawn from meaningful past impingements that fuel current behavior.

We know from the social psychologists that nobody "tells it like it happened." It is only in the telling that we discover something about the referential system of the teller. Were it not that he experiences events in a unique and repetitious way, there would not be a need for psychoanalysis. We would be closer to a behaviorist's construct than a human being. What we take hold of is the telling and the retelling. The medium of expression does not matter. It is the redundancy of the base referred to, the fantasy defended against, that is represented in many guises.

In my patient, a little girl who can pee further than the boy, dreams about phallic women, anxiety in looking under the tent, problems with impotence, concern about good girls and bad girls, all point insistently to a thoroughgoing problem representing an anxiety that was stimulated when he did not know any better about the safety of his valued sexual organ. Freud (1937) said, in his paper on Constructions, "It might have happened." His archeological models, that some take such pleasure in criticizing, involve the idea that what is reconstructed from that sham or sherd must have an imaginative element to it, but what is new in that? That has been bread-and-butter psychoanalysis since 1899.

The need for narrative persuasion comes from a force that is related to the disturbed equilibrium created by memory. We are straining to remember the thing that made us feel so good or so bad. It is like having something on the tips of our tongues. There is indeed a causal link as well as a meaningful link between past experiences and current behavior—but we have not been able to determine prospectively which link makes a difference. Finally, if we can translate some of those causal links into hypotheses to be tested, psychoanalysis would have a place among the sciences rather than become a straw man for those who seek probity or a polysemantic set of readings that varies with the reader or the reader's context.

I hold that there are more and less compelling interpretations, and that the more compelling ones have effect, because they accurately represent in words the way the past was incorporated in the mind. They capture the wishes deriving from childhood that have been recast in the present. Meaningful systems have to be linked to motivational systems if psychoanalysis is to work. Our concepts are embedded not so much in historical truths, and here I agree with Spence (1982), but in the impact of the past on current narratives. Our stories are not made up for the analyst in the immediate sense; they are made up for the patient so that he can have a view of his life that feels reasonable and helps him to grasp his experience. Analysts help patients to discover those truths through the understanding of the symbolic transformations that accrue. If being together is all there is, and analysis of the here-and-now relationship is the only aim, why do we need the analyst? I do not mean that we should again hide behind neutrality, that would be regressive, but I do mean that we should provide the rules by which we transform experience in varying media through which such truths can be discovered.

Freud stimulated a century of intellectual furor around the subjective accretions of remembering. He was first among peers in establishing some scientific bases for notions that only poets had expressed before him. We should not relegate his discoveries to another act of literary criticism before we seriously test and examine the virtues he has provided in systematizing knowledge about *the how of remembering.*

Moreover, every act of representation distorts; so does every line on a graph describing the relation of variable X to Y. Each line is a compromise that obeys the rules of *a priori* analytic mathematical relations, but only approximates nature. Every description in words is once removed from the immediacy of experience. We must remember that words have a referential intersubjective nonmystical purpose. What they signify is embedded in a common human code. If every description of the mental terrain obeys the laws of our scientific generalizations, which include oedipal conflict, unconscious fantasy, defense, transference, then we are operating within a scientific set of constructs with generalizable laws and predictive value that increases our understanding of how the past, as stored, interacts with the present. This is nomothetic; this is discovery of what is there; this is subject to lawful categorization.

Can we say what happened? No! Can we say how what happened was internalized and recreated in the present? Yes, if we use the analytic method to undo the various forms of disavowing repression and motivated forgetting we all are guilty of.

As F. Scott Fitzgerald (1925) wrote in the last lines of *The Great Gatsby,* "So we beat on, boats against the current, borne back ceaselessly into the past."

REFERENCES

Arlow JA: Fantasy, memory, and reality testing. Psychoanal Q 38:28–51, 1969

Austin JL: How to Do Things With Words. New York, Oxford University Press, 1962

Barratt BD: Reawakening the revolution of psychoanalytic method: notes on the human subject, semiosis, and desire. Psychoanalysis and Contemporary Thought 13:139–163, 1990

Blum HP: Reconstruction in adult psychoanalysis. Int J Psychoanal 61:39–52, 1980

Bowlby J: Attachment and Loss, I. Attachment. New York, Basic Books, 1969

Bretherton I, Ridgeway D, Cassidy J: Assessing internal working models of the attachment relationship, in Attachment in the Preschool Years. Edited by Greenberg T, Cichetti D, Cummings EM. Chicago, IL, University of Chicago Press, 1990, pp 273–310

Breuer J, Freud S: Studies on hysteria (1895), in The Standard Edition of the Complete Psychological Works of Sigmund Freud [SE], Vol 2. Translated and edited by Strachey J. London, Hogarth Press, 1955

Bruner J: Actual Minds, Possible Worlds. Cambridge, MA, Harvard University Press, 1986

Clyman RB: The procedural organization of emotions: a contribution from cognitive science to the psychoanalytic theory of therapeutic action. J Am Psychoanal Assoc 39:349–382, 1991

Edelson M: The hermeneutic turn and the single case study in psychoanalysis. Psychoanalysis and Contemporary Thought 8:567–614, 1985

Erdelyi MH: Repression, reconstruction, and defense: history and integration of the psychoanalytic and experimental frameworks, in Repression and Dissociation. Edited by Singer JL. Chicago, IL, University of Chicago Press, 1990

Fitzgerald FS: The Great Gatsby. New York, Scribner's, 1925

Fivush R: The functions of event memory: some comments on Nelson and Barsalou, in Remembering Reconsidered: Ecological and Traditional Approaches to the Study of Memory. Edited by Neisser U, Winograd E. New York, Cambridge University Press, 1988, pp 277–282

Freud A: The Ego and the Mechanisms of Defense (1936). Writings, Vol 2. New York, International Universities Press, 1966

Freud S: Screen memories (1899). SE, 3:301–322, 1962

Freud S: The interpretation of dreams (1900). SE, 4, 5, 1953

Freud S: Three essays on the theory of sexuality (1905). SE, 7:159–168, 1953

Freud S: Observations on transference-love: further recommendations on the technique of psycho-analysis, III (1915). SE, 12:157–173, 1958

Freud S: An autobiographical study (1925). SE, 20, 1959

Freud S: Constructions in analysis (1937). SE, 23:255–269, 1964

Gray P: Memory as resistance, and the telling of a dream. J Am Psychoanal Assoc 40:307–326, 1992

Grossman WI, Stewart WA: Penis envy: from childhood wish to developmental metaphor. J Am Psychoanal Assoc 24(suppl):193–212, 1976

Gronbaum A: The Foundations of Psychoanalysis. Berkeley, University of California Press, 1985

Henri V, Henri C: Enquête sur les premiers souvenirs de l'enfance. L'Année Psychologique 3:184, 1897

Hoffer A: Toward a definition of psychoanalytic neutrality. J Am Psychoanal Assoc 33:771–795, 1985

Jacobs TJ: On countertransference enactments. Psychoanal Q 34:289–307, 1986

Jessen P: Versuch einer wissenschaftichen Begrundung der Psychologie. Berlin, 1855

Kandel E: Psychotherapy and the single synapse. N Engl J Med 300:1028–1037, 1979

Kantrowitz JL, Katz AL, Greenman DA, Morris H, Paolitto F, Sashin J, Solomon L: The patient-analyst match and the outcome of psychoanalysis. J Am Psychoanal Assoc 37:893–920, 1989

Kohut H: The Restoration of the Self. New York, International Universities Press, 1977

Kris E: The personal myth: a problem in psychoanalytic technique. J Am Psychoanal Assoc 4:653–681, 1956

Kris E: The recovery of childhood memories in psychoanalysis. Psychoanal Study Child 9:54–88, 1962

Loewald HW: Transference-countertransference. J Am Psychoanal Assoc 34:275–287, 1986

Loewenstein RM: Some remarks on the role of speech in psychoanalytic technique. Int J Psychoanal 37:460–468, 1956

Luborsky L: Principles of Psychoanalytic Psychotherapy: A Manual for Supportive-Expressive Treatment. New York, Basic Books, 1984

Main M, Kaplan N, Cassidy J: Security in infancy, childhood, and adulthood: a move to the level of representation, in Growing Points in Attachment Theory and Research. Edited by Bretherton I, Waters E. Chicago, IL, University of Chicago Press, 1985, pp 66–106

Masson JM: The Assault on Truth: Freud's Suppression of the Seduction Theory. New York, Penguin, 1984

Masson JM: The Final Analysis: The Making and Unmaking of a Psychoanalyst. New York, Addison-Wesley, 1990

Moskovitz S: Longitudinal followup of child survivors of the Holocaust. J Am Acad Child Psychiatry 24:401–407, 1985

Nader K, Pynoos R, Fairbanks L, Frederick C: Children's PTSD reactions one year after a sniper attack at their school. Am J Psychiatry 147:1526–1530, 1990

Neisser U, Winograd E: Remembering Reconsidered: Ecological and Traditional Approaches to the Study of Memory. New York, Cambridge University Press, 1988

Schafer R: The interpretation of transferences and the conditions for loving. J Am Psychoanal Assoc 25:335–362, 1977

Schafer R: The interpretation of psychic reality, developmental influences, and unconscious communication. J Am Psychoanal Assoc 33:537–554, 1985

Schafer R: Discussion of panel presentations on psychic structure. J Am Psychoanal Assoc 36(suppl):295–311, 1988

Schwaber EA: Psychoanalytic listening and psychic reality. Int J Psychoanal 10:379–392, 1983

Searle JR: Speech Acts: An Essay on Philosophy of Language. New York, Cambridge University Press, 1969

Shapiro T: Interpretation and naming. J Am Psychoanal Assoc 18:399–421, 1970

Shapiro T: Development and distortions of empathy. Psychoanal Q 43:4–25, 1974

Shapiro T: Varieties of oedipal distortions in severe character pathologies: developmental and theoretical considerations. Psychoanal Q 46:559–579, 1977

Shapiro T: On neutrality. J Am Psychoanal Assoc 32:269–282, 1984

Shapiro T: Nuclear conflict and the nuclear self. Psychoanalytic Inquiry 6:349–365, 1986

Shapiro T: Language structure and psychoanalysis. J Am Psychoanal Assoc 36:339–358, 1987

Shapiro T: Language structure and psychoanalysis, in The Concept of Structure in Psychoanalysis. Edited by Shapiro T. Madison, CT, International Universities Press, 1991

Spence DP: Narrative Truth and Historical Truth. New York, WW Norton, 1982

Spence DP: When interpretation masquerades as explanation. J Am Psychoanal Assoc 34:3–22, 1986

Spence DP: The Freudian Metaphor. New York, WW Norton, 1987

Spence DP: Passive remembering, in Remembering Reconsidered: Ecological and Traditional Approaches to the Study of Memory. Edited by Neisser U, Winograd E. New York, Cambridge University Press, 1988, pp 311–325

Stern DB: Unformulated experience: from familiar chaos to creative disorder. Contemporary Psychoanalysis 19:71–99, 1983

Suomi S, Harlow HF, McKinney WT: Monkey psychiatrists. Am J Psychiatry 128:927–932, 1972

Terr LC: Childhood traumas: an outline and an overview. Am J Psychiatry 148:10–20, 1991

27

HENRY F. SMITH, M.D.

INTRODUCTION

Henry F. Smith graduated from Harvard College in Cambridge, Massachusetts, in 1965 and won a coveted Fulbright Scholarship to study playwriting in London with Christopher Fry. After graduating from Harvard Medical School, he went on to do adult and child psychiatry residencies at the Massachusetts Mental Health Center under Elvin Semrad. He followed this with psychoanalytic training at the Psychoanalytic Institute of New England, East (PINE), in Boston, Massachusetts, where he is currently a Supervising and Training Analyst. In his writings and professional projects, Dr. Smith has been a key figure in focusing our systematic attention on the microprocess of the clinical hour. He was the initiator of the Analyst at Work series in *The International Journal of Psychoanalysis* and the 2-day workshops on process and technique at the meetings of the American Psychoanalytic Association.

The author of over 80 articles and book chapters, Dr. Smith is Editor of *The Psychoanalytic Quarterly.* Prior to this he was Associate Editor of *The Journal of the American Psychoanalytic Association* (*JAPA*). He has also served on the editorial boards of *The International Journal of Psychoanalysis, Psychoanalytic Inquiry,* and *The American Psychoanalyst.* A valued teacher, he has held faculty positions at numerous psychoanalytic institutes, as well as at Harvard Medical School. He was the North American Co-Chair of the Program Committee for the 1999 International Psychoanalytical Association Congress in Santiago, Chile, and for many years he has been a member of the Program Committee of the American Psychoanalytic Association.

Dr. Smith's numerous honors include the Felix and Helene Deutsch Prize of the Boston Psychoanalytic Society and Institute and the Journal Prize of *JAPA.* He was invited to give the first David L. Raphling Memorial Lecture at the Washington Psychoanalytic Institute, the Roberta Held Weis Memorial Lecture at the William Alanson White Institute, the Maurice Friend Lecture at the Psychoanalytic Association of New York, the Joseph N. Gurri Lecture at the Florida Psychoanalytic Society, and the 2004 Plenary Presentation to the Annual Meeting of the American Psychoanalytic Association in San Francisco, California.

In terms of his place in American psychoanalysis, Lawrence Friedman, in introducing the 2004 plenary presentation, called Smith

> ...a master phenomenologist, a discoverer of what happens when two minds meet in an analysis: you might say he is the William James of psychoanalytic process.

Dr. Smith himself notes that although most readers identify him as a contemporary conflict theorist, some hear a Kleinian note, others a relational one:

> I think what disturbs people is that I have been arguing that theory and practice are not as closely linked as we like to think, and that, while we need to be very clear about levels of theory and the terminology we use, some theoretical approaches—conflict theory, for one—will accommodate different types of interventions or methods without producing a mindless eclecticism.

WHY I CHOSE THIS PAPER

Henry F. Smith, M.D.

This is an abbreviated version of an article originally published in *JAPA.* I chose this paper, "Countertransference, Conflictual Listening, and the Analytic Object Relationship," as one of a series in which I spell out a fuller role for the analyst's conflicts in both facilitating and impeding analytic work than has generally been heretofore acknowledged. By conflict, I am speaking of the interaction between the analyst's desires or wishes, defenses, self-criticisms, and painful affect. Not only is it potentially harmful to assume that the analyst is free of a full conflictual engagement with the patient, but it is precisely the activation of the analyst's conflicts that allows him or her access to the patient and to a conflictual object relationship with the patient, without which an analysis will forever lie fallow. I see little value in distinguishing between the analyst's conflicts and the analyst's *neurosis,* as that term is currently defined, which is not to say that one expression of conflict is identical with another; only that, if unconscious conflict is considered to be shaping every mental event, making such qualitative distinctions is no longer so simple as it was once, and it may be foolhardy.

In a somewhat loose analogy to signal anxiety I suggest that the analyst's use of his or her conflicts in the service of the analysis might be thought of as a use of *signal conflict,* as long as this is not taken to mean that the analyst can thereby avoid simultaneously putting his or her unconscious conflict into action to one degree or another at all times. At the end of the paper I illustrate one such example of how the analyst's unconscious conflict may be both activated and stabilized during the hour at the same time as its conscious manifestation serves a useful purpose in understanding the patient. I also suggest that everything the analyst does, says, and thinks in the hour is shaped by both the analyst's conflicts and the patient's, and that, as a result, every activity on the analyst's part that moves the analysis forward simultaneously interferes with that progress. This point has been the subject of some debate.

Controversial, too, is my comment to the patient, "Perhaps Dr. Rothman can be your mother." One colleague thought it so offensive an empathic rupture he could barely bring himself to speak with me about it. Another decided that I was "trying to demonstrate how a conflict theorist could behave like an interpersonalist." Still others have found it loving and thought it might qualify for what Daniel Stern and the Boston Change Group have called a "now moment."

However accurate any of these characterizations may be, my purpose in writing this paper was not to advocate a particular technique and certainly not to suggest that the analyst can examine his or her motives *during the hour* as minutely as I do here. Writing is a laborious way to convey the multiple events that take place in every microsecond of a clinical hour. My paper is rather an experimental effort to examine the interactive and what has come to be called the intersubjective aspects of the work through the lens of conflict theory. In addition to contemporary conflict theory being a parsimonious and clinically efficacious tool, it is particularly useful in keeping the analyst honest about his or her own stake in every analysis.

COUNTERTRANSFERENCE, CONFLICTUAL LISTENING, AND THE ANALYTIC OBJECT RELATIONSHIP

HENRY F. SMITH, M.D.

ANALYTIC WORK IS ALWAYS more complex than we can convey in writing, for the observation and description of any phenomenon, while allowing the reader to see an approximation of what the writer sees, inevitably oversimplifies the working field (Smith 1997a). This is a consideration in the description or depiction of any observational field, whether it be scientific writing, imaginative writing, or the visual arts; but in analysis, where so much of the observational field is obscured from view, the writer's selectivity plays a particularly powerful role in defining what is there to be observed, and these definitions then shape the evolution of our theory and our technique.

At any given analytic moment, I find that my countertransference experience is more complex than I can ever know, and certainly more varied than any single statement about it to a reader or, for that matter, to a patient could ever convey. In my view, the principal reasons for both this complexity and this obscurity are the protean manifestations of conflict in the analyst's mental life, which serve both to advance and to retard the analytic work, and which, despite the play they are receiving in recent years, continue to be marginalized in our literature and in our understanding of the work. I find this to be true in the writings of

---

Abridged from "Countertransference, Conflictual Listening, and the Analytic Object Relationship," by Henry F. Smith, M.D., an article first published in *The Journal of the American Psychoanalytic Association*, 48:95–128, 2000.

those who consider conflict to be the central focus of psychoanalytic work, as well as in those who do not. The role of unconscious conflict is easily obscured from conscious view.

I will pass over the vast literature on countertransference, except to remind the reader that it is divided somewhat arbitrarily into two camps, those who advocate either a broad or a narrow definition of the term. Over the years we have seen an established trend toward the broader view, due to many factors, one of which developed out of the narrow camp itself, namely the delayed appreciation of the ubiquity of conflict in the analyst's mental life and the observation that every mental event on the part of the analyst is itself a compromise formation (Brenner 1982).

Indeed, if we examine the literature carefully many complexities arise. The broadest definitions seem to favor conscious over unconscious phenomena and dismiss the analyst's conflictual contributions. I am thinking, for example, of Heimann's (1950) reference to the countertransference as "the patient's creation." Narrow definitions, on the other hand, that view countertransference solely as an interference in the work, seem inevitably to broaden, as we can see even in the work of Annie Reich, who by the end of her seminal 1951 paper is led by her own clinical observations to a broader view of countertransference than the one for which she is customarily known.

An exception to this confusion is the cogent and lucid writing of Jacob Arlow. Drawing on the analogy to transference, Arlow, from the narrower perspective, suggests that countertransference designates only those situations in which the patient "represents for the analyst an object of the past" (Arlow 1979, p. 198), or the analyst "takes the patient as the object of his emotional response" (Arlow 1997a), adding, "The patient has to be the object of a persistent unconscious fantasy wish on the part of the analyst to call it countertransference" (Arlow 1997a).

In his customarily incisive fashion, Arlow calls our attention here to what I would regard as essential subsets of countertransference experience. My difficulty arises when I try to make such mutually exclusive differentiations in practice, or to use Arlow's definition to distinguish certain analytic moments from any others. Whenever I examine any moment of any analysis I find that my reaction to the patient is shaped in part by what we might call my own transference experience; to one degree or another I am always "taking the patient as an object" from my past, my view of the patient variously shaped by "persistent unconscious fantasy wishes." A crucial distinction may rest on the quantitative factor, reflected in the force and the form of expression of the analyst's wishes, but as I look at it, I cannot think of a moment without countertransference, even if we define it as strictly as Arlow does. Furthermore, I do not think it is possible to separate out those countertransference phenomena that interfere with the process from those that facilitate it. All countertransference does both, all the time. With Brenner (1982) I would say, as transference is a manifestation of the patient's object relations as they appear in reaction to the analyst, so countertransference is a manifestation of the analyst's object relations as they appear in reaction to the patient. I would add that in this respect the analytic relationship is no different from any other intimate relationship.

I mention in passing another controversy, long since buried but still implicit in contemporary work, namely the presence of what Tower (1956) called "countertransference structures" and she and others referred to as a "countertransference neurosis." While I find the latter term to be anachronistic and confusing, I do believe the analyst's experience with every patient includes persistent and continuous neurotic patterns, brought by the analyst and shaped by each dyad; these neurotic patterns inform the work and provide much of the fuel for the ongoing and shifting understanding of the patient's conflicts as well as for the analyst's interventions.

CONFLICTUAL LISTENING AND SIGNAL CONFLICT

I would like to turn now to my own use of the countertransference. In so doing I will attempt to illustrate a view of countertransference as a continuous, ambivalent phenomenon, both facilitative and obstructive, one shaped both by the patient and by the analyst—that is, by the analyst's experience of the patient and by his or her own conflictual solutions.

Countertransference, defined broadly to include all of the specific conscious and unconscious responses aroused in the analyst by the specific qualities of the patient, is, for many analysts, one of two primary sources of data about the patient. The other is the more deliberate examination of the patient's words, affect, and action. I would add that I regard countertransference to be a source of data but not a source of evidence. To the extent that true evidence is attainable, only the careful examination of the patient's material can provide evidence for the conjectures that derive in part from countertransferential data.

The accumulation of data from both sources is massive, and data from one area can be used to make conjectures about the other. In listening simultaneously to both the patient and to him or herself, the analyst is in fact attending to three modalities of communication: words or thoughts, affect, and action. All three are both apperceptive and communicative modalities. Patients use their words, affect, and action to communicate to the analyst, and we as analysts receive those communications by reading not only the patient's communications but also our own affect, propensity for action, and the thoughts and words that are generated within us. While some analysts rely more upon one modality than another, I find that all three modalities are involved in all analytic communication and that, of the three, affect is the most powerful.

Although he adopts a narrow view of countertransference, the methodology of the analyst's use of him or herself is most comprehensively described by Arlow (1997b) when he writes that "unless the analyst is... completely distracted by some personal concern of his at the time, every thought, every action that occurs to him is some *commentary* on the patient's material."

As I see it, analyst and patient are engaged in an intense mutually responsive relationship. Each of them stirs associations in the other. Each stirs conflict in the other. Conflicts stirred in the analyst become his or her eyes and ears. As analysts our associations represent elicited or awakened conflict within ourselves and are in themselves compromise formations; that is, they are shaped by conflict and are themselves conflictual solutions. Whether focusing on our own responses or on the patient's material, analysts, in a state of what we might call countertransference readiness, can make observations only through their own conflictual organization. The analyst's responses are stimulated both by the patient's conflicts and by his or her own. I believe Sandler (1976) was speaking to this process in his seminal paper on role responsiveness when he wrote, "I want to suggest that very often the irrational response of the analyst... may... be usefully regarded as a compromise-formation between his own tendencies and *his reflexive acceptance of the role which the patient is forcing on him*" (p. 46, italics original). While I would prefer to reserve the term compromise formation to signify a more purely intrapsychic phenomenon, I would suggest that for analysts in their ordinary working mode, *every* thought, feeling, or action is the outcome of something stirred by the patient and their own conflictual issues.

If all of the analyst's responses are indeed compromises resulting from internal conflict, then it follows that the analyst's conflicts, his or her neurosis, if you will, *is* the listening instrument. Analytic listening is conflictual listening. And if our conflicts always influence our perceptions, it remains crucial to what extent as analysts we can observe and use our own conflictual responses as data. I have come to think of this capacity in the analyst somewhat loosely as a capacity for *signal conflict.*

Just as signal anxiety initiates compromise and defense, so signal conflict, which is essential to the analyst's apperceptive processes, elicits unpleasure in the analyst in the form either of anxiety or depressive affect, even as it initiates and sustains analytic work. Accordingly the work of analysis inevitably serves a defensive function for the analyst (Smith 1995, 1997a).

Beres and Arlow (1974) have previously described the analyst's affect as a form of "signal affect, a momentary identification with the patient which leads to the awareness, 'This is what my patient may be feeling'" (p. 35). While I agree wholeheartedly with their clinical observation, affect, as I see it, is just one part of the conflict activated in the analyst. The analyst's response is a compromise formation and as such contains all the components of conflict. Hence the activated signal conflict contains not only affect but also wish, defense, and fear of punishment. Where Beres and Arlow, then, are describing simple momentary signal affect states, I am suggesting that these momentary states are themselves more complex in nature and that they are part of an ongoing, conflictual responsiveness on the part of the analyst that contains, like the momentary states, not only affective signals but all the components of conflict.

THE ANALYST'S USE OF IDENTIFICATION AND PROJECTION

In listening to the patient, then, the analyst enters into a willing suspension of disbelief, akin to reading a novel or watching a film. We may speak of trial identifications to describe moment by moment shifts from immersion to observation, but there is an extended state of immersion and identification that must be established if the process is to happen at all. We have been reluctant to speak of the analyst's use of projection, but it is my impression that the state of immersion on the part of the analyst means that the analyst's interaction with the patient is shaped by mutual projective capacities, or, as some might think of it, mutual projective identifications. When we identify with something in the patient that feels familiar, our experience of the familiar, it seems to me, is in actuality a projection. This is true of all identifications. In every instance we are identifying with a fantasy or a representation of a person (Schafer 1968), a fantasy ultimately of our own making, and in this sense all identifications can be thought of as "projective" identifications. In fact, the analyst's identifications *with* the patient and his or her projections *onto* or *into* the patient may be the fundamental way the analyst has of learning *about* the patient. This extended state of immersion results in the experience that interpretations often seem to pertain to both parties, and at times the analyst's use of the patient takes on a kind of parasitic quality.

A patient is angry at his male lover. He is not there and should be. If I catch his loneliness I may speak to it. I know that feeling. I might say, "You feel so lost without him," and I could be speaking to myself as well. In fact my sense of his being lost comes from my observation and identification *with* him and my projection of my own experience *onto* him. I have not really found *him* but rather a mix of him and me. But remember the patient has said he is angry, and I notice that I also have been feeling irritated with him. He is lost in his sense of mistreatment. He feels abandoned by his partner, and I feel abandoned by *him*. Notice that I am identifying here with him as the abandoned one and at the same time feeling abandoned by him. His annoyance annoys me, as I suspect it has his partner. More conceptually, we might say that I am identifying in both concordant and complementary ways simultaneously, in Racker's (1968) terms. You remember, concordant identifications denote the analyst's empathy with the patient, complementary identifications are identifications with the patient's objects. I would suggest that rather than divide these forms of identification into separate phenomena, they are simultaneously present in a dynamic balance in the analyst, as in the patient, at all times. That is, the analyst is continuously identifying with both parties in the object relationship, whether we view that relationship as one formed by the patient and his objects, by the patient and the analyst, or, ultimately, by the patient's self and object representations.

Let me illustrate the complex pulls of countertransference with another example, which will also show the simultaneously facilitating and interfering nature of countertransference. This same patient is describing his sexual activity with his partner but does so in the most general of terms. I ask about his vagueness. He says, "What would be the point of being more specific?" It is a familiar response from him. He used to be afraid he would excite me but seemed to have overcome that fear. I remind him that there have been occasions when he wasn't so cautious about telling me the details. He says he remembers once he spoke about the details, but at that time he thought he must be upsetting me because I was more silent than usual. Here he is indicating both his own discomfort at telling me these details and his wish that I be a more active partner. But there is something more. I remember that silence of mine. It was indeed a response to what he was telling me. In my silence I was thinking about all the reactions his descriptions stirred in me, puzzlement, curiosity, surprise, and at moments—it is true—a certain excitement and discomfort.

My point here is that this is a typical mix of countertransference feelings, which the patient perceives incompletely but in part correctly. Because we all have within us the capacity to match the patient's expectations of us (Hoffmann 1983), we create multiple brief actualizations of the patient's fantasies all the time, which, in my view, fuel the progress of the work as we try to observe and articulate what is transpiring. For while the patient's perception may match part of the analyst's experience, the two are not synonymous (Smith 1990), and the analysis of the patient's conflicts continues both facilitated and obstructed by these momentary enactments. In my view much of the literature on enactment oversimplifies the complexity of countertransference experience with the result that retrospective self-disclosures, either in the literature or in practice, often assume a compliant or factitious quality, which misrepresents the analytic work and, in practice, initiates another phase of the continuous process of enactment.

Returning to my patient on a later occasion, we find him again reluctant to speak in detail about his sexual activity. This time I find myself a bit irritated. I ask if he is afraid he will excite me. He says, no, he is afraid I will be uncomfortable and get mad at him. This time I am not aware of feeling uncomfortable, but I am irritated at his evasiveness. I know about his struggles with his brutal father and might ask about his wish to recreate them with me now, but I wait, and soon he is telling me how angry his father used to get at him and his sense that his erotic attraction to his father made his father uncomfortable. My point here again is that there are many things happening concurrently, but my irritation, which may on the one hand have contributed to his resistance, seems also to have fueled a piece of the transference and thus facilitated another aspect of the reconstruction of his sadomasochistic, erotic, object tie to his father.

THE BENIGN NEGATIVE COUNTERTRANSFERENCE

Although it may seem crude or impolitic to speak of it, I have come to find a certain adversarial quality, especially manifest in a hint of irritation, to be a familiar accompaniment of the analysis of the patient's resistance. Rather than simply being an obstruction, which it is in part, I have often found it to be facilitative of the work. In fact I have come to think it as a kind of *benign negative countertransference.* I may be speaking here of an aspect of my work unique to my own character structure, but I do not think so. The analyst's aggression is always near at hand, as are his loving impulses.

In my view one can trace much of the development of Freud's clinical theory to his frustration—or irritation—with his patients' resistances. I have found with certain patients who have developed strong narcissistic defenses against involvement in the transference that my irritation may be the first sign of a more erotically engaged relatedness, which usually, as with my patient above, prefigures an emerging sadomasochistic object tie (Smith 1997b). But my irritations are often near at hand when patients retreat from engagement, and they stem both from my own characterological impatience with such distance and my wish that the patient achieve a fuller sense of relatedness. They are shaped by my own history and my history with the patient.

So if my irritation stems from my own conflicts and lends a conflictual element to my perception of the patient, one for which I must account, I have found it to be a useful signal about the current state of the relationship and, in particular, the patient's level of relatedness. And when I pay attention to what in the patient may be eliciting my irritation, I often find the patient is acting within the transference to close me out, to use my words as part of an action sequence rather than being able to hear them as words, and to define a particular kind of object tie. Rather than looking solely for the patient's experience in the transference, I have come to think of our experience *together* as constituting the transference (Smith 1997b). Here transference and countertransference become inseparable.

There are dangers in not paying attention to my irritation. In order to deal with the experience of being shut out and the aggression it stirs, I may become even more distracted or sleepy; I may adopt what might be called masochistic forms of listening or become gratuitously empathic. What interests me in such moments is a particular aspect of aggression in the countertransference and how it might be used productively.

AN EXTENDED CLINICAL ILLUSTRATION

I am thinking of a woman who runs her own business. She is 9 years older than myself, and at the time of the hours in question I had been seeing her for just over a decade. Abandoned at birth and adopted at 4 months, she came to me when her adoptive mother was dying because she could feel no sadness about it. More recently she has had a bout with cancer and is afraid she herself will die, although her prognosis is good. She has a persistent fear of suffocation, which sometimes increases when she lies down on the couch. Her fear has many determinants, including her developing emphysema, but it is most noticeable when she fears that she will choke on her own affect, and at such moments she sits up on the couch.

There is another component, however, in her sitting up, one which I detect first through my countertransference irritation. It is a provocative, oppositional one, and it not only defines a particular sadomasochistic tie with me but defends against her fuller expressions of affect and the more genuine relationship they subtend. At such moments she arrives and sits on the couch, looking for some response from me. I barely know what it is that is irritating me. In time she says, as if speaking to a tyrant, "I *will* lie down in a minute." I can feel myself to be a participant in an argument scripted by another. I say, "You seem to be arguing with someone." She says, "I know I'm *supposed* to lie down." Generally I am unconcerned about whether a patient is sitting or lying; what is important is its meaning. But with this patient it matters to me. For a variety of reasons I *want* her to lie down.

Notice that my countertransference irritation fits the role of the insistent tyrant with whom she is arguing. She used to get into many such struggles with her mother, whom she felt never loved her and whom she never loved. Beneath these struggles with her mother and with me lies a terror of object loss and abandonment, and within them we come back repeatedly to the projection and denial of her own rage.

Both of us are implicated in the struggle against loss and abandonment, but for all the "uses" of my irritation and its "co-creation," it is also fully mine, a defensive cover for the momentary sense that I have lost her. I feel betrayed, and I have an internal set of object relationships of my own by which I can understand my affective state.

What is curious and clinically significant is that when in time she does lie down, the provocative, oppositional posture fades, and she enters a different place in the work, more accessible to the past, to self-reflection and to her feelings, a different relationship with me and with herself. In short when she lies down she can think more effectively, and I find that I can too.

Inevitably my countertransference shifts when she lies down and puts away her provocativeness. I thought for a time we were simply playing out another version of the struggle over compliance and control. Over time I learned that it is painful for her to lie down because she feels much more alone. Sitting up, she can see me; she can engage me; and she engages me partly through her provocative oppositional behavior. But I have also learned that the more painful affect she experiences when she lies down seems to organize her, and that the very action of her lying down challenges her fantasy that she will suffocate, or disappear in compliance, or that I will disappear when she can no longer see me. Her lying down then becomes a necessary part of her working through. So we have learned many things about this positional phenomenon, but I have come overall to feel that her lying down signals her willingness to be engaged with me and with her own affect at a deeper level, to enter into a fuller object tie.

Let me take you through an ordinary hour with this patient. In it I will try to show how my shifting cognitive and affective states, including my irritations, follow like a barometer her shifting states, her transferences, the nature of the object relationship she is creating and recreating with me, and her resistance to a more genuine relatedness. I will also try to indicate how my responses, rather than being simple affect signals, are part of a complex conflictual engagement with the patient.

It is a Monday morning in September, 2 days before Rosh Hashanah and my first hour of the week. It has been raining hard outside. She is 7–8 minutes late. I note that I feel pleased I have had a few minutes to myself. I have been working in the office and straightened it up, aware of how she notices everything. Thus the enactment is in place before the patient arrives. I greet her in the waiting room and think she looks like a lost, drenched child. Her breathing is labored. She looks at me needfully. I feel the pull to take care of her and a certain reluctance to do so. It reminds me of someone familiar to me; the asking through action; the anger that lies behind it. We walk upstairs to my office. My patient used to pause outside the door, insisting on being invited in, even though the door would be open and I tromping up the stairs behind her. We have looked many times at her wish to enter another's world; her wish to see it all; her wish and fear of intruding into forbidden rooms and places. She looks at the desk with its pile of papers, straining unsuccessfully to read the title of a book there. I know she is deciding whether to ask me about it, or to resign herself to being shut out. I feel exposed and somewhat annoyed. I can't use my own desk without her making an issue of it. She is, I think, bristling with irritation of her own. But she is used to eliciting irritation from others, especially from her not so loving mother, and now I think she expects to find it in me. This is the "countertransference structure" to which I return day after day and out of which spring many of my interventions.

She sits on the far end of the couch and says, "My mouth is dry." This too is a point of contention for her. I have tried to interpret the moments when she feels she must go and get a cup of water. She usually hears it as a reprimand. Now she says, "My doctor says it is from the radiation," a remark designed, I think, to absolve herself of responsibility, to mark the topic as off limits for analysis, and to make me feel chastened. It succeeds, even though I know her thirst and her terror of confinement long preceded the radiation. I picture the radiation machine, large and frightening, her doctor beside it, and, identifying with him, I think about the pathophysiology of her dry mouth. I notice I am arguing with him, challenging, without any basis, the radiologist's opinion. I suspect she enjoys these two men fighting over her, but I am not ready to say this to her. She says, "I saw Dr. Rothman on Friday. I'll get the results of that. . . ." I lose track of what she is saying. She is speaking in a way that sounds forced, automatic, controlling, asking for a response but expecting none. She isn't *in* it, not talking with me. I think, "My mother used to talk that way; I wonder if she sounds like *her* mother." Sometimes I would say, "I don't feel as if you are talking to *me*. Could it be someone else you are speaking to?"

There are in fact a number of ways this woman reminds me of my mother, including her cancer, her emphysema, her needfulness, her terror of dying. And this echo shapes my uneasiness with her erotic attachment to me and my irritation at her distance. Although I am only aware of it in retrospect, this hour takes place, almost to the day, on the tenth anniversary of my mother's death, a time when my patient was first seeing me in psychotherapy, just before beginning analysis. My mother died on Rosh Hashanah, and I had to leave a hurried note on my door, canceling this patient's hour, who had already left for my office. My patient, who observes the holidays, was furious with me then, unaware of the circumstances, and remains angry about it to this day. In a real sense the spectre of death and abandonment hangs over the hour for both of us, as we both struggle to defend against it.

Now she is saying, "Dr. Rothman always treats you well. You always say—*we* always say—I expect more from my doctors." I think she is wanting something more from me. For a brief moment I feel less irritated because it seems perhaps "we" can talk about it, but I quickly think better of my optimism as she puts on her glasses and stares once more at the material on my desk. I am caught between annoyance, again, and amusement. She says, "I still can't see it." She smiles at me. Another surge of annoyance. I feel toyed with. I'm tired of it. I think, leave me alone. My irritation builds to a crescendo. For a brief moment I hate her. Before I have time to feel guilty about it, I think of her hatred of her mother, and her mother's hatred of her. I hear her say, "I said to Dr. Rothman, 'If you develop a relationship with a patient it must feel awful when they die.'" She looks at me challengingly, "I said that to him. It must be a presumption of a relationship. Am I supposed to feel guilty at that or ashamed that I talk to him that way—he's my kid's age—to relate to him that way, that I have complete faith in his medical judgment and yet I can...." She lies down. I am surprised. I miss a few words. "So I guess I wonder about that." She sounds calmer. Less angry. I feel myself relaxing. She says, "So I left and said, 'You know, Mike, I really love you.'" And then to me, "I don't want to feel ashamed of that. He grinned." She has occasionally told me, "You know, Smith, I really love you," usually just as she leaves the office. Now she is giving her love to another and, as if acknowledging the implicit communication, she adds, "I wanted to talk with you about that."

Notice how unstable my affect is during this sequence, as it traces the outlines of her struggle with the level of her relatedness. And notice in what follows that the first clue that things are changing is another shift in my affect. She tells me that Friday evening, after we met, she went to someone's house, someone named Coleman. I think of someone I knew as a child by that name. He was hard to reach, always smiling; it made me feel lonely then and now. She is saying, "Everyone got to singing. It was enormous fun, enormous pleasure." It sounds forced to me. I don't believe her. I think she is covering up. Is it her loneliness or mine? I think she feels left out. To be sure I feel left out, both *by* her and in identification *with* her. She has, I believe, made me feel what she does not want to feel. I picture songfests as a child at holiday time, usually happy memories for me. Now they feel empty. She says, "I gave out a card to someone; I hope he will call." She is reaching out to a stranger. She says, in a way that sounds almost hypomanic, "I saw the lunatic that took me to Handlebar Harry's." A bar. Harry is my nickname. From reaching out to mocking in an instant, just as she is doing with me. Ordinarily I might comment on this defensive shift. She barrels on, "I can't believe I was up that late and now at 7:20 in the morning I'm complaining to you. I was tired. I thought maybe I should stay up late because if you deprive depressed people of sleep they do very well." I notice she is breathing more easily. "Paula and I went to the Lyric Stage." And then more self-reflectively, "I'm filling you in on the weekend; I'm not sure why this is. The only thing I'm questioning is the thing with Dr. Rothman. I suppose the other thing is my kids. What distance is appropriate between people and what isn't." This is her question, and of course it is my question too.

I say—and this is my first comment in the hour—"What distance is appropriate, and how resentful you feel when the other person doesn't behave the way you want them to, how lonely and left out." I have taken my affect and what I infer to be hers to make this remark. I am still thinking of her look at my desk, but I am hedging my bets between resentment and loneliness, which seem to be shadowing each other during the hour.

"I started to think about my conversation with Paula." She begins to sound whiney; I think she feels scolded by me and is playing the injured child. It irritates me a bit more. I suspect we are in for a mother-daughter battle. "She said she was out of sync with her kids when the baby-sitter called and said she couldn't make it. I thought what she needed was a mother." This is an old theme between us, and it is what I have been thinking *she* wants from me and from Dr. Rothman, now displaced onto Paula.

Thinking of her question about Dr. Rothman and by-passing her defense, I say, "Perhaps Dr. Rothman can be your mother." I am a little startled by my comment, which emerges impromptu, and realize it is designed in part to startle *her.* If all interventions draw on the analyst's aggression and include in their determinants the analyst's countertransference, to advance both the resistance and the deepening insight, for the moment I seem to have joined with her in the provocative, erotic interaction she is crafting, and in supporting her playful "manic" defense.

As analysts we have paid too little attention to the role of action in our own psychology. No doubt its importance varies markedly from analyst to analyst, but I find that sometimes it is only in listening to one's *spoken* thoughts that unspoken thoughts, unfelt affects, and hence aspects of the countertransference become consciously known. Speech is by definition part of a relationship and as such carries all the communicative tonality of the relationship with the patient. Speech also communicates aspects of intrapsychic experience that can be made conscious only in action; as analysts, we may be able to locate aspects of ourselves, and hence of the patient, only after hearing ourselves speak.

My comment, "Perhaps Dr. Rothman can be your mother," reminds me for a moment of my own analyst, his playfulness, and the surprise that his comments sometimes elicited from me. Am I bringing him into the room for assistance? She says, "Oh *shit*, Smith" so loudly that I jump, "are we in that again? Yeah, probably I do. I feel like that stupid book, are *you* my mother, are *you* my mother? I think it's true that if you don't get your mothering right, you don't do it right later." She speaks of a friend who was brought up by maids, a "poor little rich boy," but she is still not really in the room with me, and I wonder if I have simply fueled her resistance. Then she tells me about a close friend who said to her, "You don't remember how much your husband loved you and the good years you had with him." Her husband died several years ago. Her friend is picking up on the same resistance I am; perhaps my patient finds my voice less threatening in the person of her friend. "She said to me, 'He really adored you.' I know it's true." For the first time she sounds more fully present with me, with herself and with her affect. Has this been facilitated by my comment?

She continues, "Did I make him my mother? Probably I got a lot of holding and comforting and protecting." I am beginning to feel that we are in a conversation together for the first time in the hour. Now she speaks of a child starting college whose parents are coming in for parents' weekend. She mentions some relatives, whom I do not recognize, using their first names only, as if I were part of the family. She says, "We bought kazoos for everybody." She sounds more joyful, less frenetic.

I say, "You'd like to have somebody buying kazoos with you and sometimes you'd like it to be me. At least I could tell you the name of the book so you wouldn't have to strain." That book and her making me part of the family are joined in my mind, glued together by my affective reaction to her wish to be included in my work, in my life, and in her mother's life.

"I didn't see it. Maybe I will when I get up." She has taken my comment as an invitation. I am annoyed with myself.

Using her response and mine, I press on, "You have to steal these things from me that I don't give you—with your nose pressed up against the glass." I stare at the clock and think of my father, now also dead. He long outlived his cancer. My sense of estrangement from him, from his body, his cancer, *her* cancer. I think of a body riddled with it. This must be how she pictures *her* body. I start to feel more content with her.

She says with complete and transparent conviction, "Yes. That is exactly the way I feel." So I have used my affect to find her, even as my annoyance has shaped my intervention. She continues, "But somehow I haven't made my world at this point what I would want it to be. I'm upset. Ann and Jane (her daughters-in-law who do not like each other) cannot be together. I'm really upset with the way that works. It takes my family time and cuts it to pieces. I'm truly sorry I could not take them to the Cape for this weekend because they couldn't get along."

I start to say, "It deprives *you,*" think better of it, afraid she will hear it too critically for this point in the hour, and then, to my surprise, hear her say it herself: "I feel deprived of that immediate pleasure of being with my grandchildren and giving them a really nice holiday."

I join her, "You feel deprived of the wonderful family weekend you might have had."

She speaks of pushing herself into other people's families and then sits up. "Oh, Smith," she says, putting her head on her knees, "I feel like such a fucking orphan half the time." She did in fact spend 4 months in an orphanage before she was adopted. At the start of the analysis she had brought in her adoption papers, on which was written, as the reason for adoption, the single word *abandonment.* Her sense of abandonment, by both her biological and adoptive mothers, as well as by me, has occupied our attention for many years.

I say, "It makes you very angry."

"Did you say angry? It makes me sad. It *does* make me angry," the two affects still playing hide and seek, as they have in her and in me throughout the hour. "I don't want to be all over my kids. I want my own life." Now she looks at the book on my desk, puts on her glasses and looks again. It is Betty Joseph's (1989) *Psychic Equilibrium and Psychic Change;* I have just started work on this paper. "Looks like fun reading," she mocks and leaves.

DISCUSSION OF THE HOUR

I present this hour not as a model of technique but to illustrate with a particularly lively patient, who, like all patients, comes and goes in the engagement with me, how my countertransference, especially my irritation, which is a manifestation of what we might call signal conflict, traces the variations in her presence and absence like a barometer. I have also tried to demonstrate how my thoughts, behavior, and more especially my affect, run as a commentary on her affect, her shifting level of resistance, and the fluctuating nature of the object tie she is continually making and remaking with me, as we struggle together to find the affect beneath her provocations and some truer affective engagement with each other.

Bear in mind that this hour, like any report, is an artifact of reconstruction, subject to both invention and omission. For example, I have not sufficiently emphasized my cognitive attention to the patient's associative drift, nor my more conscious examination of her shifting defensive patterns. These are casualties of selection. At the same time, in filling in some of my countertransference responses, many of which would usually take place just outside my awareness, the hour sounds busier with conscious self-reflection than it should. Even so, the hour can only hint at the degree of complexity I am trying to demonstrate, the continuous conflictual engagement with the patient that serves both to advance and to retard the work.

To further demonstrate the analyst's ongoing conflictual involvement, one can take any single moment and examine the analyst's part in it as one ordinarily would the patient—put the analyst on the couch, so to speak. Every technical choice an analyst makes, every aspect of his or her behavior, opens into a conflictual network of associations. In the hour I have just presented, my own conflicts are clearly present in my moments of irritation, but so are they in every other moment.

Take my comment, "Perhaps Dr. Rothman can be your mother." In the session it reminded me of my own analyst, and I ask myself if I am calling on him for assistance. Soon after I think of my father, his body, his cancer, and it brings me to a more fuller understanding of what I imagine to be my patient's experience of her body. But if I examine this moment more carefully there is more. I have said that this patient reminds me of my mother, her illness, her anxiety, her needs, and her erotic desires; at moments in turn my patient treats me like one of her sons. The erotic component of the transference stirs my own oedipal anxiety in an attenuated, barely conscious form, and I feel for brief moments like a small boy unable to stem the course of my patient's illness or take care of her overwhelming needs and wishes. Hence I reach in my thoughts to my father. Maybe he can help. Maybe he can manage this woman's needs and erotic desires. In other words there is a familiar oedipal anxiety and retreat. And as I bring my father into the room, my state shifts and I can hear my patient more attentively, less anxiously. My thought of him, in addition to leading me to something specific about my patient, helps to sustain my analyzing function. The thought of my father, then, like the thought of my analyst, stems from my conscious and unconscious attention to my patient's concerns as well as from my anxiety raised by those concerns, and it seems both to calm me and to direct me back to the patient. Thus the thoughts I have and the actions I take are multiply determined by many aspects of the material and by my own conflict-stabilizing needs.

So is this countertransference interference or countertransference facilitation? I hope that by now, viewed at this level of detail the bipolar nature of the question becomes meaningless. I suggest that all such moments are mixtures of both, in countless variations, and that, given the ubiquity of conflict, it does little good to speak about either in such absolute terms. If the analyst is engaged in the work with the patient and there is therefore an object relationship that has been established, that engagement will necessarily be a conflictual one. In fact it may only be when the relationship has become *consciously* conflictual, when the analyst is aware of a countertransference response to the patient's resistance, for example, that it becomes clear an object relationship has indeed been established and an analytic process is under way. It will be up to the analyst to what extent he or she can use this awakened conflict consciously and unconsciously to the benefit of the patient's analysis. In this light we can see that even the empathic pursuit of the patient's point of view is a complex conflictual phenomenon.

CONCLUSION

The analyst at his or her best is not simply responding affectively and cognitively to the patient's material, but enters into a complex conflictual engagement with the patient that includes all the components of conflict, including anxiety or depressive affect; defense; fear of punishment; and erotic and aggressive wishes. It is these components, which define the analyst's ongoing object relationship with the patient, that have largely been overlooked in the literature, except as pathological interferences.

The analyst's conflicts are expressed in affect, thought, and action. They lead the analyst toward, as well as away from, the patient, and they help to sustain, as well as to interfere with, the analyst's effectiveness. Together with the patient's conflicts, they define an analytic relationship that in its fundamental conflictual structure is no different from any other object relationship.

REFERENCES

Arlow JA: The genesis of interpretation. J Am Psychoanal Assoc 27(suppl):193–206, 1979

Arlow JA: Discussion from the floor, panel on "Countertransference, Self-Examination, and Interpretation," Midwinter meeting, American Psychoanalytic Association, New York, December 19, 1997a

Arlow JA: Personal communication, 1997b

Beres D, Arlow J: Fantasy and identification in empathy. Psychoanal Q 43:26–50, 1974

Brenner C: The Mind in Conflict. New York, International Universities Press, 1982

Heimann P: On countertransference. Int J Psychoanal 31:81–84, 1950

Hoffmann IZ: The patient as interpreter of the analyst's experience. Contemp Psychoanal 19:389–422, 1983

Joseph B: Psychic Equilibrium and Psychic Change. London, Routledge, 1989

Racker H: Transference and Countertransference. New York, International Universities Press, 1968

Reich A: On Countertransference. Int J Psychoanal 32:25–31, 1951

Sandler J: Countertransference and role responsiveness. Int Rev Psychoanal 3:43–48, 1976

Schafer R: Aspects of Internalization. New York, International Universities Press, 1968

Smith HF: Cues: the perceptual edge of the transference. Int J Psychoanal 71:219–228, 1990

Smith HF: Analytic listening and the experience of surprise. Int J Psychoanal 76:67–78, 1995

Smith HF: Resistance, enactment, and interpretation: a self-analytic study. Psychoanalytic Inquiry 17:13–30, 1997a

Smith HF: Richard and Cyrano: narcissistic resistances to transference love. Presented at the 40th IPA Congress, Barcelona, July 1997b

Tower LE: Countertransference. J Am Psychoanal Assoc 4:224–255, 1956

28

DANIEL N. STERN, M.D.

INTRODUCTION

Daniel Stern was educated at Harvard University in Cambridge, Massachusetts, and Albert Einstein College of Medicine in New York and did his residency at the New York Psychiatric Institute and his analytic training at the Columbia Psychoanalytic Center in New York. He has, at various times, held the positions of Associate Professor of Psychiatry at Columbia College of Physicians and Surgeons, Professor of Psychiatry at Cornell Medical College, Professor of Psychiatry and Human Behavior at Brown University in Providence, Rhode Island, and Professor of Psychology at the University of Geneva, Switzerland. In the course of a career dedicated to research in infant and child development, he has undertaken missions to orphanages in Romania and Bulgaria, has served in several roles at the National Institute of Mental Health, and has taught in settings throughout the world.

It is some indication of the significance and merit of Dr. Stern's contributions that he has received an extraordinary number of awards, including the David M. Levy Award of the Association for Psychoanalytic Medicine, First Prize in the American Medical Writers' Association, Honorary Doctorate from Université de Mons-Hainault, Belgium, the Sigmund Freud Prize and Lectureship at the Frankfurter Psychoanalytic Institute, the International Sigmund Freud Award for Psychotherapy of the City of Vienna, Austria, Honorary Doctorate at the University of Palermo, Sicily, and Honorary Doctorate at the University of Copenhagen, Denmark. He has delivered the Freud Memorial Lecture in London, the

Rene A. Spitz Memorial Lecture in Denver, the Karen Horney Memorial Lecture in New York, the Helen Ross Lectureship at the Institute for Psychoanalysis, Chicago, the Sigmund Freud Lecture at the Anna Freud Center, London, the Sandor Rado Lecture at the Columbia Psychoanalytic Center, and the John Bowlby Lecture in London, to name but a few. His six books have been translated into more than 10 languages and include *The First Relationship: Infant and Mother, The Interpersonal World of the Infant: A View from Psychoanalysis and Developmental Psychology, The Journal of a Baby,* and *The Present Moment in Psychotherapy and Everyday Life.* He is the author of several hundred journal articles and chapters.

For more than 30 years, Dr. Stern has worked at the interface between research and practice, between developmental psychology and psychodynamic psychotherapy, between infant observation and experimentation in the clinical reconstruction of early experience, and between the interpersonal and intrapsychic perspectives. His work has served a bridging and integrating function, informing the developing consensus of contemporary psychoanalysis. He has been a pioneer in direct study of mother-infant interaction, demonstrating in film and in papers and books the complex attachment that develops in the very earliest phases of infant life. He has cast new light on our understanding of attunement and our processing of experiences.

WHY I CHOSE THIS PAPER

Daniel N. Stern, M.D.

I chose "Some Implications of Infant Observations for Psychoanalysis" for inclusion in this volume because it pulls together so many of the strands of all my work but makes the implications for psychoanalysis more clear.

The implications of the intersubjective view, when fully embraced, are enormous. The interpersonal becomes as important as the intrapsychic, a two-person psychology starts to replace a one-person psychology, the notion of an objective and neutral stance on the part of the psychoanalyst starts to be questionable, transference and countertransference are no longer periodic phenomena but become a special subset of the ongoing intersubjectivity. This view, which is more and more widely held (e.g., by the "relational psychoanalysts"), approaches the status of a paradigm shift. It is for this reason I have tried to examine the basis and ontogeny of intersubjectivity to better evaluate it.

The second major theme is "implicit relational knowing." The roads leading to the focus on this come directly from a career as an infant watcher and the amazement at all that infants know and learn well before language (i.e., as implicit knowing). The major implication of this for psychoanalysis is that it creates a new category of the unconscious, which is not dynamic in the sense of being repressed but simply in a different mental system, largely unavailable to be verbalized, yet containing valuable clinical information. We must become more sensitive to this domain of the unconscious and realize that it is not retrievable with defense analysis because it is not defended against. Other techniques must be used that are compatible with the analytic frame, if possible.

SOME IMPLICATIONS OF INFANT OBSERVATIONS FOR PSYCHOANALYSIS

DANIEL N. STERN, M.D.
BOSTON CHANGE PROCESS STUDY GROUP

THIS CHAPTER WILL EXPLORE two concepts: intersubjectivity and implicit knowledge. These two have been chosen because there has been much fascinating recent progress in understanding them, especially in early development, and because these findings have directly or indirectly influenced and will continue to influence the course of psychoanalysis. Our emphasis will be on presenting the relevant developmental background material and then pointing out some implications for psychoanalysis.

INTERSUBJECTIVITY

There has been a pendulum swing from the intrapsychic side to the intersubjective/relational side—that is, from the individual to the social.

The members of the Boston Change Process Study Group are, alphabetically: Nadia Bruschweiler-Stern, Karlen Lyons-Ruth, Alec Morgan, Jeremy Nahum, Lou Sander, and Daniel Stern.

This general trend is not unique to psychoanalysis but has been occurring in many diverse fields such as philosophy, language acquisition, literary criticism, and even "social neuroscience." In fact, one can ask whether it is only a pendulum swing or is instead a paradigm shift. Infancy studies have contributed to this change for several reasons. The most obvious is that infants cannot talk about their intrapsychic experience and thus it must be inferred from overt interpersonal behaviors. Once the focus is placed on interactive behavior, the perspective naturally becomes social, and many different findings and views about babies' relational capacities are revealed.

There is yet a deeper reason: infancy studies have forced us to reconceptualize the breadth, depth, and ontogeny of the domain of intersubjectivity. We are led to believe, from a variety of sources, that we develop and live in an intersubjective matrix. The implications of this for issues of self/other differentiation, phases of development, empathy, identification, and internalization will become clearer as we go along.

What then is the intersubjective matrix? Our nervous systems are constructed to be captured by the nervous systems of others, so that we can experience others as if from within their skin as well as from within our own. A direct feeling route into the other is potentially open and we resonate with and participate in the other's experiences, and the other in ours. We have always known this, but now we have a new evidence base that we will describe below.

Other people are not just another object but are immediately recognized as a special kind of object—an object like us, available for sharing inner states. In fact, our minds naturally work to seek out the experiences in others that we can resonate with. We naturally parse others' behavior in terms of the inner states that we can grasp, feel, participate in, and thus share. When we put all this together, a certain intersubjective world emerges. We no longer see our minds as so independent, separate, and isolated. We are no longer the sole owners, masters, and guardians of our subjectivity. The boundaries between self and others remain clear but are more permeable. In fact, a differentiated self is a condition of intersubjectivity. Without it, there would be only fusion. (Rochat and Morgan 1995; Stern 1985). We live in a surround of others' intentions, feelings, and thoughts, which interact with our own. Our *intentions* are modified or born in a shifting dialogue with the felt intentions of others. Our *feelings* are shaped by the intentions, thoughts, and feelings of others. And our *thoughts* are co-created in dialogue (even when it is with our several selves acting as others).

In short, our mental life is co-created. This continuous co-creative dialogue with other minds is what we are calling the *intersubjective matrix*.

The perspective sketched above has become more dominant, with particular importance for viewing therapy both clinically and theoretically. The ideas of a one-person psychology or of purely intrapsychic phenomena are no longer tenable in this light. Current thinking in psychoanalysis has moved a great distance in the recent past, from a one-person to a two-person psychology (Renik 1993). This movement is evident from the rapid growth of the intersubjective and relational schools of psychoanalysis (Aron 1996; Beebe and Lachmann 2002; Benjamin 1995, 2004; Ehrenberg 1982, 1992; Jacobs 1986; Knoblauch 2000; Lichtenberg 1989; Mitchell 2000; Ogden 1994; Stolorow and Atwood 1992; Stolorow et al. 1994). We are suggesting here that we move even further. We used to think of intersubjectivity as a sort of epiphenomenon that arises occasionally when two separate and independent minds interact. Now, we view the intersubjective matrix as the overriding crucible in which interacting minds take on their current form. Two minds create intersubjectivity. But equally, intersubjectivity shapes the two minds. The center of gravity has shifted from the intrapsychic to the intersubjective.

Similarly, intersubjectivity in the clinical situation can no longer be considered only as a useful tool, or as one of many ways of being with another that comes and goes as needed. Nor can it be seen as arising only in the therapist or only in the patient. Rather, the therapeutic process will be viewed as occurring in an ongoing intersubjective matrix. All physical and mental acts will be viewed as having an important intersubjective determinant because they are embedded in this intersubjective tissue. Of course, some material comes from the repertoire (past and present) of one individual, but even then, its moment of appearance on the scene, the exact final form it takes, the coloration of its meaning, are fashioned in the intersubjective matrix.

What then is the evidence for such an intersubjective matrix? We will go into this at some length because of its potential importance for psychoanalytic thinking.

One crucial finding is the discovery of *mirror neurons*. These provide possible neurobiological mechanisms that underpin the following phenomena: reading other people's states of mind, especially intentions; resonating with another's emotion; experiencing what someone else is experiencing; capturing an observed action so one can imitate it; empathizing with another and establishing intersubjective contact; identification; and internalization (Gallese and Goldman 1998; Gallese et al. 1996; Rizzolatti and Arbib 1998; Rizzolatti et al. 2001).

Mirror neurons sit adjacent to motor neurons in the premotor cortex. They fire in an observer who is doing nothing but watching another person behave (e.g., reaching for a glass or making a face). And the pattern of firing in the observer mimics the exact pattern that the observer would use if reaching for that glass or making that face him- or herself. In brief, the visual information received when watching another act gets mapped on to the equivalent motor representation in our own brain by the activity of these mirror neurons. It permits us to directly participate in another's actions, without having to imitate them. We experience the other as if we were executing the same action or feeling the same emotion. These *as if* mechanisms have been described by Damasio (1999) and Gallese (2001). This "participation" in another's mental life creates a sense of feeling/sharing with/understanding the other, and in particular the other's intentions and feelings. Here the term *feelings* is used purposely instead of *affects* so as to include sentiments, sensory sensations, and motor sensations, along with classical Darwinian affects.

There is another feature of this system: It is particularly sensitive to goal-directed actions (i.e., movements with a readily inferable intention). Even more, the perception of an attributable intention seems to have its own brain localization—a sort of intention-detecting center (Blakemore and Decety 2001). For example, the intention-detector brain center will get activated if the action, in its context, seems to have an intention. If the exact same movement is seen in a different context where no intention can be attributed, the brain center will not activate.

The long-standing idea of a human tendency of mind to perceive and interpret the human world in terms of intentions (desires, wishes) is strengthened by such findings. And the reading of others' intentions is cardinal to intersubjectivity.

There is another finding that may serve as a neural correlate for intersubjectivity. To resonate with someone, the two of you may have to be in synch, out of awareness. You could move in synchrony, as lovers may do when they sit across a coffee table and trace a dance as they simultaneously approach and withdraw their faces from one another or start to move their hands together at the same instant. Or you could coordinate the speed and rate of change of your movements to jointly create an everyday practical pas de deux—for example, one person washing the dishes and the other drying them. The wet washed dish is handed from the washer to the dryer in one smooth joint motion with no pause in between. And the two are regarding one another only with peripheral gaze. Some mechanisms must be available for this dyadic coordination.

The discovery of adaptive oscillators may provide a clue. These oscillators act like clocks within our body. They can be reset over and over, and their rate of firing can be adjusted to match the rate of an incoming stimulation. These inner clocks use the real-time properties of incoming signals (e.g., from someone handing you a dish) to "set" your adaptive oscillators so that they immediately bring their own rate of neural firing into synch with the periodicity of the incoming signal (Port and van Gelder 1995; Torras 1985). The result is that the outreaching arm of the person drying the dishes is perfectly coordinated in time with the outreaching hand of the person handing over the dish.

The need for some such mechanism is evident when one thinks about the extraordinary temporal coordination human beings are capable of. Think how easy it is for us to kick a moving soccer ball while we are running or to catch a fly ball on the run. In interpersonal interactions the problems of temporal coordination may be even more complex because we alter trajectories more rapidly and unpredictably than moving balls do. Even so, when two people move their heads together for a kiss, even for a first-time, sudden, passionate kiss, they rarely end up breaking their front teeth. There is usually a soft landing.

The essential point is that when people move synchronously or in temporal coordination, they are participating in an aspect of the other's experience. They are partially living from the other's center, as well as from their own.

So far, all of this evidence is applicable to one-way intersubjectivity ("I know what you are feeling"). But what about two-way or full intersubjectivity? An apparent redundancy? ("I know that you know that I know what you are feeling, and vice versa"). This requires another step. Could the mechanisms described above be sufficient? At least two "readings" of the other are required for two-way intersubjectivity. The first is to know what the other is experiencing. The second is to know how the other is experiencing your experience of him or her. There is a recursive or reiterative reading going on. The role of context is crucial here. The presence of one-way intersubjectivity is the determining context in which the second reading of the other must be interpreted to arrive at full intersubjectivity. Still, something more than a resonant mechanism, even reiterated, may be needed. We will address this below as a developmental issue.

There is a problem. If these mechanisms work well so that we live completely in an intersubjective matrix, why are we not constantly captured by the nervous systems of others and permeated by their experience (like yawning)? Now that clear mechanisms exist to permit intersubjectivity, the question becomes, not how do we *do* it, but how do we *stop?* Clearly the system needs brakes. In fact, three sets of brakes. The first is selection. There must be a gating of attention so that the other is sufficiently taken in and engaged by the mind, or is excluded from the process. Another set is needed to make sure the activation of mirror neurons does not spill over to trigger corresponding motor neurons with the result of automatic or reflexive imitation as seen in dementia patients with echopraxia and "imitative behavior" (cited in Gallese 2001). A third set is needed to inhibit, or more accurately, to dose the degree of resonance with the other. This is an area of great potential, both neuroscientifically and clinically. Recall that many psychiatric disorders are characterized in part by a lack of empathy and an inability to adopt the other's point of view. We are referring here not to the extreme case of autism, but to narcissistic, borderline, and antisocial personalities, where this lack can be striking and causes patients the problems that bring them to psychotherapy.

Even within the normal range, people differ greatly in the manifestation of certain forms of intersubjectivity. Are their basic mechanisms for resonance compromised? Or are their systems of braking and inhibiting their intersubjective immersion overworking? And what is the role of experience during development in setting these parameters? Much research is needed here.

The developmental evidence for early intersubjectivity is growing rapidly. Early forms of intersubjectivity can be seen in infants beginning right after birth. This argues for the fundamental nature of the intersubjective matrix in which we develop. Several researchers have described intersubjective behaviors in preverbal, presymbolic infants. This very early manifestation of intersubjectivity speaks to the issue of innateness. Beatrice Beebe and colleagues (2003) provided an excellent review and comparison of three parallel approaches to early intersubjectivity.

Colwyn Trevarthen found primary intersubjectivity in very young infants by observing the tight mutual coordination of infant and mother behavior in free play: the timing of their movements, the onset of their facial expressions, and their anticipation of the intentions of the other (Trevarthen 1974, 1979, 1980; Trevarthen and Hubley 1978). For instance, in one experiment, the mother and infant interact via a television setup, so that they are actually in separate rooms but see and hear each other on a monitor as if sitting face to face. If a split-second delay in the sound or sight of the behaving mother is experimentally introduced, the infant quickly notices and the interaction breaks up. Correspondence is already expected in interhuman contact. Correspondence is the key word that leads Trevarthen to speak of "primary intersubjectivity."

Early imitation has been another major route to proposing early forms of intersubjectivity (Kugiumutzakis 1998, 1999, 2002; Maratos 1973; Meltzoff 1981, 1995, 1999; Meltzoff and Gopnik 1993; Meltzoff and

Moore 1977). Meltzoff and colleagues began by focusing on neonates imitating actions seen on an experimenter's face (e.g., sticking the tongue out). How could one explain such behaviors when the infant did not know he had a face or tongue—when he only saw a visual image of the experimenter's act—yet responded with a motor act guided by his own proprioceptive (not visual) feedback? And when there had been no previous learning trials to establish such an (invisible) imitation? The answer lay in an early form of intersubjectivity based on cross-modal transfer of form and timing, most probably based on mirror neurons. Other such examples of early imitation have been found. Meltzoff and colleagues concluded that infants take in something of the other in the act of imitation, which solidifies the sense that the other is "like me" and "I am like them." He further speculates that for an infant to learn about (make internal representations of) inanimate objects she must manipulate or mouth them, but to learn about (and represent) people she must imitate them. The infant's mind uses different channels for people.

We (Stern 1977, 1985, 2000; Stern et al. 1984) have taken a third route. We have been more interested in how the dyad can let the other know about their inner feeling states. For instance, if an infant emitted an affective behavior after an event, how could the mother let the infant know that she grasped not simply what the infant did but also the feeling the infant experienced that lay behind what he did? The emphasis has shifted from the overt behavior to the subjective experience underlying it. We proposed *affect attunement,* a form of selective and cross-modal imitation, as the path to sharing inner feeling states, in contrast to faithful imitation as the path to sharing overt behavior.

Jaffe and colleagues (2001) added another piece of suggestive evidence. They showed how preverbal infants (4 and 12 months) and mothers precisely time the starting, stopping, and pausing of their vocalizations to create a rhythmic coupling and bidirectional coordination of their vocal dialogues. This implies that they not only control their own timing but have "captured" that of the other as well.

The issue of coordinated timing is obviously central for synchronicity and the access to another's experience. Watson (1994) and Gergely and Watson (1999) have found a fascinating way that the infant becomes sensitive to the behavior and timing of others. They propose that we, and infants, have "innate contingency detection analyzers." Such modules measure the extent to which someone's behavior is exactly synchronous with your own. They find that before 3 months, infants are more interested in events that are perfectly contingent with their behavior. This would make babies most sensitive to themselves (but still able to discriminate self from other). Between 4 and 6 months there is a shift.

Infants become more interested in events that are highly but imperfectly contingent with their own behavior. That is exactly what an interacting other person does. They now become more interested in the behavioral timing of others, using themselves as the standard.

The work of many others also bears significantly on these issues (e.g., Emde and Sorce 1983; Klinnert et al. 1983; Sander 1977, 1995; Stern and Gibbon 1978; Tronick 1989; Tronick et al. 1979). Most significant, all of these authors agree that infants are born with minds that are especially attuned to other minds as manifest through their behavior. This attunement is based in large part on the detection of correspondences in timing, intensity, and form that are intermodally transposable. The result is that from birth on, one can speak of a psychology of mutually sensitive minds.

Further, these researchers agree that during preverbal infancy, babies are especially sensitive to the behavior of other humans. They use different perceptual and expectational capacities in interpersonal interactions than they do in interactions with themselves or inanimate objects. They treat and expect others to be similar to them but not identical. They form presymbolic representations of others or of being-with-others. They can participate in another's mind state. In short, an early form of intersubjectivity is present.

No studies of mirror neurons or adaptive oscillators have been as yet attempted in infants of this age, for ethical reasons. Yet such oscillators, or something very like them, must be present.

After roughly 7 to 9 months, the scene changes somewhat. The infant becomes capable of a more elaborate form of intersubjectivity, what Trevarthen and Hubley (1978) have called "secondary intersubjectivity" (see also Stern 2000, new introduction). These forms of intersubjectivity, too, are being put in place well before the infant is verbal or symbolic. The sharable mental states start to include goal-directed intentions, focus of attention, affects and hedonic evaluations, and, as before, the experience of action. Each is a partially separate domain of intersubjectivity. The participation in the other's feelings is only one such domain. There is far more work going on concerning the sharing of the focus of attention in order to triangulate an object, where the infant "passes through the other" to reach the object. This is a more cognitive aspect of intersubjectivity necessary for symbolization and language (e.g., Hobson 2002).

Our interests are more in the feeling/experiencing domain of intersubjectivity. In this domain, the reading of intentions deserves a special mention, because intentions are central to the forms of intersubjectivity that will most interest us clinically. The argument, to summarize in advance, is that the ability to read intentions appears very early to the infant.

In all perspectives on motivated human activity, intention is central. Some psychological element is needed to push, pull, activate, or somehow put events in motion. Intentions go under many guises and variations. In folk psychology, using the examples of journalism and gossip, it is the motive—the *why?*—that propels the tale. In psychoanalysis it is the wish or desire. In ethology it is the activated motivation. In cybernetics it is the goal and its value. In narrative theories it can be the desire, or belief, or goal, or motive, or trouble. Intentions, in one form or another, and in one state of completeness or another, are always there, acting as the engine driving forward the action, story, or mind.

We see the human world in terms of intentions. And we act in terms of our own. You cannot function with other humans without reading or inferring their motives or intentions. This reading or attributing of intentions is our primary guide to responding and initiating action. Inferring intentions in human behavior appears to be universal. It is a mental primitive. It is how we parse and interpret our human surround. One who is unable to infer the intentions of others, or profoundly uninterested in so doing, will act outside of the human pale. Autistic people have been assumed to be in this position.

There is another reason to place such weight on parsing behavior into intentions as a kind of mental primitive: The perceiving/inferring of intentions in human actions begins so early in life. Meltzoff (1995; Meltzoff and Moore 1999) has described two situations in which preverbal infants grasp the intention of someone acting, even when they have never seen the intention fully enacted to the point of reaching its intended goal. In such a situation, grasping the intention requires an inference.

In one experiment, the preverbal infant watched an experimenter pick up an object and "try" to put it into a container. But the experimenter dropped the object en route, so the intended goal was not reached. Later, when the infant was brought back to the scene and given the same material, he picked up the object and directly put it into the container. In other words, he enacted the action that he assumed was intended, not the one he saw. The infant had chosen to privilege the unseen, assumed intention over the seen, actual action.

In another such experiment a preverbal infant watched an experimenter act as if he wished to pull a knob off of a dumbbell-like object, but he failed. Later, when the infant was given the object (a deferred imitation experiment), he immediately tried to pull the knob off. He succeeded and seemed pleased. If, however, the "experimenter" was a robot that performed the same failed actions as the real experimenter, the infant, when given the chance, did not try to pull the knob off. Infants seem to assume that only people, not robots, have intentions that are worth inferring and imitating.

Braten (1998a, 1998b) pulled together the above developmental evidence in the presymbolic infant by coining the term *altero-centered participation.* By this he meant that intersubjectivity is available in infancy by virtue of the innate ability to enter into the other's experience and participate in it. He suggested that the human mind is constructed to encounter "virtual others" and, of course, real others. His conclusions fit very well with the presence of underlying mechanisms of mirror neurons and adaptive oscillators.

At 9 to 12 months "social referencing" is seen (Emde and Sorce 1983; Klinnert et al. 1983) A common example is when an infant just learning to walk falls and is surprised but not really hurt. She will look to her mother's face to "know" what to feel. If the mother expresses fear and concern, the infant will cry. If she smiles, the baby will probably laugh. In other words, in situations of uncertainty or ambivalence, the affect state shown in others is pertinent to how the baby will feel.

After 18 months, when the child becomes verbal, new forms of intersubjectivity start to be quickly added (Astington 1993). As soon as the infant can herself do, feel, or think something, she can probably participate in its being done, felt, or thought by others. The breadth of the child's intersubjectivity only awaits her own development. (There is an interesting unanswered question here: Could an infant participate in another's experience even before she could do it herself? This is a legitimate question, because as a rule in development, receptive capacities appear before productive ones.)

Cognitive psychology assumes that several years later, children acquire a more general "theory of mind," developing a more formal capacity to represent mental states in others. Several versions of theory of mind in children are currently debated (e.g., Baron-Cohen 1995; Gopnik and Meltzoff 1997; Hobson 2002; Leslie 1987). A major point of contention is to what extent the ability to represent other minds is a formal cognitive process and to what extent it is one that relies on resonance or simulation to permit direct feeling access to the other's experience. Certainly, each could reinforce the other as development proceeds. But one cannot imagine any fundamental base for intersubjectivity without resonance, by whatever mechanism. In the last analysis, resonance is about feeling, not cognition (see also Widlocher 1996).

There are two other points worth mentioning. Dyadic intersubjectivity requires some kind of recursive participation in or representation of the other's mind. Theory of mind may be helpful in such considerations, at least after infancy. For instance, one-way intersubjectivity ("I know/feel that you…") may not require a theory of mind. However, the intersubjective reiteration necessary for two-way intersubjectivity ("I know that you know that I know" or "I feel that you feel that I feel") may be greatly enhanced by a theory of mind when it develops later.

In brief, the developmental evidence suggests that beginning at birth the infant enters into an intersubjective matrix. This is assured because basic forms of intersubjectivity are manifest right away. As new capacities are developed and new experiences come available the infant will be swept into the intersubjective matrix, which has its own ontogenesis. The breadth and complexity of this matrix expands rapidly, even during the first year of life when the infant is still presymbolic and preverbal. Then, as the infant reaches the second year and is capable of new experiences, such as language and the "moral" emotions of shame, guilt, and embarrassment, these are drawn into the intersubjective matrix as something he can now experience within himself and in others. Intersubjective richness expands again with the advent of more developed cognitive capacities during childhood. And again, at each phase of life course development the intersubjective matrix grows deeper and richer.

Some clinical conditions add to the picture being drawn. The world as experienced by autistic people continues to amaze. What makes autistic people appear so strange, yet still draws our attention to them with a fascination and a strong desire to understand, is that they look so completely human, but violate so much of what we expect of humanness. They appear to live outside of our familiar intersubjective matrix. There are several moving accounts of this condition. Some, such as Temple Grandin's (1995) autobiographical picture with an introduction by Oliver Sacks, concern adults with Asperger's syndrome, a higher-functioning subcategory of the autistic spectrum. These accounts are perhaps the most telling, because with Asperger's syndrome the clinical picture is less cluttered with incapacities and other pathological forms seen in many other forms of autism when some degree of pervasive developmental disorder is present.

Other accounts focus more on children with various forms of autism (e.g., Baron-Cohen et al. 1995; Happé, 1998; Hobson 1993; Nadel and Butterworth 1999). But there, too, these children's' avoidance of eye contact (the window into the other's subjectivity); their relative unresponsiveness to human contact, physical and psychological; and their disinterest in or inability to communicate verbally or nonverbally (except in instrumental ways) are invariably commented on. Concerning this last point, an example serves. When infants toward the end of the first year of life start to point, two kinds of pointing are distinguished: pointing to get something and pointing to show something that is interesting or novel. Only the second kind of pointing is intersubjective in the sense that the intention is to share the same experience with another. Some autistic children point, but only to get something they want, very rarely to share experience.

What strikes one most about autistic people is that they are not immersed in an intersubjective matrix. There appears to be a failure of "mind reading." Even more, one receives the impression that there is no interest in reading another's behavior or mind, as if it had no special attractions or possibilities, no more than an inanimate object. Others, like Francis Tustin (1990), claim that this "disinterest" and nonattention to things human is defensive, to protect them from painfully low thresholds for human stimulation. Even if this explanation is correct, in whole for some cases or in part for others, the result is the same. The human world is not treated as special and "like them."

There is a massive failure of intersubjectivity in autistic people. They appear to be "mind blind." It is this that make autists often appear odd, or from "another world," as Sacks puts it in describing Temple Grandin as "an anthropologist from Mars" who struggles to understand the other humans that surround her. There is no intellectual impairment here; she is a Ph.D. and world-renowned in her specialty. Yet she has to remember to ask if someone is hungry or thirsty because it does not come to her directly, empathically, but rather as a logical probability given the circumstances. One of the human events that most mystifies her is watching children play. She doesn't understand what happened that all of a sudden made them all laugh or fight. She does not engage in intimate social friendships. They are too complicated and incomprehensible.

Braten (1998b) provides an illuminating clinical anecdote on this point. When a mother puts up her hands, palms out, her normal infant is likely to do the same and put up his hands so that their palms touch (preliminary to pat-a-cake games). Is that an imitation? Yes, in the sense that the infant has done what the mother did. Yet the infant is seeing the mother's palms, not the back of her hands. Why doesn't he put the back of his hands against the palms of her hands and in that way be able to see his own palms just as he saw hers? That is what many autistic children do. Normal infants have imitated from within the mother's point of view, which they participated in. Autistic children have imitated from their own point of view, with only partial participation in the mother's experience.

The existence of autism is not in itself evidence for the intersubjective matrix. However, the picture of people living without being immersed in an intersubjective matrix gives a perspective on the matrix we normally live in. This matrix is like oxygen. We breathe it all the time without noticing its presence. When confronted with autism, we can sense the world without oxygen, and it is a shock.

Historically, we, in the modern, scientifically oriented West, have isolated the mind from the body, and from nature, and from other minds. Our experience of our body, nature, and other minds has to be constructed privately and perhaps quite idiosyncratically within our own mind. Until recently this view has been dominant and largely unchallenged except by philosophers.

We are now experiencing a revolution. This revolution has been inspired largely by the work of the philosopher of phenomenology Edmund Husserl (1913, 1930a, 1930b, 1931, 1964). The phenomenological approach has been revitalized by contemporary philosophers and incorporated by some scientists into current alternative views of human nature that are rapidly gaining strength (e.g., Damasio 1994, 1999; Freeman 1999; Sheets-Johnstone 1999; Stern 2004; Thompson 2001; Varela 1996).

This new view assumes that the mind is always embodied in and made possible by the sensorimotor activity of the person, that it is interwoven with and co-created by the physical environment that immediately surrounds it, and that it is constituted by way of its interactions with other minds. The mind takes on and maintains its form and nature from this open traffic. The mind emerges and exists only from the ongoing interaction of intrinsic self-organizing brain processes with the environment, including other minds. Without these constant interactions there would be no recognizable mind.

One of the consequences of this phenomenological view of "embodied cognition" is that the mind is, by nature, "intersubjectively open," since it is partially constituted through its interaction with other minds (Husserl 1931; Thompson 2001; Zahavi 2001). What this means is that human beings possess a mental primitive described as "the passive (not voluntarily initiated), prereflected experience of the other as an embodied being like oneself" (Thompson 2001, p. 12).

Neurobiologically speaking, this prereflected experience of intersubjective openness can be seen as emerging from mechanisms such as mirror neurons, adaptive oscillators, and other similar processes likely to be soon found. But at the experiential level, this intersubjective openness creates the conditions for the primary intersubjectivity (synchrony, imitation, attunement, etc.) seen in early infancy, and for the manifestations of secondary intersubjectivity (such as "true" empathy) seen later. It is in this sense, we believe, that Stein Braten (1998b) wrote of the infant's being made by nature to encounter "virtual others." We are pre-prepared to enter into the intersubjective matrix, which is a condition of humanness.

Any consideration of the process of psychotherapy must take into account the above premises. The existence of an intersubjective matrix defines the psychological context in which the therapeutic relationship takes form. Transference and countertransference are only special cases of a constant process. The idea of a one-person psychology is unthinkable in this situation.

SOME IMPLICATIONS FOR PSYCHOANALYSIS OF THE SHIFT TO INTERSUBJECTIVITY

The Nature and Conception of the Therapeutic Process

The well commented upon movement from a one-person psychology to a two-person psychology is accelerated by the above-mentioned work. It has become clear that the human mind not only develops, but is maintained in an environment of traffic with other minds. To paraphrase Winnicott, there is no such thing as a single mind alone. And we have come to accept the notion in contemporary psychoanalysis that no one's mind can be known "objectively" in psychoanalytic therapy. It is this realization that has given rise to the schools of intersubjective and relational psychoanalysis. One of the more interesting and radical intersubjectivist positions views the psychoanalytic session as the interplay of two subjectivities that co-create intersubjective phenomena that are the real subject matter of psychoanalysis. Such phenomena have been referred to in different ways. They are similar to the psychoanalytic object of Aron (1999), to the psychoanalytic "third" of Benjamin (2004), and to the emergent properties of the Boston Change Process Study Group (2002, 2005a). The idea of an emergent property that is co-created (besides being inspired by dynamic systems theory) owes some debt to the observations of infants with their parents. One of the wonders of parent-infant play is to watch dyadic affective states emerge, fade, strengthen, and progress into sequences, while the two are interacting with only a loose agenda but in a structured frame. What is also remarkable is that each change in intersubjective state is largely unpredictable. This turns out to be similar to the unpredictability that obtains when one is in the middle of an analytic session. One does not know with certainty what the patient, or even oneself, will say next. After the session is over and one can look back, the flow of the session takes on coherence, even inevitability. But while it is being lived (i.e., co-created), its immediate course is unpredictable.

This is a curious situation. When the session is reviewed after it is over, the process appears to be linear and causal. But when one is in the *middle,* it is largely unpredictable and cannot be described or explained by a linear causal model. Rather, a model taken from dynamic systems theory that can deal with high degrees of complexity and unpredictability is needed. The move to intersubjectivity also requires a move to a different model of description. In reality, a mixture of the two models may be needed. Stretches of a session are adequately described with a linear causal model, but for other stretches a dynamic systems model must be called on. All of this is necessary because of the spontaneous, immediate co-creativity of the intersubjective process.

This view from the middle of the session not only is necessary for a therapist but would be extremely useful for a candidate learning about psychoanalysis.

Self/Other Differentiation

There is no intersubjectivity if there is not some degree of self/other differentiation. Imitation requires two subjectivities. Yet we see it in newborns. The idea of a very early self/other differentiation, essentially from birth, has been put forward before (Stern 1985), based on the evidence that infants can identify synchronicity, coherence, continuity, and the match of volition and effect that characterizes agency. All of these are different when the self is acting or experiencing than when an other is. This is a constructionist approach to the problem, where various pieces of self versus other are established and then assembled in a sense of a core self that would be evident to the infant. Philosophers (e.g., Zahavi 1999) have taken a more global approach which, in short, proposes that it is part of the human condition to sense that you are the experiencer of what is on your mental stage or in your sensorimotor experience. Future neuroscience will most probably support this more global view, which the present authors now share.

This view, along with all the evidence of neonates reaching out for and perceiving the external world, especially people, presents an unsolvable problem for Mahler's description of "normal autism" (Mahler et al. 1975) or for the idea of an exclusively narcissistic preoccupation in the beginning of life. It also throws into question the idea of a subsequent phase of "normal symbiosis." If these two phases are no longer tenable, then the need for a phase of separation-individuation is left hanging.

In the present view, the self and the other are forming from the beginning, one as the inevitable foil for the other. In other words, attachment/"being with" and separation/individuation are continuous simultaneous tasks that run throughout the entire life span in parallel. Each takes developmental leaps when new capacities become available and, perhaps, has a sensitive period—but in themselves, they do not constitute a phase.

Phases and Stages in General

The problems raised by infancy research that beset the traditional stages of self/other differentiation create similar problems for the stages of infantile psychosexual development that were so crucial to Freud's view of both development and psychopathology (Freud 1905, 1915, 1916–17). A hundred years after Freud's formulation of infant sexuality, there is no confirming evidence of such stages coming from systematic infant observations or experimentation. And psychic energy that invests one bodily zone and later another is now a largely an abandoned concept. This is not to say that orality, anality, and so forth do not exist clinically. They are clearly visible in children and adults of any age in different forms of pathology or character. But there are no special phases of development during which these are laid down, or charged with more psychic energy, or more vulnerable to trauma or distortion. In essence, the ground has been taken away from the pathogenic model of fixation/regression as it applies to psychosexual stages of development, since there are no predesigned natural phases to get fixated to or to regress to. Nonetheless, trauma at any developmental age can serve as a point of fixation/regression. And as a general rule, the earlier the trauma, the greater its effect. But the elegant developmental specificity of Freud's original idea is lost.

Early oral activity is a good case in point. One sees a great deal of oral behavior in the first months of life. Freud's formulations of this into a stage acted to blind many (for decades) to noticing that there is a great deal of visual and aural exploration of the world at the same time. Erik Erikson stated in 1978 (at the first meeting of what is now the World Association of Infant Mental Health) that in preparation for the Congress he had decided to look at some newborns and young infants, since he had not done so for a long time. What struck him was how fiercely the infants ate up the world with their eyes—a different observation than he had made in the 1950s.

More recently, an entirely different slant on "orality" has emerged. Meltzoff and his colleagues, as previously mentioned, have suggested that when the infant wants to learn about inanimate objects, she mouths them or manipulates them. When she wants to learn about people, she imitates them, in reality or virtually via mirror neuron activity (Meltzoff and Moore 1999). The place now given to imitation in learning about things human has been greatly expanded (see Gallese 2001; Nadel and Butterworth 1999; Reddy 2002).

Many psychoanalysts today would say that we are fighting past battles here. We find that is only partially true. Although many of the original ideas of psychoanalysis are passé, they continue to circulate and are used clinically at times, even when the basic idea is no longer held. In short, they continue as underlying but un(re)examined concepts.

THE IMPLICIT NONCONSCIOUS AND THE DYNAMIC UNCONSCIOUS

One of the more important results of infancy research in general and of attachment research in particular has been to contribute to the concept of implicit knowledge. It has been found that infants remember and form representations of complicated social and affective situations long before they have available to them the explicit domain of verbal and symbolic functioning. It thus has become obvious that implicit relational knowing goes well beyond the exclusively sensorimotor core of "procedural" knowledge.

As the Boston Change Process Study Group (2005 and in press), we advance the view, consistent with current scientific views of mind and brain function, that implicit relational knowing is a separate form of representation from language-based explicit knowledge. Implicit relational knowing does not change with the acquisition of language, nor is it transformed into language when language arrives. It is a separate domain of represented experience that continues to develop throughout the life span, as does explicit semantic knowledge. Implicit relational knowing is not confined to anticipations of relational actions alone, but includes their associated feelings and intention cues. The richness of implicit knowing is one of the most important findings of the last decades of infant observation. These findings have made it clear that implicit relational knowing is one vehicle through which the past is carried into the present. Implicit relational knowing cannot express anything but the past (as personally experienced), and the present moment contains everything from the past that organizes the person's response now (see also Stern 2004).

Analysts must consider the possibility that the most important levels of psychodynamic meaning can be carried, enacted, and expressed through nonsymbolizing processes. Perhaps the confusion that this assertion generates stems from a belief that meaning can be generated only through symbolization. Michael Basch (1975) defined *meaning* as "a dispositional effect on action." This definition applies to both explicit and implicit meanings, but it is a particularly good description of implicit forms of meaning. The relationally imbedded meanings that are exchanged through rapid affective communications during lived experiences are the ones that most fundamentally organize one's directions, and these are central to psychoanalysis. Therefore, we dispute the idea that each human seeks meaning through the mediation of semiotic systems shared with other humans.

While semiotic systems are unquestionably important, they are merely a part of a much more inclusive intersubjective system that begins with the sharing of affective and intentional orientations toward one another and toward the world, and such sharing of orientations is at the heart of interpersonal exchange and the generation of meaning. We believe it is a fundamental error that has been carried forward in psychoanalytic thinking to base meaning (and mediation) in semantic meaning. Language and abstract forms of thought build on earlier modes of making and representing meaning, but these earlier modes are not symbolic, nor are they superseded by the symbolic. Although the infant is biologically prepared to develop the ability to use symbols, a large cognitive and neuroscience literature supports the view that the kinds of generalized expectations that the infant elaborates, as well as the generalized perceptual prototypes that emerge from repeated experiences with different exemplars of objects, are not to be equated with their eventual symbolic representations.

We would not agree, then, that it is through symbolic or protosymbolic processes that a rich, discriminated set of experiences comes to be remembered and expected. Instead, the processes involved rest on different cognitive and perceptual capacities from those that support symbolic functioning (e.g., see Sabbagh 2004 for the dual neural sites involved in representing the thoughts and feelings of others). Indeed, symbolic functioning does not become available until the middle of the second year. This does not mean that the infant is not thinking. Thought and symbol use are not synonymous, nor are they isomorphic.

IMPLICATIONS OF IMPLICIT KNOWLEDGE FOR PSYCHOANALYSIS

The Extent of Implicit Knowledge

Because of the scope and importance of the implicit domain, the space of the unconscious must be adjusted. Let us call the entire territory of the topographically unconscious, the *nonconscious*. The nonconscious can then be divided for clinical and theoretical purposes into three areas: a) the *dynamic unconscious,* which is kept out of consciousness by defenses, particularly repression; b) the *preconscious,* which is kept out of or revealed to consciousness by shifts in attention; and c) the *implicit,* which is not conscious because it resides in a different system that is nonsymbolic and nonverbal, but not under repression.

The implicit domain holds everything that was learned about human relatedness until the infant was about 18 months old. This basic relational knowledge of what to do with your eyes when gazing at someone, how to fashion and nuance facial expressions, how to read them on other's faces, how to read tone of voice and modulate your own depending on the situation, what affects are appropriate and how to dose them, how to orient your head and body when relating, how to adjust depending on the relationship, how a family Sunday dinner unfolds, what it is like to be with grandmother, with uncle Jim, and so on. This wealth of implicit knowledge continues to grow and get richer, more nuanced, and more flexible after 18 months and continues to do so throughout the life span. It represents a very large segment of our nonconscious. It comes into play the minute the patient first walks into the consulting room. It guides the manifestations of the transference; in fact, it helps to constitute the transference.

Psychodynamic Material in the Implicit Domain

The Boston Change Process Study Group (in press) is trying to bring greater attention to the implicit domain as a vast and clinically important part of the nonconscious, and to emphasize how much of what is "psychodynamic" is nonconscious not because of repression, but because it is organized implicitly. As we have elaborated in a previous paper (Lyons-Ruth 1999), defensive infant behaviors around attachment needs are precisely the evidence we need to locate the onset of defensive processes in implicit (nonreflective, nonsymbolic) affective processes available prior to the mediation of semiotic systems. (See also evidence for the relation of early forms of dialogue to later dissociative processes in Lyons-Ruth 2003 and Ogawa et al. 1997.) In our view, nonconflicted affective exchanges, as well as the more conflicted defensive stances that may be a part of those exchanges, are grounded in implicit or procedural forms of representation of lived experiences with others. With development, verbal exchanges increasingly become a part of interactions with others; however, the "rules" governing those interactions are negotiated through affect cues from the beginning of life and are rarely raised to the level of conscious verbal description. Instead, they remain a part of our implicit relational knowing. Such rules for interaction include expectations about what forms of affective relatedness can be expressed openly in the relationship and what forms need to be expressed only in "defensive" ways—that is, in distorted or displaced forms. As with the syntax governing language use, we begin deriving and using these rules very early in life, as part of our procedural knowledge, long before we are capable of generating any conscious verbal descriptions of them.

In short, the dynamic unconscious is only one important source of psychodynamic material. Implicit relational knowing is another.

The Role of the Analysis of Defenses

Some of the traditional schools of psychoanalysis have focused on the importance of the analysis of defenses. Although the analysis of defenses may be necessary to uncover the dynamic unconscious, it is not appropriate for bringing the implicit nonconscious into consciousness. Other techniques are needed—in particular, those with a greater emphasis on empathy and the creation of a holding environment. Since both forms of nonconscious material will necessarily exist in the same patient, some flexibility and judgment are needed to know which kind of nonconscious material one is faced with and how to deal with it.

What Is "Deep" and What Is "Superficial"

Psychoanalysis traditionally privileges the explicit, verbalizable meaning of psychodynamic forces that are interpretable. This level provides the "deep" meaning. The "superficial" or "surface" level is considered to be the local level of small, second-by-second behaviors that have implicit or intrinsic meanings (silences, facial expressions, gestures, positional shifts, and, very importantly, the implicit meanings of words that rearrange the intrapsychic space). The nonverbal implicit meanings are considered to be only the manifestation of the deeper level—that which gets instantiated at the local level.

In our view (Boston Change Process Study Group, in press), previous work in psychoanalysis has conceptually reversed what should be considered the deeper level of meaning and what should be considered the more superficial. The deepest level of meaning—from which all later forms of meaning emerge and to which they refer—is the level of lived engagements with others around central developmental needs, as these engagements are represented in implicit, procedural forms of memory. The central implication of what we are saying is that the traditional view of what is "profound" or "deep" and what is "superficial" must be turned on its head. Our suggestion is that conflict, defense, and unconscious fantasy originate in the implicit knowing of lived interactions. We consider the local level to provide the raw material, the foundation, for the grasping of the psychodynamics that then will be responded to implicitly and rendered interpretively by the analyst. It is here, at the local level, that the past is carried forward into the present. The concepts of conflict, defense, and so on, as explicated in language, are useful abstractions that arise from the lived experiencing of conflict and defense in the interaction that is encoded in the implicit. In this sense, these abstractions are secondary. One of the reasons for this misunderstanding is that in analysis, one talks about these issues many times over, so that one loses sight of the fact that the explicit version comes from an original implicit experience.

Although relational transactions have been considered the surface level of meaning in previous analytic theorizing, this level of enactive representation encodes the most profound aspects of human experience, including their elements of conflict, defense, and affective resistance. Therefore, this level can no longer be considered "surface" or superficial.

We hope that ongoing and future infancy research will continue to pose useful questions to psychoanalysis.

REFERENCES

Aron L: A Meeting of Minds: Mutuality in Psychoanalysis. Hillsdale, NJ, Analytic Press, 1996

Aron L: Clinical choices and the relational matrix. Psychoanalytic Dialogues 9:1–30, 1999

Astington JW: The Child's Discovery of the Mind. Cambridge, MA, Harvard University Press, 1993

Baron-Cohen S: Mindblindness: An Essay on Autism and Theory of Mind. Cambridge, MA, MIT Press, 1995

Basch M: Toward a theory that encompasses depression, in Depression and Human Existence. Edited by Anthony EJ, Benedek T. Boston, MA, Little, Brown, 1975, pp 485–534

Beebe B, Lachmann F: Infant Research and Adult Treatment: Co-constructing Interactions. Hillsdale, NJ, Analytic Press, 2002

Beebe B, Knoblauch S, Rustin J, Sorter D: I. Introduction: a systems view. Symposium on intersubjectivity in infant research and its implications for adult treatment. Psychoanalytic Dialogues 13:743–776, 2003

Benjamin J: Like Subjects, Love Objects. New Haven, CT, Yale University Press, 1995

Benjamin J: Beyond doer and done to: an intersubjective view of thirdness. Psychoanal Q 73:5–46, 2004

Blakemore S-J, Decety J: From the perception of action to the understanding of intention. Nat Rev Neurosci 2:561–567, 2001

Boston Change Process Study Group: The "something more than interpretation": sloppiness and co-construction in the psychoanalytic encounter. Int J Psychoanal 83:1051–1062, 2002

Boston Change Process Study Group: The "something more" than interpretation revisited: sloppiness and co-creativity in the psychoanalytic encounter. Report Number 4. J Am Psychoanal Assoc 53:693–729, 2005

Boston Change Process Study Group: Response to reviewers of "The 'Something More' Than Interpretation: Revisited." J Am Psychoanal Assoc (in press)

Braten S: Infant learning by altero-centric participation: the reverse of egocentric observation in autism, in Intersubjective Communication and Emotion in Early Ontogeny. Edited by Braten S. Cambridge, UK, Cambridge University Press, 1998a

Braten S (ed): Intersubjective Communication and Emotion in Early Ontogeny. Cambridge, UK, Cambridge University Press, 1998b

Damasio A: Descartes' Error: Emotion, Reason, and the Human Brain. New York, Putnam, 1994

Damasio A: The Feeling of What Happens: Body and Emotion in the Making of Consciousness. San Diego, CA, Harcourt, 1999

Ehrenberg DB: Psychoanalytic engagement: the transaction as primary data. Contemporary Psychoanalysis 10:535–555, 1982

Ehrenberg DB: The Intimate Edge. New York, WW Norton, 1992

Emde RN, Sorce JE: The rewards of infancy: emotional availability and maternal referencing, in Frontiers of Infant Psychiatry, Vol 2. Edited by Call JD, Galenson E, Tyson RL. New York, Basic Books, 1983, pp 17–30

Freeman WJ: How Brains Make Up Their Minds. London, Weidenfeld and Nicholson, 1999

Freud S: Three essays on the theory of sexuality (1905), in The Standard Edition of the Complete Psychological Works of Sigmund Freud [SE], Vol 7. Translated and edited by Strachey J. London, Hogarth Press, 1953, pp 159–168

Freud S: Repression (1915). SE, 14:141–158, 1957

Freud S: Introductory lectures on psychoanalysis (1916–17). SE, 15/16, 1961, 1963

Gallese V: The "shared manifold" hypothesis: from mirror neurons to empathy. Journal of Consciousness Studies 8(5–7):33–50, 2001

Gallese V, Goldman A: Mirror neurons and the simulation theory of mind reading. Trends Cogn Sci 2:493–501, 1998

Gallese V, Fadiga L, Fogassi L, Rizzolatti G: Action recognition in the premotor cortex. Brain 119:593–609, 1996

Gopnik A, Meltzoff AN: Words, Thoughts and Theories (Learning, Development, and Perceptual Change). Cambridge, MA, MIT Press, 1997

Grandin T: Thinking in Pictures. New York, Doubleday, 1995

Happé F: Autism: An Introduction to Psychological Theory. Cambridge, MA, Harvard University Press, 1998

Hobson P: Autism and the Development of Mind. Hillside, NJ, Lawrence Erlbaum, 1993

Hobson RP: The Cradle of Thought. London, Macmillan, 2002

Husserl E: Ideas Pertaining to a Pure Phenomenology and to a Phenomenological Philosophy (1913). First Book, General Introduction to Pure Phenomenology. Translated by Gibson B. New York, Collier, 1962

Husserl E: Ideas Pertaining to a Pure Phenomenology and to a Phenomenological Philosophy, Second Book (1930a). Translated by Rojcewicz R, Schuwer A. Dordrecht, Germany, Kluwer Academic, 1989

Husserl E: Ideas Pertaining to a Pure Phenomenology and to a Phenomenological Philosophy, Third Book: Phenomenology and the Foundation of the Sciences (1930b). Translated by Klein TE, Pohl WE. The Hague, Netherlands, Martinus Nijhoff, 1980

Husserl E: Cartesian Meditations (1931). Translated by Cairns D. The Hague, Netherlands, Martinus Nijhoff, 1960

Husserl E: The Phenomenology of Internal Time-Consciousness. Translated by Churchill JS. Bloomington, Indiana University Press, 1964

Jacobs TJ: On countertransference enactments. J Am Psychoanal Assoc 34:289–307, 1986

Jaffe J, Beebe B, Feldstein S, Crown S, Jasnow, M: Rhythms of Dialogue in Early Infancy. Monographs of the Society for Research in Child Development, Vol 66, No 2, Serial No 264, 2001

Klinnert MD, Campos JJ, Sorce JF, Emde RN, Svejda M: Emotions as behavior regulators: social referencing in infancy, in Emotion: Theory, Research, and Experience. Edited by Plutchik R, Kellerman H. New York, Academic Press, 1983, pp 57–86

Knoblauch S: The Musical Edge of Therapeutic Dialogue. Hillsdale, NJ, Analytic Press, 2000

Kugiumutzakis G: Neonatal imitation in the intersubjective companion space, in Intersubjective Communication in Early Ontogeny. Edited by Braten S. Cambridge, UK, Cambridge University Press, 1998, pp 63–88

Kugiumutzakis G: Genesis and development of early human mimesis to facial and vocal models, in Imitation in Infancy. Edited by Nadel J, Butterworth G. Cambridge, UK, Cambridge University Press, 1999, pp 36–59

Kugiumutzakis G: On human development, education and culture. Paper presented at the symposium "We Share, Therefore We Are" in honor of Jerome Bruner. Crete, Greece, October 2002

Leslie AM: Pretence and representation: the origins of "theory of mind." Psychol Rev 94:412–426, 1987

Lichtenberg JD: Psychoanalysis and Motivation. Hillsdale, NJ, Analytic Press, 1989

Lyons-Ruth K: The two-person unconscious: intersubjective dialogue, enactive relational representation, and the emergence of new forms of relational organization. Psychoanalytic Inquiry 19:576–617, 1999

Lyons-Ruth K: Dissociation and the parent-infant dialogue: a longitudinal perspective from attachment research. J Am Psychoanal Assoc 51:883–911, 2003

Mahler MS, Pine F, Bergman A: The Psychological Birth of the Human Infant. New York, Basic Books, 1975

Maratos O: The origin and development of imitation in the first six months of life. Unpublished doctoral dissertation, University of Geneva, Switzerland, 1973

Meltzoff AN: Imitation, intermodal coordination and representatioin in early infancy, in Infancy and Epistemology. Edited by Butterworth G. Brighton, UK, Harvester Press, 1981, pp 85–114

Meltzoff AN: Understanding the intentions of others: re-enactment of intended acts by eighteen month-old children. Dev Psychol 3:838–850, 1995

Meltzoff AN, Gopnik A: The role of imitation in understanding persons and developing a theory of mind, in Understanding Other Minds: Perspectives From Autism. New York, Oxford University Press, 1993, pp 335–366

Meltzoff AN, Moore MK: Imitation of facial and manual gestures by human neonates. Science 198:75–78, 1977

Meltzoff AN, Moore MK: Persons and representations: why infant imitation is important for theories of human development, in Imitation in Infancy. Edited by Nadel J, Butterworth G. Cambridge, UK, Cambridge University Press, 1999, pp 9–35

Mitchell S: Relationality: From Attachment to Intersubjectivity. New York, Analytic Press, 2000

Nadel J, Butterworth G (eds): Imitation in Infancy. Cambridge, UK, Cambridge University Press, 1999

Ogawa JR, Sroufe L, Weinfield NS, Carlson EA, Egeland B: Development and the fragmented self: longitudinal study of dissociative symptomatology in a nonclinical sample. Dev Psychopathol 9:855–879, 1997

Ogden T: Subjects of Analysis. Northvale, NJ, Jason Aronson, 1994

Port R, van Gelder T (eds): Mind as motion: explorations in the dynamics of cognition. Cambridge, MA, MIT Press, 1995

Reddy V, Williams E, Vaughan A: Sharing humor and laughter in autism and Down's syndrome. Br J Psychol 93 (pt 2):219–242, 2002

Renik O: Analytic interaction: conceptualizing technique in the light of the analyst's irreducible subjectivity. Psychoanal Q 62:553–571, 1993

Rizzolatti G, Arbib MA: Language within our grasp. Trends Neurosci 21:188–194, 1998

Rizzolatti G, Fogassi L, Gallese V: Neurophysiological mechanisms underlying the understanding and imitation of action. Nat Rev Neurosci 2:661–670, 2001

Rochat P, Morgan R: The function and determinants of early self-exploration, in The Self in Infancy: Theory and Research. Edited by Rochat P. Advances in Psychology No 112. Amsterdam, North-Holland/Elsevier, 1995, pp 395–415

Sabbagh MA: Understanding orbitofrontal contributions to theory-of-mind reasoning: implications for autism. Brain Cogn 55:109–219, 2004

Sander LW: Infant and caretaking environment: investigation and conceptualization of adaptive behavior in a system of increasing complexity, in Explorations in Child Psychiatry. Edited by Anthony EJ. New York, Plenum, 1975, pp 129–166

Sander LW: The regulation of exchange in the infant-caretaker system and some aspects of the context-content relationship, in Interaction, Conversation and the Development of Language. Edited by Lewis M, Rosenblum LA. New York, Wiley, 1977, pp 133–156

Sander LW: Paradox and resolution: from the beginning, in Handbook of Child and Adolescent Psychiatry. Edited by Noshpitz JD. New York, Wiley, 1997, pp 153–160

Sheets-Johnstone M: The Primacy of Movement. Philadelphia, PA, John Benjamins, 1999

Stern DN: The First Relationship: Infant and Mother. Cambridge, MA, Harvard University Press, 1977

Stern DN: The Interpersonal World of the Infant. New York, Basic Books, 1985

Stern DN: New Introduction to The Interpersonal World of the Infant: A View From Psychoanalysis and Developmental Psychology. New York, Basic Books, 2000

Stern DN: The Present Moment in Psychotherapy and Everyday Life. New York, WW Norton, 2004

Stern DN, Gibbon J: Temporal expectancies of social behavior in mother-infant play, in Origins of the Infant's Social Responsiveness. Edited by Thoman EB. Hillsdale, NJ, Lawrence Erlbaum, 1978, pp 409–429

Stern DN, Hofer L, Haft W, Dore J: Affect attunement: the sharing of feeling states between mother and infant by means of intermodal fluency, in Social Perception in Infancy. Edited by Field T, Fox N. Norwood, NJ, Ablex, 1984, pp 249–268

Stolorow RD, Atwood GE: Contexts of Being: The Intersubjective Foundations of Psychological Life. Hillsdale, NJ, Analytic Press, 1992

Stolorow RD, Atwood GE, Bandschaft B (eds): The Intersubjective Perspective. Northvale, NJ, Jason Aronson, 1994

Thompson E: Empathy and consciousness. Journal of Consciousness Studies 8(5–7):1–32, 2001

Torras C: Temporal-Pattern Learning in Neural Models. Amsterdam, Springer-Verlag, 1985

Trevarthen C: Conversations with a two-month-old. New Scientist 2:230–235, 1974

Trevarthen C: Communication and cooperation in early infancy: a description of primary intersubjectivity, in Before Speech: The Beginning of Interpersonal Communication. Edited by Bullowa MM. New York, Cambridge University Press, 1979, pp 321–348

Trevarthen C: The foundation of intersubjectivity: development of interpersonal and cooperative understanding in infants, in The Social Foundation of Language and Thought. Edited by Olson D. New York, WW Norton, 1980, pp 316–342

Trevarthen C, Hubley P: Secondary intersubjectivity: confidence, confiders and acts of meaning in the first year, in Action, Gesture and Symbol. Edited by Lock A. New York, Academic Press, 1978, pp 183–229

Tronick EZ: Emotions and emotional communication in infants. Am Psychol 44:112–119, 1989

Tronick EZ, Als H, Adamson L: Structure of early face-to-face communicative interactions, in Before Speech: The Beginning of Interpersonal Communication. Edited by Bullowa M. New York, Cambridge University Press, 1979, pp 349–370

Tustin F: The protective shell in children and adults. London, Karnac, 1990

Varela FJ: Neurophenomenology. Journal of Consciousness Studies 3:230–249, 1996

Watson JS: Detection of self: the perfect algorithm, in Self-Awareness in Animals and Humans: Developmental Perspectives. Edited by Parker S, Mitchell R, Boccia M. Cambridge, UK, Cambridge University Press, 1994, pp 131–149

Widlocher D: Les nouvelles cartes de la psychanalyse. Paris, Odile Jacob, 1996

Zahavi D: Self-Awareness and Alterity: A Phenomenological Investigation. Evanston, IL, Northwestern University Press, 1999

Zahavi D: Beyond empathy: phenomenological approaches to intersubjectivity. Journal of Consciousness Studies 8:151, 2001

29

ROBERT D. STOLOROW, PH.D.

INTRODUCTION

Robert Stolorow received his B.A. in Biology and Ph.D. in Clinical Psychology from Harvard University in Cambridge, Massachusetts, and his analytic training at the Postgraduate Center for Mental Health in New York. He is a Founding Member of the International Council for Psychoanalytic Self Psychology as well as of the Institute of Contemporary Psychoanalysis in Los Angeles, California. He is a Fellow of the Academy of Psychoanalysis and a member of the Advisory Board of the International Association for Relational Psychoanalysis and Psychotherapy. He has served on numerous editorial boards, including those of *Psychoanalytic Inquiry, Psychoanalytic Dialogues, The International Journal of Psychoanalytic Self Psychology,* and *Psychoanalytic Review.* He is a Clinical Professor of Psychiatry at UCLA School of Medicine and a Training and Supervising Analyst at the Institute of Contemporary Psychoanalysis in Los Angeles. Dr. Stolorow is also a faculty member of the Institute for the Psychoanalytic Study of Subjectivity in New York. He is the author (with coauthors) of eight books, of which the most recent title is *Worlds of Experience: Interweaving Philosophical and Clinical Dimensions in Psychoanalysis.* He has written more than 180 journal articles.

In recognition of his work, Dr. Stolorow has received a number of significant awards, including the Outstanding Teacher Award of the Southern California Psychoanalytic Institute, the Author's Recognition Award of the Postgraduate Center for Mental Health, and the Distinguished Scientific Award from the Division of Psychoanalysis of the American Psychological Association.

Stolorow has said of himself:

> My development as a psychoanalytic thinker is coextensive with the evolution, over the course of nearly three decades, of a psychoanalytic perspective that my collaborators and I have come to call *intersubjective systems theory* (see Stolorow 2004 for a chronicling of this evolution). Having graduated in 1974 from a psychoanalytic institute not affiliated with the American Psychoanalytic Association, I was in large part marginalized by the psychoanalytic establishment during my early years as a psychoanalyst despite my having made numerous contributions to the psychoanalytic literature during this period. In the context of this marginalization, my participation in the annual self psychology conferences, beginning in 1978, was particularly important to me (despite my disagreements with a number of Kohut's ideas) because these meetings provided a forum in which I could present my ideas and dialogue with analysts from around the country and the world. Kohut's work left a lasting imprint on my clinical sensibility. However, my general theoretical framework bears a closer kinship to what is now called *relational psychoanalysis,* even though my own intersubjective perspective predated the so-called relational movement in the United States by a decade (see Stolorow et al. 1978).
>
> My impression is that my viewpoint, emphasizing the exquisite context-sensitivity and context-dependence of emotional experience, has had considerable impact on the field, being incorporated by many into their clinical thinking and practice, and being energetically criticized and debated by many others. In recent years, I have been cultivating the role of conduit between philosophy and psychoanalysis, having written several articles on the relevance of various Continental philosophies to psychoanalytic thought. I am, in my sunset years, searching for philosophical foundations for contemporary psychoanalytic theory and practice, a search that I am hoping will eventuate in a book on that subject.

WHY I CHOSE THIS PAPER

Robert D. Stolorow, Ph.D.

There are several reasons why "World Horizons" is a favorite paper for me. First, it is an example of what can result when my dear friends, George Atwood and Donna Orange, and I collaborate. The interplay among our respective experiential worlds brings out the best in each of us, and the outcome is a unique blend of philosophical questioning, theoretical understanding, and clinical sensibility.

Second, in attempting to rethink the Freudian unconscious, we seek in the paper to reconceptualize what most analysts would agree is a cornerstone of all psychoanalytic thought. The paper is the most recent of our efforts to *contextualize* differing forms of unconsciousness by situating them within formative intersubjective systems. Any such contextualization of its theoretical cornerstone will, of necessity, also contextualize virtually every other aspect of psychoanalysis. Hence, the paper became a centerpiece of our latest book, *Worlds of Experience: Interweaving Philosophical and Clinical Dimensions in Psychoanalysis*.

Third, we employ in the paper a highly evocative horizonal metaphor borrowed from Continental phenomenology to capture the contextuality of unconsciousness. For this purpose, the idea of a horizon is a particularly well-suited metaphor because we know that visual horizons constantly change as we move about in space from one context to another.

Last, the paper is the only one I know of in the psychoanalytic literature in which a treating analyst—myself—reexamines and explains a successful psychoanalysis from a theoretical perspective entirely different from the one that guided the treatment decades before. "World Horizons" thus provides a chronicle of the evolution of my psychoanalytic thinking over a span of 30 years.

REFERENCES

Stolorow RD: Autobiographical reflections on the intersubjective history of an intersubjective perspective in psychoanalysis. Psychoanalytic Inquiry 24:542–557, 2004

Stolorow RD, Atwood GE, Ross JM: The representational world in psychoanalytic therapy. Int Rev Psychoanal 5:247–256, 1978

WORLD HORIZONS

A Post-Cartesian Alternative to the Freudian Unconscious

ROBERT D. STOLOROW, PH.D.
DONNA M. ORANGE, PH.D., PSY.D.
GEORGE E. ATWOOD, PH.D.

> A mythology reflects its region.
>
> —*Wallace Stevens*

> The boundary is that from which something begins its presencing.
>
> —*Martin Heidegger*

> Sensibility does not simply record facts; it unfolds a world… from which they will not be able to escape.
>
> —*Emmanuel Levinas*

Donna M. Orange is a faculty member and Supervising Analyst at the Institute for Specialization in the Psychoanalytic Study of the Self and Relational Psychoanalysis in Rome and at the Institute for the Psychoanalytic Study of Subjectivity in New York. George E. Atwood is Professor of Psychology at Rutgers University and a founding faculty member and Supervising Analyst at the Institute for the Psychoanalytic Study of Subjectivity in New York.

"World Horizons: A Post-Cartesian Alternative to the Freudian Unconscious," by Robert D. Stolorow, Ph.D., Donna M. Orange, Ph.D., Psy.D., and George E. Atwood, Ph.D., was first published in *Contemporary Psychoanalysis*, 37(1):43–61, 2001.

FREUD'S "DISCOVERY" OF THE unconscious has been characterized as a second Copernican revolution in that it radically undermined the epistemological status of the self-conscious subject, which had been the centerpiece of Descartes' philosophy and of Enlightenment thought in general. From a Freudian perspective, Descartes' self-conscious *cogito* was exposed as a grandiose illusion; consciousness was shown to be a mere pawn of vast unconscious forces of which the subject was completely unaware. Nevertheless, the Freudian unconscious remained deeply saturated with the very Cartesianism to which it posed a challenge (Cavell 1993). Descartes' philosophy had bifurcated the subjective world into outer and inner regions, reified the resulting separation between the two, and pictured the mind as an objective entity that takes its place among other objects, a "thinking thing" that has an inside with contents and looks out on an external world from which it is essentially estranged. The Freudian unconscious and its contents are but a sealed-off, underground chamber within the Cartesian isolated mind.

Within the conversation of post-Cartesian, post-Freudian, relational psychoanalysis, what is left of "the unconscious"? Without the mechanistic and reductionistic thinking of Freudian metapsychology, we can no longer envision the dynamic unconscious as a subterranean locale from which derivatives of instinctual drives are pushing and pulling conscious experience. When we relegate the topographic model (Freud 1900) of conscious, unconscious, and preconscious to the realm of metaphor—comparable in some ways to stories of heaven, hell, and purgatory, all with gatekeepers—we lose some of the evocative power of the Freudian unconscious. Similarly, when we see the structural theory (Freud 1923) of ego, id, and superego as elaborate and pernicious reification, completely untenable once we are committed to think phenomenologically about human psychology, have we anything left from Freud's second Copernican revolution?

Perhaps we do. We have the Freudian intuition, shared by all who have ever seen value in psychoanalysis, that human experience—including our own—involves "more than meets the eye," combined with the sense that whatever this "something more" may be, it is the key to what most profoundly ails us.

THE FREUDIAN UNCONSCIOUS

Let us first consider the Freudian unconscious from his point of view, so far as this is possible from ours today. In an ironic twist on the scientific empiricism dominant in the world from which Freud so much wanted acceptance, his unconscious, not at all open to verification or measurement, was for him the absolute measure of truth. He (Freud 1915) even appealed to Kant for inspiration:

> The psycho-analytic assumption of unconscious mental activity ... [is] an extension of the corrections undertaken by Kant of our views on external perception. Just as Kant warned us not to overlook the fact that our perceptions are subjectively conditioned and must not be regarded as identical with what is perceived though unknowable, so psycho-analysis warns us not to equate perceptions by means of consciousness with the unconscious mental processes which are their object. (p. 171)

Freud further used a Kantian, or transcendental, form of argument to justify his claim that mind is in itself unconscious. Consciousness, he believed, is full of holes. It is not only troubled people in psychoanalysis who exhibit symptoms that are, at best, counterproductive and, at worst, create for their possessors a life of torture. In addition, ordinary daily experience is full of forgetting, slips of the tongue, and other parapraxes. All of us have dreams that are hard to decipher. Most of all, thought Freud, there is repression, which creates many lacunae in conscious experience and makes our lives difficult to understand. Therefore, Freud argued, we must assume that the psychically "real" is unconscious and that consciousness is only an epiphenomenon. The unconscious—by definition something that could not be directly experienced—was the result of an inference. It must exist, or we could not see the connections in our lives. It provides the missing links.

Let us consider some features of the Freudian unconscious. It is, above all, the source of truth about human nature. Orthodox Freudians (along with Kleinians) hold a profoundly pessimistic view of human nature, according to which, in their version of original sin, we are by nature filled with incestuous lust and destructive rage. These live largely in the unconscious, unknown by the subject, who represses them whenever they or their derivatives erupt into consciousness, but who nonetheless suffers from the distortions that repression creates in experience and living. Only an analyst, who possesses esoteric knowledge of the universal contents of this unconscious realm, can lead the way down into the patient's private hell, and thus back out into relief, or at least into a more conscious acceptance of the required renunciations. Or, in a Freudian metaphor for the detached expert, the patient needs a psychological surgeon who skillfully penetrates and rearranges the unconscious insides of the patient. The Freudian concept of the unconscious, with contents dictated by theoretical doctrine and already "known" by the analyst prior to any collaborative exploration, is responsible for many of the authoritarian features of traditional analysis. With privileged knowledge of the unconscious, the analyst is readily viewed as a *Besserwisser* or "know-it-all." The analyst possesses truth, the patient only distortions and unawareness.

The Freudian unconscious functions as a reified and substantialized storehouse for whatever the conscious subject cannot tolerate. Whether, as one Freudian metaphor would have it, we envision the unconscious as a seething cauldron of incestuous and aggressive instinctual desires, or as just a somewhat disorderly mental museum, this unconscious mind is a container. Granted, it contains more than a Cartesian *cogito,* and surely its contents are neither clear nor distinct. It also contains more than Lockean ideas, though these are surely there in the form of representations or mental copies of lived experiences. The Freudian unconscious contains mental pictures and drive derivatives such as wishes, impulses, and affects, all related, Freud believed, in lawful ways. Most important, the unconscious contains all that has been repressed.

The concept of repression cannot be separated from the Freudian unconscious. What is unconscious has been repressed, or will be if it ever slips into conscious awareness, and what is repressed automatically enters and lives in the unconscious. Becoming conscious of the repressed causes unpleasure in Freud's early work and psychic conflict in his later work. Always there is much to hide: originally the drive derivatives themselves and later all the compromises we have made to keep them out of awareness. Both repression and the unconscious are inherent in the Freudian view of human nature, which includes a basic sense of one's native badness and shamefulness. Familial and other developmental contexts are peripheral to the whole story of the Freudian unconscious, in that the child and his or her infantile instinctual wishes are the fundamental source of later problems. The unconscious is thus pictured as the home and source of innate, ahistorical, decontextualized evil.

While heavily steeped in Cartesian isolated-mind thinking, this vision of the unconscious can also be seen to have served powerful psychological functions for Freud. In our (Atwood and Stolorow 1993) psychobiographical study of the personal, subjective origins of Freud's metapsychology, we found that Freud protected himself from awareness of the profound emotional impact of a series of early painful disappointments and betrayals by his mother by attributing his sufferings to his own omnipotent inner badness—that is, his incestuous lust and murderous hostility—a defensive translocation that found its way into his important adult relationships, including those with Fliess and with his wife, as well as into his formulations of clinical cases. This defensive solution, a form of defensive grandiosity, Freud also imported into his theory of psychosexual development and pathogenesis, a theory in which the primary pathogens were believed to be the unruly instinctual drives buried deep within the unconscious interior of the psyche. In this theoretical vision, idealized images of the parents, especially the mother, were preserved, allowing Freud (1933), in a remarkable statement, to characterize the relationship between a mother and her son as "altogether the most perfect, the most free from ambivalence of all human relationships" (p. 133), and to apply the Oedipus myth in a manner that completely neglected the central role of the father's filicidal urge in setting the tragic course of events in motion. This same defensive principle fatefully shaped Freud's view of the psychoanalytic situation, wherein the *cordon sanitaire* that he wrapped around the parents he also wrapped around the presumptively neutral analyst, so that the patient's transference experiences could be seen as arising solely from unconscious contents within the isolated mind of the patient, rather than being codetermined by the impact and meanings of the stance and activities of the analyst.

AN ALTERNATIVE: WORLD HORIZONS

Let us now bring a set of assumptions different from Freud's to the problem of unconsciousness in human psychological life. Let us begin, not with a Cartesian isolated mind-entity equipped with conscious, preconscious, and unconscious compartments, but with the concept of a multiply contextualized experiential world—a cornerstone of our intersubjective perspective. In place of Freud's topographical and structural theories of mind we envision an organized totality of lived personal experience, more or less conscious and more or less contoured according to those emotional convictions or organizing principles formed in a lifetime of emotional and relational experiences. Instead of a container we picture an experiential system of expectations, interpretive patterns, and meanings, especially those formed in the contexts of psychological trauma—losses, deprivations, shocks, injuries, violations, and the like. Because such convictions and ordering principles usually operate outside the domain of reflective self-awareness, we have characterized them as prereflectively unconscious (Atwood and Stolorow 1980, 1984). Within such a system or world, one can feel and know certain things, often repetitively and with unshakable certainty. Whatever one is not able to feel or know falls outside the horizons (Gadamer 1975) of his or her experiential world, requiring no container. The rigidity that we associate with various kinds of psychopathology can be grasped as a kind of freezing of one's experiential horizons so that other perspectives remain unavailable. We could say that one is always organizing his or her emotional and relational experiences so as to exclude whatever feels unacceptable, intolerable, or too dangerous in particular intersubjective contexts.

Psychoanalysis, in this view, is no longer an archaeological excavation of ever deeper layers of an isolated and substantialized unconscious mind. Instead, it is a dialogic exploration of a patient's experiential world, conducted with awareness of the unavertable contribution of the analyst's experiential world to the ongoing exploration. Such empathic-introspective inquiry seeks understanding of what the patient's world feels like, of what emotional and relational experiences it includes, often relentlessly, and what it assiduously excludes and precludes. It seeks comprehension of the network of convictions, the rules or principles that prereflectively organize the patient's world and keep the patient's experiencing confined to its frozen horizons and limiting perspectives. By illuminating such principles in a dialogic process, and grasping their life-historical origins, psychoanalysis aims to expand the patient's experiential horizons, thereby opening up the possibility of an enriched, more complex, and more flexible emotional life.

We turn now to some further theoretical and clinical implications of our conception of unconsciousness in terms of the limiting horizons of an experiential world. First and foremost, unlike the repression barrier, which Freud viewed as a fixed intrapsychic structure within an isolated mind, world horizons, like the experiential worlds they delimit, are conceptualized as emergent properties of ongoing dynamic, relational systems (Stolorow 1997). Forming and evolving within a nexus of living systems, experiential worlds and their horizons are recognized as being exquisitely context-sensitive and context-dependent. The horizons of awareness are thus fluid and ever-shifting, products both of the individual's unique intersubjective history and of what is or is not allowed to be known within the intersubjective fields that constitute his or her current living. Our conception of world horizons as emergent features of intersubjective systems bears a kinship to Gerson's (1995) idea of a "relational unconscious" and Stern's (1997) discussion of "unformulated experience." Stern, whose views, like our own, have been strongly influenced by Gadamer's philosophical hermeneutics, claims as we do that it is the relational field that "structures the possibilities of knowing—the potential for what we can say and think and what we cannot" (p. 31).

Our ideas about world horizons have developed over the course of more than two decades from our attempts to describe the intersubjective origins of differing forms of unconsciousness (Atwood and Stolorow 1980, 1984; Stolorow and Atwood 1989, 1992). Our evolving theory rested on the assumption that the child's conscious experience becomes progressively articulated through the validating attunement of the early surround. Two closely interrelated but conceptually distinguishable forms of unconsciousness were pictured as developing from situations of massive malattunement. When a child's experiences are consistently not responded to or are actively rejected, the child perceives that aspects of his or her own experience are unwelcome or damaging to the caregiver. These regions of the child's experiential world must then be sacrificed in order to safeguard the needed tie. Repression was grasped here as a kind of negative organizing principle, always embedded in ongoing intersubjective contexts, determining which configurations of conscious experience were not to be allowed to come into full being. In addition, we argued, other features of the child's experience may remain unconscious, not because they have been repressed, but because, in the absence of a validating intersubjective context, they simply never were able to become articulated. This form of unconsciousness would seem to be closely similar to Stern's (1997) concept of unformulated experience—uninterpreted "material that has never been *brought into* consciousness" (p. xii). With both forms of unconsciousness, the horizons of awareness were pictured as taking form in the medium of the differing responsiveness of the surround to different regions of the child's experience. This conceptualization was seen to apply to the psychoanalytic situation as well, wherein the patient's "resistance" can be shown to fluctuate in concert with perceptions of the analyst's varying receptivity and attunement to the patient's experience.

During the preverbal period of infancy, the articulation of the child's experience is achieved through attunements communicated in the sensorimotor dialogue with caregivers. With the maturation of the child's symbolic capacities, symbols gradually assume a place of importance alongside sensorimotor attunements as vehicles through which the child's experience is validated within the developmental system. Therefore, we argued, in that realm of experience in which consciousness increasingly becomes articulated in symbols, unconscious becomes coextensive with unsymbolized. When the act of articulating an experience is perceived to threaten an indispensable tie, repression can now be achieved by preventing the continuation of the process of encoding that experience in symbols.

Interestingly, the foregoing description of repression bears a close similarity to Stern's view of dissociation, which he defines as a "refusal to interpret" (p. xii) experience, a defensive "avoidance of verbal [symbolic] articulation" (p. 114). He, in turn, equates dissociation with unformulated experience. We think it would be better to speak here of *dysformulated* experience, thereby distinguishing the active aborting of a symbolizing process believed to be too dangerous from a situation wherein a symbolizing process did not occur in the first place.

What seems particularly interesting, though, is that, whereas historically psychoanalysts have attempted to distinguish sharply between repression and dissociation, Stern has used the word *dissociation* to designate virtually the same process—the aborting of symbolization—that we have called *repression.* What can this mean? We think it means that in a post-Cartesian philosophical world, with no subject-object bifurcation, no cognition-affect split, and no isolated unconscious mind-entities containing contents, it is no longer so necessary or compelling to make the sharp distinctions implied in such terms as *repression, dissociation, splitting, denial,* and *disavowal.* From a contextualist viewpoint, we can recognize such terms as referring to all the varieties of limiting world horizons, of disclosure and hiddenness, which reflect patterns of organizing activity formed and maintained within living, intersubjective systems.

A CASE OF UNCONSCIOUSNESS REVISITED

To illustrate our view of unconsciousness in terms of contextualized experiential worlds and their limiting horizons, we revisit a dramatic instance of unconsciousness illuminated during an analysis conducted nearly 30 years ago by one of us while he was a candidate in training (Stolorow 1974). At the time of the treatment, the case was formulated according to the assumptions of Freudian ego psychology, which included the characteristics of the Freudian unconscious that we described earlier. Here we first present an abridged summary of the case as it was understood then, excerpted from a published report (Stolorow and Lachmann 1975). Then we take another look from an intersubjective systems perspective.

When Anna began her 4-year analysis she was 31 years old. She had been married for 12 years and worked as an executive. She complained of both diffuse anxiety and states of acute panic, the content of which centered around fantasies that her husband would leave her for another woman.

Anna was born in Budapest where, in her early years, she lived through the horrors of World War II and the Nazi occupation. When she was 4 years old, her father was taken to a concentration camp where he eventually died. During an analytic session, while exploring the ways in which she kept aspects of her relationship with her father alive in her current experiences with men, Anna made a startling discovery that proved to be pivotal in her treatment. She suddenly realized that she had never accepted the reality of her father's death. Indeed, she exclaimed that she believed even now, with a feeling of *absolute conviction,* that her father is still alive. Much of the remainder of her analysis was concerned with uncovering the genetic roots and characterological consequences of this firmly embedded conviction.

At age 4, Anna had not yet developed the cognitive capacities that would have enabled her to comprehend on her own the meaning of the terrible events that were taking place around her, especially the sudden and inexplicable disappearance of her father. The surviving adults in Anna's environment, particularly her mother, failed to provide sufficient assistance to her in the task of integrating the grim realities of the war and her father's incarceration and death. The mother falsified the reality of the war, telling Anna that the exploding bombs were just doors slamming. She also pretended to Anna that the father was not taken to a concentration camp and tacitly perpetuated the myth that he was alive by never directly discussing his death with Anna and never openly mourning his loss. These experiences left Anna with a feeling of confusion about what was real and what was unreal, a feeling that was reactivated in her analysis with the discovery of her unconscious conviction that her father was still alive. It was left to Anna's own fantasy life to fill the vacuum left by maternal omissions and falsifications, in order to make some sense of these incomprehensible and tragic events and regain some feeling of mastery:

> I had to find some reason. It all seemed so crazy. I couldn't accept that such things could happen and there was nothing you could do. I was trying to understand what was happening. None of the adults would tell me. No one sat down with me and told me my father was in a concentration camp or dead. So I made up my own explanations.

The specific content of the fantasies that Anna elaborated to "explain" her father's disappearance and continued absence developed as the complex consequence of several factors, including her level of ego development, the particular circumstances surrounding her father's disappearance, and her level of psychosexual development at the time of his loss.

With regard to ego development, there is evidence that a child at age

4 has not yet attained the abstract concept of death as a final and irreversible cessation of life. To the extent that a death is acknowledged at all, it is typically conceived of as a potentially reversible departure to a distant geographical location. A common element in all of the conscious fantasies with which Anna explained her father's absence was the notion that he was living somewhere in Russia and might some day return to her. Throughout her childhood and on into adulthood, at first consciously and later unconsciously, she "waited and waited" for him to come back to her and feared that she might "miscalculate" or "do something wrong" that would make her miss her "last chance" to see him.

Consistent with this level of ego and superego development, Anna in her fantasy explanations blamed herself for her father's departure and continued absence. The particular circumstances surrounding his departure contributed to the content of her fantasies. It was actually Anna herself who had found and brought to her father the notice instructing him to report to a concentration camp. She did not understand what it was and so took it very lightly. She even felt excited about the opportunity to deliver something to her father. When she gave the notice to him, she danced around him in a very happy and excited mood. Later she discovered that the notice meant her father would have to go away, and she felt she had done a terrible thing to him by being so happy. After he was gone, she developed a fantasy that he hated her for being happy when she delivered the notice because her happiness meant she did not care about him. She further fantasized that if only she had demonstrated her love and devotion by becoming "hysterical enough" about the notice, then he would have returned to her.

The final elements for Anna's fantasy explanations of her father's disappearance—perhaps the most fateful ones for her characterological development—were provided by the vicissitudes of her psychosexual development. Because her father had been taken away when she was 4 years old, Anna's explanations of his absence contained derivatives of both castration anxiety and the oedipal stage. She developed fantasies that her father stayed away because she was defective, repulsive, and totally valueless to him. And she developed further fantasies that he stayed away because he had met another woman in Russia and had chosen to stay there and live with her: if Anna could just win him away from the woman who had stolen him, he would return.

Material that unfolded in the course of her analysis suggested that castration derivatives played the more prominent role in her interpretation of her father's absence. The loss of her father intensified and "fixated" the feelings of narcissistic mortification characteristic of the castration anxiety phase, a time when Anna looked to her father for a feeling of wholeness and self-worth. The importance of castration anxiety in Anna's reaction to the loss of her father was supported by the important role that a clear-cut illusory penis played in her development. From her early childhood, Anna had maintained a fully conscious conviction that a small penis protruded from her vulva, a conviction that obviously held disastrous consequences for her developing self-image and sense of sexual identity.

It is questionable whether the various explanatory and restitutive fantasies discussed so far technically fall within the category of defensive denial fantasies. Primarily, they seem to represent attempts on the part of a 4-year-old child to adapt to a state of cognitive insufficiency; that is, to fill in with phase-specific fantasy elaborations the cognitive vacuum left by an immature ego inadequately supported by the surviving adults in her environment.

At some point after the war, during her latency period, when cognitive and ego maturation and expanded sources of information had enabled Anna to begin to register and comprehend the realities of her father's incarceration and death, she indeed began to construct an elaborate defensive denial-in-fantasy system which, until its dissolution by analysis, functioned to keep her father alive. Her efforts at this later point can properly be described as a denial that warded off the mourning process of which she was now becoming developmentally capable. The denial was promoted by the libidinal, the aggressive, and the self-preservative components of her complex, ambivalent attachment to him.

In constructing the denial-in-fantasy system, Anna made ample use of the ready-made fantasies by which she originally had explained her father's absence. In order to deny his death, she now had to cling to both the castration derivatives and fantasies of oedipal defeat. To maintain this denial system, she had to select and cling to negative memories of her father's devaluing, rejecting, and excluding her, and repress all positive memories of his loving, caring for, and valuing her, lest they contradict and jeopardize her denial fantasies. In her adult life, Anna further buttressed her denial system by clinging to real or imagined experiences in which a father surrogate devalued or rejected her or was devoted to another woman. This, in turn, reinforced her conviction that her father was rejecting of her or chose another woman but was still alive. Furthermore, she warded off experiences of feeling loved, valued, or chosen by a man so that her denial fantasies and her devotion and loyalty to her father would not be jeopardized.

It was between the age of 10 and early adolescence that circumstances necessitated the final consolidation of Anna's denial fantasies into a static and unassailable system. When Anna was 10, her mother remarried, and Anna's denial fantasies dovetailed with a host of oedipal-competitive and sexual conflicts, greatly intensified and complicated by Anna's hope that her stepfather would substitute for her lost father. At this point Anna, in reality a bright and pretty child, began to feel ugly, stupid, defective, and "freaky" and became obsessively preoccupied with her illusory penis—symptoms that remained with her until they were removed by the analysis.

The mother's remarriage represented to Anna the first tacit acknowledgment of her father's death by the adults in her environment. This threatened abruptly to obliterate her denial fantasies. Hence Anna was forced to redouble her efforts at denial and restitution and to fortify all of the mechanisms by which she was keeping her father alive. Moreover, she had to mobilize feelings of being totally unloved and abused by her stepfather, because to recognize and accept his affection and caring would mean accepting that her father too had loved and valued her and was therefore absent because he was dead. By warding off the stepfather with various castration derivatives, Anna insured that she would not "miscalculate" by accepting her father's death and accepting her stepfather, and that she, unlike her mother, would be ready and waiting for her father when he returned.

The final consolidation of her denial system occurred during Anna's early adolescence as her pubertal development exacerbated the threat of overt sexual activity with her stepfather. In response to her stepfather's sexual intrusiveness and seductiveness, Anna would think to herself, "My real father would never do such things" and wistfully yearn for her real father's return. She elaborated fantasies in which he would return from Russia, her mother would choose to stay with the stepfather, and Anna would remain with her real father and enjoy his care and protection. This necessitated a final consolidation of the denial fantasies, through which she kept her father alive, into a static defensive system with all its unfortunate consequences for Anna's self-image, self-esteem, and patterns of relating to men.

Much of the above history was of course recapitulated in the transference. During the period when the analytic work consisted of active confrontations with the denial fantasies and encouragement for Anna to accept the reality of the father's death, she became immersed in rage-filled transference struggles in which she cast the analyst in the image of the sexually intrusive stepfather who threatened to destroy her devotion and loyalty to her real father.

The therapeutic alliance withstood the impact of these transference storms, and Anna was eventually able to work through the transference and to give up her denial system. The most immediate consequence was that she experienced a belated mourning process as she permitted herself to imagine the horrors and prolonged, tortured death her father must have suffered at the hands of the Nazis. (At this point she also began to fear the analyst would die.) Coincident with this unfolding mourning process was Anna's dramatic recovery of positive memories of a loving father; along with these memories, she also retrieved repressed memories of loving devotion from various other men. Anna now clearly recognized that she had elaborated a complex denial system in which she viewed herself as defective and sacrificed her memories of her father's and other men's love in order to spare her father the terrible, agonizing death she now realized he must have experienced. Just as the sacrifices she endured to keep him alive were a measure of her great love for her father, so now was her pain in belatedly imagining how he died.

Predictably, as Anna accepted and mourned the death of her father, she also began to give up the feelings of being defective and undesirable. The working through of her denial system and her father's death had made possible the uncovering and reintegration of the repressed split-off imago of the loving father. This in turn resulted in marked and lasting improvements in her self-image and self-esteem and in increasingly strong feelings of being valued and desired by men in her current life. (Stolorow and Lachmann 1975, pp. 600–609)

The foregoing case report demonstrates that the Freudian unconscious provides a coherent and compelling explanatory account of a dramatic instance of unconsciousness, so long as one leaves unchallenged the Cartesian, isolated-mind assumptions that saturate Freudian theory. How is our understanding of the case altered if we rethink it from an intersubjective systems viewpoint? Can we thereby arrive at a more comprehensive theoretical explanation of the therapeutic process and its results?

For one thing, the psychosexual fantasies—that is, the recurring images of genital defectiveness and rivalrous defeat—that pervaded this analysis can no longer be viewed as manifestations of an innate, decontextualized, instinctual bedrock, a hard-wired epigenetic masterplan presumed to predetermine the developmental trajectories of all human beings. Instead, we view such concrete imagery as dramatic symbolizations of the themes that came to dominate Anna's experiential world, themes that crystallized in the patterns of intersubjective transaction that took place between Anna and her caregivers over the course of her psychological development. These relational patterns and resulting principles of organization were, of course, themselves influenced by the historical, cultural, and linguistic contexts in which they were embedded.

Even Anna's so-called cognitive capacities at the time of her father's death, which contributed heavily to her interpretations of this tragic event, must be contextualized. What Anna could know of her father's death was codetermined by her sense of what her caregivers could and could not permit her to know. The "maternal omissions and falsifications" mentioned in the published case report were not simply a failure to assist Anna in the task of integrating the grim realities of the war and her father's death. They were also powerful messages to Anna as to what perceptions and knowledge were not permissible and tolerable within the developmental system. Anna's "inability" to know her father's death and her later denial of it can be understood, in part, as compliance with her mother's requirement that she not know, a compliance that became tightly woven into the fabric of Anna's perceptual world, fixing the experiential horizons that so sharply limited her self-esteem and sense of herself in relationships with men.

A further contextualization of Anna's unconsciousness is achieved when we focus on her affectivity. A shift from instinctual drive to affect as the central motivational principle for psychoanalysis is one of the hallmarks of intersubjectivity theory. This shift is of great theoretical importance because unlike drives, which originate deep within the interior of the isolated Freudian unconscious, affectivity is something that from birth onward is regulated, or misregulated, within an ongoing intersubjective system (Stolorow and Atwood 1992). Thus the shift from drive to affect automatically entails a contextualization of both human motivation and unconsciousness.[1]

A prominent affect state pervading Anna's experiential world was omitted from the published case report even though it appeared abundantly in the clinical process notes—namely, what Anna called her "nameless terror." This affect state, which came to be grasped as overwhelming feelings of aloneness, vulnerability, and helplessness in a dangerous, annihilating world, was frequently revived in the analysis as she remembered and pictured the horrors of the war years and Nazi occupation and, especially, her father's incarceration and death. For our purposes here, the most important characteristic of these traumatized states is that the terror was "nameless." How is this to be understood?

---

[1]As Aron (1996) has noted, a focus on affect has been characteristic of much contemporary psychoanalytic theory. The contextualizing implications of such a focus were anticipated in Sullivan's (1953) discussion of the contagion of anxiety that can occur between a mother and her child.

Clearly, the "maternal omissions and falsifications" discussed earlier not only curtailed Anna's knowing; they had a powerfully aborting impact on her affective development as well. She portrayed her mother as being oblivious to Anna's emotional experience in general. Surely a mother who needed to falsify the horrors occurring around her family on a daily basis could not provide articulating, validating attunement to her daughter's terror and other painful feelings. Hence, until articulated in analysis, the most painful and frightening regions of Anna's affectivity remained incompletely symbolized, "nameless." Additionally, it seems likely that she experienced her mother's falsifications as an indication that Anna's painful feelings were unwelcome, an injunction not to feel or name her own affective pain, to keep her most unbearable emotional states outside the horizons of symbolized experience. Hence, yet another source—perhaps the most important—of the denial system that kept her father alive was Anna's compliance with her mother's requirement that she not feel or utter her own grief.

Let us now reconsider further Anna's psychosexual fantasies from an experiential-world perspective. Anna's world was shattered by a traumatic loss that could not be assimilated, not only because it was surrounded by unspeakable horror but also because no one acknowledged it. Her fantasies can be grasped as desperate attempts to reassemble an experiential world from the shards of disaster, in the face of her mother's lies. She needed to make sense of the glaring disparity between her own experience of loss and others' denial. This sense-making required evermore elaborate efforts to fill in the missing pieces of her traumatically destroyed life. Her fantasies are no longer seen as derivatives of unconscious instinctual drives, but rather as a creative expression of the fundamental need to organize her experience. Given enough traumatic shock, which, as we have written, includes the contexts of denial, indifference, and invalidation, such fantasies can become rigid and, as seen with Anna, quite crippling. Yet, no matter how bizarre they may appear to be, they can be understood as attempts to name what is nameless.

Lastly, let us contextualize the gains that Anna achieved in her analysis by considering another crucial element left out of the published report: the analyst's transference relationship with his patient, which he explored in his own analysis. The analyst had loved his own mother dearly and, throughout his childhood and adolescence, had yearned to find ways to unlock the emotional aliveness he believed was encased behind the wall of her chronic wooden depression. These feelings were strongly revived in his relationship with Anna, for whom he cared deeply. Once Anna's denial of her father's death had been revealed, the analyst quickly saw her aborted grief as the key that could unlock her shackled affective vitality. If he could reach her grief, then he could do for Anna what he had never been able to do for his mother. Unlike Anna's mother, who could not tolerate her daughter's grief, the analyst wanted and welcomed it, and this, we believe, was a powerfully therapeutic element that helped her give up the denial system and embrace a view of herself as a desired, valued, and loved woman.

The widening of Anna's experiential horizons that was taking place within the therapeutic relationship was concretized in a dramatic revision of her life history that occurred during the period in which she was letting go of the denial system and beginning to grieve for her father. She began a session by reminding the analyst of the "cruddy old yellow doll carriage" her father had given her that for so long had remained a symbol of her father's lack of love for her. Then she said she had remembered something she had "completely forgotten": that originally her father had bought her a "brand new, really beautiful" pink doll carriage. In the session, she remembered overhearing her family discussing a tricycle as a possible gift for her, but her father objected, insisting that a pretty little girl should have a beautiful doll carriage. She recalled further that one day she took her precious carriage to a playground and let another girl use it, and that the latter walked away with it, and it was never found again. Her father had bought the cruddy yellow carriage as a replacement for the one that had been lost.[2] She said she now understood that "forgetting" the first beautiful carriage, a symbol of her father's love, served the fantasies through which she kept him alive by "explaining" why he failed to return to her, and she soon remembered many other instances of her father's loving her. The recovery of the beautiful doll carriage also symbolized the process that was occurring in the relationship with her analyst, in whom she found both a mother who could help her grieve and the lost loving father of her childhood. Like constricting world horizons, expanding horizons of awareness too can only be grasped in terms of the intersubjective contexts within which they take form.

Anna's analyst created with her a hospitable place for her nameless terror. His recognition of her need to grieve allowed her to know, to name, and to reorganize the horror of an early traumatic loss in which

---

[2]It has occurred to us that the memory of the beautiful doll carriage being stolen and replaced by a cruddy *yellow* one may have been a screen memory metaphorically encoding the devastating impact of Anna's experiences of anti-Semitic persecution.

she had remained painfully trapped. This loss, outside the horizons of the world her mother could permit her, required the creative work of fantasy, but these fantasies became calcified because they remained insulated from dialogue and questioning. Such questioning dialogue is indispensable if a psychological world is to develop and expand. And it is this questioning dialogue, not the excavation of an isolated unconscious mind, that constitutes the quintessential work of psychoanalysis.

In reaction to our reconceptualization of Anna's analysis, colleagues have posed the question: How would this new understanding have altered the conduct of Anna's treatment? The conceptual shift with the clearest therapeutic implications concerns Anna's inability to know her father's death, which we now see less as a product of her limited cognitive capacities at the time of the loss and more as a compliance with her mother's requirement that Anna's grief remain unnamed. Leaving aside the considerable difficulties involved in postdicting a change in the course of an analysis conducted 30 years ago, it seems to us that the different understanding of Anna's unconsciousness might have significantly altered the analytic approach to her "rage-filled transference struggles" during the period when her analyst actively confronted her denial fantasies and encouraged her to accept her father's death. With the aid of this new understanding, he might have inquired, repeatedly throughout the period of these struggles, whether Anna feared that he would be intolerant of her emerging grief as her mother had been, and whether she was responding to anything from him that lent itself to such an expectation. Was she thus experiencing his confrontations and encouragement as invitations to disaster for the therapeutic relationship? The illumination of this emotional conviction organizing Anna's experience of the analytic exchange might have significantly deepened the therapeutic bond and expanded even further her capacity to grieve and, more broadly, to experience, name, and integrate painful affect.

Upon further reflection, however, the foregoing hindsight must be tempered by the realization that at the time of the analysis a change was already beginning to take place in the analyst's perspective. Anna's young analyst was already working contextually with her, even though his guiding framework, still in germinal form, was as yet unformulated, prereflective, nameless. It was only years later, when the communitarian context of *his* thinking could permit a widening of *his* world horizons, that this pretheoretical aspect of his developing clinical style could be articulated and named as an intersubjective systems perspective on pathogenesis and the therapeutic process. It is our belief that any such expansion of an analyst's theoretical horizons will have a salutary impact on therapeutic outcome, to the degree that such expansion enhances the analyst's capacity to grasp features of the patient's experiential world hitherto obscured. Yet, insofar as the analytic dyad functions as a complex, nonlinear, dynamic system (Stolorow 1997), the specific therapeutic impact of change in any one of its elements (such as the analyst's theory) cannot be precisely forecasted. When we first began to develop our ideas about the role of the intersubjective context in the analytic process (Stolorow et al. 1978), we could not have predicted all of the ramifications of this enlarging perspective for therapeutic practice and effectiveness—in the treatment of psychotic states, for example (Stolorow et al. 2002). The attitude we bring to our theories of therapeutic action is thus a fallibilistic one (Orange et al. 1997), holding them lightly rather than tightly. Within the changing horizons of our current psychoanalytic world, much is yet unknown.

REFERENCES

Aron L: A Meeting of Minds. Hillsdale, NJ, Analytic Press, 1996

Atwood GE, Stolorow RD: Psychoanalytic concepts and the representational world. Psychoanalysis and Contemporary Thought 3:267–290, 1980

Atwood GE, Stolorow RD: Structures of Subjectivity: Explorations in Psychoanalytic Phenomenology. Hillsdale, NJ, Analytic Press, 1984

Atwood GE, Stolorow RD: Faces in a Cloud: Intersubjectivity in Personality Theory, 2nd Edition. Northvale, NJ, Jason Aronson, 1993

Cavell M: The Psychoanalytic Mind: From Freud to Philosophy. Cambridge, MA, Harvard University Press, 1993

Freud S: The interpretation of dreams (1900), in The Standard Edition of the Complete Psychological Works of Sigmund Freud [SE], Vol 4–5. Translated and edited by Strachey J. London, Hogarth Press, 1953, pp xxiii–751

Freud S: (1915), The unconscious. SE, 14:159–204, 1957

Freud S: The ego and the id (1923). SE, 19:3–66, 1961

Freud S: New introductory lectures on psycho-analysis (1933). SE, 22:5–182, 1964

Gadamer H-G: Truth and Method (1975). Translated by Weinsheimer J, Marshall D, 2nd Edition. New York, Crossroads, 1991

Gerson S: The analyst's subjectivity and the relational unconscious. Paper presented at the spring meeting of the Division of Psychoanalysis, American Psychological Association, Santa Monica, CA, 1995

Orange DM, Atwood GE, Stolorow RD: Working Intersubjectively: Contextualism in Psychoanalytic Practice. Hillsdale, NJ, Analytic Press, 1997

Stern DB: Unformulated Experience: From Dissociation to Imagination in Psychoanalysis. Hillsdale, NJ, Analytic Press, 1997

Stolorow RD: A neurotic character structure built upon the denial of an early object loss. Graduation paper, Psychoanalytic Institute of the Postgraduate Center for Mental Health, New York, NY, 1974

Stolorow RD: Dynamic, dyadic, intersubjective systems: an evolving paradigm for psychoanalysis. Psychoanal Psychol 14:337–346, 1997

Stolorow RD, Atwood GE: The unconscious and unconscious fantasy: an intersubjective-developmental perspective. Psychoanalytic Inquiry 9:364–374, 1989

Stolorow RD, Atwood GE: Contexts of Being: The Intersubjective Foundations of Psychological Life. Hillsdale, NJ, Analytic Press, 1992

Stolorow RD, Lachmann FM: Early object loss and denial: developmental considerations. Psychoanal Q 44:596–611, 1975

Stolorow RD, Atwood GE, Ross JM: The representational world in psychoanalytic therapy. Int Rev Psychoanal 5:247–256, 1978

Stolorow RD, Atwood GE, Orange DM: Worlds of Experience: Interweaving Philosophical and Clinical Dimensions in Psychoanalysis. New York, Basic Books, 2002

Sullivan HS: The Interpersonal Theory of Psychiatry. New York, WW Norton, 1953

30

ROBERT S. WALLERSTEIN, M.D.

INTRODUCTION

Robert Wallerstein graduated from Columbia College and Columbia University College of Physicians and Surgeons in New York and did his psychiatric training at Mount Sinai Hospital and the Menninger School of Psychiatry. He did his analytic training at the Topeka Institute for Psychoanalysis, where he was appointed a Training and Supervising Analyst. He also served as Director of Research for the Menninger Foundation in Topeka. After moving to San Francisco, he became Chief of Psychiatry at the Mount Zion Hospital in San Francisco and subsequently Professor and Chairman of the Department of Psychiatry at the University of California, San Francisco, School of Medicine. He has also served as a Training and Supervising Analyst at the San Francisco Psychoanalytic Institute.

Dr. Wallerstein is the winner of many awards and honors for his roles in psychiatric and psychoanalytic research and education. These have included the Heinz Hartmann Award of the New York Psychoanalytic Institute, the I. Arthur Marshall Distinguished Alumnus Award of the Menninger School of Psychiatry, the J. Elliott Royer Award of the University of California, San Francisco, the Gold Medal Award of the Mount Airy Foundation and Psychiatric Center, and the Mary S. Sigourney Award for Outstanding Contributions to Psychoanalysis. He was twice a Fellow at the Center for Advanced Study in the Behavioral Sciences at Stanford, California, and also a Fellow at the Rockefeller Foundation Study Center, at Bellagio, Lake Como, Italy. He has been visiting professor at universities around the world and has served as trustee or on the Advisory Board of the Anna Freud Center, the Menninger Foundation, and the Center for Advanced Study in the Behavioral Sciences.

Dr. Wallerstein has been President of the American Psychoanalytic Association, President of the International Psychoanalytical Association (IPA), and North American Editor of *The International Journal of Psychoanalysis* and has served on the advisory boards of many other journals, to mention but a few of the positions that he has held. He is author or coauthor of 16 books, including *The Teaching and Learning of Psychotherapy, Forty-Two Lives in Treatment: A Study of Psychoanalysis and Psychotherapy, The Talking Cures: The Psychoanalyses and the Psychotherapies,* and *Lay Analysis: Life Inside the Controversy.*

Both as a researcher and a leader, Dr. Wallerstein has been a seminal figure in the development of American and international psychoanalysis. He has resisted narrow theoretical labels and has embraced the multiple theoretical perspectives that now characterize psychoanalysis in America. Wallerstein has said of himself:

> Actually, I have had two roles: the first has been as a formal and systematic empirical researcher, both in developing and carrying over its lifetime the 30-year-long Psychotherapy Research Project of the Menninger Foundation and, as a consequence of that, also becoming an advocate for and promoter of psychoanalytic research within organized psychoanalysis (chairing the American's Committee on Training for Research, chairing its Committee on Scientific Activities, chairing its Fund for Psychoanalytic Research, etc., along with a similar role in the IPA) and consulting with psychoanalytic research programs around the world.
>
> My second role in psychoanalysis in America has been in having been fortunate to become a central part of "the establishment" through my organizational work within the American Psychoanalytic Association, where I have been in a position to advocate for the causes that were important to me and to know that I have been listened to and heard, even though those causes were not always universally popular. They have included a more progressive organization of the hierarchy within the American, bringing the almost century-long contentious issue of the place of "lay analysis" within organized psychoanalysis to appropriate resolution, the promotion of the research enterprise worldwide, exerting what I hoped was a unifying perspective both intellectually and organizationally—both/and rather than either/or positions, again whether in theoretical discourse or in the organizational structure.
>
> I guess I have been fortunate in my psychoanalytic career in that I have had a part in promoting activities that I felt would be important to our discipline over the long haul, with more success than many others have experienced.

WHY I CHOSE THIS PAPER

Robert S. Wallerstein, M.D.

I think this paper may be the most influential of all my contributions to the psychoanalytic world. Although obviously I have written a lot more about psychoanalytic research, and have devoted my professional life centrally to both doing and promoting psychoanalytic research, I think that for better or for worse (I mean for worse) my research contributions have made a lesser impact on the totality of psychoanalysis than has my thinking about the issue of the psychoanalytic pluralism with which we live, and our search within that pluralism for the common ground that holds us together as adherents of a shared discipline. That's why I chose "One Psychoanalysis or Many?"—which was, after all, my plenary address as President of the IPA to the Montreal Congress of 1987—for inclusion in this volume.

ONE PSYCHOANALYSIS OR MANY?

ROBERT S. WALLERSTEIN, M.D.

THE PRIVILEGE, AS PRESIDENT, of addressing the IPA Congress in an opening-day plenary session is tempered by the corresponding obligation to select a topic of sufficient importance to the worldwide psychoanalytic community, in the hope that a dialogue about it initiated or furthered here can enhance our shared psychoanalytic understanding and commitment. Such a topic, I think, is the one I have selected today, that of our increasing psychoanalytic diversity, or pluralism as we have come to call it, a pluralism of theoretical perspectives, of linguistic and thought conventions, of distinctive regional, cultural, and language emphases; and what it is, in view of this increasing diversity, that still holds us together as common adherents of a shared psychoanalytic science and profession.

Psychoanalysis was not always characterized by this pluralism; in fact, quite the opposite. Perhaps more than any other branch of human knowledge psychoanalysis has been uniquely the singular product of the creative genius of one man, Sigmund Freud. His lifetime of productive work was extraordinarily prodigious and if the totality of psychoanalysis consisted of nothing more than the corpus of Freud's work, *die Gesammelte Werke,* I think we could readily agree that all the fundamental principles and the essential fabric of a fully operating scientific and professional activity would be available to us as students and as practitioners.

Presented at the 35th International Psychoanalytical Association (IPA) Congress, Montreal, July 1987.

And Freud made strenuous efforts throughout his lifetime to define the parameters of his new science of the mind, and to hold it together as a unified enterprise against both destructive or diluting pressures or seductions from without and also against fractious human divisivenesses from within. To him psychoanalysis was not only a science and a profession, but also a Movement with all the calls to a dedicated and disciplined allegiance that that word connotes. When divergent tendencies threatened to splinter the unified edifice that Freud was trying to build, he created the famous Committee of the seven ring holders to try to guarantee the stability of his central psychoanalytic doctrines. And we all know the story, which Freud chronicled in 1914, in "On the History of the Psychoanalytic Movement," of how that first wave of close co-workers who began to differ with him in major ways, Adler and Stekel and Jung, each found it necessary to leave psychoanalysis over the 3-year span from 1910 to 1913.

Freud from his side declared the psychological deviations of these dissidents to be totally incompatible with the fundamental postulates of psychoanalysis as he had established them to that point, and when they left the Movement over these differences, he professed himself to be satisfied that they should pursue any psychological and psychotherapeutic bent that they wished so long as they did not claim it to be psychoanalysis. Two of them did establish schools or movements of their own; Adler called his "Individual Psychology" and Jung took the name "Analytical Psychology." Of these two new theoretical systems Freud felt Adler's to be the more important (p. 60) and potentially the more enduring and in this his prediction proved to be faulty. It is the Jungian movement, which has more recently even reappropriated for itself the designation psychoanalysis, which has endured worldwide as an alternative therapeutic system—and I will return later to its potential current relationship to the psychoanalysis represented within the ranks of the IPA.

Freud did declare that both Adler and Jung had brought valuable new contributions to analysis, Adler to the psychology of the ego and its role in adaptation and to the recognition of the importance of the aggressive drives in mental life, and Jung to tracing the way infantile impulses are used to serve our highest ethical and religious interests. But Freud felt that each of these two in his own way had at the same time abandoned the central psychoanalytic concepts of the unconscious and repression, of resistance and transference, and that they had therefore placed themselves outside the definitional statement that Freud made for psychoanalysis in this selfsame History of his Movement—actually the first, the most succinct, and the best known of the several such statements that Freud enunciated over the long span of his writings. As we all know so well he said there, "the facts of transference and of resistance. Any line of investigation which recognizes these two facts and takes them as the starting-point of its work has a right to call itself psycho-analysis, even though it arrives at results other than my own. But anyone who takes up other sides of the problem while avoiding these two hypotheses will hardly escape a charge of misappropriation of property by attempted impersonation, if he persists in calling himself a psycho-analyst" (Freud 1914a, p. 16). Of course we must add here that the key words *transference* and *resistance* also imply the concepts of the unconscious, of psychic conflict, and of defense, the key building stones of our shared psychoanalytic edifice.[1] Since then, of course, several of Adler's central conceptions—like those of the ego and adaptation or of the motive power of aggression—have been actively reincorporated into the main body of psychoanalysis, first by Freud and then by others who came after, like Hartmann, and perhaps that is related to the near collapse of Adlerian psychology as a separate therapeutic enterprise. There have been lesser but nonetheless still substantial reincorporations also from Jungian psychology, or at least cognate developments within the psychoanalytic framework, like Erikson's life span focus with its shift in emphases to the coequal concern with the second half of the life span, or like our focus on unconscious fantasy systems as guides to understanding motivation and behavior—albeit in a different way than the Jungians—and this somewhat lesser reappropriation of concepts from Jung's theoretical system may relate to its continuing greater vigor as a separate psychology and therapy than its Adlerian counterpart.

Within another decade, after the departures of Adler and Stekel and Jung, psychoanalysis was threatened with new deviations, those of Ferenczi and of Rank, partly linked together in their monograph *The Development of Psycho-analysis* (Ferenczi and Rank 1924), and partly developing in differing, albeit related, directions, Ferenczi in his Active Therapy and Rank later in his Will Therapy. Actually despite the severe

[1] Freud himself made the point of this addendum of mine quite explicit further along in the very same "History." He said at this further point, "The first task confronting psycho-analysis was to explain the neuroses; it used the two facts of resistance and transference as starting-points, and, taking into consideration the third fact of amnesia, accounted for them with its theories of repression, of the sexual motive forces in neurosis and of the unconscious" (Freud 1914a, p. 50). He just does not specifically mention the word *conflict,* but it is totally inherent; the concepts mentioned don't hang together otherwise.

strains aroused by these theoretical and technical developments, Ferenczi never left psychoanalysis, though Rank ultimately did and developed a new school in America more influential in social work than within psychoanalysis, the so-called functional school of social work, but that Rankian deviation and outgrowth has like Adler's psychology mostly now faded into history.

But that same decade of the 20s also saw the origin of the first major new theoretical direction within psychoanalysis that at the same time fought fiercely to maintain its sense of direct descent from the psychoanalysis of Freud, that indeed in some respects, like its unswerving acceptance of Freud's most problematic and controversial theorizing—the introduction of the death instinct theory in "Beyond the Pleasure Principle" in 1920—and the making of it a central building block in its own theoretical conceptual development, that in this it could even claim a closer adherence to the persona and the mind of Freud than those of the Viennese school who while closer to Freud personally yet split sharply on the value to psychoanalysis of this particular theoretical turn of Freud's. I refer here, of course, to Melanie Klein and the development of Kleinian analysis.

Riccardo Steiner (1985) in his published review of the British Society's so-called "Controversial Discussions" of 1943 and 1944 traces clearly the political history of the Kleinian theoretical development in England; the original invitation to Melanie Klein to come from Berlin to London to lecture on her new ideas about theory and technique that had developed out of her work with children, the interest aroused by these ideas in the British group, the invitation then to come permanently to London and the early support and adherence to the Kleinian views by Jones and a distinguished group of the first generation British analysts, and the adversarial letters around this between Jones and Freud with Jones supporting Melanie Klein and Freud supporting his daughter Anna in the growing controversy over the proper theoretical and technical development of child psychoanalysis seen as an unhappy divergence between Kleinian and Anna Freudian views or between what was called the London and Vienna positions, representing at that time the two main centers of psychoanalytic influence in Europe and actually in the world.

The fundamental difference here, however, was that the Kleinian development did not lead to a split and departure from the organized body of institutional analysis, the IPA. Rather the Kleinians insisted, as I have stated, on their even more impeccable psychoanalytic credentials and their movement remained within the British organizational framework and therefore within the IPA although the exact terms under which the British Society would henceforth operate with a Kleinian group and a Freudian group, and in between, an independent or middle group, these terms were not settled until the year-long Controversial Discussions which took place 4 to 5 years after Freud's death.

My point here is that the Kleinian development, still within Freud's lifetime and when his personal leadership in psychoanalysis was, of course, unquestioned, nonetheless represented the beginnings of the gradual transition of psychoanalysis from being—at least in appearance—a thoroughly unified theoretical structure evolved around the creative intellectual corpus of its founding genius, Sigmund Freud, a gradual transition from that into the present-day worldwide theoretical diversity in which we have existing now side by side the American ego psychological (and by now post-ego psychological) school, the Kleinian, the Bionian, the (British) object-relational sometimes narrowed down to the Winnicottian, the Lacanian (largely outside but to a considerable extent in Europe and in Latin America inside our official ranks), and even in the United States, so long the stronghold of the unquestioning monolithic hegemony of the ego psychological metapsychology paradigm of Hartmann and Rapaport, where we have, however, recently witnessed the rise of Kohut's self psychology as a major alternative psychoanalytical theoretical perspective and, to a lesser extent as new schools, Mahler's developmental approach and Schafer's new voice or new idiom for psychoanalysis.

And, of course, these varying *theoretical* perspectives do not exhaust the diverging conceptual developments within our field. We have all the advocates of our traditional natural science approach to the nature of the psychoanalytic enterprise with its requirements ultimately for evidence and validation in our inferential and predictive processes in accord with the canons of empirical science, albeit, of course, in ways fully consonant with the subjectivistic nature of our primary data, the transactional exchanges in our consulting rooms; all this as against those who see psychoanalysis as a social or historical science that is somehow different in the logic of its theory, in its epistemological base, and in its methods of discovery and validation, a different *kind* of science, in Harrison's (1970) words, "our science" meaning our "peculiar" science; and all the way from this to those who see psychoanalysis as not any kind of science at all but rather a hermeneutical discipline like literary criticism or the Biblical exegetical interpretation from which the term "hermeneutics" derived in the first place, a psychology that is based only on reasons, on the "why" of human behavior, and not at all like a science which is based on causes, on the "how" of human behavior. Though the natural science perspective has its main strongholds in

America and in Britain and the hermeneutical perspective with such names as Gadamer (1975), Habermas (1968), and Ricoeur (1970) is centered in Germany and France, there are indeed passionate advocates of each of these polar opposed positions everywhere, and within the hermeneutic camp there are all varieties of hermeneutic, phenomenological, exclusively subjectivistic and/or linguistically based conceptualizations of our field. All these issues of the *nature* of psychoanalysis as a discipline I have dealt with at length elsewhere in my Freud Anniversary Lecture in New York (Wallerstein 1986) and need not elaborate further for my purposes here today.

But I do want to call attention in this context to yet another array of distinctivenesses that characterizes organized psychoanalysis worldwide. I am referring to all the regional and cultural and language emphases that make French (or francophone) analysis, quite aside from Lacan, into a different analytic "voice" than Anglo-American (or anglophone) analysis. This is what Bergeret in France has in mind when he calls for an official Scientific Council under the auspices of the IPA that would extend the contending conceptions about the nature of our discipline as a science beyond the "English language cultural model" with its particular linguistic and thought conventions that can tend to constrain analysis into one predominant mold, not responsive to what he calls "*all* the currents of thought existing in the psychoanalytic world" (J. Bergeret, "Reflections on the Scientific Responsibilities of the International Psycho-Analytical Association," unpublished manuscript, 1986). It is also what the recently inaugurated meetings between French and American analysts—the first was in Paris in the spring of 1983—have been about, to give the Americans present a "sampling of the range of ideas of French analytic thought" (Poland and Major 1984, p. 145), and of course vice versa, and hopefully in ways that would enable each side to the dialogue to transcend the prevailing stereotypes concerning the other. These differences that were explored are not just stylistic but also perspectival and therefore value laden with, for example, the differential allegiances, as values, to fluid and expressive freedom of discourse by metaphor and poetic allusion as against precision of meaning with careful denotation of explicit thought boundaries. All of this, of course, underlines what Steiner (1984) said in his review of the English-language book *Psychoanalysis in France*, edited by Lebovici and Widlöcher (1980), that "despite the universality of the process of the unconscious, psychoanalysis is considerably influenced by the historical, cultural and social context in which it is developing. This can be regarded as a negative or as a positive phenomenon according to one's point of view, but it is a reality which cannot be easily refuted" (p. 233).

It should not be thought, however, that this transition which I have traced to this point from the theoretical unity of psychoanalysis that Freud tried to embody and enforce in his conception of a shared intellectual movement built around the intellectual charisma of his leadership, from that to the broad theoretical diversity with which we are today variously easily or uneasily content, was a smooth or uneventful journey. The interpolated momentous event for psychoanalysis, given the nature of our discipline and its origins, was the death of Freud and the burden thereupon thrust upon analysts to have to carry their field beyond the consummate genius of the one man who had so adventurously single-handedly brought it into being on to what now had to become a discipline and a science, that, true, built on its past, but rested on the from-now-on independent work of its collectivity.

This was for psychoanalysis a truly wrenching task. Freud's name and work had come to mean so much and not just to psychoanalysts. As the literary critic Alfred Kazin (1957) expressed it in his assessment of the Freudian revolution, "His name is no longer the name of a man; like "Darwin," it is now synonymous with a part of nature. This is the very greatest influence that a man can have. It means that people use his name to signify something in the world of nature which, they believe, actually exists.... Every hour of every day... there are people who cannot forget a name, or make a slip of the tongue, or feel depressed; who cannot begin a love affair, or end a marriage, without wondering what the 'Freudian' reason may be" (p. 15).

It is perhaps then small wonder that though Freud died in 1939, almost a half century ago, we have still collectively not yet fully come to terms with his transience and his death (Wallerstein 1983a). We still use his monumental contributions as the benchmarks against which to measure our progress as in this very Congress built around the reconsideration 50 years later of his last great clinical paper, "Analysis Terminable and Interminable" (Freud 1937). For so many of us Sigmund Freud still remains our lost object, our unreachable genius, whose passing we have perhaps never properly mourned, at least not in the emotional fullness that leads to intellective accommodation. Knight (1953) put it thus: "Perhaps we are still standing too much in the shadow of that giant, Sigmund Freud, to permit ourselves to view psychoanalysis as a science of the mind rather than as the doctrine of a founder" (p. 211). Gombaroff, in a recent paper on our training issues, has called Freud "the father who does not die" (M. Gombaroff, "Considerations of the Psychoanalytic Institution," unpublished manuscript). What this persisting feeling, of course, adds up to is that, unlike other sciences, psychoanalysis has not yet been able really to accept Whitehead's famous dictum: "A science that hesitates to forget its founders is lost." Witness our common habit established by Freud's first followers of clinching our arguments by reciting a relevant passage from his papers; witness the curricula of our Institutes built so centrally still around the corpus of Freud's writings, usually studied chronologically. And we all know well the galvanizing impact of Lacan's battle cry, "back to Freud," as the rallying point of the Lacanian movement, the point of pride in differentiating themselves from all the rest of us who by implication have not as fully kept this personal (and personality) faith.[2]

It would be a digression here to try to trace the multiple consequences for our discipline of this unique continuing historic and mythic relationship to our founder as a fantasied continuing presence amongst us. I want now only to speculate about its relationship to my own central theme in this presentation, the dialectic between the effort to maintain the theoretical unity of psychoanalysis through a process of extrusion of those like Jung and Adler and others in subsequent generations whose new theoretical proposals, whatever their putative value, were, or seemed to be, linked to a major dilution if not a full abandonment of central psychoanalytic concepts, as against the contrapuntal effort at accommodation of diverging theoretical perspectives within a more generous and elastic overall definitional framework for psychoanalysis—albeit one that somehow can define what nonetheless we all do share and keeps us together as analysts (and differentiates us from non-analysts), despite, amongst ourselves, our diversity in theory, in perspective, and in cultural and language emphasis and thought convention.

The main thrust of our developmental dynamic following upon Freud's death could have tilted in either of these two opposed directions, either of an ever tighter circle of orthodoxy, or required adherence to one mainstream psychoanalytic doctrine, or of an expanding diversity of theory that could ultimately pose bewildering problems of boundaries, of deviation, of what is then "wild analysis," and of what is altogether beyond analysis, problems which all seemed simpler of

---

[2]J. Sandler made this identical point well in his prepublished paper for the 1983 IPA Congress in Madrid: "Freud's ideas are seen as the core of existing theory, and acceptable later developments are viewed as amplifications and additions which are consistent—or at least not inconsistent—with Freud's thoughts. Those who think in these terms will, when they disagree with other writers, do so on the grounds that the others have misunderstood, misinterpreted or misapplied Freud, and will turn back to Freud's writings to find supporting evidence for their own ideas" (p. 35).

resolution in Freud's day. In practice and for a long time after Freud's death—until the 1970s in fact, the tilt was in *both* directions, toward diversity in Europe and by extension also in Latin America, and toward maintained unity within one "mainstream" in the United States.

The philosophy and the justification of the European development toward an acceptance of diversity was spelled out by Susan Isaacs (1943) in her response to the discussion of her paper "The Nature and Function of Phantasy" during the British Society's Controversial Discussions in 1943. She said, "Listening to the selective accounts of Freud's theories offered by some of the contributors to this discussion, and noting their dogmatic temper, I cannot help wondering what would have happened to the development of psychoanalytic thought, if for any reason Freud's work had not been continued after 1913, before his work on Narcissism and Mourning and Melancholia; or after 1919, before *Beyond the Pleasure Principle* and the *Ego and the Id*. Suppose some other adventurous thinker had arrived at these profound truths and had dared to assert them! I fear that such a one would have been treated as a backslider from the strict path of psychoanalytic doctrine, a heretic whose views were incompatible with those of Freud, and therefore subversive of psychoanalysis" (p. 151). Certainly Isaacs' heartfelt cry can be read as a Kleinian plea for tolerance of diverse theoretical viewpoints *within* the body of psychoanalysis, each equally sincerely—and perhaps with equally good reason—feeling itself to be in a direct and logical developmental line from the overall corpus of Freud's work, each in emphasis perhaps centering itself more in one than in another of the main theoretical conceptions for the understanding of the human mind offered by Freud over the span of his life's work, and not all of these conceptions easily reconciled with each of the others.

Sparked then by the success of this Kleinian development in England even within Freud's lifetime, a success consolidated in the outcome of the so-called "Controversial Discussions" shortly thereafter, and sparked perhaps also by the natural national and language diversity of the European continent, from rather early on, the psychoanalytic development in Europe was diverse and pluralistic. The Kleinian movement spread to other parts of Europe, as far away as India and Australia, and most significantly became the dominant theory in the original growth of psychoanalysis all over the South American continent. The role of the British Society with its powerful Kleinian group as a main training center for so many of the psychoanalytic pioneers in these various countries has been, of course, a central element in that development.

But the post-World War II decades have also seen the rise and flowering of the differing theoretical work of Lacan and his followers in

France, of the extensions of Kleinian thought by Bion in England, and of the whole development of the British independent group of the object relational perspectives in psychoanalysis pioneered by Suttie and Fairbairn and Guntrip and further developed by Balint and Bowlby and Winnicott and a host of others. It is this pluralistic theoretical development, to which can be added in Europe the various other distinctive and differentiating perspectives to which I have already alluded, the natural science versus hermeneutical, as well as the varying cultural and linguistic emphases—it is all this that has, despite our usually professed desire to see psychoanalysis as a body of theory which is expected to be consonant with some unifying perspective on Freud's writings—it is all this that has rather eventuated in our present-day pluralism of perspectives with varyingly inconsistent psychoanalytic theoretical structures to which we differentially adhere, depending mostly, it should be added, not on grounds of inherent appeal, plausibility or heuristic usefulness, but rather on where and how we were trained, and where we then live and practice. And in a tour that Dr Weinshel and I made of the various Latin American psychoanalytic societies last summer it became clear to us how that whole region, once thought to be a monolithic center of Kleinian analysis, has become home to each and every one of the theoretical developments in analysis emanating from centers in Europe, and from the United States as well.

By contrast to these developments in Europe in the post-war decades, psychoanalysis in the United States for a long time took a different course. With the rise of Hitler and the collapse of the main psychoanalytic strongholds in central Europe, the main bulk and intellective power of psychoanalysis was transplanted to the United States though, of course, some went to the periphery of the European continent, to England, and to South America. And in America the post-war historical tilt, different from that elsewhere in the world, was in the direction of a unitary and unifying "mainstream"—the heir in that way of the political-administrative ambitions of Freud, epitomized in his conception of the role of the seven ring holders and expressed in the development and fruition in America of the ego psychology metapsychological paradigm, which under the aegis of Hartmann and Kris and Loewenstein and Rapaport and Jacobson and a host of others for long maintained a monolithic hegemony over the psychoanalytic domain in an arena which contained in those earlier postwar years at least half the world's psychoanalysts.

And when divergent theoretical directions emerged in the United States as they did elsewhere, as early as the forties—and here the names of Horney and Fromm and Thompson and Sullivan as well again of many others come to mind, all associated under the loose rubrics of either the interpersonal or the culturalist schools of psychoanalysis—when these divergences arose, the resulting controversy led in America just as it had in Freud's day in Vienna to a forced leaving of the affiliation with organized psychoanalysis and the founding of independent schools and training centers, though some like Fromm-Reichmann and Rado and Kardiner did manage to remain within the American Psychoanalytic Association and even to found new institutes and societies within it. But overall the turmoil and the leavings of the forties in America were indeed reminiscent of the turmoil and the leavings of Adler and Stekel and Jung three decades earlier in Vienna.

However, this uniform character of the defined psychoanalytic mainstream was in the end no better able to survive intact in post-World War II America than in post-World War I Europe. The ego psychological metapsychology edifice has itself, though it is still the main focal strength of American psychoanalysis, nonetheless been gradually transformed into what some today call the post–ego psychological age, and object relations perspectives have been varyingly incorporated into it by such workers as Zetzel and Modell and Kernberg. The natural science model of psychoanalysis has been vigorously attacked including by some of its once staunchest adherents with a variety of hermeneutical, phenomenological, totally subjectivistic, and/or linguistically based perspectives like those offered by George Klein and Gill and Schafer and Spence. And, of course, aside from the decades-long work of Mahler and her followers who have used their child development observations to fashion an explicitly developmental perspective into psychoanalytic theory and praxis—which has never quite become a school of its own, however—aside from this there has been the evolution within America starting in the seventies of the self psychology of Kohut and his many followers, a psychology with a distinctive metapsychology of the bipolar self and the vision of Tragic rather than Guilty Man, very much an alternative psychoanalytic theory, a psychoanalytic school of its own.

All this has now led to a situation of diverse and diverging developments within American psychoanalysis in recent years that though it is not yet comparable to the established pluralism of psychoanalysis in Europe and in Latin America is perhaps fast getting there. This indeed led a representative of one of the outside groups in the United States to comment at a recent panel of the American Psychoanalytic Association devoted to this current growing diversity of theoretical perspectives within American analysis to say that it would be a fine thing if the split of 50 years ago in America could be healed, so that all American analysts could discuss their different views within a single scientific and professional organization. For after all, he said, "the differences of Silverberg, Rado, Sullivan and Horney from orthodox psychoanalytic views are not materially greater—in fact, less so—than those of Kohut and Schafer, both of which, and others, are today comfortably contained within the American Psychoanalytic Association" (Post 1986, p. 21).

Which brings me to the crux of the dilemma, or if not dilemma, the issue that I am proposing for consideration by us all. Psychoanalysis, despite all the efforts of Sigmund Freud, its founding father, and despite the like-minded efforts of many of his most gifted followers, which actually succeeded for so many more years in the United States than anywhere else in the world in maintaining an integrated and overall uniform perspective on psychoanalysis, called (and cherished as) the mainstream, that despite all this, psychoanalysis worldwide today and all within the organizational framework of the IPA consists of multiple (and divergent) theories of mental functioning, of development, of pathogenesis, of treatment, and of cure.

If this is so, that, to advert to the title of my presentation, we do indeed have several, or even many psychoanalyses today, and not one, then we are faced with two formidable questions, questions for any discipline, any body of theory or derivatively body of praxis, that strives to organize and give meaning to a coherent and discrete segment of human experience. The first question is what do these diverse theories all have in common that they are all recognizably psychoanalysis in terms of fundamentally shared assumptions? The second question, perhaps the other side of the same coin, is what differentiates them together from all the other, the unpsychoanalytic theories of mental life, for surely not every psychology of human behavior is psychoanalytic, and there is only intellectual destructiveness in a posture that "anything goes" or that anything, anything mental that is, can somehow be construed as psychoanalytic.

To begin with, what they all *do* have in common are our shared definitional boundaries of psychoanalysis. Here we do, I think properly, revert to Freud and his definitional statement of 1914 on "the facts of transference and of resistance" which I quoted at the beginning of this talk. There are any number of ways to try to capture in a single statement the central conception of Freud's revolutionary way of understanding mental life. Certainly though I think we can all agree that Freud's fundamental discovery was that human beings have thoughts and feelings that they don't know they have, and that these constitute an unconscious mental life expressed in unconscious fantasy and unconscious conflict—and that this set of conceptions is not only contained within but is the distinguishing feature of each and every psychoanalytic psychology of mental life. In Ernst Kris's famous aphoristic definition, psychoanalysis is "nothing but" human behavior considered from the point of view of conflict.[3]

Considered this way the decision about whose work and whose theoretical views then belong within psychoanalysis is not a political-administrative issue of who remained within the organized institutional psychoanalytic framework of the IPA like Fromm-Reichmann and Alexander and who left it like Fromm and Horney (and, of course, there are Lacanians in significant numbers both inside and outside the IPA). Nor can that decision be based just on whether one claims Freud's heritage, as the adherents of both Melanie Klein and Kohut do, or disavows it, as Jung did in creating his Analytical Psychology. In fact, Jungian analysis is a case in point as in recent years its followers have reappropriated the label psychoanalysis, calling themselves Jungian psychoanalysts and implying that only political and organizational issues, reflections of bygone struggles, keep them in a world apart from the psychoanalysis operating within the IPA. I am myself not in a position to have an adequately informed opinion on the psychoanalytic credentials of Jungian theory. Here I would only quote Goodheart (1984), a Jungian analyst in America, who in a detailed disquisition on Jung's doctoral dissertation published in 1902, in which Jung's first clinical material and clinical formulations were presented, demonstrates impressively how Jung avoided seeing the interactional dynamic, the evidence of psychic conflict, seeking out instead a mechanical (and

---

[3]I include in this conception of who and what is properly psychoanalytic Kohut's self psychology even though it avows itself to be centrally a psychology of the supraordinate self and its developmental struggle for cohesion, with a psychopathology and a therapy based on conceptions of deficit and of restoration rather than primarily of conflict and its resolution. I do this on the basis of my reading of the clinical material presented by Kohut and other self psychologists and my view of the clinical data that are presented as indeed dealing planfully with the interplay of conflicted transferences (and countertransferences); I present my reading of these reported clinical interactions in the several critiques I have published (Wallerstein 1981, 1983b, 1985) on self psychology and its relation to American mainstream ego psychology and post-ego psychology. I therefore view self psychology as a new and variant theoretical school of psychoanalysis and not as a species of nonanalytic psychotherapy which some of its critics have declared it to be (see particularly Wallerstein 1985).

nonpsychological) explanatory framework of autonomous psychic productions—the autonomous psyche that was ultimately expressed in the collective unconscious existing apart from personal experience or meaning. Goodheart describes how at several points in his dissertation Jung came close to the Freudian notions of conflict but then each time backed away and how finally, "Jung skipped away from his own proposals and inserted the abruptly aborting conclusion that all this "must remain unanswered." This is actually the first Freud–Jung split" (p. 12). All this is written by a Jungian analyst and is describing Jung's thinking even before he ever met Freud. Goodheart took it to presage the ultimate actual break with Freud. It is on the basis of evidence of this kind that I would in the end answer for myself whether Jung's psychology is truly a *psychoanalytic* psychology or not; clearly such a perspective as Goodheart's would first have to be substantiated by other thoughtful and knowledgeable students of Jung's scientific corpus.

All this, of course, creates for us another dilemma or issue. Living with the pluralism of psychoanalysis not only creates what Cooper (1984) called "porous boundaries" (p. 255) for our field, but at the same time makes it much more difficult today than it seemed for Freud (1910) to try to define "wild" analysis. Schafer (1985) made just this point in an article entitled "Wild Analysis." When Freud wrote on the subject in 1910 psychoanalysis was indeed simpler, it was more one thing, and it was easier to say what departed from it, what was "wild" analysis. Today with our pluralistic conceptions, our varying theoretical perspectives and models of the mind, what may be conventional or proper analysis within one perspective may well be wild within another. To deal with this issue Schafer introduced the phrase "comparative analysis" and said of it, "The appropriate name for my method of reexamining wild analysis is comparative analysis, that is to say, seeing how things look from within the perspective of each system" (p. 276) and he undertook to compare from this point of view the theoretical systems of Melanie Klein, Kohut, and Gill. One can wonder, incidentally, in this connection how much Glover's (1931) conceptions of inexact interpretation, incomplete interpretation, and incomplete analysis would be relevant in this context.

Given the acceptance of these realities then, of a polytheoretical psychoanalysis, how can we understand what we all know as a commonplace everyday observation, that we all, adherents of whatever theoretical position within psychoanalysis, all seem to do reasonably comparable clinical work and bring about reasonably comparable clinical change in the (comparable enough) patients that we deal with? An example drawn from Kohut's last book (1984) puts this question as well as anyone has. In that book Kohut gives a detailed account (pp. 92ff) of an interchange with a Kleinian colleague from Latin America who told him how she had responded interpretively to a patient's silent withdrawal from the analytic work in the hour immediately after notification of the planned cancellation of a session in the near future. The interpretation had followed the presumed standard Kleinian format, that the patient's basic perception of the analyst had been abruptly altered by the announcement, that the analyst had shifted from being a good, warm, feeding breast to becoming a bad, cold, withholding one, and that the patient had responded with sadistic rage against the analyst *qua* bad breast, a rage that was defended against through a general inhibition, with a particular inhibition of oral activity, of "biting words."

Kohut, in his account, expressed surprise that this (to him) "far-fetched interpretation" (Kohut 1984, p. 92), albeit given in a "warmly understanding tone of voice" (p. 92) nonetheless elicited a very favorable response from the patient. He went on to say that the analyst could equally have couched an interpretation within ego psychological, conflict-drive-defense terms (i.e., the cancellation experienced as an abandonment by the oedipal mother locking the child-patient out of the parental bedroom), or, for that matter, within Kohutian self psychological terms (the loss of a self-sustaining selfobject leaving the patient feeling empty and not fully alive). What Kohut made of all this was that the clinical context given by his Kleinian colleague was insufficient to decide which interpretation would be closest to the mark in this instance and so he called all three, examples, potentially, of "wild analysis"—until proven otherwise. What I will make of it—as I shall make clear further on—is that the clinical context, by itself, will never determine which interpretation, within which theoretical framework, is closest to the mark, that in fact, put in those terms, the issue is totally miscast.

At this point I only want to add that the lesson that Kohut drew from the patient's favorable response, however, was that though the (Kleinian) *content* of the interpretation may have been wrong, off the mark (in Kohut's sense), it was nevertheless a therapeutically effective "inexact interpretation" in Glover's (1931) sense, since it was "in its essence more right than wrong" (p. 97) since the analyst was conveying (indeed in any of the three alternative interpretive forms presented, could have been conveying) her understanding that the patient was sorely troubled over the announced cancellation and was understandably reacting unhappily to it. Again, my framework for understanding the patient's favorable response will differ significantly from that of Kohut, but here there will also be points of convergence.

To make clear what I have in mind, and how I would understand and interpret the whole sequence outlined by Kohut, I will turn first to some fresh perspectives on familiar conceptions proposed by Joseph and Anne-Marie Sandler in their papers on the past unconscious and the present unconscious. As elaborated in this sequence of papers (J. Sandler and A.-M. Sandler 1983, 1984; J. Sandler 1986), "the *past unconscious* can be conceived of as containing the whole gamut of immediate, peremptory wishes, impulses, and responses of the individual that have been formed early in his life" (Sandler and Sandler 1984, p. 369); these are clearly stated to be "more than instinctual wishes...they also include the immediate and spontaneous modes of reacting in any given psychological situation, at any given moment, in any particular set of internal or external circumstances" (p. 369). That is, they "may be instinctual but need not necessarily be so. Thus, for example, solutions to conflict devised or elaborated in early childhood acquire a peremptory quality, as do all sorts of responses aimed at avoiding dangerous situations and preserving safety" (p. 370). In sum total the past unconscious represents the "child within the adult" (p. 370), the totality of the mental life roughly "corresponding, from a developmental point of view, to the first 4 to 6 years of life" (p. 371). It is all this which is essentially sealed off by the repression barrier which covers the infantile amnesia and "which is for the most part only reconstructed in analysis, reconstruction which is usually reinforced by those scattered memories that are available from the first years of life, but which memories can only be understood in the light of later reconstruction" (p. 371).

Granted that this "past unconscious is active in the present, and is stimulated by internal or external events occurring in the here-and-now, what...[the Sandlers] have termed the *present unconscious* is conceived of as a very different organization.... Whereas the past unconscious acts and reacts according to the past, the present unconscious is concerned with maintaining equilibrium in the present and regards the impulse from the past unconscious as intrusive and upsetting" (Sandler and Sandler 1984, p. 372). And, "While it is itself...the product of the past development of the individual, it [the present unconscious] is orientated, *not to the past, but to the present,* in order to prevent the individual from being overwhelmed by painful and uncontrollable experiences. It constantly creates conflict-solving compromises and adaptations that help to keep an inner balance. Foremost among these is the continual creation or recreation of current *unconscious fantasies and thoughts.* These have a function in the present, are constantly being modified and orientated to the present, although they will, of course, reflect their history in the past" (J. Sandler 1986, p. 188). In the clinical situation the prime example of such fantasies, of course, are the unconscious transference fantasies about the analyst.

It, of course, follows from all of this that the central interpretive work in the analytic situation is with the unconscious transference fantasies that are the direct representations of the activities of the present unconscious. And since "the *present unconscious,* contains present-day, here-and-now fantasies and thoughts that are after all current adaptations to the conflicts and anxieties evoked by the contents of the *past unconscious*" (J. Sandler 1986, p. 191), it is clear that via the analysis of the fantasies of the present unconscious, centrally the transference fantasies of the present unconscious, we can and do reach an understanding of the originating infantile past, what the Sandlers call the past unconscious. The mechanism of that understanding, they remind us, is a creative act of *reconstruction,* abetted by whatever fragmentary memories have survived the childhood amnesia, but these memories, too, being given meaning only via the act of reconstruction that puts them into coherent context.

All of this stated in this somewhat new language is, of course, recognizable to us as a vivid description of our everyday work of analysis. How does it all relate to my central theme of the *pluralism* of the theoretical frameworks within which we do our *consensually shared* psychoanalytic work and to my case example drawn from Kohut's account as the paradigm illustration of my theme? I would submit that the thrust of the present unconscious in the patient described by Kohut as conveyed in the analyst's transference interpretation (albeit clothed within the analyst's Kleinian theoretical language which as Kohut indicated could have alternatively been equally well embedded in an ego psychological or a Kohutian self psychological explanatory language), that the transference fantasy of the present unconscious was centered in the meaning—common to all the three possible theoretical explanatory languages presented—that the patient was acutely distressed over the coming cancellation and was reacting unhappily and resentfully to that announcement. Here we are dealing in the actual observables of the analytic interaction, in the clinical data of the consulting room fashioned into the low-level and experience-near "clinical theory" that in George Klein's (1976) perspective is all the theory that psychoanalysis needs and is indeed all the theory that its data can truly sustain and can test.

When we reach beyond the interactions of the analytic consulting room, beyond the elucidation of the present unconscious, beyond, that is, the clinical phenomena captured in and explained by our *clinical* theory, to a more encompassing, more generally explanatory, more causally developmental accounting of mental life from its earliest fathomable origins, we are getting into the other realm that George Klein called the unnecessary *general* theory that we should sever and cast out by an action he dubbed "theorectomy," the realm that the Sandlers call the *reconstructed* past unconscious, the realm of our pluralistic theoretical perspectives in psychoanalysis, the ego psychological, the object relational, the Kleinian, the Lacanian, etc. These, as Kohut illustrated so well with his vignette, can *each* be invoked and each used to explain the same clinical interaction, i.e., to put its specific into a framework of general meaning within an overall theoretical context. And each of these theoretical explanatory contexts, the Kleinian, the ego psychological, and the self psychological will be persuasive indeed to the adherents of that viewpoint who in fact will look at it as *the* useful and natural way in which to understand the phenomenon, the clinical interaction.

What I am suggesting by all this is that our *data* are the data of the present unconscious and their interpretation that carries real meaning is embedded in our clinical theory, the theory of transference and resistance, of conflict and defense, i.e., the original fundamental elements of Freud's 1914 definition of psychoanalysis with which I began this presentation and which I have underlined as the consensual understanding that unites us all as psychoanalysts. What I am further suggesting is that our pluralism of theoretical perspectives within which we try to give overall meaning to our clinical data in the present (in the present unconscious) and to *reconstruct* the past out of which the present developed (the past unconscious), that this pluralism of perspectives represents the various scientific *metaphors* that we have created in order to satisfy our variously conditioned needs for closure and coherence and overall theoretical understanding.

The Sandlers had already approached this same conception in their statement that deep interpretations into the infantile past could be viewed as but metaphoric reconstructions. For example, "It is our firm conviction that so-called 'deep' interpretations can have a good analytic effect only because they provide metaphors that can contain the fantasies and feelings in the second system. The patient learns to understand and accept these metaphors, and if they provide a good fit, both cognitively and affectively, then they will be effective. This view gives us a way of understanding the interpretive approach of some of our colleagues" (Sandler and Sandler 1983, p. 424). Or, "In terms of the model we have put forward, we would say that Kleinian interpretations that are affectively and cognitively 'in touch,' when formulated in terms of the most primitive processes and fantasies, provide 'past unconscious' *metaphors* for processes in the present unconscious" (Sandler and Sandler 1984, p. 392). I would only broaden and extend this thinking to the conception that all our theoretical perspectives, Kleinian, but also ego psychological, and all the others are but our chosen explanatory *metaphors*, heuristically useful to us, in terms of our varying intellectual value commitments, in explaining, i.e., making sense of the primary clinical data of our consulting rooms, the realm of our present unconscious in the Sandlers' terms, or the realm of our clinical theory, in George Klein's terms. Put most simply this conceptualization makes all our grand general theory (and all of our pluralism of general theory) nothing but our chosen array of metaphor.

In order to make sure that my meanings are not misunderstood as an assault upon the credentials of psychoanalysis as a science, I should at this point state my perspective on the relationship of metaphor to science or, better put, the role of metaphor *in* science. Metaphor is, of course, usually regarded as the province of poetry and art and therefore the antithesis of science. When it finds a place in scientific theorizing, and Freud—along with many others, it should be added—was famous for his use of metaphor, it is characteristically ascribed to the immaturity of the particular scientific undertaking that will in due time be able to replace the metaphor by theory linked operationally to observable phenomena that can be manipulated and studied within an experimental setting or some other of almost equal rigor and with analogous control. And some psychoanalytic theorists, like Schafer, have dedicated themselves to a relentless quest to extirpate metaphor from our theory statements.

Let me here propose a different perspective on metaphor and science. I want to follow here with Wurmser (1977) in his vigorous defense of the place of metaphor in theory formation in psychoanalysis. Wurmser's position is that rather than trying to eschew and uproot metaphor as a tool for theorizing within psychoanalysis, we should unequivocally accept that "No science can operate without metaphors" (p. 472) and he quotes the physicist Heinrich Hertz who tried to derive all the physics of his time from the basic concepts of time, space, and mass. Hertz was particularly explicit about metaphor, declaring, "the basic concepts of *every* science, the means by which it poses its questions and formulates its solutions, appear not as passive copies of a given being, but as self-created intellectual symbols," i.e., metaphors (p. 472, my italics). Wurmser goes on himself to declare that "What is crucial is that our science, like any other science, is woven of the warp of observations and held together by the intricate woof of symbolism, of many layers of abstractions, of stark and faded metaphors which 'interpret' for us ('explain' to us) the 'direct' facts which, as we know, are never really direct" (pp. 476–477). And even more that, "Metaphors, taken literally are unscientific. But Metaphors, understood as symbols, are the only language of science we possess, unless we resort to mathematical symbols" (p. 483).

In the end Wurmser comes to the statements: "Metaphors (unless reified . . . and treated as if they were 'substance,' not 'function') are indispensable for scientific generativity. They are not evil and to be shunned; they are to be sought and applied. . . . We do not have too many metaphors in psychoanalysis; we have too few. We should not eliminate parts of our theory because they are too metaphorical; we should respect them as such and enlarge them" (p. 491). However, far-ranging as this defense of the vital role of metaphor in our theory formation is, I would still like to extend beyond it, and to develop more explicitly what is only implicit in Wurmser when he states, for example, that "our interest is *whether and in what forms and on what levels we choose symbolic representatives* for the specific experiences gained by the psychoanalytic method and the scientific inquiry based on this method" (p. 482).

What I would like to suggest in my extension of this thinking is that I view the role of metaphor differently (both in its scope and in its developmental place) in regard to what Rapaport and George Klein have designated the clinical theory of psychoanalysis—the clinically near theory of conflict and compromise, of resistance and defense, of transference and countertransference, in which we all of us who are psychoanalysts relate to our patients with common intent and common impact—than I view its role in regard to what they have designated the general theory of psychoanalysis—all the different metapsychologies that distinguish our different theoretical perspectives in psychoanalysis, our theoretical pluralism. In regard to the clinical theory, I view the theory formation, aided though it is in its conceptualizations by the symbolisms of our metaphoric constructions, as nonetheless sufficiently experience-near, anchored directly enough to observables, to the data of our consulting rooms, that it is amenable to the self-same processes of hypothesis formation, testing, and validation as any other scientific enterprise, albeit, of course, by methods adapted to the peculiar subjectivistic nature of the essential data from the psychoanalytic situation. For on this, our whole claim to be a discipline of the mind that is also a science of the mind does—and must—rest, and this, the nature of psychoanalysis as a science, is something on which I have written affirmatively at length elsewhere (Wallerstein 1976, 1986).

But in regard to our general theory or theories, our metapsychologies—and here I interpolate a reminder of Freud's metaphoric commentary, our *witch* metapsychology (Freud 1937, p. 225)—our different and distinguishing theoretical positions, ego psychological, Kleinian, object relational, etc., that mark our psychoanalytic pluralism, in regard to all these I see them, at least at this stage of our historic developmental dynamic, as primarily metaphors, our large-scale explanatory metaphors, or symbolisms, which we use to give a sense of coherence and closure to our psychological understandings and therefore to our psychoanalytic interventions. They are therefore the metaphors we live by, that are our pluralistic psychoanalytic articles of faith, and that I feel in our current developmental stage to be essentially beyond the realm of empirical study and scientific process.[4] This, of course, is not meant to draw an all-or-none line between our clinical theory and our general theory and certainly some aspects of what I call our large-scale explanatory general theories may already be linked enough to observables as to come within the scope of scientific testing. Nor does it preclude that future developments—in psychoanalytic observation and psychoanalytic theorizing—may yet bring us to a much further evolved general theory formation that can pass beyond metaphoric symbolism, but by then we would have witnessed the processes of accommodation and translation that would have brought a coalescence of our current disparate theories and our theoretical pluralism into an overarching consensually accepted general theoretical structure. That day is not yet and at this point looks far away. My current vision of psychoanalysis then is of a unitary clinical theory that is empirically testable—a theory which binds and unifies us as psychoanalysts—and of a pluralistic general theory, the explanatory symbols, i.e., the metaphors, which embody our intellectual commitments and values and to which we differentially adhere.

That life values are distinctly involved in our choice of theoretical perspectives has been clearly articulated by Gedo (1984), though perhaps not in a form with which we would all agree. He has said on this issue, "Each of these conceptual schemata [the various psychoanalytic theories] encodes one or another of the primary meanings implicit in human existence—unfortunately, often to the exclusion of all other meanings. Thus, the view of man embodied in the libido theory, especially in the form it took prior to 1920, attributed primary significance

---

[4]Freud made much the same point in regard to the relationship between the observational base and the theoretical structure of psychoanalysis in his famous statement in the paper on narcissism (Freud 1914b): "For these ideas [the theory] are not the foundations of science, upon which everything rests: that foundation is observation alone. They are not the bottom but the top of the whole structure, and they can be replaced and discarded without damaging it" (p. 77). He made very similar statements in "Instincts and Their Vicissitudes" (Freud 1915, p. 117) and in the "Two Encyclopaedia Articles" (Freud 1923, p. 253, paragraph entitled "Psycho-Analysis an Empirical Science").

to the satisfaction of the appetites. By contrast, Melanie Klein's psychoanalytic system teaches the need to make reparation for man's constitutional wickedness.... In the 1970s Heinz Kohut promulgated views that give comparable emphasis to the unique healing power of empathy while acknowledging man's entitlement to an affectively gratifying milieu.... Let me hasten to add that I am emphatically in agreement with the need to satisfy appetites, to curb human destructiveness, and to provide an affectively gratifying environment for our children. And I am for other desiderata to boot! Isn't everyone?" (p. 159).[5]

I would like now to close with two cautionary implications of what I have been saying today, one related to issues of therapy and technique,

---

[5]This same point, that our theoretical positions in psychoanalysis are inevitably embedded in fundamental social, political, and moral value dispositions has been strongly made as the closing statement in Greenberg and Mitchell's (1983) book on object relations perspectives in psychoanalysis traced developmentally and historically through critical discussion of the work of the various major object relations theorists starting with such diverse contributors as Melanie Klein, W.R.D. Fairbairn, and Harry Stack Sullivan. The summarizing point that they make at the end of their book is that the drive theory perspective and the relational theory perspective are linked to differing views of the essential nature of human experience: Drive theory is linked philosophically to the positions of Hobbes and Locke, that man is an essentially individual animal and that human satisfaction and goals are fundamentally personal and individual; the role of the state rests on the concept of "negative liberty," that the state adds nothing essential to individual satisfaction as such, but just ensures the possibility of personal fulfilment: Relational theory is linked philosophically to the positions of Rousseau, Hegel, and Marx, that man is an essentially social animal and that human satisfactions and goals are realizable only within a community; the role of the state here rests on the concept of "positive liberty," to provide an indispensable "positive" function by offering its citizens that which they cannot provide for themselves in isolation. Greenberg and Mitchell state in relation to this that "The drive/structure and the relational/structure model embody these two major traditions within Western philosophy in the relatively recently developing intellectual arena of psychoanalytic ideas" (p. 402). And in this context they quote Thomas Kuhn (1977), the well-known philosopher and historian of (natural) science, that "communication between proponents of different theories is inevitably partial.... What each takes to be facts depends in part on the theory he espouses, and ... an individual's transfer of allegiance from theory to theory is often better described as *conversion* than as choice" (p. 338, my italics).

the other to issues of theory and science, and then with a final general statement. The first caution on the matter of technique is in response to Cooper's (1977) view in regard to the modern-day pluralism of our theories which he presents as a very welcome transition in the history of analysis. He has said of this, "Because we have more than one mode of conducting psychoanalysis [i.e., more than one theoretical framework], it is incumbent upon us to make sufficiently accurate diagnosis to decide which mode is best suited for the given patient" (pp. 20–21). I would disagree with this conclusion since to me *each* theoretical framework essays to be a comprehensively adequate explanatory system within which the whole range of psychoanalytically amenable psychopathology can be understood and treated—and in practice, of course, they all try to do just that. We have different theories, that is, to deal with the *same* patients; our explanatory and therapeutic psychologies do not change with our patients' diagnostic categories.

The second caution on the matter of science is in response to Edelson's (1985) view that since Freudian, Adlerian, and Jungian theorists all claim that the data of the consulting rooms support their hypotheses, that this argument in theory can and should be tested by the methods of science. He has said of this, "If incompatible inferences about an analysand, based on different theories, are made by different psychoanalysts, then the same kinds of scientific arguments about the relation between rival or alternative hypotheses and evidence I shall describe further on ... in this paper must be used to decide which inference or hypothesis is to be provisionally accepted over another" (p. 584). Here, too, I would disagree since our general (metapsychological) theories that constitute our pluralism of explanatory frameworks are in my view but our grand and very experience-distant symbolisms or metaphors, and therefore far from the realm of empirical testing which can operate at this point only in the realm of our experience-near clinical theory encompassing the interactional phenomena of our engagements with our patients' present unconsciouses.

My concluding general statement can be understood in either scientific or political terms. Psychoanalysis has developed a pluralism of theoretical perspectives in order preferentially to explain the essence of mental development and human psychology, what I have conceptualized as our variety of symbolisms or metaphors designed to grasp and to give coherence to our own internal unknowables, our past unconsciouses. In that very real sense there are today many psychoanalyses. At the same time psychoanalysts in their daily work deal with the shared phenomena of our consulting rooms employing interactional techniques built around the dynamic of the transference and the countertransference, as we try empathically to reach our patients' present unconsciouses, the psychic pressures that disturb their current lives and bring them to us. In that equally real sense there is but one discipline of psychoanalysis. I trust that the International Psychoanalytical Association can represent proudly and well both our diversity of theoretical viewpoint and our unity of clinical purpose and healing endeavor.

SUMMARY

This paper describes the historic development of psychoanalysis, the singular product of the genius of one man, Sigmund Freud, and which he made such strenuous efforts through his lifetime to maintain as a unified enterprise, defining out dissidents (like Adler, Jung, etc.), into what has become in the almost half-century since his death a science and a discipline characterized by an increasing diversity or pluralism, of theoretical perspectives, of linguistic and thought conventions, and of distinctive regional, cultural, and language emphases.

I discuss both the understanding of this theoretical diversity and what, in the face of it, holds us together as common adherents of a shared psychoanalytic science and profession. My thesis is that what unites us is our shared focus on the clinical interactions in our consulting rooms, the phenomena encompassed by the "present unconscious" (the Sandlers) or the "clinical theory" (George Klein). When we look beyond that to an explanatory structure within which to conceptualize the genetic-developmental process, normal and abnormal mental functioning, psychopathology and its reversal (cure) i.e., the realm of the "past unconscious" or the "general theory," we posit our various theoretical, linguistic or thought perspectives, i.e.—at this stage of our historical development—our *metaphors* or our various explanatory symbolisms. Some implications of this viewing of our various theoretical perspectives in psychoanalysis (ego psychological, object-relational, self-psychological, Kleinian, Bionian, Lacanian, etc.) as but metaphoric expressions, are reviewed.

REFERENCES

Cooper AM: Clinical psychoanalysis: one method or more—the relation of diagnosis to psychoanalytic treatment. Presented at the fall meeting, American Psychoanalytic Association, 1977

Cooper AM: Psychoanalysis at one hundred years: beginnings of maturity. J Am Psychoanal Assoc 32:245–267, 1984

Edelson M: The hermeneutic turn and the single case study in psychoanalysis. Psychoanalysis and Contemporary Thought 8:567–614, 1985

Ferenczi S, Rank O: The Development of Psychoanalysis (1924). Madison, CT, International Universities Press, 1986

Freud S: "Wild" psycho-analysis (1910), in The Standard Edition of the Complete Psychological Works of Sigmund Freud [SE], Vol 11. Translated and edited by Strachey J. London, Hogarth Press, 1957, pp 159–168

Freud S: On the history of the psycho-analytic movement (1914a). SE, 14:7–66, 1957

Freud S: On narcissism: an introduction (1914b). SE, 14:67–102, 1957

Freud S: Instincts and their vicissitudes (1915). SE, 14:109–140, 1957

Freud S: Beyond the pleasure principle (1920). SE, 18:7–64, 1955

Freud S: Two encyclopaedia articles (1923). SE, 18:233–259, 1955

Freud S: Analysis terminable and interminable (1937). SE, 23:211–253, 1964

Gadamer HG: Truth and Method. New York, Seabury Press, 1975

Gedo J: Psychoanalysis and Its Discontents. New York, Guilford, 1984

Glover E: The therapeutic effect of inexact interpretation. Int J Psychoanal 12:397–411, 1931

Goodheart WB: C.G. Jung's first "patient": on the seminal emergence of Jung's thought. Journal of Analytical Psychology 29:1–34, 1984

Greenberg JR, Mitchell SA: Object Relations in Psychoanalytic Theory. Cambridge, MA, Harvard University Press, 1983

Habermas J: Knowledge and Human Interests (1968). Translated by Shapiro JJ. Boston, MA, Beacon Press, 1971

Harrison SI: Is psychoanalysis "our science"? Reflections on the scientific status of psychoanalysis. J Am Psychoanal Assoc 18:125–149, 1970

Isaacs S: Conclusion of Discussions in 1943 on her paper "The nature and function of phantasy" (1943). Sci Bull Br Psychoanal Soc 17:151, 153, 1967. Quoted in Steiner 1985, p 49

Kazin A: The Freudian revolution analyzed, in Freud and the 20th Century. Edited by Nelson B. New York, Meridian Books, 1957, pp 13–21

Klein GS: Psychoanalytic Theory: An Exploration of Essentials. New York, International Universities Press, 1976

Knight RP: The present status of organized psychoanalysis in the United States. J Am Psychoanal Assoc 1:197–221, 1953

Kohut H: How Does Analysis Cure? Chicago, IL, University of Chicago Press, 1984

Kuhn T: The Essential Tension. Chicago, IL, University of Chicago Press, 1977

Lebovici S, Widlöcher D: Psychoanalysis in France. New York, International Universities Press, 1980

Poland WS, Major R (eds): French psychoanalytic voices. Psychoanalytic Inquiry 4:145–311, 1984

Post S: Psychoanalytic rapprochement: a correspondence. Academy Forum (of the American Academy of Psychoanalysis) 30(2):21, 1986

Ricoeur P: Freud and Philosophy: An Essay on Interpretation. Translated by Savage D. New Haven, CT, Yale University Press, 1970

Sandler J: Reflections on some relations between psychoanalytic concepts and psychoanalytic practice. Int J Psychoanal 64:35–45, 1983

Sandler J: Reality and the stabilizing function of unconscious fantasy. Bulletin of the Anna Freud Centre 9:177–194, 1986

Sandler J, Sandler A-M: The "second censorship," the "three box model," and some technical implications. Int J Psychoanal 64:413–425, 1983

Sandler J, Sandler A-M: The past unconscious, the present unconscious, and interpretation of the transference. Psychoanalytic Inquiry 4:367–399, 1984

Schafer R: Wild analysis. J Am Psychoanal Assoc 33:275–299, 1985

Steiner R: Review of Psychoanalysis in France. Edited by Lebovici S, Widlöcher D. Int J Psychoanal 65:232–233, 1984

Steiner R: Some thoughts about tradition and change from an examination of the British Psycho-Analytical Society's Controversial Discussions (1943–1944). Int Rev Psychoanal 12:27–71, 1985

Wallerstein RS: Psychoanalysis as a science: its present status and its future tasks, in Psychology versus Metapsychology: Psychoanalytic Essays in Memory of George S. Klein. Edited by Gill MM, Holzman PS. Psychological Issues, Monogr No 36, Vol 9, 1976, pp 198–228

Wallerstein RS: The bipolar self: discussion of alternative perspectives. J Am Psychoanal Assoc 29:377–394, 1981

Wallerstein RS: Reflections on the identity of the psychoanalyst, in The Identity of the Psychoanalyst. Edited by Joseph ED, Widlöcher D. New York, International Universities Press, 1983a, pp 265–276. [Also available in French as: Réflexions sur le symposium, l'identité du psychanalyste. Paris, Presses Universitaires de France, 1979, pp 273–283]

Wallerstein RS: Self psychology and "classical" psychoanalytic psychology: the nature of their relationship, in The Future of Psychoanalysis. Edited by Goldberg A. New York, International Universities Press, 1983b, pp 19–63. Reprinted in Psychoanalysis and Contemporary Thought 6:553–595, 1983

Wallerstein RS: How does self psychology differ in practice? Int J Psychoanal 66:391–404, 1985

Wallerstein RS: Psychoanalysis as a science: a response to the new challenges. Psychoanal Q 55:414–451, 1986

Wurmser L: A defense of the use of metaphor in analytic theory formation. Psychoanal Q 46:466–498, 1977

INDEX

*Page numbers printed in **boldface** type refer to tables or figures.*